Practical Critical Care in Cardiology

FUNDAMENTAL AND CLINICAL CARDIOLOGY

1. *Drug Treatment of Hyperlipidemia*, edited by Basil M. Rifkind
2. *Cardiotonic Drugs: A Clinical Review, Second Edition, Revised and Expanded*, edited by Carl V. Leier
3. *Complications of Coronary Angioplasty*, edited by Alexander J. R. Black, H. Vernon Anderson, and Stephen G. Ellis
4. *Unstable Angina*, edited by John D. Rutherford
5. *Beta-Blockers and Cardiac Arrhythmias*, edited by Prakash C. Deedwania
6. *Exercise and the Heart in Health and Disease*, edited by Roy J. Shephard and Henry S. Miller, Jr.
7. *Cardiopulmonary Physiology in Critical Care*, edited by Steven M. Scharf
8. *Atherosclerotic Cardiovascular Disease, Hemostasis, and Endo-thelial Function*, edited by Robert Boyer Francis, Jr.
9. *Coronary Heart Disease Prevention*, edited by Frank G. Yanowitz
10. *Thrombolysis and Adjunctive Therapy for Acute Myocardial Infarction*, edited by Eric R. Bates
11. *Stunned Myocardium: Properties, Mechanisms, and Clinical Manifestations*, edited by Robert A. Kloner and Karin Przyklenk
12. *Prevention of Venous Thromboembolism*, edited by Samuel Z. Goldhaber
13. *Silent Myocardial Ischemia and Infarction: Third Edition*, Peter F. Cohn
14. *Congestive Cardiac Failure: Pathophysiology and Treatment*, edited by David B. Barnett, Hubert Pouleur, and Gary S. Francis
15. *Heart Failure: Basic Science and Clinical Aspects*, edited by Judith K. Gwathmey, G. Maurice Briggs, and Paul D. Allen

16. *Coronary Thrombolysis in Perspective: Principles Underlying Conjunctive and Adjunctive Therapy*, edited by Burton E. Sobel and Désiré Collen
17. *Cardiovascular Disease in the Elderly Patient*, edited by Donald D. Tresch and Wilbert S. Aronow
18. *Systemic Cardiac Embolism*, edited by Michael D. Ezekowitz
19. *Low-Molecular-Weight Heparins in Prophylaxis and Therapy of Thromboembolic Diseases*, edited by Henri Bounameaux
20. *Valvular Heart Disease*, edited by Muayed Al Zaibag and Carlos M. G. Duran
21. *Implantable Cardioverter-Defibrillators: A Comprehensive Textbook*, edited by N. A. Mark Estes III, Antonis S. Manolis, and Paul J. Wang
22. *Individualized Therapy of Hypertension*, edited by Norman M. Kaplan and C. Venkata S. Ram
23. *Atlas of Coronary Balloon Angioplasty*, Bernhard Meier and Vivek K. Mehan
24. *Lowering Cholesterol in High-Risk Individuals and Populations*, edited by Basil M. Rifkind
25. *Interventional Cardiology: New Techniques and Strategies for Diagnosis and Treatment*, edited by Christopher J. White and Stephen R. Ramee
26. *Molecular Genetics and Gene Therapy of Cardiovascular Diseases*, edited by Stephen C. Mockrin
27. *The Pericardium: A Comprehensive Textbook*, David H. Spodick
28. *Coronary Restenosis: From Genetics to Therapeutics*, edited by Giora Z. Feuerstein
29. *The Endothelium in Clinical Practice: Source and Target of Novel Therapies*, edited by Gabor M. Rubanyi and Victor J. Dzau
30. *Molecular Biology of Cardiovascular Disease*, edited by Andrew R. Marks and Mark B. Taubman
31. *Practical Critical Care in Cardiology*, edited by Zab Mohsenifar and P. K. Shah
32. *Intravascular Ultrasound Imaging in Coronary Artery Disease*, edited by Robert J. Siegel

ADDITIONAL VOLUMES IN PREPARATION

Saphenous Vein Bypass Graft Disease, edited by Eric R. Bates and David R. Holmes

Practical Critical Care in Cardiology

edited by

Zab Mohsenifar
P. K. Shah
Cedars-Sinai Medical Center
and University of California, Los Angeles, School of Medicine
Los Angeles, California

MARCEL DEKKER

MARCEL DEKKER, INC.   NEW YORK • BASEL • HONG KONG

ISBN: 0-8247-0097-X

The publisher offers discounts on this book when ordered in bulk quantities. For more information, write to Special Sales/Professional Marketing at the address below.

This book is printed on acid-free paper.

Marcel Dekker, Inc.
270 Madison Avenue, New York, New York 10016
http://www.dekker.com

Current printing (last digit):
10 9 8 7 6 5 4 3 2 1

Printed in the United States of America

Series Introduction

Marcel Dekker, Inc., has focused on the development of various series of beautifully produced books in different branches of medicine. These series have facilitated the integration of rapidly advancing information for both the clinical specialist and the researcher.

My goal as editor-in-chief of the Fundamental and Clinical Cardiology series is to assemble the talents of world-renowned authorities to discuss virtually every area of cardiovascular medicine. In the current monograph, *Practical Critical Care in Cardiology*, Zab Mohsenifar and P. K. Shah have edited a much-needed and timely book. Other contributions to this series include books on molecular biology, interventional cardiology, and clinical management of such problems as coronary artery disease and ventricular arrhythmias.

Samuel Z. Goldhaber

Preface

Approximately two years ago, we were invited to chair a symposium on critical care issues of importance to cardiologists and related specialists at the American Heart Association meeting in Anaheim, California. The symposium focused on topics pertinent to intensive care management that are not usually emphasized in general cardiology training. Following this successful symposium, a number of the attendees approached us about writing a textbook that would focus on noncardiology critical care issues likely to be encountered in cardiac intensive care units. Thus, the seeds of this textbook were planted that afternoon in Anaheim.

The field of critical care has blossomed tremendously over the last 10 years and, indeed, a variety of major disciplines such as pulmonary medicine, surgery, anesthesiology, and pediatrics, have recognized critical care as a distinct subspecialty. In order to keep pace with new developments in this rapidly broadening field, it is prudent for the cardiologist to be aware of critical care issues that may be encountered in the care of patients. This text is intended to provide the practicing cardiologist and physicians in related fields (e.g., cardiac surgeons) with cogent, evidence-based, science-enhancing, yet practical information to assist them in dealing with numerous and important noncardiac problems that may complicate the progress of a patient in the cardiac care unit. A better grasp of noncardiac critical care issues may both minimize the need for noncardiology consultants and refine the use of appropriate referral and consultation. The editors have ensured that chapters are comprehensive, state-of-the-art reviews, written in a clear and practical style.

Mechanical ventilation is an intervention that cardiologists have traditionally shied away from. The text addresses this topic in detail and provides sufficient knowledge and adequate tools to assist the physician in practical, simple ventilator management, as well as the background and skills necessary for weaning from mechanical ventilation in an expeditious manner. The text also deals with a number of other important clinical problems, such as pulmonary embolism, gastrointestinal bleeding, and coagulopathies, emphasizing clinical background and management principles. The function of respiratory muscles may be compromised in a variety of settings likely to be encountered in the cardiac ICU. Respiratory muscle performance and other important settings in cardiac patients are discussed. Furthermore, the subject of sleep-related disorders is addressed in detail. A comprehensive review of pertinent infectious disease topics (nosocomial infections, cardiac-related infections, etc.) of interest to cardiologists is included. A comprehensive, practical, easy-to-read review of the complex area of diabetic ketoacidosis, an issue that periodically becomes challenging in the coronary care unit, is also provided. And the text provides a comprehensive and detailed understanding of the dynamics of postoperative cardiac patients and a practical approach to these highly important management issues. Critical care pharmacology, an ever-expanding field, is also covered, in a thorough review of drug interactions in the cardiac care environment. Finally, imaging techniques pertinent to critically ill cardiac patients are reviewed in detail.

In our time, managing critically ill patients has become highly complex and sophisticated, requiring knowledge beyond the traditional bounds of the field of cardiac care. And in this environment of increasing managed care and limited resources, it behooves the physician to be more of a "Renaissance man" than merely a subspecialist. The many contributors to this textbook have done a sterling job in presenting state-of-the-art material in a very readable and practical format. The editors are grateful for the hard work and teamwork of many experts in producing an outstanding final product.

Zab Mohsenifar
P. K. Shah

Contents

Contributors

Khaja R. Ahmed, M.D. Assistant Professor, Department of Medicine, University of California, Los Angeles, School of Medicine, Los Angeles, California

Philip Barnett, M.D., Ph.D. Director, Diabetes Program, Division of Endocrinology and Metabolism, Cedars-Sinai Medical Center, and Associate Professor, University of California, Los Angeles, School of Medicine, Los Angeles, California

Samuel A. Berkman, M.D., F.A.C.P. Clinical Professor, Division of Hematology/Oncology, Department of Medicine, University of California, Los Angeles, School of Medicine, Los Angeles, California

Julien Bohé, M.D., Ph.D. Centre Hospitalier Lyon-Sud, Lyon, France

Bojan Cercek, M.D. Director, Coronary Intensive Care Unit, Cedars-Sinai Medical Center, and Associate Professor of Medicine, University of California, Los Angeles, School of Medicine, Los Angeles, California

Caroline Chia-Lin Chow, M.D. Assistant Professor, Department of Diagnostic Radiology, University of Maryland Medical Center, Baltimore, Maryland

Eric S. Daar, M.D. Assistant Professor of Medicine, University of California, Los Angeles, School of Medicine, and Medical Director, AIDS and Immune Disorder Center, Division of Infectious Diseases, Department of Medicine, Cedars-Sinai Medical Center, Los Angeles, California

Sven de Vos, M.D. Department of Medicine, Cedars-Sinai Medical Center, Los Angeles, California

Andrea T. Feinberg, M.D. Senior Pulmonary/Critical Care Fellow, Department of Medicine, Cedars-Sinai Medical Center, and University of California, Los Angeles, School of Medicine, Los Angeles, California

Paula L. Gaut, M.D. Assistant Medical Director, AIDS and Immune Disorders Center, Division of Infectious Diseases, Department of Medicine, Cedars-Sinai Medical Center, and Assistant Clinical Professor of Medicine, University of California, Los Angeles, School of Medicine, Los Angeles, California

Sanjay Kaul, M.D. Attending Cardiologist, Division of Cardiology, Department of Medicine, Cedars-Sinai Medical Center, Los Angeles, California

Jonathan D. Kaunitz, M.D. Professor, Department of Medicine, University of California, Los Angeles, School of Medicine, Los Angeles, California

Steven S. Khan, M.D. Associate Professor, Divisions of Cardiology and Cardiothoracic Surgery, Department of Medicine, Cedars-Sinai Medical Center, and University of California, Los Angeles, School of Medicine, Los Angeles, California

Charles F. Lacy, Pharm.D. Drug Information Coordinator, Pharmacy Services, Cedars-Sinai Medical Center, Los Angeles, California

Michael I. Lewis, M.D. Director, Respiratory Intensive Care Unit, Pulmonary and Critical Care Division, Department of Medicine, Cedars-Sinai Medical Center, and University of California, Los Angeles, School of Medicine, Los Angeles, California

Vias Markides, M.B., M.R.C.P. St. Thomas' Hospital, London, England

Sylvia Martin, Pharm.D. Drug Utilization Evaluation Pharmacist, Pharmacy Services, Cedars-Sinai Medical Center, Los Angeles, California

Zab Mohsenifar, M.D. Director, Pulmonary and Critical Care Division, Cedars-Sinai Medical Center, and Professor of Medicine, University of California, Los Angeles, School of Medicine, Los Angeles, California

A. Rekha K. Murthy, M.D., F.R.C.P.(C) Associate Professor of Medicine, University of California, Los Angeles, School of Medicine, and Director, Hospital Epidemiology, Cedars-Sinai Medical Center, Los Angeles, California

Minhtri Nguyen, M.D. Director, Renal Fellowship Training Program, Division of Nephrology, Department of Medicine, University of California, Los Angeles, School of Medicine, Los Angeles, California

Mehmet Pekerol, M.D. Division of Infectious Diseases, Department of Medicine, Cedars-Sinai Medical Center, Los Angeles, California

Anderson Rowe, M.D. Division of Gastroenterology, Department of Medicine, University of California, Los Angeles, School of Medicine, and Division of Gastroenterology, Department of Medicine, Cedars-Sinai Medical Center, Los Angeles, California

Stefan Schneider, M.D. Division of Infectious Diseases, Department of Medicine, Cedars-Sinai Medical Center, Los Angeles, California

Jeremy Schwieger, M.D. Assistant Clinical Professor of Medicine, Department of Internal Medicine, University of California, Los Angeles, School of Medicine, Los Angeles, California

Guy W. Soo Hoo, M.D. Associate Clinical Professor of Medicine, Pulmonary and Critical Care Section, New West Los Angeles Veterans Affairs Medical Center, and University of California, Los Angeles, School of Medicine, Los Angeles, California

Jay Udani, M.D. Chief Resident, Department of Internal Medicine, Cedars-Sinai Medical Center, Los Angeles, California

Charles S. White, M.D. Associate Professor, Department of Diagnostic Radiology, University of Maryland Medical Center, Baltimore, Maryland

Adrian J. Williams, M.B., F.R.C.P. St. Thomas' Hospital, London, England

Practical Critical Care in Cardiology

1

Noninvasive Mechanical Ventilation in Cardiac Care Units: Use in Patients With Congestive Heart Failure

GUY W. SOO HOO

New West Los Angeles Veterans Affairs Medical Center and University of California, Los Angeles, School of Medicine, Los Angeles, California

I. INTRODUCTION

The past decade has seen increasing use of noninvasive mechanical ventilation in the management of acute respiratory failure. This refers to ventilatory support that does not require placement of an endotracheal or tracheostomy tube. It is not a new approach, but resurgence of management was first described over 50 years ago in patients with pulmonary edema supported noninvasively with positive pressure ventilation delivered via a face mask (1,2). The advent of the endotracheal tube and mechanical ventilation in the 1950s supplanted this use with continued application limited to a few centers.

The use of nasal continuous positive airway pressure (CPAP) to treat patients with obstructive sleep apnea in the 1980s led to the extension of noninvasive ventilation to other types of respiratory failure. Initial experience was limited to patients with neuromuscular respiratory failure or severe chronic obstructive pulmonary disease (COPD) who were considered poor candidates for intubation and mechanical ventilation. A major impetus behind noninvasive ventilation has been to limit intubation and mechanical ventilation and eliminate its attendant complications. Subsequent experience has led to its application for all types of respiratory failure and increasing acceptance as initial therapy. The following will review the rationale and indications for noninvasive ventilation in coronary care units as well as guidelines to ensure its successful application.

II. RATIONALE FOR USE

Subjects with congestive heart failure (CHF) have marked changes in ventilatory function which corresponds to the development of pulmonary congestion and interstitial and alveolar edema (3–6). Pulmonary vascular congestion produces peripheral airway compression with an increase in airway resistance and decrease in lung compliance. The decreased compliance is most evident at low lung volumes. The development of interstitial edema produces further peripheral airway compression, and with increasing alveolar edema there are further increases in airway resistance. Initial peripheral airway compression produces an obstructive ventilatory defect. As interstitial and alveolar fluid increases, lung volumes decrease producing a restrictive ventilatory defect. These alterations have been confirmed with serial pulmonary function tests in patients recovering from episodes of decompensated congestive heart failure. In addition, animal studies suggest that there is decreased diaphragmatic strength and increased fatigability in congestive heart failure (6). With progressive pulmonary edema, patients become more hypoxemic and hypercapnic, and develop a metabolic acidosis and life-threatening respiratory failure (7).

Patients usually respond to treatment with supplemental oxygen, diuretics, morphine sulfate, and nitrates. However, patients with worsening gas exchange, increasing respiratory fatigue, or obtundation may require ventilatory support. This can be provided with just positive airway pressure delivered either as positive end-expiratory pressure (PEEP) or continuous positive airway pressure (CPAP). This is not positive pressure *ventilation*, although the beneficial effects of PEEP or CPAP to the cardiopulmonary system are the same as achieved with positive pressure ventilation.

Improvement in ventilatory mechanics with positive airway pressure is achieved as follows (8,9) and is summarized in Figure 1. PEEP or CPAP increases functional residual capacity, and shifts tidal breathing to a more compliant portion of the lung's pressure-volume curve. This allows generation of a larger tidal volume for the same amount of distending pressure, or, alternatively, less pressure is needed to achieve the same tidal volume. With increases in transpulmonary pressure, there are increases in airway caliber. This decreases airway resistance. Alveoli that may have been previously closed are recruited, allowing for improvement in gas exchange and ventilation/perfusion relationships. The positive airway pressure also prevents fluid formation in the alveoli, and maintains the surface tension-reducing benefits of pulmonary surfactant. The sum of these effects is improved oxygenation, improved ventilation, and partial unloading of the respiratory muscles; this procedure also reduces the work of breathing. These benefits have been reported with pressures in the 5 to 18 cm H_2O range. Although higher pressures may also be beneficial in some patients, adverse effects on alveolar

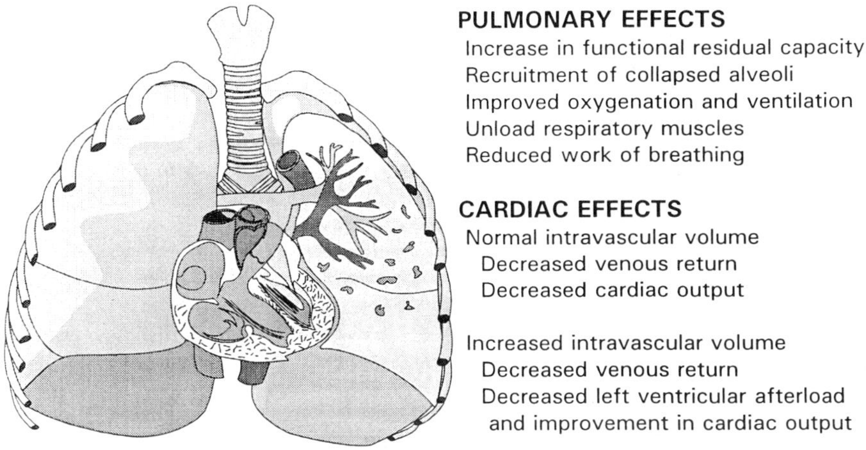

Figure 1 Cardiac and pulmonary effects of positive pressure ventilation. See text for details.

distension and cardiac depression may limit its effectiveness. Positive pressure ventilation has the same effects on the pulmonary system.

The effects of positive airway pressure or positive pressure ventilation on cardiac function are well recognized. In subjects with normal intravascular volume, there are reduction of venous return and restriction of ventricular filling, leading to decreased cardiac output and arterial pressure (10,11). Based on animal and human investigations, there are benefits in subjects with left ventricular dysfunction exposed to positive intrathoracic pressures (12–18). Positive intrathoracic pressure decreases transmural systolic left ventricular pressure. The decreased transmural pressure results in a reduction in the afterload to the left heart, with resultant improvement in left ventricular emptying and cardiac output. The reduction in venous return also decreases left ventricular preload. This has a salutory effect in patients with pulmonary edema who are effectively volume-overloaded. It is important to note that the beneficial afterloading effects of positive airway pressure are present as long as preload is elevated or maintained by volume infusion. With a significant decline in preload, the detrimental effects of positive pressure on venous return will outweigh the beneficial effects on left ventricular function.

These studies and the bulk of the clinical confirmation of the beneficial effects of positive pressure ventilatory support have involved patients ventilated through an endotracheal tube with a bedside ventilator. However, it is important to realize that these observations can also be generalized to patients receiving noninvasive positive pressure ventilatory support. Therapy can be delivered with a variety of patient-ventilator interfaces (masks) and devices of varying degrees of sophistication.

The most rudimentary configuration to deliver positive airway pressure involves a tight-fitting face mask attached to a breathing circuit with one-way valves and an expiratory resistance creating PEEP. The circuit can be modified to provide positive airway pressure during both inspiration and expiration, or CPAP. This can be accomplished with continuous gas flow or a demand valve that generates flow with patient efforts. CPAP can also be delivered using a portable air compressor attached to either a nasal or a face mask. These units are used primarily to treat patients with obstructive sleep apnea and function as a pneumatic splint to prevent airway collapse. They can be used to provide ventilatory assistance for patients, but patients must be spontaneously breathing with an adequate respiratory drive, as these devices cannot ventilate apneic patients. CPAP is available on portable and bedside ventilators to be used alone or in conjuction with other ventilatory modes. In this fashion, it is synonymous with PEEP, and positive airway pressure is generated by adjustment of a variety of expiratory valves.

Subjects with an erratic respiratory drive or who require full ventilatory support can be supported noninvasively using either volume-, pressure-, or time-cycled bedside ventilators and a multitude of ventilatory modes. Although the assist control (AC) mode is most commonly used, successful support has been reported with synchronized intermittent mandatory ventilation (SIMV), pressure support (PS), or pressure control (PC) with or without PEEP. However, a microprocessor-based bedside ventilator is not necessary; many of these patients can be supported with portable ventilators. There are portable devices that provide bilevel positive airway pressure (BiPAP), allowing manipulation of the inspiratory positive airway pressure (IPAP) and expiratory positive airway pressure (EPAP).

III. NONINVASIVE VENTILATION IN CLINICAL USE

A. Pulmonary Edema

Patients presenting with acute cardiogenic pulmonary edema are generally treated with medications directed at improving myocardial function and reducing myocardial workload. This includes agents that decrease preload (diuretics, nitrates) and afterload (arterial vasodilators) and that improve cardiac contractility (digoxin, dobutamine). Therapy is also directed at conditions that may further depress cardiac function (hypoxemia, dysrhythmias, etc.). Most patients respond rapidly to aggressive directed therapy; it is the minority that require invasive ventilatory support. In a series of 50 consecutive patients admitted with acute cardiogenic pulmonary edema, only six (12%) required intubation and mechanical ventilation (7). Over half of the patients were either eucapnic or hypercapnic, and all had a significant metabolic acidosis. Four were intubated upon presentation, and two after begining therapy for their pulmonary edema. The initial arterial blood gases of these patients were pH = 7.15 ± 0.10; $PaCO_2$ = 69 ± 22 mm Hg; PaO_2 = 41 ± 5 mm Hg.

The previously described cardiopulmonary benefits of positive airway pressure support its use as an adjunct to medical therapy in cardiogenic pulmonary edema. The complications associated with intubation and mechanical ventilation are legion even if in place for only a short duration. Therefore, noninvasive ventilation would be an important therapeutic option which could avert intubation as well as provide treatment for pulmonary edema. Indeed, several investigators have reported the successful treatment of cardiogenic pulmonary edema with noninvasive ventilation. Noninvasive ventilation includes patients treated with CPAP and the bulk of the experience with noninvasive ventilation in cardiogenic pulmonary edema has been with CPAP. The first reported patients responded to 3 and 7 cm H_2O of CPAP delivered through either a mouthpiece or a face mask (1). There are numerous anecdotal reports of mask CPAP used to treat patients with cardiogenic pulmonary edema (19–22). These patients are grouped with patients with other etiologies of respiratory failure and the overall experience supports its use.

There are only three studies, two from Finland and one from Australia, that have critically assessed the use of mask CPAP in acute cardiogenic pulmonary edema. All have delivered CPAP by using high-flow breathing circuits with an external valve to provide CPAP at 10 cm H_2O. The first Finnish study randomly assigned CPAP and medical therapy to 20 patients and compared their response to 20 medically treated patients (23). Patients were subjected to a minimum of 10 min and up to 3 h of CPAP. Changes were evident after only 10 min of CPAP, with patients experiencing a decline in their respiratory rate, heart rate, blood pressure, and $PaCO_2$ and improvement in oxygenation. These changes persisted during the 3-h period. There was a marked if not statistically significant difference in the intubation rate, with 60% of the medically treated patients eventually intubated compared to 30% of the CPAP patients. These investigators subsequently performed another trial in 40 patients in which CPAP was alternated with increased supplemental oxygen applied in random order for 10 min (24). Again, they noted a decline in respiratory rate, heart rate, and blood pressure with an improvement in oxygenation, which was greater with CPAP than with increasing supplemental oxygen.

The most compelling support for CPAP is found in a prospective randomized trial from Australia of 39 patients with severe cardiogenic pulmonary edema (25). After 30 min of face mask CPAP, patients had a significantly greater decline in respiratory rate and hypercapnia, with improvement in pH and PaO_2/FIO_2 ratio. These patients were in severe pulmonary edema, with a mean pH of 7.18 ± 0.08 and $PaCO_2$ of 58 ± 8 mm Hg. There was also a significant reduction in the intubation rate, with no patient treated with CPAP requiring intubation, as compared to seven (35%) medically treated patients. There was no reduction in the length of hospital stay or mortality.

More detailed investigations of the hemodynamic effects of CPAP in patients with CHF have been reported using nasal mask CPAP applied with a portable CPAP device. Bradley and colleagues evaluated nasal CPAP at 5 cm H_2O in 22 patients with idiopathic cardiomyopathy undergoing endomyocardial biopsy (26). Only subjects with an elevated pulmonary capillary wedge pressure (PCWP) $\geq$ 12 mm Hg demonstrated a response to CPAP, with an average improvement in cardiac index of 17% and stroke volume index of 24%. Baratz and colleagues evaluated increasing levels of nasal CPAP in 13 patients admitted to an intensive care unit with exacerbations of underlying CHF (27). Nasal CPAP was increased at 20-min intervals from 5 to 15 cm H_2O in subjects with PCWP readings $\geq$ 20 mm Hg. Seven of the 13 patients demonstrated about 16% improvement in cardiac index, and stroke volume at the highest tolerated CPAP level. Most of the subjects could tolerate 10 cm H_2O of CPAP, but only four of 13 completed the trial at 15 cm H_2O. Of interest, when nasal CPAP was discontinued, the changes in hemodynamic parameters reverted to initial levels, providing additional evidence that the changes were due to CPAP and not other concomitant therapy.

Noninvasive ventilation using either volume-cycled or pressure-cycled ventilators to treat cardiogenic pulmonary edema has not had as focused an experience as CPAP. Most reported series include a few patients with cardiogenic pulmonary edema along with other causes of respiratory failure. A recent review of noninvasive ventilation identified only 10 patients in four series with congestive heart failure as the cause of their respiratory failure (28). Success usually defined by correction of respiratory failure and prevention of intubation was 70% in the review. Wysocki and colleagues reported a randomized comparison of face mask pressure support ventilation with conventional therapy in 41 nonCOPD patients (29). Fourteen patients were felt to have cardiogenic pulmonary edema as the cause of their respiratory distress. No differences were noted in the intubation rate, length of ICU stay, or death rate between those treated with noninvasive ventilation or conventional therapy. Post hoc analysis suggested that hypercapnic patients ($PaCO_2$ > 45 mm Hg) were more likely to benefit from noninvasive ventilation than eucapnic patients. The actual response of patients with cardiogenic pulmonary edema was not characterized in this report.

Two recent abstracts from France have reported experience in patients with cardiogenic pulmonary edema treated with face mask pressure support ventilation (30,31). Both report the use of pressure support in the 12 to 20+ cm H_2O range and PEEP of 3 to 5 cm H_2O with success rates of 77% and 87%, respectively. Of note, their successfully treated patients were hypercapnic (mean $PaCO_2$ > 45 mm Hg) and acidemic (mean pH < 7.25) whereas their failures were hypocapnic (mean $PaCO_2$ = 32 mm Hg). This experience suggests that there may have been an element of respiratory muscle fatigue in these patients and may identify a subgroup of patients more amenable to noninvasive ventilation.

In a randomized comparison between BiPAP and CPAP in pulmonary edema, BiPAP-treated patients had more rapid resolution of respiratory symptoms, but there were no differences in outcome measures (duration of hospital stay, intubation rate, mortality rate) and BiPAP was associated with a higher myocardial infarction rate. There was no clear explanation for this unexpected complication (31a).

In summary, the cardiopulmonary benefits of noninvasive positive pressure ventilation make it an ideal adjunct in the management of acute cardiogenic pulmonary edema. Additional clinical indications for noninvasive ventilation are summarized in Table 1. Although most of the experience has been with CPAP, any type of positive pressure ventilation that can be tolerated by the patient should be beneficial. It appears that as little as 5 to 10 cm H_2O of CPAP applied for as short a time as 5 min can improve oxygenation and decrease respiratory distress. The success rate exceeds 70%, and hypercapnia may be a predictor of success.

B. Postextubation Respiratory Failure

In addition to acute respiratory failure, noninvasive mechanical ventilation has gained increasing use in patients developing respiratory distress following extubation (32,33). This is a particularly vulnerable period, and postextubation respiratory insufficiency and failure may occur in as many as 20% of patients. A number of pathophysiological mechanisms may contribute singly or in unison to difficulty with discontinuation of mechanical ventilation. The removal of positive airway pressure after mechanical ventilation may allow an increase in left ventricular preload and afterload, which may worsen cardiac failure and lead to respiratory failure as previously described. Respiratory muscle weakness or fatigue and

Table 1 Indications for Noninvasive Ventilation in Cardiac Care Units

Cardiogenic pulmonary edema
Respiratory distress (tachypnea, accessory muscle use, abdominal paradox)
Hypercapnic respiratory failure
Hypoxemic respiratory failure
Postextubation respiratory failure
Cardiogenic pulmonary edema
Upper airway obstruction
Hypercapnic respiratory failure
Hypoxemic respiratory failure
Sleep disorders and congestive heart failure
Obstructive sleep apnea
Cheyne-Stokes breathing

failure as previously described. Respiratory muscle weakness or fatigue and increased work of breathing are common. Other mechanisms leading to failure included increased CO_2 production, upper airway obstruction, and inadequate ventilatory drive. These are manifest as either hypercapnic or hypoxemic respiratory failure.

The possibility of upper airway obstruction postextubation is particulary intriguing. Upper airway edema and trauma are acknowledged complications of prolonged endotracheal intubation, although the incidence and time frame for resolution are not well characterized. In patients intubated an average of 7 days, Nathan and colleagues noted increased work of breathing postextubation (35,36). Their most stiking finding was that of a sawtooth pattern on flow volume loops suggestive of upper airway abnormalities similar to those seen in patients with obstructive sleep apnea. This has been attributed to redundant upper airway tissue and may represent upper airway or laryngeal edema in these patients. It was felt that the increased work of breathing was related to these upper airway abnormalities and would be amenable to therapy with CPAP. This hypothesis remains to be confirmed, but there are several investigators who have successfully treated patients with postextubation respiratory failure with noninvasive ventilation.

Meduri and colleagues reported successful use of face mask pressure support ventilation in seven patients with COPD, congestive heart failure, or pneumonia who developed respiratory distress postextubation (32). Pennock and colleagues had an almost 80% success rate in 22 postoperative patients with both hypoxemic and hypercapnic respiratory failure using a nasal mask and a BiPAP device (33). Fifteen (68%) of these patients had cardiac surgery. The average settings were an IPAP of 10 cm H_2O (range 7.5–16) and EPAP of 5 cm H_2O (range 4 to 10). Duration of ventilation ranged from as little as 2 h to as long as 6 days. Wysocki and colleagues successfully treated five of six patients who developed postextubation respiratory failure with face mask pressure support delivered using a bedside ventilator (34). Cardiogenic pulmonary edema was felt to be the cause of respiratory failure in one patient, and upper airway obstruction the cause in most of the others.

In summary, noninvasive ventilation appears to be an acceptable alternative to reintubation in patients who develop postextubation respiratory failure. Common causes of postextubation respiratory failure—in particular, cardiogenic pulmonary edema and upper airway obstruction—appear to be ideally suited for noninvasive ventilation. These entities are usually short-lived and patients may need only a brief period of support before their resolution. The current reported experience suggests an 80% success rate. However, these findings will need corroboration by comparison with standard medical therapies and much larger numbers of subjects.

C. Sleep Disturbances and Congestive Heart Failure

Although noninvasive ventilation has been primarily directed at the treatment of respiratory failure, there is increasing evidence to support its use in patients with

CHF and sleep-related breathing disorders. Although patients with sleep-related breathing disorders usually do not require admission to a critical care unit, sleep-related breathing disorders are well recognized in patients with severe CHF. These patients are usually admitted to critical care units, and treatment of patients' sleep disturbance may help their cardiac function. In addition, patients may present with severe cardiac abnormalites including pulmonary hypertension, cardiac dysrhythmias, and pulmonary edema, which are the result of severe sleep apnea and which respond to treatment of the sleep apnea (37,38). It may be difficult to separate the primary disturbance (cardiac vs. sleep), but the approach would be to treat the sleep disturbance with nocturnal nasal CPAP.

This problem has been approached primarily by identifying and treating the sleep-related breathing disorder in patients with CHF. Bradley and colleagues have been at the forefront of these investigations (39–41). They were able to demonstrate improvement in left ventricular ejection fraction (LVEF) in 8 patients with dilated cardiomyopathy and severe obstructive sleep apnea after four weeks of daily nocturnal nasal CPAP. These patients had a mean nadir in nocturnal oxygen saturation of 85% with esophageal pressure swings ranging from −25 to −90 cm H_2O. This would represent an extraordinary increase in left ventricular afterload during sleep. Subjects had an increase in mean LVEF of 37 ± 4% to 49 ± 5% with CPAP, which subsequently declined after therapy was discontinued. They also demonstrated improvement in their functional status with improvement of at least one New York Heart Association (NYHA) classification level.

They have extended their observations to patients with Cheyne-Stokes respirations, which is characterized by periodic breathing, multiple episodes of central apneas, hypoxemia, and arousals from sleep. The presence of Cheyne-Stokes respirations in subjects with CHF is important, as it defines a group of patients with advanced heart disease and high mortality (42). Nasal CPAP is successful in eliminating the apneas and correcting the oxygen desaturation. In one study, they evaluated five patients with CHF and Cheyne-Stokes respirations. After only 4 weeks of nasal CPAP in the 8.5 to 12 cm H_2O range, patients had improvement in the left ventricular ejection fraction (LVEF) and NYHA class (40). This led to a prospective randomized comparison of nasal CPAP and medical therapy in 29 similar patients over a 3-month trial (41). Twenty-four patients completed the study, with equal numbers in each group. The treated subjects had a mean increase in LVEF of 8% from a baseline of 20% as well as an improvement in NYHA class. This compares favorably with vasodilator therapy in which improvement in LVEF has been in the 2% to 4% range. It should be noted that these findings have not been corroborated by other investigators although the severity of the cases, duration of therapy, and degree of support are not truly comparable (43,44).

In summary, noninvasive ventilation administered as nocturnal nasal CPAP may be a useful adjunct to treat patients with severe CHF and sleep-related breathing disorders. Both obstructive sleep apnea and Cheyne-Stokes respirations are amenable to treatment that improves cardiac function and functional status.

There is potential for improvement in the both morbidity and mortality associated with CHF; however, questions with respect to patient selection, duration, and intensity of treatment remained to be defined by future and larger studies.

IV. GUIDELINES FOR APPLICATION

A. Patient Selection

Appropriate patient selection is crucial for the successful application of noninvasive ventilation. Key points are summarized below and in Table 2. Patients must be able to cooperate with mask fitting and be able to coordinate with the ventilator. They can be lethargic, but must be awake enough able to cooperate and provide

Table 2 Guidelines for Instituting Noninvasive Ventilation

Patient selection	
Requirements	Contraindications
Mental status: lethargic, arousable at worst	Comatose or barely arousable
Cooperative, able to follow instructions	Unable to follow instructions
Able to protect airway; intact gag reflex	Inablity to protect airway
Able to control secretions	Excessive secretions or inability to control secretions
Lack of other significant comorbidity	Comorbidity including Hypotension or hemodynamic instability Cardiac dysrhythmias or ischemia Active gastrointestinal bleeding Status epilepticus or uncontrolled seizures Facial deformity preventing mask fit
Mask selection	
Features favoring nasal marks	Features favoring face masks
Less acutely ill, more cooperative patient	More acutely ill, less cooperative patient
Less dead space	Edentulous patient
Allows easier communication	Mouth breathing pattern
Less aspiration risk if patient with emesis	Pursed-lips breathing pattern
May be better tolerated in claustrophobic patients	
More comfortable for long-term (weeks) use	

feedback. This would eliminate any comatose or uncooperative patient. This also eliminates any patient who would need immediate intubation because of respiratory failure. In addition, setup and initiation of noninvasive ventilation requires a greater time commitment from nursing and respiratory therapy staff than endotracheal intubation. Maintenance of noninvasive ventilation also requires additional vigilance. Adequate support staff is essential for the success of noninvasive ventilation; their role and importance cannot be overestimated.

In a coronary care unit, acute cardiogenic pulmonary edema would be the most common condition that would be amenable to noninvasive ventilation. Given the beneficial effects of positive airway pressure on cardiac function, it could conceivably be of benefit in nearly all patients with pulmonary edema. In practice, it is usually reserved for patients with respiratory distress, but who do not need immediate intubation. Patients may have evidence of increased work of breathing such as tachypnea, accessory muscle use, or abdominal paradox during inspiration. Based on the experience with face mask CPAP, patients may be quite hypoxemic with PaO_2/FIO_2 ratios < 150, hypercapnic with both metabolic and respiratory acidosis, and a pH averaging 7.18 ± 0.08 (25). Because of the rapidity in which pulmonary edema may clear with both medications and noninvasive ventilation, these values may not even represent the lower limit of successful noninvasive ventilation. Experience with other types of respiratory failure has not been able to define the lower threshold of successful noninvasive ventilation (45–47). However, it appears that hypercapnic patients (>45 mm Hg) fare better than eucapnic or hypocapnic patients. Most studies in other types of respiratory failure have also limited application to patients with a pH $\geqslant 7.25$, but these causes of respiratory failure do not have the potential for as rapid a reversal as acute pulmonary edema. Their findings may not be uniformly generalized to patients with pulmonary edema, but they lend insight into factors that influence successful outcome. Variables that may predict unsuccessful noninvasive ventilation include a greater severity of illness defined by an APACHE II score, encephalopathy, and azotemia. It is important to identify factors that may help to identify patients most likely to be successfully treated with noninvasive ventilation to avoid delays in marginal patients better served by intubation and mechanical ventilation.

In addition, the ideal patient's presentation should be limited to pulmonary edema and respiratory distress. Because of the frequent attention to noninvasive ventilation required for its success, patients with severe comorbid conditions requiring ongoing active therapy are best treated with endotracheal intubation. Patients are best ventilated with the head of the bed elevated at a 45° angle or greater. This eliminates from consideration hypotensive patients or those who are hemodynamically unstable. Patients with other comorbid conditions such as cardiac dysrhythmias or ongoing ischemia, gastrointestinal bleeding, seizures, or other conditions that require airway protection are also not candidates for noninvasive ventilation. This would include patients who pose an aspiration risk because of altered neuromuscular function or decreased level of consciousness.

The bane of noninvasive ventilation is mask leaks. The ability to fit the nasal or face mask properly is crucial for success. This would exclude patients who have facial deformities and those with significant facial defects following extensive head and neck surgery, which would prevent proper placement and seating of the mask over the nose and/or face. Patients with beards are a little more difficult because of mask leaks due to the beard, but presence of a beard is not a contraindication to noninvasive ventilation. Leaks around the mask can be corrected by adjustment of the mask or placement of gauze at leakage sites.

Edentulous patients have a particularly difficult time with nasal mask ventilation (45). It is more difficult for them to maintain a proper mouth seal. During noninvasive ventilation, there are several anatomic barriers to mouth leaks. The positive airway pressure displaces the soft palate anteriorly against the tongue to form a seal. The teeth form another barrier, and the lips provide the final barrier against mouth leaks. In addition, the loss of teeth make fitting the mask over the upper lip more difficult, because of the loss of the upper mandibular ridge. If available, dentures help with minimizing mouth leaks. A chin strap can be used as well. If there are excessive leaks with a nasal mask, the face mask provides an alternative interface.

Once the mask has been properly fitted, then patients must be able to synchronize with the ventilator. This is less of a problem with CPAP ventilation. In some patients, the nearly immediate relief of dyspnea and decreased work of breathing during noninvasive ventilation help facilitate patient-ventilator synchrony and ventilation. In others, however, the mask, especially the face mask, may create a claustrophobic sensation and worsen dyspnea (48). Some patients with extreme dyspnea are unable to allow any support by the ventilator. Patients with a pursed-lips breathing pattern may comprise another group unable to tolerate nasal ventilation. Excess secretions or pneumonia also pose a problem. Patients are unable to expectorate during noninvasive ventilation, and the secretions interfere with proper patient-ventilator synchrony. Some patients are extremely anxious and it has been tempting to consider sedatives and anxiolytics to facilitate their adaptation to noninvasive ventilation. The risks of respiratory depression and aspiration during noninvasive ventilation make this problematic; very anxious patients are probably better served by sedation and endotracheal intubation.

B. Masks

Noninvasive ventilation is delivered through either a clear nasal mask or a face mask. A clear face mask is important in the event of emesis. There are several manufacturers offering a wide range of sizes, including the ability to customize the fit of nasal masks for individual patients. Patients ventilated with the two types of masks are shown in Figure 2. Problems with fitting, leaks, and pressure points have been ameliorated with sealing flaps, air, or foam cushions. The masks are

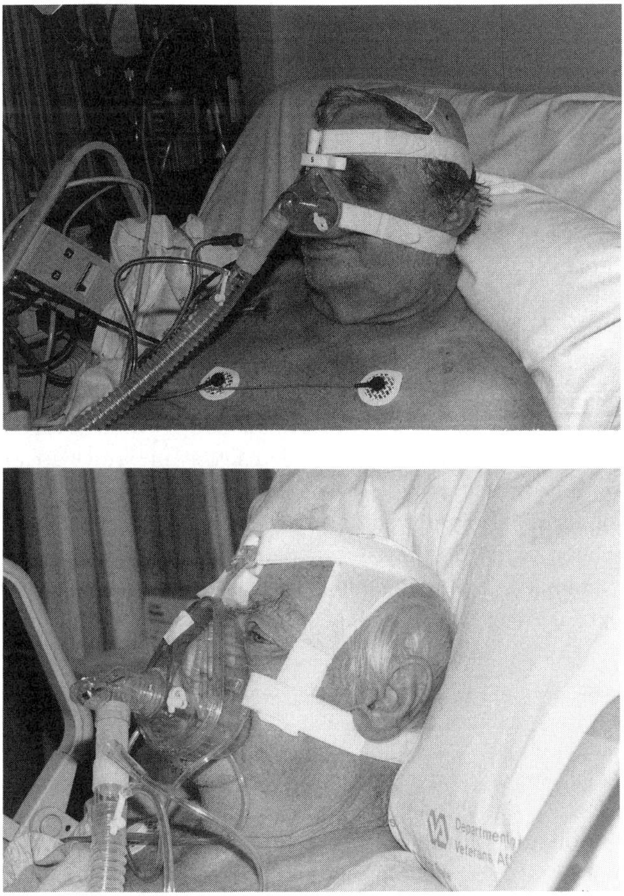

Figure 2 Photograph of patient treated with nasal mask noninvasive ventilation. A portable ventilator was used, and supplemental oxygen was supplied just distal to the end of the nasal mask (top). Photograph of patient treated with face mask noninvasive ventilation (bottom). Note the nasogastric tube that is inserted through the left nostril. This was used to administer medications and not needed to relieve gastric distension.

held in place with either rubber or Velcro head straps, and there is the option for head caps and chin straps. The masks also have ports which allow either monitoring of expired gases or administration of low-flow oxygen. Some are designed with release straps which allow rapid removal of the mask. There are also adaptors that will accommodate and anchor a nasogastric tube. Both disposable and reusable masks are available.

It is unlikely that one type of mask is clearly superior to the other. There are reports that support one over the other, but study biases obscure their conclusions. One study compared the two types of mask using a group of patients who were regulary ventilated using a nasal mask (49). The other assessed a group of patients who could not tolerate nasal masks (50). For most patients, the nasal mask is more comfortable and less obtrusive, has less dead space, and allows easier communication. Claustrophobia may be less of a problem with the nasal mask. On the other hand, the nasal mask does require a little more coordination by the patient. Patients must be able to maintain a mouth seal; if unable to prevent mouth leaks (edentulous, mouth breathing pattern), patients are better suited for the face mask. It makes sense that less acutely ill patients may be more likely to tolerate and be successfully ventilated with a nasal mask. In earlier studies, concern with gastric insufflation during noninvasive ventilation prompted routine nasogastric tube placement in patients treated with face mask ventilation. However, it has become evident that gastric insufflation is not a problem provided airway pressures do not exceed the 25 cm H_2O opening pressure of the lower esophageal sphincter (51). A nasogastric tube is no longer routinely placed during face mask ventilation. The nasal mask is probably better tolerated if long-term ventilatiion (weeks) is necessary or anticipated. In summary, if properly fitted, effective ventilation can be accomplished using either a nasal or face mask interface. Personal preference may dictate the final choice.

C. Ventilators

Noninvasive ventilation can be delivered with a wide spectrum of ventilatory assist devices. Both bedside and portable ventilators have been successful utilized. Crucial differences and individual advantages are summarized in Table 3. The bedside ventilator has more ventilatory options and can allow a mix of modalities including assist control (AC), SIMV, PS, PC, CPAP, and PEEP as well as control over flow rates and FIO_2. However, it may not be as tolerant of leaks as the portable ventilator, and alarms may need frequent adjustment. There is no other modification of the bedside ventilator necessary for noninvasive ventilation, and the same humification and breathing circuits can be used.

Portable or home ventilator devices are less expensive and are also suitable for noninvasive ventilation. They are usually equipped with fewer alarms and may therefore be more tolerant of system leaks. Some devices, specifically the BiPAP devices, also compensate for leaks much better than bedside ventilators. Humidifiers are not standard equipment and have to be attached, especially if noninvasive ventilation is used for extended periods of time. The high flow rates can cause drying and discomfort of mucosal airways. Although some portable ventilators allow adjustment of FIO_2, supplemental oxygen must be added in others, specifically those designed primarily to provided only CPAP or BiPAP. This is done by attaching oxygen tubing either to the ventilator tubing or to the mask. In addition,

Table 3 Ventilators in Noninvasive Ventilation

Ventilators	
Features favoring bedside ventilators	Features favoring portable or home ventilators
Wider array of options	Less expensive
Ability to provide higher levels of pressure support	Fewer alarms
No need to add humidification or oxygen	More tolerant of system leaks
No risk of CO_2 rebreathing	Portable; can be used in transition from hospital to home
Hospital staff more familiar with operation	
Ventilator modes	
Advantages of volume ventilation	Disadvantages of volume ventilation
Most familiar to staff	Requires most coordination by patient
Ability to provide precise minute ventilation	May be subject to high inspiratory pressures
Advantages of pressure support ventilation	Disadvantages of pressure support ventilation
Patient-initiated, patient-controlled	Risk of prolonged inspiratory cycle if with large mask leaks
May be better tolerated by patients	
Advantages of BIPAP ventilation	Disadvantages of BiPAP ventilation
Portable, less expensive	IPAP limited to 22 cm H_2O (some models)
Able to compensate for leaks	Risk of CO_2 rebreathing
Same advantages as pressure support (above)	
Advantages of CPAP	Disadvantages of CPAP
Simplest device	Higher levels not well tolerated
Can be delivered by alterations of breathing circuit	
Can be delivered in conjunction with volume or pressure support ventilation (PEEP)	

these devices are designed to deliver pressure through a single tube with an exhalation port or connector which allows a venting of expired gas and CO_2. In most patients, there is sufficient expiratory time to allow dissipation of expired gases. However, if the expired flow rates exceed the leak rate of the vent or if expiratory times are short and inadequate to allow proper venting of expired gases, CO_2 rebreathing will occur. This can be clinically significant, as both increased work of breathing and failure to correct hypercapnia have been attributed to this mechanism in patients under study conditions (52,53). This problem can be corrected by using a valve that adds a small amount of PEEP to the circuit. Alternatively, it appears that a EPAP level in the 5 to 8 cm H_2O range would also correct this potential problem. In addition, there are differences in the inspiratory trigger sensitivity and flow acceleration between bedside and different portable ventilators. There does not appear to be any difference in ventilation (tidal volume, respiratory rate) of patients at the same level of pressure support with these devices, but there can be as much as a 30% increase in measure of work of breathing with the portable device (54). Some portable devices are also limited to 22 cm H_2O as the maximal amount of pressure support (or IPAP) that can be delivered. This might be a problem in patients with either noncompliant lungs or very severe pulmonary edema, and this group may be better served with support supplied by a bedside ventilator. Newer models can deliver up to 30 cm H_20 IPAP. However, it should be noted that in spite of these potential shortcomings, the clinical experience with these devices has been excellent with results comparable to or better than those achieved with other ventilatory devices.

Noninvasive ventilation can be delivered using either volume-cycled or pressure-cycled modes with no clear-cut treatment advantage of one mode over the other (55–58). There are study data that support one mode over the other with respect to work of breathing, patient ventilator synchrony, or air leakage, but this has yet to translate into a clinically significant advantage. Volume ventilation does allow for a more precise minute ventilation and can actually provide controlled ventilation. It also requires more coordination by the patient with the ventilator. Pressure support is patient-initiated and allows the patient more control of the ventilatory pattern including inspiratory time and breathing frequency. There is less coordination required of the patient, and pressure support is probably better tolerated. As with the masks and ventilators, personal preference and experience greatly influence the ventilatory mode utilized.

Once the decision has been made on the mode of ventilation and the mask has been properly fitted, the patient can be attached to the ventilator in the same manner as intubated patients. The ventilator settings are very similar to those used in intubated patients. Using volume ventilation, the tidal volume should be in the 10 to 12 ml/kg range, inspiratory flow rate of 60 L/min, and a respiratory rate of 12 breaths/min. If the patient remains dyspneic, the rate or inspiratory flow rate can be increased with further adjustments as dictated by patient comfort. Peak inspiratory pressures are usually low and should not exceed 25 to 30 cm H_2O. If the peak pressures are too high, adjustments can be made in the tidal volume or inspiratory flow rate. Leaks can be assessed manually by placing hands around the mask and feeling the air leak. Leaks around the eyes are particulary uncomfortable and need to be minimized. Mask leaks are to be expected (defined by the difference between inspiratory and expiratory volumes), but with adequate mask fitting should not exceed 100 ml. It is also important that head straps not be excessively tightened, as this can be uncomfortable and lead to pressure necrosis of the skin. Goals include maintance of oxygen saturation above 90%, elimination of accessory muscle use, and reduction in respiratory rate and heart rate.

Subjects who are able to synchronize with the ventilator often experience immediate relief. There are rapid reduction in hypercapnia and correction of hypoxemia. A significant correction of respiratory acidosis is usually seen within an hour or 2 of institution of therapy and can be used as an indicator of patient-ventilator synchrony and predictor of successful ventilation. One advantage of noninvasive ventilation is its intermittent application. Patients are encouraged to undergo noninvasive support, usually in 4-h blocks with 1-h breaks over the first 24 h. Some patients are able to tolerate much longer periods (8 to 12 hours) at a time. Breaks are utilized for facial skin care, feeding, and communication. In patients with nasogastric tubes, some investigators have instituted enteral feedings during noninvasive ventilation.

The same technique of instituting noninvasive ventilation can be used with pressure support (59). Pressure support settings are adjusted to achieve a tidal volume more in the 7 to 10 ml/kg range. Pressure support ventilators can better compensate for minor leaks, although it is important to eliminate large leaks to prevent a prolonged inspiratory cycle. The initial pressure support level should be 10 cm H_2O with increments of 2 to 3 cm H_2O every 15 to 20 minutes until tidal volume and oxygenation goals are achieved. PEEP is optional but is usually added at 5 cm H_2O and can also be increased by 2 to 3 cm H_2O, especially if there is hypoxemic respiratory failure. Patients can tolerate fairly high levels of pressure support, but the possibility of gastric insufflation places a limit of pressure support at 22–25 cm H_2O. Most patients cannot tolerate more than 10 cm H_2O of PEEP. If a BiPAP device is used, the initial settings include an IPAP of 10 cm H_2O and and EPAP of 5 cm H_2O, especially given the potential for rebreathing CO_2.

With CPAP, an initial pressure as low as 5 cm H_2O may be beneficial. This can be increased in increments of 3 to 5 cm H_2O up to 15 cm H_2O. Past experience suggests that 10 cm H_2O is the optimal and best-tolerated level, with many fewer patients able to tolerate 15 cm H_2O. However, the level for each patient needs to be adjusted individually based on response and tolerance.

There is a significant time requirement for staff (60,61). The first hour usually requires the most intensive attention to the patient and is crucial for success. Patients often require prompting, especially with nasal ventilation and mouth leaks. Mask leaks may be uncomfortable and require adjustment of straps or placement of gauze. There is also a significant learning curve for all health care staff (physicians, nursing, respiratory therapy), the importance of which cannot be overestimated. The time commitment was a significant concern during the initial experience with noninvasive ventilation. But as staff have gained experience, more recent reports note no difference in time commitment or difficulty in management as compared to medically treated controls or intubated patients for nursing staff. There was an increased time committment for respiratory staff, but only for the first 8 h and was actually less for noninvasive ventilation with time.

D. Duration of Ventilation

The duration of noninvasive ventilation should be dictated by the patient's response to therapy, resolution of respiratory failure, and tolerance of treatment. Patients with cardiogenic pulmonary edema were successfully treated with only 9.3 ± 4.9 h of CPAP. Subjects with other types of respiratory failure have been treated for as long as 23 days, but most reports note successful resolution of respiratory failure with noninvasive support in less than 4 days. Some patients who require continued support can be converted to nocturnal ventilation. Appropriate end points include correction of hypercapnia and respiratory acidosis using a pH $\geqslant 7.35$. Since noninvasive ventilation is intermittently applied, the need for continued support can be assessed with each break in ventilation. Therefore, there is no need for an extended "weaning" period. Patients with respiratory muscle fatigue and impending failure may require only a brief period of respiratory muscle rest, which can be achieved with noninvasive ventilation. Each break can be viewed as a trial of ventilatory support, with noninvasive ventilation reinstituted if there are any signs of respiratory distress. This approach results in the use of noninvasive ventilation for a relatively short duration as compared to endotracheal intubation and ventilation. This translates into shorter ICU and hospital stays with decreases in morbidity and mortality, which is directly related to the prevention of mechanical ventilation and its attendant complications.

Alternatively, there must also be close monitoring for signs of failure of noninvasive ventilatory support. Even in the best of circumstances, the success rate in only in the 70% to 80% range. As outlined earlier, patient selection in crucial for success with comorbidities, uncorrectable mask leaks, or an inability to synchronize with the ventilator early signs of failure. Many investigators have noted marked improvement in respiratory acidosis defined as either $\geqslant 15\%$ decline in $PaCO_2$ or improvement of pH to $\geqslant 7.30$ within 1 to two h of instituting therapy (32,45). The rapidity of correction helps identify successfully treated patients and serves as a marker of patient ventilator synchrony. It should be noted, though, that the improvement may be more gradual in other patients. The lack of improvement without accompanying evidence of further progression of respiratory distress or indications for intubation should not be viewed as an automatic indication for discontinuation of noninvasive ventilation. Some investigators have noted that resolution of respiratory failure and respiratory acidosis may require upwards of 36 h.

There are several criteria that have been used to help define an adequate trial of noninvasive ventilation. Some response or nonresponse to therapy can be seen in most patients within 30 min, and this time frame would constitute a minimal trial of noninvasive ventilation. This underscores the need for near-constant surveillance by staff during the first hour of therapy. Failure to correct gas exchange abnormalities, respiratory distress or dyspnea, an inability to tolerate the mask or progression of symptoms, are self-evident criteria of failure. Investigators have further divided criteria into major and minor categories and are often viewed as intubation criteria (62). Any major criteria including respiratory arrest, respiratory pauses with loss of consciousness or gasping, psychomotor agitation requiring sedation, a heart rate < 50 beats per minute (BPM) with decreased level of alertness, or hemodynamic instability with a systolic blood pressure < 70 mm Hg would be an indication of failure of noninvasive ventilation and need for intubation. Any two minor criteria, defined as a respiratory rate > 35 breaths per minute and increase from admission, pH < 7.30 with a decline from admission, PaO_2 < 45 mm Hg despite supplemental oxygen, or increase in encephalopathy score, were used to halt noninvasive ventilation and proceed with intubation. In addition, others have included tidal volumes < 5 ml/kg, $PaCO_2$ increase of 10 mm Hg or pH decline of 0.08, oxygen saturation < 90% despite supplement oxygen, ischemic ECG changes or dysrhythmias, blood pressure changes characterized as a rise or fall of 20 mm Hg systolic or fall of 10 mm Hg diastolic, or inability to manage secretions as discontinuation criteria (63). These changes may be noted not only during institution of therapy, but also at any time during noninvasive ventilation. These are suggested guidelines, of course, and the decision to intubate or terminate noninvasive ventilation requires some individual consideration.

V. COMPLICATIONS

There are relatively few complications reported with noninvasive ventilation (51). The most common problem is skin necrosis at the mask contact sites. The bridge of the nose is the most common site and undoubtedly related to tightening of the mask to minimize air leaks. Gauze or foam can be used to relieve pressure, and some masks do have protective foam. Portable BiPAP ventilators can better compensate for leaks, and patients do not require as tight-fitting a mask with these devices. Repositioning the mask and head straps to relieve pressure points may help, and may provide periodic breaks from noninvasive ventilation. The risk of skin necrosis increases with duration of ventilation and may also increase in patients requiring higher airway pressures. Other complications include conjunctivitis, aspiration, and pneumothorax and gastric distension. The overall complication rate is about 10%, which compares very favorably with intubation and mechanical ventilation where the complication rate may exceed 50% and complications are much more serious (e.g., nosocomial pneumonia, gastrointestinal bleeding, intubation-associated airway trauma, etc.) (64).

VI. SUMMARY

Noninvasive ventilation is a well-tolerated and effective method of providing ventilatory support in patients with respiratory distress and failure. It is uniquely suited as an adjunct to cardiogenic pulmonary edema because of its beneficial cardiac effects. Keys to successful application include patient selection, proper mask fitting, and patient cooperation. Use of noninvasive ventilation will increase as the medical community gains experience with the technique and as its role in the management of respiratory failure becomes more defined.

REFERENCES

1. Poulton PE. Left-sided heart failure with pulmonary oedema: its treatment with the "pulmonary plus pressure machine." Lancet 1936; 2:981–983.
2. Barach AL, Martin J, Eckman M. Positive pressure respiration and its application to the treatment of acute pulmonary edema. Ann Intern Med 1938; 12:754–795.
3. Hogg JC, Agarwal JB, Gardiner AJS, Palmer WH, Macklem PT. Distribution of airway resistance with developing pulmonary edema in dogs. J Appl Physiol 1972; 32:20–24.
4. Sharp JT, Griffith GT, Bunnell IL, Greene DG. Ventilatory mechanics in pulmonary edema in man. J Clin Invest 1958; 37:111–117.
5. Light RW, George RB. Serial pulmonary function in patients with acute heart failure. Arch Intern Med 1983; 143:429–433.
6. Supinski G, DiMarco A, Dibner-Dunlap M. Alterations in diaphragm strength and fatiguability in congestive heart failure. J Appl Physiol 1994; 76:2707–2713.
7. Aberman A, Fulop M. The metabolic and respiratory acidosis of acute pulmonary edema. Ann Intern Med 1972; 76:173–184.
8. Hopewell PC, Murray JF. Effects of continuous positive-pressure ventilation in experimental pulmonary edema. J Appl Physiol 1976; 40:568–574.
9. Katz JA, Marks JD. Inspiratory work with and without continuous positive airway pressure in patients with acute respiratory failure. Anesthesiology 1985; 63:598–607.
10. Cournand A, Motley HL, Werko L, Richards DW. Physiological studies on the effects of intermittent positive pressure breathing on cardiac output in man. Am J Physiol 1948; 152:162–174.
11. Luce JM. The cardiovascular effects of mechanical ventilation and positive end-expiratory pressure. JAMA 1984; 252:807–811.
12. Buda AJ, Pinsky MR, Ingels NB, Daughters GT, Stinson EB, Alderman EL. Effect of intrathoracic pressure on left ventricular performance. N Engl J Med 1979; 301: 453–459.
13. Jardin F, Farcot J-C, Boisante L, Curien N, Margairaz A, Bourdarias J-P. Effect of positive end-expiratory pressure on left ventricular performance. N Engl J Med 1981; 304:386–392.
14. Grace MP, Greenbaum DM. Cardiac performance in response to PEEP in patients with cardiac dysfunction. Crit Care Med 1982; 6:358–360.

15. Pinsky MR, Summer WR, Wise RA, Permutt S, Bromberger-Barnea B. Augmentation of cardiac function by elevation of intrathoracic pressure. J Appl Physiol 1983; 54:950–955.
16. Pinsky MR, Summer WR. Cardiac augmentation by phasic high intrathoracic pressure support in man. Chest 1983; 84:370–375.
17. Pinsky MR, Matuschak GM, Klain M. Determinants of cardiac augmentation by elevations in intrathoracic pressure. J Appl Physiol 1985; 58:1189–1198.
18. Pinsky MR, Marquez J, Martin D, Klain M. Ventricular assist by cardiac cycle-specific increases in intrathoracic pressure. Chest 1987; 91:709–715.
19. Greenbaum DM, Millen JE, Eross B, Snyder JV, Grenvik A, Safar P. Continuous positive airway pressure without tracheal intubation in spontaneously breathing patients. Chest 1976; 69:615–620.
20. Covelli HD, Weled BJ, Beekman JF. Efficacy of continuous positive airway pressure administered by face mask. Chest 1982; 81:147–150.
21. Hoff BH, Flemming DC, Sasse F. Use of positive airway pressure without endotracheal intubation. Crit Care Med 1979; 7:559–562.
22. Perel A, Williamson DC, Modell JH. Effectiveness of CPAP by mask for pulmonary edema associated with hypercarbia. Intens Care Med 1983; 9:17–19.
23. Rasanen J, Heikkila J, Downs J, Nikki P, Vaisanen I, Viitanen A. Continuous positive airway pressure by face mask in acute cardiogenic pulmonary edema. Am J Cardiol 1985; 55:296–300.
24. Rasanen J, Vaisanen IT. Continuous positive airway pressure and supplemental oxygen in the treatment of cardiogenic pulmonary edema. Chest 1987; 92: 481–485.
25. Bersten AD, Holt AW, Vedig AE, Skowronski GA, Baggoley C. Treatment of severe cardiogenic pulmonary edema with continuous positive airway pressure delivered by face mask. N Engl J Med 1991; 325:1825–1830.
26. Bradley TD, Holloway RM, McLaughlin PR, Ross BL, Walters J, Liu PP. Cardiac output response to continuous positive airway pressure in congestive heart failure. Am Rev Respir Dis 1992; 145:377–382.
27. Baratz DM, Westbrook PR, Shah PK, Mohsenifar Z. Effect of nasal continuous positive airway pressure on cardiac output and oxygen delivery in patients with congestive heart failure. Chest 1992; 102:1397–1401.
28. Meyer TJ, Hill NS. Noninvasive positive pressure ventilation to treat respiratory failure. Ann Intern Med 1994; 120:760–770.
29. Wysocki M, Tric L, Wolff MA, Millet H, Herman B. Noninvasive pressure support ventilation in patients with acute respiratory failure: a randomized comparison with conventional therapy. Chest 1995; 107:761–768.
30. Rusterholtz T, Kempf J, Gayol S, et al. Is low $PaCO_2$ a factor of failure of facial mask pressure support ventilation (FMOSV) during acute cardiogenic pulmonary edema (ACPE)? Am J Respir Crit Care Med 1996; 153:A606.
31. Bollaert PE, Weber M, Lucchelli JP, et al. Noninvasive pressure support ventilation (NIPSV) for acute cardiogenic pulmonary edema: a case control study. Am J Respir Crit Care Med 1996; 153:A609.
31a. Mehta S, Jay GD, Woolard RH, et al. Randomized, prospective trial of bilevel versus

continuous positive airway pressure in acute pulmonary edema. Crit Care Med 1997; 25:620–628.
32. Meduri GU, Abou-Shala N, Fox RC, Jones CB, Leeper KV, Wunderink RG. Noninvasive face mask mechanical ventilation in patients with acute hypercapnic respiratory failure. Chest 1991; 100:445–454.
33. Pennock BE, Kaplan PD, Carlin BW, Sabangan JS, Magovern JA. Pressure support ventilation with a simplified ventilatory support system administered with a nasal mask in patients with respiratory failure. Chest 1991; 100:1371–1376.
34. Wysocki M, Tric L, Wolff MA, Gerner J, Millet H, Herman B. Noninvasive presssure support ventilation in patients with acute respiratory failure. Chest 1993; 103: 907–913.
35. Nathan SD, Ishaaya AM, Koerner SK, Belman MJ. Prediction of minimal pressure support during weaning from mechanical ventilation. Chest 1993; 103:1215–1219.
36. Ishaaya AM, Nathan SD, Belman MJ. Work of breathing after extubation. Chest 1995; 107:204–209.
37. Ferguson KA, Fleetham JA. Consequences of sleep disordered breathing. Thorax 1995; 50:998–1004.
38. Chaudhary BA, Ferguson DS, Speir WA. Pulmonary edema as a presenting feature of sleep apnea syndrome. Chest 1981; 82:122–124.
39. Malone S, Liu PP, Holloway R, Rutherford R, Xie A, Bradley TD. Obstructive sleep apnea in patients with dilated cardiomyopathy: effects of continuous positive airway pressure. Lancet 1991; 338:1480–1484.
40. Takasaki Y, Orr D, Popkin J, Rutherford R, Liu P, Bradley TD. Effect of nasal continuous positive airway pressure on sleep apnea in congestive heart failure. Am Rev Respir Dis 1989; 140:1578–1584.
41. Naughton MT, Liu PP, Benard DC, Goldstein RS, Bradley TD. Treatment of congestive heart failure and Cheyne-Stokes respirations during sleep by continuous positive airway pressure. Am J Respir Crit Care Med 1995; 151:92–97.
42. Findley LJ, Zwillich CW, Ancoli-Israel S, Krike D, Tisi G, Moser KM. Cheyne-Stokes breathing during sleep in patients with left ventricular heart failure. South Med J 1985; 78:11–15.
43. Buckle P, Millar T, Kryger M. The effect of short-term nasal CPAP on Cheyne-Stokes respiration in congestive heart failure. Chest 1992; 102:31–35.
44. Davies RJO, Harrington KJ, Ormerod OJM, Stradling JR. Nasal continuous positive airway pressure in chronic heart failure with sleep-disordered breathing. Am Rev Respir Dis 1993; 147:630–634.
45. Soo Hoo GW, Santiago S, Williams AJ. Nasal mechanical ventilation for hypercapnic respiratory failure in chronic obstructive pulmonary disease: determinants of success and failure. Crit Care Med 1994; 22:1253–1261.
46. Ambrosino N, Foglio K, Rubini F, Clini E, Nava S, Vitacca M. Non-invasive mechanical ventilation in acute respiratory failure due to chronic obstructive pulmonary disease: correlates for success. Thorax 1995; 50:755–757.
47. Wysocki M, Girard T, Chevret S, Wolff MA, Millet H, Herman B. Noninvasive ventilation in patient with acute exacerbation of COPD: multivariate analysis of predicted factors of failure. Am J Respir Crit Care Med 1995; 151:A236.

48. Soo Hoo GW, Williams, AJ. Noninvasive face-mask ventilation in patients with acute hypercapnic respiratory failure. Chest 1993; 103:1304–1305.
49. Reid PT, Mikelsons C, Bott JB, Wedzicha JA. Comparison of face and nasal masks for non-invasive ventilation in COPD patients. Thorax 1994; 49:1063P.
50. Criner GJ, Tavaline JM, Brennan KJ, Kreimer DT. Efficacy of a new full face mask for noninvasive positive pressure ventilation. Chest 1994; 106:1109–1115.
51. Abou-Shala N, Meduri GU. Noninvasive mechanical ventilation in patients with acute respiratory failure. Crit Care Med 1996; 24:705–715.
52. Ferguson GT, Gilmartin M. CO_2 rebreathing during BiPAP ventilatory assistance. Am J Respir Crit Care Med 1995; 151:1126–1135.
53. Lofaso F, Brochard L, Touchard D, Hang T, Harf A, Isabey D. Evaluation of carbon dioxide rebreathing during pressure support ventilation with airway management system (BiPAP) devices. Chest 1995; 108:772–778.
54. Lofaso F, Brochard L, Hang T, Lorino H, Harf A, Isabey D. Home versus intensive care pressure support devices: experimental and clinical comparison. Am J Respir Crit Care Med 1996; 153:1591–1599.
55. Brochard L, Isabey D, Piquet J, et al. Reversal of acute exacerbations of chronic obstructive lung disease by inspiratory assistance with a face mask. N Engl J Med 1990; 323:1523–1530.
56. Ambrosino N, Nava S, Bertone P, Fracchia C, Rampulla C. Physiologic evaluation of pressure support ventilation by nasal mask in patients with stable COPD. Chest 1992; 101:385–391.
57. Vitacca M, Rubini F, Foglio K, Scalvini S, Nava S, Ambrosino N. Non-invasive modalities of positive pressure ventilation improve the outcome of acute exacerbations in COLD patients. Intens Care Med 1993; 19:450–455.
58. Meecham-Jones DJ, Paul EA, Grahame-Clarke C, Wedzicha JA. Nasal ventilation in acute exacerbations of chronic obstructive pulmonary disease: effect of ventilator mode on arterial blood gas tensions. Thorax 1994; 49:1222–1224.
59. Pennock BE, Crawshaw L, Kaplan PD. Noninvasive nasal mask ventilation for acute respiratory failure: institution of a new therapeutic technology for routine use. Chest 1994; 105:441–444.
60. Chevrolet J-C, Jolliet P, Abajo B, Toussi A, Louis M. Nasal positive pressure ventilation in patients with acute respiratory failure: difficult and time consuming procedure for nurses. Chest 1991; 100:775–782.
61. Kramer N, Meyer TJ, Mehard J, Cece RD, Hill NS. Randomized, prospective trial of noninvasive positive pressure ventilation in acute respiratory failure. Am J Respir Crit Care Med 1995; 151:1799–1806.
62. Brochard L, Mancebo J, Wysocki M, et al. Noninvasive ventilation for acute exacerbation of chronic obstructive pulmonary disease. N Engl J Med 1995; 333:817–822.
63. Schuster D. A physiologic approach to initiating, maintaining and withdrawing mechanical ventilatory support during acute respiratory failure. Am J Med 1990; 88:268–278.
64. Stauffer JL, Olson DE, Petty TL. Complications and consequences of endotracheal intubation and tracheostomy. A prospective study of 150 critically ill adult patients. Am J Med 1981; 70:65–76.

2

Respiratory Muscles in Critically Ill Patients

ANDREA T. FEINBERG and MICHAEL I. LEWIS

Cedars-Sinai Medical Center and University of California, Los Angeles, School of Medicine, Los Angeles, California

I. INTRODUCTION

The respiratory muscles constitute the vital "ventilatory pump" of the chest, and as such may contribute significantly to both the morbidity and/or mortality of critically ill patients. The following chapter reviews an enormous body of literature, with an emphasis on respiratory muscle dysfunction likely to be encountered in patients treated in a cardiac (medical) or cardiothoracic (surgical) intensive care unit environment. The review is divided into three sections: an introduction to respiratory muscle structure and pathophysiology; clinical problems; and management principles.

A. Functional Anatomy of the Respiratory Muscles (1)

The diaphragm (DIA) is the most important primary inspiratory muscle and separates the chest wall into rib cage and abdominal compartments. The dome is composed mainly of the central tendon, while the cylindrical portion is composed of muscle fibers which insert on the upper margins of the lower six ribs and the xiphoid process. The DIA fibers apposed to the inner aspect of the lower rib cage comprise the zone of apposition and covers ~25% to 30% of the total ribcage surface area. As the abdominal contents are relatively incompressible, the piston-like descent of the DIA is resisted, and there is a rise in abdominal pressure and outward excursion of the anterior abdominal wall. The positive intra-abdominal

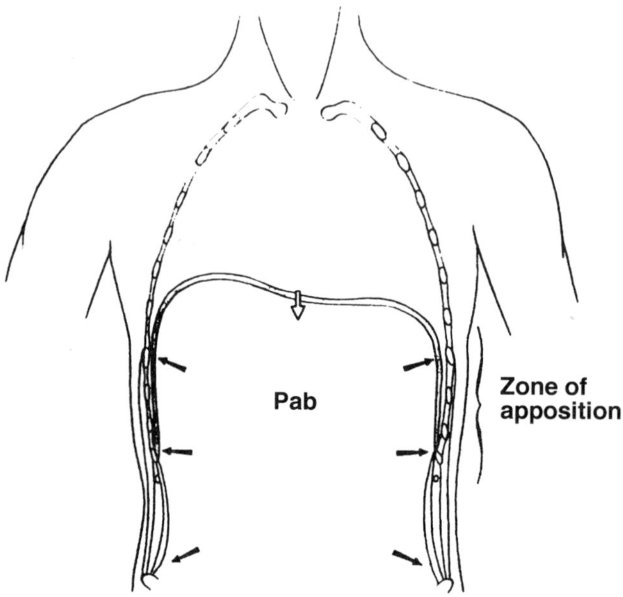

Figure 1 Appositional component of diaphragm action. From: De Troyer A, Estenne M. Functional anatomy of the respiratory muscles. Clin Chest Med 1988; 9:175–193; with permission.

pressure is transmitted through the apposed DIA to expand the lower ribcage (appositional action; Fig. 1). In addition, with contraction of DIA fibers, the forces exerted on the lower ribs are directed cranially in the direction of the muscle fibers, which lifts and outwardly rotates the lower ribs (insertional action). The appositional forces of DIA contraction may be diminished or virtually negated by a highly compliant abdominal wall (e.g., tetraplegia with DIA intact) or lung hyperinflation due to a reduction or elimination of the zone of apposition and attenuated rise in intra-abdominal pressure. With severe hyperinflation, the orientation of the DIA fibers may also be altered so that the insertional forces are directed inward, with a paradoxical inward (expiratory) movement of the lower rib cage (Hoover's sign). The DIA is innervated by the right and left phrenic nerves which arise from cervical roots 3, 4, and 5.

The parasternal intercostals are the interchondral portion of the internal intercostals and are considered important primary inspiratory muscles. On the other hand, the external intercostals and levator costae (muscle fibers run from the transverse process of the vertebra to the angle of the rib) function primarily as an inspiratory reserve system (i.e., accessory role) under conditions of increased load or ventilatory demand. The internal interosseous intercostals are expiratory in function. The intercostal muscles are innervated by the intercostal nerves.

The scalenes are also primary inspiratory muscles in man. They originate from the transverse processes of cervical vertebrae, insert on the first two ribs, and are innervated by cervical nerves C4 to C8. The scalenes are responsible for increasing the anteroposterior and transverse diameters of the upper rib cage and elevating the sternum. The sternocleidomastoids, by contrast, have an accessory role in that they are not recruited during resting ventilation. Motor innervation is from the XI cranial nerve.

The abdominal muscles are not phasically recruited during resting ventilation. However, they exert phasic expiratory influences on the rib cage when the ventilatory pump is subject to increased loads or is facing increased ventilatory demands (e.g., exercise). Abdominal muscle recruitment may serve to reduce inspiratory muscle work by allowing the DIA to passively descend at the onset of inspiration with relaxation of abdominal muscle effort. The abdominals are innervated by branches of T7 to T12.

1. Motor Units, Fiber Types, and Myosin Heavy Chain Phenotypes

A recent, well-referenced, comprehensive review by Sieck is an excellent resource for further reading (2). In brief, DIA motor units are comprised of the phrenic motor neuron and the muscle fibers it innervates. As noted in Figure 2, while type S (slow) motor units produce the lowest levels of force, they are the most fatigue-resistant. By contrast, type FF motor units, while producing the greatest levels of force, are most fatigable. DIA motor units are likely recruited in an orderly fashion (i.e., S → FR → Fint → FF). During resting ventilation, recruitment of only type S and some FR units at relatively low firing frequencies (e.g., 8 to 16 Hz) usually suffices. Increased ventilatory demand results in the recruitment of other fast motor units and/or higher firing rates (i.e., frequency coding), but the limitation in this circumstance is the recruitment of more fatigable motor units, which cannot sustain the increased force requirements. The most common histochemical scheme for classifying muscle fibers is based on the pH lability of myofibriller ATPase staining. Muscle fibers may be classified as type I (slow) and type II (fast). Type II fibers may be subclassified as IIa, IIb, IIc, and a more recently determined fiber type, IIx. Type S motor units compose type I fibers, while FR, Fint, and FF motor units comprise IIa, IIx, and IIb fibers, respectively. Myosin heavy chains (MHC) comprise a series of important contractile proteins responsible for many of the physiologic characteristics of the constituent muscle fibers. In adult respiratory muscle, the following MHC isoforms have been identified: MHC slow, 2A, 2B, 2X. Coexpression of MHC isoforms within a single muscle fiber may occur under normal or, more likely, pathologic states (e.g., following denervation).

B. Concepts of Respiratory Muscle Weakness and Fatigue

A number of excellent review articles are available on this complex and extensive subject (3–6). In brief, a recent NHLBI workshop on respiratory muscle fatigue,

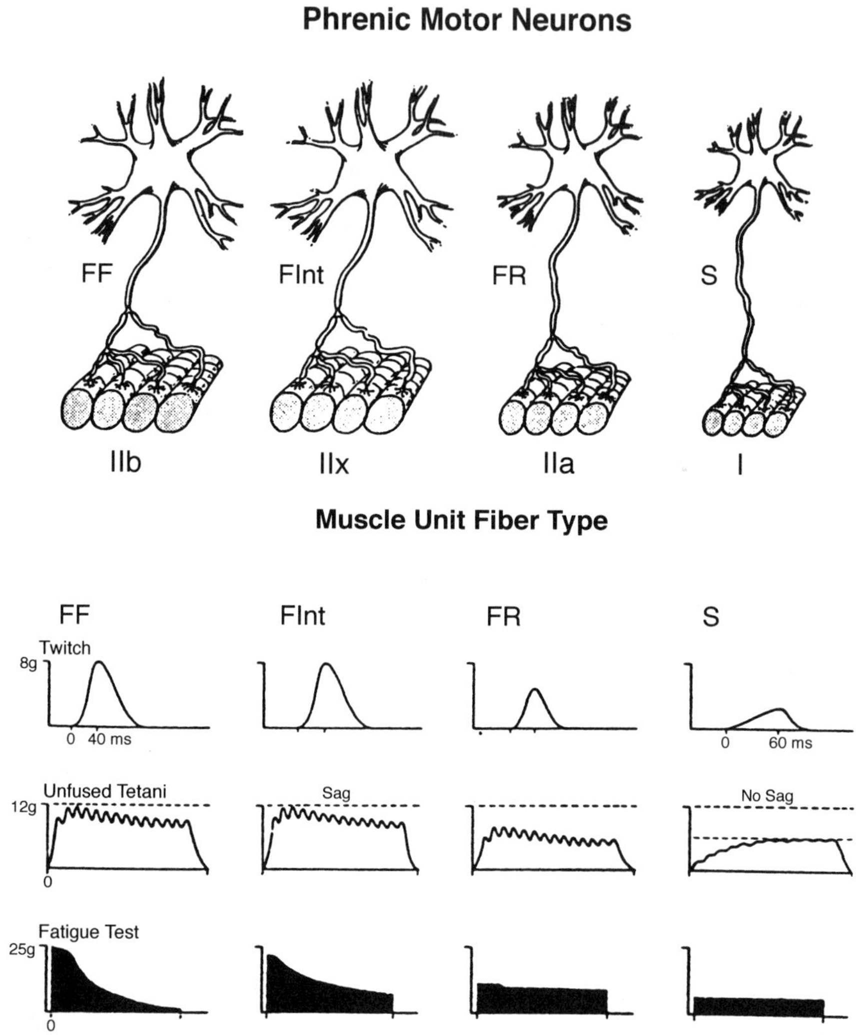

Figure 2 Diaphragm motor units comprising the phrenic motoneuron and the muscle fibers innervated. Twitch force, presence or absence of "sag" during unfused tetany, and a fatigue test are used to distinguish the different motor unit types. Muscle unit fibers can be subclassified histochemically as types I, IIa, IIb, and IIx. From: Sieck G. Organization and recruitment of diaphragm motor units. In: Roussos C, ed. The Thorax. 2nd ed. New York: Marcel Dekker, 1995:783–820, with permission.

defined *muscle fatigue* as "a condition in which there is loss in the capacity for developing force and/or velocity of a muscle, resulting from muscle activity under load and which is reversible by rest." Clinically, respiratory muscle fatigue may therefore be viewed as a condition in which the ability of the respiratory muscles to generate pressure and/or airflow is impaired. The latter is the result of heightened contractile activity of the respiratory muscles relative to strength and/or a decrease in energy supply. Finally, the impairment of respiratory muscle function would be expected to be improved by rest (i.e., complete unloading) or a decrease in the activity level of the muscles (i.e., partial unloading). By contrast, *muscle weakness* was defined as "a condition in which the capacity of a rested muscle to generate force is impaired" (8). Two other important concepts were highlighted: firstly, the fatiguing process may ensue prior to the inability to generate the required force despite maximal efforts; and secondly, that this point of exhaustion or task failure is dependent on a defined end point which in turn depends on the balance between pump capacity and load (Fig. 3). From the clinical perspective, task failure of the respiratory muscle pump may be viewed as the onset of ventilatory failure. The factors responsible for excessive load and diminished capacity of the inspiratory muscles are listed in Table 1.

Respiratory muscle fatigue has been classified as peripheral fatigue (includes contractile fatigue and neurotransmission fatigue) or central fatigue. Contractile fatigue refers to impaired contractile function of the muscle related to mechanisms

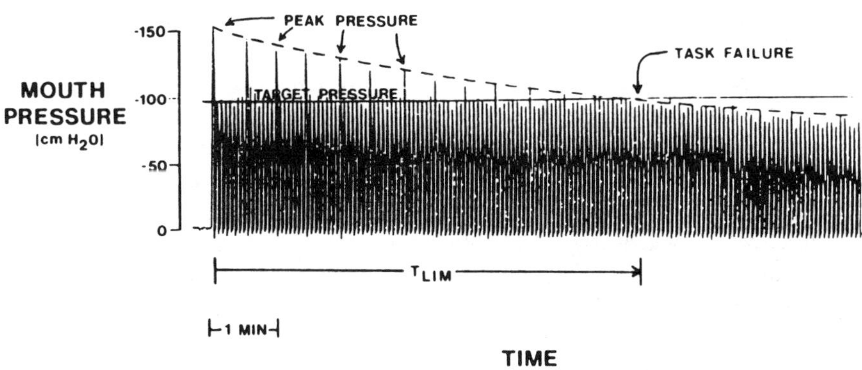

Figure 3 Changes in the capacity to generate pressure during a submaximal endurance run at a target pressure of 67% of peak pressure, measured prior to the endurance challenge. Note that peak pressure measured every 30 sec falls progressively during the endurance run indicating that a "fatiguing process" is under way. The point of task failure is defined in this endurance run as the inability to generate the target pressure (i.e., maximum efforts now fall below the target pressure). From: Grassino A, Clanton T. Respiratory muscle fatigue. Semin Respir Med 1991; 12:305–321, with permission.

Table 1 Factors Predisposing to Inspiratory Muscle Fatigue

Excessive load
- Increased work of breathing (minute ventilation, frequency, tidal volume, inspiratory time, compliance, resistance)

Reducing capacity
- *Weakness* (nutritional status, atrophy, neuromuscular distress, prematurity, lung volume)
- *Limited energy supply and stores*
  - —Reduced muscle blood flow (cardiac output, distribution of perfusion, intensity of contraction)
  - —Reduced content of arterial blood (O_2 saturation, Hb concentration)
  - —Reduced blood substrate concentration (glucose, free fatty acids)
  - —Reduced ability to utilize oxygen and substrates (sepsis)
  - —Reduced energy stores (muscle glycogen, ATP, phosphocreatanine)

Source: Roussos C et al. Respiratory muscle fatigue. In: Roussos C, ed. The Thorax. New York: Marcel Dekker, 1995:1405–1461 (with permission).

operating within the muscle fibers themselves. These include disturbances in the sarcolemma, metabolic aberrations such as accumulation of H+ and Pi, critical substrate depletion, and alterations in excitation—contraction coupling mediated by mechanical or chemical factors producing minor muscle injury (7).

Clinically, contractile fatigue of respiratory muscles may be longlasting (9). Neurotransmission fatigue refers to a reduction in the amplitude of action potentials mediated by axonal branch point conduction failure or impaired release, binding, or reuptake of the neurotransmitter at the neuromuscular junction. Myasthenia gravis, characterized by acetylcholine receptor antibodies and reduced number of acetylcholine receptors, is a classic example (10). Central fatigue refers to a diminution in force generation secondary to a reduction in central neural respiratory drive. The contractile response, however, can be restored by nerve stimulation (nonmotivational) or voluntary supereffect (motivation). Central fatigue has been viewed as a protective mechanism to preserve muscle integrity and prevent any undue contractile failure. It is clear, therefore, that multiple factors may contribute to the fatiguing process, which, depending on respiratory muscle capacity, imposed load, and modulating influences, may ultimately lead to task failure (i.e., ventilatory failure).

C. Assessment of Respiratory Muscle Function

A number of clinical signs may indicate a response of the respiratory muscles to increased load. These include a rapid shallow breathing pattern (11), respiratory alternans (12) (i.e., alternation between rib cage and abdominal breathing), paradoxical abdominal motion (13), and accessory muscle and/or abdominal muscle recruitment (14). While these signs are useful indicators of load and may occur as part of the fatiguing process, they do not necessarily imply the presence of respiratory muscle fatigue (13).

The maximal inspiratory pressure (MIP or PI_{max}) measured at RV or FRC is a useful test of global inspiratory muscle strength (15,16). Maximum expiratory pressure (MEP or PE_{max}) is measured at TLC and is a global measure of expiratory muscle strength. The major drawbacks in measuring MIP are that the test is effort-dependent and requires patient cooperation and is nonspecific with regard to distinguishing muscle weakness from fatigue or poor effort. In critically ill patients, the variances can be wide within patients (17). Lesser variances may be evident by measuring esophageal pressure (Pes) following a maximal sniff, but this procedure requires the use of an esophageal balloon catheter (18). Transdiaphragmatic pressure (Pdi) is measured as the difference between gastric pressure (Pga) and Pes (i.e., Pdi = Pga − Pes). Pdi provides specific data regarding DIA strength. A number of different techniques have been reported to produce a maximal Pdi (Pdi_{max}). These include a maximal static inspiratory effort (Mueller maneuver) (19), a Mueller maneuver combined with an abdominal expulsive effort (20), and the Pdi generated with a maximal sniff effort (sniff Pdi) (21). In addition, unilateral or bilateral phrenic nerve stimulation may be used to determine twitch Pdi responses using either electrical (surface or needle electrodes) (22) or cervical magnetic stimulation (23), thus providing objective data not influenced by patient effort. Furthermore, phrenic nerve conduction time (normally <9.5 msec) can be assessed to determine the possibility of phrenic nerve trauma or neuropathy (24). Normal values for the above tests are presented in Table 2. The maximum relaxation (MRR) is the percentage of force loss in 10 msec measured from voluntary or stimulated contractions. Slowing of the MRR may occur with respiratory muscle loading; the clinical applicability of such measurements are currently under investigation (25,26).

The concepts underlying a sustainable level of force/load by respiratory muscles are useful in understanding the factors determining the functional force reserve and endurance capacity of the respiratory pump. Skeletal muscles, including the respiratory muscles, can sustain repetitive loads for prolonged periods or indefinitely, provided the forces generated are below a critical/threshold percentage of the maximum force capacity. For example, Roussos and Macklem reported that the critical Pdi above which DIA fatigue occurred in normal subjects breathing against inspiratory resistive loads was 40% of Pdi_{max} (27). Thus, if the maximum force generating capacity of a muscle is reduced for any reason, the muscle will under basal conditions be operating at a higher percentage of maximum force, which may approach or, with added loads, exceed the critical ratio, resulting in task failure. Bellemare and co-workers reported that the tension time index of the DIA (TTdi) was strongly related to endurance, DIA blood flow, and oxygen consumption (28–30). The TTdi is the product of (Pdi/Pdi_{max}) and duty

Table 2 Normal Ranges for Tests of Respiratory Muscle Performance

Test		Male	Female	Reference
PI_{max}	(tube MP)	−123 ± 21	−87 ± 15	15
(cm H_2O)	(flanged MP)	−106 ± 30	−73 ± 21	16
PE_{max}	(tube MP)	232 ± 42	152 ± 56	15
(cm H_2O)	(flanged MP)	148 ± 34	93 ± 16	16
Sniff Pes (cm H_2O)		−105 ± 25	−89 ± 21	21
Snif Pdi (cm H_2O)		148 ± 24	121 ± 25	21
Maximum Static Pdi (Mueller) (cm H_2O)		108 ± 30	65 ± 31	21
Pdi (combined Mueller/ expulsive technique) (cm H_2O)		180 ± 14		20
Bilateral twitch Pdi		34 ± 10		22
(cm H_2O)		22 ± 4		60
Phrenic conduction time (ms) (R or L)		<9.5	<9.5	24

Key: MP = mouthpiece; Pi_{max} = maximum inspiratory mouth pressure; Pe_{max} = maximum expiratory mouth pressure; Pes = esophageal pressure; Pdi = transdiaphragmatic pressure. Values are mean ± SD.

cycle (Ti/Ttot), where Ti = inspiratory time and Ttot = total respiratory time. In normal subjects, the resting TTdi is about 0.02. A TTdi of 0.15 to 0.18 proved to be a fatiguing threshold, beyond which respiratory muscle fatigue ensued in less than 30 min (Fig. 4).

II. RESPIRATORY MUSCLE DYSFUNCTION IN THE ICU: CLINICAL APPLICATIONS

A. Congestive Heart Failure

It has become increasingly apparent in recent years that impaired respiratory muscle performance in patients in cardiac failure can potentially contribute to symptoms of dyspnea, impaired exercise capacity, and reduced functional force reserve of the respiratory pump.

1. Animal Studies

The structure and function of the DIA have been evaluated in chronic animal models of pacing-induced congestive cardiomyopathy. Supinski and co-workers (31) reported that the maximum specific force of the DIA (i.e., force per unit cross-

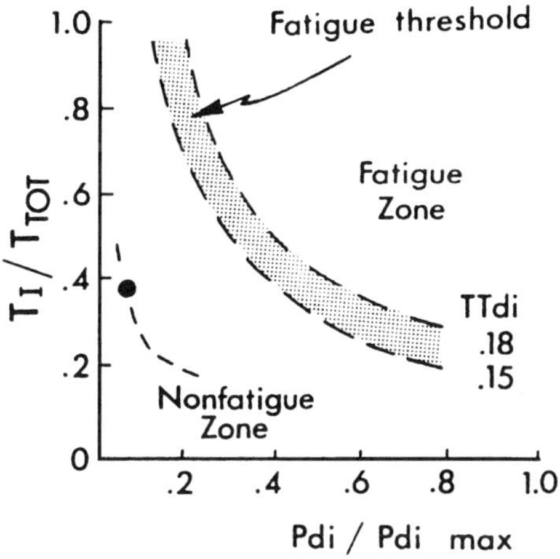

Figure 4 Relationship between duty cycle (Ti/Ttot) and mean spontaneous Pdi expressed as a percentage of Pdi_{max}. The fatigue threshold and fatigue zone are depicted. Any breathing pattern resulting in a TTdi of ≥0.15 will result in a defined limitation to sustained efforts. In addition to the parameters depicted in the figure, endurance capacity of the ventilatory pump may also be influenced independently by either lung volume or flow rate. From: Bellemare F, Grassino A. Effect of pressure and timing of contraction on human diaphragm fatigue. J Appl Physiol 1982; 53:1190–1195, with permission.

sectional area) measured in situ was significantly reduced in dogs when congestive heart failure (CHF) had been induced, compared to control dogs (Fig. 5). Similarly, Howell and colleagues (32) demonstrated significantly reduced Pdi's in an in vivo minipig model of CHF, following bilateral phrenic nerve stimulation (Pdi reduced by ~40% at low frequencies of stimulation and by 60% at high frequencies). In addition, enhanced fatigability of the DIA was observed in CHF dogs compared to controls, following repetitive stimulation over a 30-min period (31) (Fig. 5). Blood flow studies in CHF dogs revealed an altered phrenic arterial hyperemic response to transient occlusion and significantly reduced phrenic arterial flow during fatiguing contractions (31) (Fig. 5). Pericardial tamponade induced experimentally in dogs produced respiratory muscle fatigue and ventilatory failure (33). Despite reduced cardiac output and hypotension, blood flow to the respiratory muscles increased 361% (i.e., 21% of cardiac output). Despite this, the respiratory muscles failed as pressure generators as the energy demands exceeded the supply and respiratory failure ensued. Mechanical ventilation reduced respiratory muscle demands such that blood supply to the respiratory muscles was reduced to 3% of the cardiac output. This served to redistribute needed blood flow and oxygen supply to other vital organs (34).

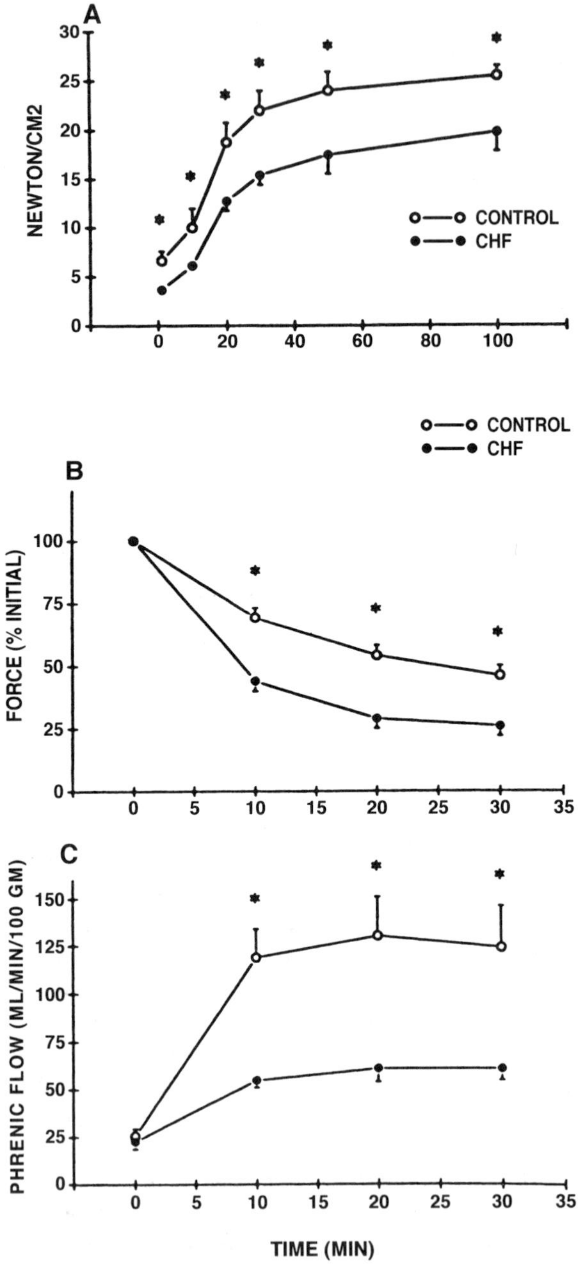

Figure 5 (A) Force/frequency relationships of the diaphragm in control and congestive heart failure (CHF) dogs. Note a significant reduction in specific forces at all frequencies in CHF dogs. (B) Fatigue trial depicting enhanced fatigability of the diaphragm in CHF dogs compared to control. (C) Phrenic arterial flow during fatigue trial. Note significantly reduced phrenic arterial flow throughout the fatigue run in CHF dogs. Values are means

Histochemical studies in minipigs with CHF revealed atrophy of type I (slow), IIa, and IIb/x (fast) DIA muscle fibers (32). The proportion of type I fibers increased while the proportion of type IIa fibers decreased. Thus, the relative contribution of type I fibers to total DIA area increased. Oxidative capacity, as measured by succinate dehydrogenase activity (SDH), was increased in fast fibers (IIa, IIb/x). Studies performed on the latissimus dorsi revealed less intrinsic adaptive changes than the DIA (32).

2. *Human Studies*

Inspiratory and expiratory mouth pressures, as well as sniff Pdi's, have been reported to be significantly reduced in patients with CHF, compared to age-matched controls (35–38). In addition, MIP (PI_{max}) was significantly correlated with both cardiac index (CI) and maximum oxygen consumption ($\dot{V}O_2$ max) (37). By contrast, Evans et al. (38) reported that CI did not correlate with mouth pressures, but rather with sniff Pdi. Furthermore, McPharland and co-workers reported that mouth pressures were significantly correlated with dyspnea during daily activity (35). Exercise studies in patients with CHF also revealed significant linear correlation between ratings of perceived dyspnea and mouth pressures (39). In addition, dyspnea correlated with the TTdi of the DIA (which was significantly greater in patients with CHF both at rest and at peak exercise) and measures of accessory muscle deoxygenation, which were determined using near-infrared spectroscopy (39). By contrast, Evans et al. (38) failed to show a relationship between exertional dyspnea and exercise time and measures of respiratory muscle force in patients with CHF.

3. *Mechanisms of Respiratory Muscle Dysfunction*

Reduction in DIA force with CHF may be accounted for in part by significant atrophy of DIA fibers (i.e., less muscle mass) (32). In addition, the increased relative contribution of type I fibers to total DIA area in CHF minipigs may in part explain the reduced specific force of the DIA (32), as type I fibers have a lower specific force than type II fibers (40). A variety of mechanisms may underlie the atrophy of muscle fibers. These include reduced regional blood flow, altered vascular reactivity due to abnormal endothelial production of vasoactive substances (e.g., endothelin, NO), vessel wall edema, or alterations in the neurohumoral milieu accompanying CHF (e.g., catecholamines, renin-angiotensin system, tumor necrosis factor, etc.) (41–43). Other factors affecting DIA structure and function could include malnutrition effects (cardiac cachexia), electrolyte aberrations, deconditioning, and a generalized myopathic process (44,45). Recent clinical studies in patients with CHF revealed no significant correlation between inspiratory muscle force and nutritional status, electrolyte levels, or limb muscle

---

± SE. From: Supinski G, DiMarco A, Dibner-Dunlap M. Alterations in diaphragm strength and fatigability in congestive heart failure. J Appl Physiol 1994; 76:2707–2713.

strength (46). The latter argues against the reduced inspiratory muscle forces being explained as part of a generalized myopathic process.

4. Clinical Implications

The reduced specific force of the DIA coupled with atrophy of muscle fibers would reduce the total force-generating capacity of the DIA. Thus the DIA would be operating at a greater percentage of its maximum even under basal conditions. With any added load (e.g., increased pulmonary venous congestion; pulmonary edema), the contracting DIA may approach or exceed the critical ratio above which fatigue may ensue. Thus the functional force reserve and endurance capacity of the DIA would be severely curtailed, and task failure (i.e., respiratory failure) may develop. In keeping with this concept, Mancini and co-workers reported that the TTdi of the DIA increased significantly in patients with CHF during exercise and approached levels known to induce fatigue (39). In addition, any alteration in electrolyte status, blood gas exchange, or nutritional compromise during acute exacerbations of the condition may contribute further respiratory muscle weakness and further diminish their reserve capacity.

Respiratory muscle weakness may also contribute to the sensation of dyspnea (35,39). Indeed, Mancini et al. (39) reported that respiratory muscle strength, work, and oxygenation in patients with CHF were significantly correlated with the ratings of perceived dyspnea. This is in keeping with the work of Bradley et al. (47), who reported that there was a very strong correlation between inspiratory effort sensation and esophageal pressure (Pes) expressed as a percentage of maximal Pes (i.e., Pes/Pes max %).

B. Phrenic Nerve Injury After Open Heart Surgery

DIA dysfunction secondary to phrenic nerve injury following open heart surgery has been well-characterized in recent years with a reported incidence of 10% to 73%, depending on surgical considerations, preventive measures, and methods of detection (48–50). In more recent studies, the incidence of phrenic neuropathy ranged from 26% to 36% when ice slush topical hypothermia was utilized (51,52). The prevalence of clinically significant severe diaphragmatic dysfunction, however, was reported by Diehl and colleagues (53) to be significantly lower in a large cohort of patients (i.e., 2.1% when ice slush with no insulation measures was used, and 0.5% when to topical cooling was utilized). In children undergoing cardiac surgery, the frequency of phrenic neuropathy has been estimated to range from 0.5% to 7% (radiologic criteria) to as high as 10% (phrenic conduction studies) (54,55).

1. Pathogenesis

Most cases are likely related to cold-induced phrenic nerve injury (phrenic "frostbite"). Dureuil and co-workers (56) evaluated the effects of phrenic nerve cooling in dogs and reported the development of complete phrenic nerve conduction block within ~100 ms of cold exposure. The speed and extent of conduction block recovery depended on the duration of cold exposure. A significant reduction in Pdi was noted following cold exposure with phrenic stimulation at frequencies up to 100 Hz. Clinically, the use of ice slush appears to enhance the risk of phrenic injury more than other cold solutions (50,57). In addition, harvesting of the internal mammary artery appears to increase the incidence of phrenic neuropathy (57). Nerve traction injury and vascular compromise of the phrenic nerve may also contribute to injury. It is unlikely, however, that direct surgical damage to the phrenic nerve plays a role.

2. *Clinical Features*

The clinical presentation may be acute or subacute, with the diagnosis in the latter case commonly missed and clinical signs and symptoms attributed to other causes (58). The need for prolonged mechanical ventilation following surgery is an important clue, especially in the absence of other abnormalities such as cardiac dysfunction, noscomial pneumonia, sepsis, etc. (53). Severe and persistent orthopnea is an important symptom indicative of severe DIA weakness/paralysis. This may be accompanied by paradoxical abdominal motion (i.e., inward motion of the abdominal wall on inspiration) with spontaneous breathing efforts during weaning attempts following extubation, especially in the supine posture (Fig. 6) (53,57). Respiratory failure and/or respiratory arrest may complicate the clinical course following early/premature extubation (53). Indeed, clinically relevant/severe DIA

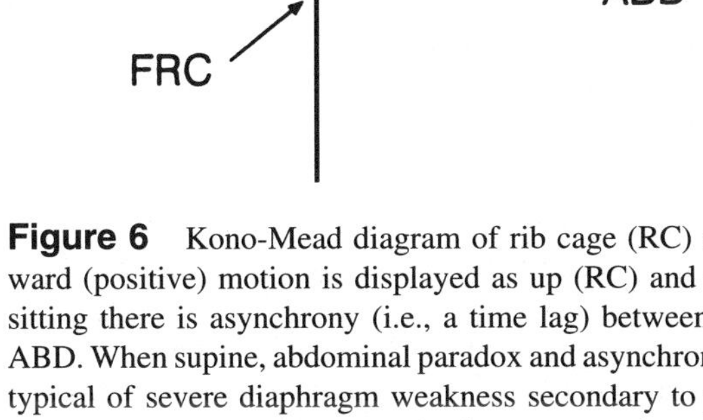

Figure 6 Kono-Mead diagram of rib cage (RC) and abdominal (ABD) motion. Outward (positive) motion is displayed as up (RC) and to the right (ABD). Note that while sitting there is asynchrony (i.e., a time lag) between outward movement of the RC and ABD. When supine, abdominal paradox and asynchrony are clearly evident. These plots are typical of severe diaphragm weakness secondary to phrenic injury following open heart surgery. From: Olopade C et al. Time course of recovery from frostbitten phrenics after coronary artery bypass graft surgery. Chest 1991; 99:1112–1115, with permission.

dysfunction following cardiac surgery may result in significant morbidity and/or mortality (53,59). Of 13 patients with severe DIA weakness following cardiac surgery, Diehl and co-workers (53) reported cardiorespiratory arrest following early extubation in 38%, prolonged mechanical ventilation in all (48 ± 41 days), the development of nosocomial pneumonia in 73%, and a fatal outcome in 23%. In patients with less severe impairment, sleep disturbances (including desaturation, disturbed sleep, and insomnia) and excessive daytime somnolence have been reported, related in part to the profound inhibition of intercostal muscle activity during sleep—particularly REM sleep. Chest radiographs may reveal an elevated left hemidiaphragm often accompanied by left lower lobe atelectasis and effusion. It should be noted, however, that only 20% or less of atelectases noted in postcardiac surgery patients can be attributed to phrenic nerve damage and DIA weakness (48,52). In addition, bilateral DIA involvement is rare (<5% of cases) (58). While isolated unilateral or bilateral DIA weakness/paralysis may be clinically well-compensated in other, more subacute or chronic conditions, the presence of an associated cardiopulmonary disorder substantially reduces the reserve of the respiratory pump (60,61).

3. *Diagnostic Tests*

The chest radiograph, while sensitive, is not specific. Assessment of DIA motion can be performed fluoroscopically or by real-time ultrasound at the bedside with the patient breathing spontaneously in a supine posture (51). Diminished excursion or paradoxical motion of the DIA may be noted. In the upright position, active recruitment of the abdominal muscles may result in passive DIA descent with inspiration (i.e., false positive). The vital capacity can also be measured at the bedside. With severe DIA weakness, a significant fall in the vital capacity may be noted in the supine posture (~37% fall [bilateral] vs. ~16% [unilateral]) (52,60). Tests of respiratory and/or DIA strength are useful in quantifying the degree of weakness. Reduction in pressures will be more marked with bilateral than unilateral involvement. MIP, for example, is moderately reduced with severe bilateral DIA weakness (~40 ± 15% of predicted), while MEP is preserved. By contrast, maximal sniff Pdi is markedly reduced with severe bilateral DIA weakness (8.7% of predicted) (60). Data from patients with clinically significant DIA dysfunction are displayed in Figure 7 (53). The ratio of ΔPga/ΔPdi during inspiration is a good, nonvolitional index of DIA contribution to inspiratory pressure swings, with a negative ratio indicating DIA weakness or paralysis. It is of interest that the TTdi of the DIA in the group with phrenic nerve injury is close to the critical fatiguing threshold. Thus, with any added load, ventilatory failure is likely (53).

Phrenic nerve conduction, considered by some to be the "gold standard," can be measured following phrenic stimulation. Prolongation (i.e., > 9.5 msec) indicates phrenic nerve damage (24,51,52,63). The amplitude of the evoked action potential may be variable; however, a recent study suggested that the amplitude

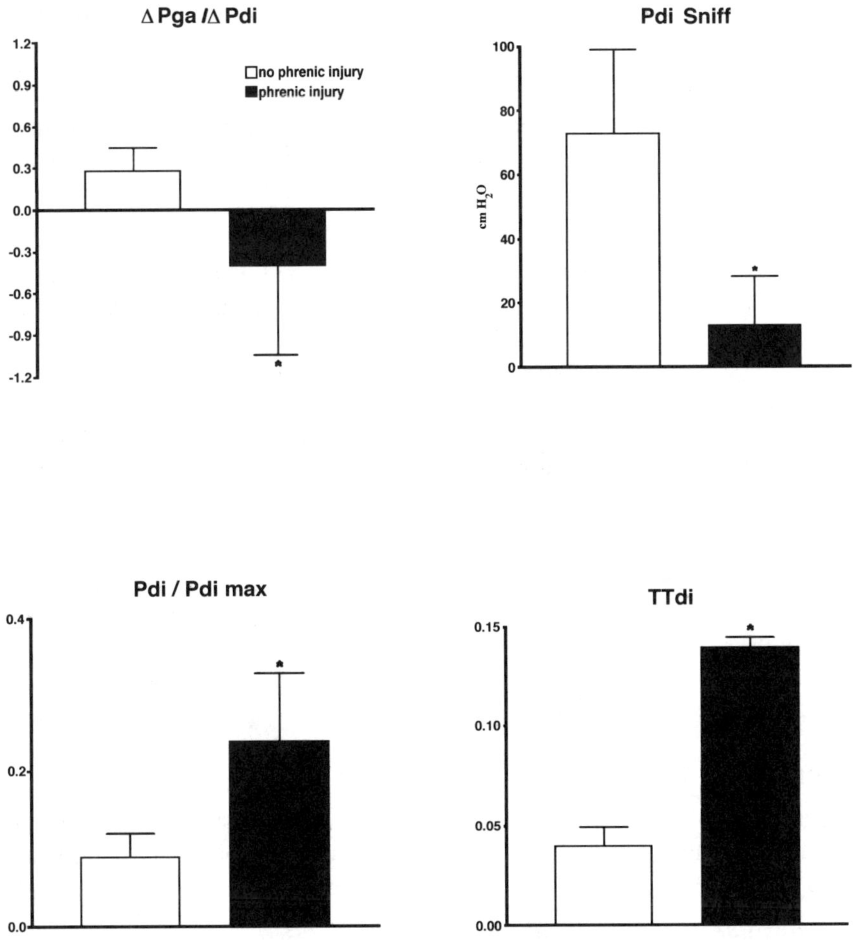

Figure 7 Data depicting diaphragm muscle performance in patients with significant diaphragm dysfunction following open-heart surgery. See text for details. Pga = gastric pressure; Pdi = transdiaphragmatic pressure; TTdi = tension time index of the diaphragm. Figures drawn from data reported in Diehl JL, Lofaso F, Deleuze P, Similowski T, Lemaire F, Brochard L. Clinically relevant diaphragmatic dysfunction after cardiac operations. J Thorac Cardiovasc Surg 1994; 107:487–498. Values are means ± SD.

and area of the evoked response may be a sensitive indicator of phrenic damage (64).

4. *Natural History*

Most patients can expect a full recovery of function. While full recovery can take as long as 1 or 2 years, the majority of patients will recover within 3 to 6 months (51,65).

5. *Modes of Treatment*

While severely affected patients may require prolonged mechanical ventilation (53), less invasive measures have been used in non-ventilator-dependent but symptomatic patients following extubation. These include the use of noninvasive positive pressure ventilation, negative pressure ventilation, rocking beds, and the use of pneumo belts (66–68). Such measures may be necessary until patients are able to assume a supine posture without dyspnea. Patients with prolonged neuropathy have also been successfully treated with surgical DIA plication (69,70).

6. *Preventive Measures*

A variety of insulation devices placed between the heart and pericardium have been reported to significantly reduce or eliminate DIA dysfunction (71,72). Likewise, avoiding the use of topical cooling has been reported to eliminate or significantly reduce the incidence of clinically relevant phrenic injury (53,57). Recently, "warm heart" surgery was reported in a randomized, controlled trial to eliminate the presence of DIA dysfunction (73).

C. Sepsis and the Respiratory Muscles

The pathophysiologic changes affecting the respiratory muscles in sepsis are key to a full appreciation of the complex pathophysiologic and biochemical sequelae of this disorder (74).

1. *Sepsis and Ventilatory Failure*

Hussain and colleagues (75) evaluated the effect of endotoxemia in dogs on DIA performance. All animals in which endotoxin was administered died as a consequence of ventilatory failure and respiratory arrest (75). The latter was secondary to peripheral fatigue of the DIA (and other respiratory muscles), which eventually failed as pressure generators (Fig. 8) (75). While the mean inspiratory flow and Pdi increased initially with a concomitant fall in PCO_2, a subsequent progressive rise in PCO_2 to hypercapnic levels was accompanied by a marked reduction in mean inspiratory flows and Pdi, despite enhanced drive to the respiratory muscles (DIA EMG [Edi] increased to 350% of control values) (Fig. 8). Mechanical ventilation of the endotoxemic dogs would clearly have offset the demands on the ventilatory pump, preventing respiratory arrest. Clinically, such a strategy may be necessary in patients with severe sepsis and/or septic shock.

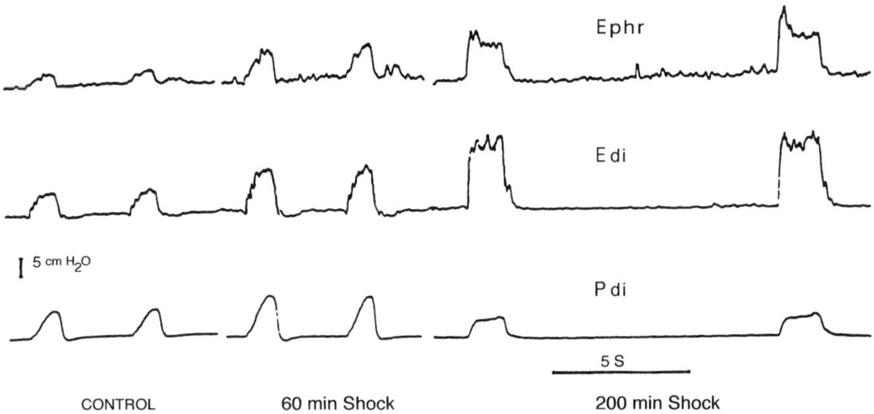

Figure 8 Simultaneous tracings of Ephr (integrated phrenic neurogram), Edi (integrated diaphragm EMG), and Pdi (transdiaphragmatic pressure) recorded from a dog during the course of endotoxic shock. Note that after 200 min following induction of endotoxemia, Pdi is markedly reduced despite significant increases in Edi and Ephr, indicating failure of the diaphragm as a pressure generator. From: Hussain S, Simkus G, Roussos C. Respiratory muscle fatigue: a cause of ventilatory muscle failure in septic shock. J Appl Physiol 1985; 58:2033–2040, with permission.

a. Respiratory Muscle Blood Flow and Sepsis. During septic shock, increased ventilation and respiratory muscle work must be met by an increased blood flow and improved oxygen extraction by the ventilatory pump, if fatigue and task failure are to be prevented. Dog studies during induced endotoxic shock revealed a marked increase in blood flow to the respiratory muscles which accounted for 8.8% of the cardiac output (Fig. 9A) (76). Because total blood flow was limited, blood flow to vital organs decreased significantly, often to levels inducing ischemic injury (e.g., cerebral blood flow) (Fig. 9B). With the institution of mechanical ventilation, respiratory muscle blood flow dropped to 1.9% of the cardiac output, and blood flow was diverted to other organs, with significant increases in cerebral, gut, and skeletal muscle flow (Fig. 9B). Despite a significant increase in DIA blood flow following endotoxic shock in spontaneously breathing dogs (76), relative limitations in DIA blood supply and/or oxygen extraction resulted in local lactate production and glycogen depletion in the DIA muscle (77). This is substantiated by more recent studies by Kim et al. (78), in which the maximum oxygen extraction of the DIA in endotoxemic dogs was significantly reduced compared to saline controls. In addition, the critical oxygen delivery required to sustain DIA oxygen consumption was significantly elevated in the endotoxic animals (78). Furthermore, Boczkowski and co-workers (79) reported that the percentage of

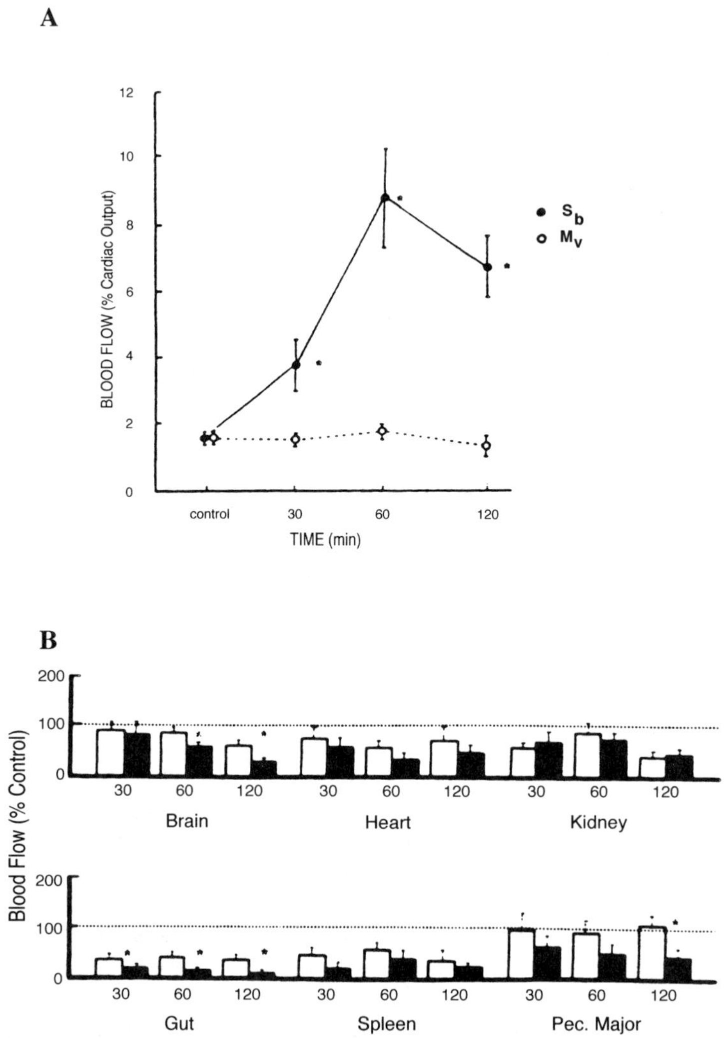

Figure 9 (A) Graph depicting total respiratory muscle blood flow during endotoxic shock in spontaneously breathing (Sb) and mechanically ventilated (Mv) dogs. Note the significant increment in respiratory muscle blood flow during Sb which was reversed with Mv. (B) Graphs depicting blood flow to various organs at 30, 60, and 120 min of endotoxic shock (referenced as a percentage of control values). Filled bars indicate blood flow with Sb; open bars depict blood flow with MV. See text for details. From: Hussain S, Roussos C. Distribution of respiratory muscle and organ blood flow during endotoxic shock in dogs. J Appl Physiol 1986; 60:486–493, with permission.

nonperfused DIA capillaries was significantly increased in septic rats compared to controls, despite similar levels of arterial blood pressure. Mechanical (e.g., endothelial swelling, granulocyte obstruction) and/or mediator-induced factors may account for the functional decrement of DIA capillaries in the septic animals (80).

Treatment regimens employed in the dog endotoxic shock model provide useful data with clear clinical implications. Hussain and colleagues (81) administered either fluids (saline and dextran) or norepinephrine infusions to endotoxic dogs and reported that despite normalization of arterial blood pressure, total body $\dot{V}O_2$ did not change, compared to untreated animals. However, the partition of total $\dot{V}O_2$ was such that DIA $\dot{V}O_2$ ($\dot{V}O_2$ di) was significantly reduced in the two treatment groups, despite similar minute ventilation and respiratory muscle work. This implies that more oxygen would be available to vital and other organs with treatment, and that during hypoxemia, the efficiency of the DIA was compromised, as it required a higher $\dot{V}O_2$ to sustain similar pressure. Norepinephrine has also been reported to augment contractility of the fatigued DIA in hypo- and nomotensive states, likely secondary to an increased DIA blood flow (82,83). Dobutamine and dopexamine proportionally increased blood flow to vital organs in endotoxemic rats with no disproportionate redistribution of blood flow to any organ (84). Finally, the administration of vasopressors (dopamine, norepinephrine) to sustain arterial pressure in septic rats (cecal ligation and spillage) failed to improve survival, while the institution of mechanical ventilation did improve survival, emphasizing the importance of unloading the respiratory muscles and a multimodal approach to management (85).

b. Acute Respiratory Distress Syndrome (ARDS). Sepsis remains one of the most important causes of ARDS. Magdar and co-workers (86) studied an oleic acid model of ARDS in dogs in whom cardiac output and blood pressure was unaltered by the intervention. Respiratory muscle work and blood flow increased significantly, with blood flow amounting to 11.4% of the cardiac output. Blood flow to the kidney, spleen, and gut was significantly reduced, while cerebral and cardiac blood flow rates were preserved. The reduced renal and splanchnic blood flow may have important clinical sequelae in terms of ischemic injury to the kidney and gut, the latter promoting bacterial translocation and endotoxemia.

c. Effects of Sepsis on Respiratory Muscle Function. In the early stages of sepsis, a variety of factors may interact to impair DIA contractility, including the effects of hypotension, excessive demands on the respiratory pump, metabolic acidosis, and derangement of blood gas exchange. If these factors are controlled for, DIA force generation may initially be preserved (87). Leon et al. (88) evaluated Pdi following acute endotoxin administration in mechanically ventilated rats, and reported reduced Pdi at high frequencies of stimulation (50 to 100 Hz) and reduced endurance capacity. While respiratory muscle work was unloaded, the experimental animals remained hypotensive.

The consequences of prolonged sepsis (i.e., effects following 2 or 3 days) have been reported and have clear and important clinical implications. Boczkowski et al. (89) studied rats 3 days following pneumococcal inoculation and reported that both DIA strength and endurance capacity were significantly curtailed (Fig. 10). No changes in DIA mass were evident (89). Similarly, in vitro studies of hamster DIA revealed reduced DIA forces at all frequencies of stimulation and increased fatigability (i.e., decreased fatigue resistance) of the DIA muscle 2 days following endotoxin administration (90).

Clinically significant reductions in MIP and MEP were observed in patients with naturally acquired upper respiratory tract infections, compared to healthy controls (91). The fall in mouth pressures was maximal between 3 and 7 days following the onset of the illness; this returned to normal within 16 days. The mechanisms underlying this transient dysfunction include a viral myositis or the sequelae of cytokine-mediated proteolysis (92). These data have obvious implications for patients with chronic cardiac or pulmonary disorders in whom respiratory muscle function may already be compromised.

2. *Influence of Mediators and Therapeutic Implications*

Oxygen-derived free radicals are thought to play a major role in mediating respiratory muscle dysfunction and fatigue in a variety of settings, including

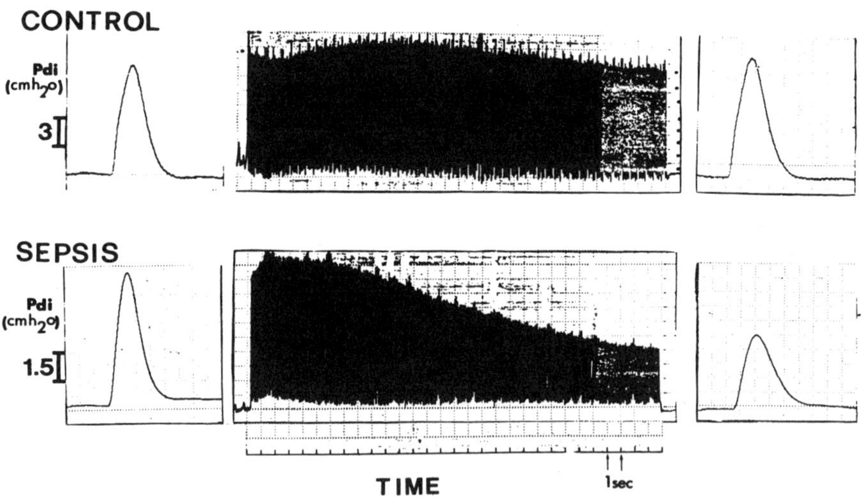

Figure 10 Tracing depicting changes in transdiaphragmatic pressure (Pdi) during a 30-sec fatigue trial in control and septic rats. Note enhanced fatigability in the septic animals. From: Bockowski J, Dureuil B, Branger C, et al. Effects of sepsis on diaphragmatic function in rats. Am Rev Respir Dis 1988; 138:260–265, with permission.

sepsis (93). Free radicals can induce lipid peroxidation (i.e., fragmentation of lipid membranes and generation of reactive lipid peroxides), resulting in further membrane and protein damage and enzyme inhibition. DNA damage, increased intracellular Ca^{2+}, and reduced glycolysis and ATP generation may also occur. The impact of free radical scavengers on DIA and intercostal muscle forces in endotoxic hamsters were evaluated in vitro after 2 days (90,94). Administration of PEG-superoxide dismutase (SOD; scavenges superoxide), PEG-catalase (hydrogen peroxide), and dimethylsulfoxide (DMSO; hydroxyl scavenger) markedly attenuated the reductions in forces noted with endotoxin administration alone (90,94). In addition, the increased levels of malondialdehyde (MDA; an index of lipid peroxidation) noted in the DIAs of endotoxic animals was not observed in endotoxic animals given PEG-SOD (90). Similarly, N-acetylcysteine (accelerates reduced glutathione biosynthesis) prevented the reduced DIA strength and endurance and increase in DIA MDA in endotoxic rats (95). Finally, the adverse effects on DIA strength and fatigability induced by an ischemia-reperfusion model in dogs was reversed with the administration of DMSO.

Nitric oxide (*NO*) is a small, lipophilic, short-acting transcellular messenger that is synthesized from L-arginine by the enzyme NO-synthase (NOS) of which there are three isoforms—neuronal constitutive (nc), endothelial constitutive (ec), and inducible (i). NO is now considered a normal physiologic regulator of DIA contractile function (inhibits) and vascular tone, and mediates its effects via the second messenger, cGMP (97). As endotoxin may upregulate iNOS; NO may contribute to DIA dysfunction in sepsis/endotoxemia. Indeed, the DIA of *E. coli* endotoxic rats showed increased cGMP and NOS activity, and the administration of a NOS inhibitor (L-NMMA) reversed the reduced DIA force with endotoxin alone (98). Similar results were reported by Shindoh et al. (99). In addition, Hussain (100) demonstrated that enhanced NO production in endotoxic dogs plays a major role in vascular dilatation and dysregulation in the DIA which could be reversed by the administration of a NOS inhibitor.

Cytokines including *tumor necrosis factor* (*TNF*) are important inflammatory regulators that may contribute to respiratory muscle dysfunction in sepsis. Lipopolysaccharide-stimulated monocyte supernatant (containing TNF and IL-1) impaired the contractile function of the hamster DIA in vitro (101). The effects of TNF alone on DIA function in vitro are variable, and may reflect the bath concentrations used (102,103). Recently, Wilcox and co-workers (104) reported early impaired DIA contractility in dogs in vivo following TNF administration. A reduction in DIA compound action potential suggested impaired neurotransmission (104). A recent study suggested that impaired DIA force in vitro following TNF incubation was mediated by NO (105).

Prostaglandins and other *eicosanoid products* may be generated during endotoxemia. Inhibition of prostaglandin synthesis (indomethacin) prevented the reduction in DIA strength in vivo in rats given endotoxin (106). Indomethacin may also prevent proteolysis and muscle wasting in septic states (107). It is likely that, in the future, complex interactions among the various mediators may be uncovered that may further clarify the key pathways mediating muscle injury in sepsis.

D. Ventilatory Failure and the Respiratory Muscles

Respiratory failure has traditionally been viewed as a process characterized by either impairment of gas exchange and hypoxemia and/or impairment of ventilation characterized by hypercapnia. The latter may be related to ventilatory pump failure, alterations in respiratory timing and pattern of breathing, and abnormal gas exchange (108,109). Ventilatory pump failure may be secondary to impaired central respiratory drive (e.g., during overdose of depressant drugs such as opiates or barbiturates), respiratory muscle weakness, or excessive respiratory loads (110). In critically ill patients, respiratory muscle weakness may be caused by a variety of diverse etiologies (e.g., acidosis, electrolyte deficiencies, sepsis, hypotensive states, hypercatabolic states, malnutrition, corticosteroids, and neuromuscular disorders such as Guillain-Barré, myasthenia gravis, critical illness polyneuropathy, etc.). Excessive loads may be due to flow resistive factors, elastic loads, mass loading (obesity), and threshold loads (auto PEEP).

The pressure time index (PTI) is the product of the ratio of P_{breath} (i.e., the mean pressure generated during inspiration) to PI_{max} and the duty cycle. As the latter is similar in normal subjects and in patients with a variety of disease states (111), major changes in the PTI are related to alterations in the P_{breath}/PI_{max} ratio, where P_{breath} is a reflection of the loads imposed and PI_{max} is a reflection of the "force reserve" of the respiratory pump. P_{breath}/PI_{max} during normal resting ventilation is 0.05. A ratio of 0.4 cannot be sustained indefinitely, while a ratio $\geqslant$ 0.6 rapidly results in task failure (112). The factors influencing the ratio and thus endurance capacity are depicted in Table 3.

The alveolar ventilation equation (113) states that

$$PCO_2 = \frac{\dot{V}CO_2 \cdot K}{\dot{V}A}$$

where $\dot{V}CO_2 = CO_2$ production, $\dot{V}A$ = alveolar ventilation, and K = 0.863 (constant of proportionality). As $\dot{V}A = \dot{V}E(1-fVd/fVt)$, the equation can be rewritten as:

$$PCO_2 = \frac{\dot{V}CO_2 \cdot K}{VT \cdot f(1 - Vd/Vt)}$$

where VE = total minute ventilation, Vt = tidal volume, f = respiratory frequency, and Vd/Vt = dead space fraction (ratio).

PCO_2 will rise if $\dot{V}CO_2$ is elevated or VA falls (Vd increases, Vt falls, or both, with or without a decrement in $\dot{V}E$).

Table 3 Factors Influencing the Fatiguing Process

Accelerate fatigue onset[a]	
• Increase in P_{breath}	Larger tidal volume
High resistance	
Low compliance	
• Decrease in PI_{max}	Muscle weakness
	Mechanical disadvantage
Retard fatigue onset	Smaller tidal volume
• Decrease in P_{breath}	Restore muscle contractility
• Increase in PI_{max}	

[a]P_{breath}: pressure needed to inspire a breath; PI_{max}: maximal inspiratory pressure.

Source: Rochester D. Respiratory muscle fatigue and respiratory failure. Semin Respir Med 1992; 13:7–13 (with permission).

Changes in respiratory timing and pattern of breathing may contribute to hypercapnia. As previously mentioned, rapid shallow respiration is a common response of the respiratory muscles to added ventilatory loads (11). The following scenario or sequences of events may therefore induce hypercapnia in the absence of overt peripheral respiratory muscle fatigue (110). Inspiratory loads and/or respiratory muscle weakness results in a change in breathing pattern characterized by a shortened inspiratory time, which reduces Vt and therefore P_{breath} and PTI (i.e., reduces energy demands). The reduced Vt results in an increment in Vd/Vt and is compensated for by an increased f. If $\dot{V}E$ is not augmented sufficiently, hypercapnia will ensue. Under these circumstances, ventilatory failure is accompanied by a high respiratory drive. Clinically, overt respiratory muscle fatigue is not necessarily the final common pathway in established acute ventilatory failure, because of central and other modifying influences imposed, once a fatiguing pattern of contraction ensues. Of interest, Efthimiou and co-workers (114) reported data suggestive of overt fatigue of the sternomastoid muscle in 10% of patients with COPD admitted to hospital because of acute exacerbations of their condition. While these data are of interest, it is unclear what the significance of these findings are for the respiratory pump and to what extent other respiratory muscles might be susceptible to overt fatigue under the loaded conditions.

Recently, the magnitude of the loads imposed on the inspiratory muscles in patients with acute respiratory failure of varying etiologies were quantified (115). This study demonstrated the presence of intrinsic PEEP and dynamic hyperinflation following discontinuation of mechanical ventilatory support in patients with acute respiratory failure. The latter imposed an inspiratory threshold load as sufficient inspiratory force needed to be generated to overcome the positive recoil pressures at end expiration, prior to the initiation of airflow. The P_{breath}/PI_{max} ratio was high (0.42 ± 0.11), and the PTI was significantly greater than normal, clustered around or exceeded a critical threshold isopleth (Fig. 11) (115). These data suggest, but do not prove, that the potential for inspiratory muscle fatigue exists in such patients. In addition, in critically ill patients, a complex array of factors may be present that impose continued high energy demands and/or limit or further reduce energy supply to the working respiratory muscles. These factors severely tax the respiratory pump such that the load compensating strategies described above, which serve to limit contractile fatigue and sense of dyspnea, may fail. The precise role of the respiratory muscles in the genesis of ventilatory failure in critically ill patients certainly needs further research efforts and clarification.

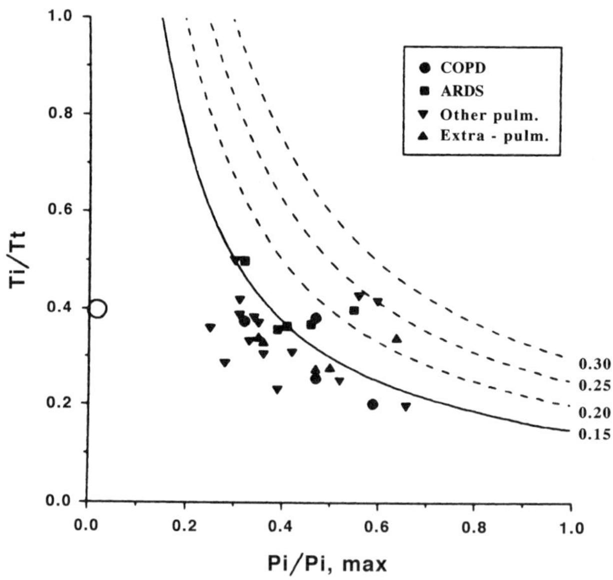

Figure 11 Relationship between duty cycle (Ti/Ttot) and ratio of inspiratory pressure (Pi) and maximum inspiratory pressure (Pi_{max}). The isopleths depicted refer to pressure-time indices (PIT) of varying degrees. Note that in patients with acute respiratory failure, the PTI following disconnection from the ventilator clustered around or exceeded a critical threshold. From: Zakynthinos SG, Vassilakopoulos T, Roussos C. The load of inspiratory muscles in patients needing mechanical ventilation. Am J Respir Crit Care Med 1995; 152:1248–1255, with permission.

III. MANAGEMENT OF RESPIRATORY MUSCLE DYSFUNCTION IN THE ICU

The general principles underlying management of respiratory muscle dysfunction in critically ill patients are directed toward improving the balance between energy demands and energy supply, so as to optimize pump capacity. In the presence of incipient or overt fatigue, effects should be directed initially toward resting or appropriately unloading the respiratory muscles. In addition, a multitude of factors may contribute to the development of respiratory muscle weakness in critically ill patients, which need to be reversed. Lastly, specific therapeutic measures may be applied that aim to improve respiratory muscle strength and/or endurance capacity.

A. Rest and Unloading of the Respiratory Muscles

1. Rationale and Clinical Implementation

In the presence of established or impending acute ventilatory failure accompanied by overt or incipient respiratory muscle fatigue, initial respiratory muscle rest using mechanical ventilation is an appropriate therapeutic measure. As overt peripheral muscle fatigue (i.e., contractile fatigue) is longlasting (9), appropriate rest or unloading might be necessary for the first 24 to 48 hours. The advantages of initial respiratory muscle rest/unloading during the acute phase are to prevent further muscle injury and longlasting contractile fatigue (116,117), improve or relieve dyspnea, divert needed blood supply and oxygen to other vital and nonvital organs (76), and improve blood gas composition and acid-base status (see below). Every effort should be made to optimize the mechanical ventilatory mode used and to prevent patient-ventilator dyssynchrony. It is now well established that lengthening contractions of the DIA (i.e., eccentric contractions) may induce DIA fiber injury (116). A number of factors can predispose to eccentric respiratory muscle injury, which include active abdominal muscle recruitment (14), persistent inspiratory muscle contraction throughout the respiratory cycle (117), and discoordination between patient efforts and ventilator-delivered breaths.

Changes in the power spectrum of the DIA EMG may signal undue loading and a fatiguing pattern of contraction, signified by a shift in the power from high to low frequencies and a fall in the high-low (H/L) ratio. Brochard and co-workers (14) evaluated the H/L in patients with difficulty weaning from mechanical ventilation. In the majority of patients, the H/L fell immediately when ventilatory support was withdrawn, but returned to baseline with the provision of appropriate levels of pressure support (114). Figure 12, from their study, is an excellent example of loading and unloading of the DIA, and emphasizes the need to tailor the level of pressure support required in each individual patient.

Recently, much emphasis has been placed on the use of noninvasive ventilatory modes in order to avoid intubation and conventional mechanical ventilation.

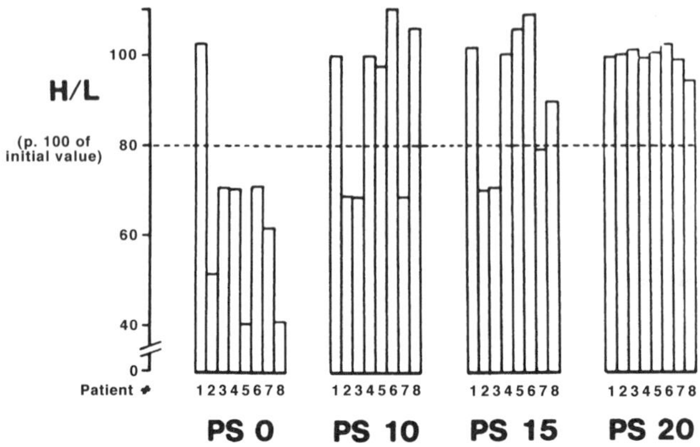

Figure 12 Bar graphs depicting the high/low ratio (H/L) of the diaphragm EMG at different levels of pressure support (PS). The reduction in the H/L to 80% of the initial value was regarded as significant (dashed line). See test for further details. From: Brochard L, Haarf A, Lorino H, Lemare F. Inspiratory pressure support prevents diaphragmatic fatigue during weaning from mechanical ventilation. Am Rev Respir Dis 1989; 139:513–521, with permission.

Three randomized controlled studies have been reported using noninvasive positive pressure ventilator modes (NIPPV) delivered via nasal or face masks (118–120). In these studies, most of the experience reported was with hypercapnic COPD patients during acute exacerbations. In this subset of patients, the results were encouraging. For example, Kramer et al. (119) reported that while 67% of patients receiving standard medical therapy required conventional mechanical ventilation, 9% of those receiving NIPPV were subsequently intubated. Reduced morbidity and mortality were also reported (118,120). Unfortunately, experience with NIPPV for other causes of acute respiratory failure is much more limited, with little high-grade evidence reported in terms of controlled clinical trials (122). Further trials are clearly indicated to identify appropriate patient populations, signs of impending success or failure, the most appropriate modes and interfaces, and cost-effectiveness of NIPPV for diverse patient populations.

Intrinsic (auto) PEEP (PEEPi) develops because of insufficient expiratory time for the lungs to exhale to the normal relaxation volume of the respiratory system prior to the delivery of the subsequent mechanical breath (121). This results in dynamic hyperinflation and positive end-expiratory alveolar pressure, which places the DIA at a mechanical disadvantage and imposes elastic and threshold loads on the respiratory muscles. The latter increases the work of breathing as the respiratory muscles must generate sufficient force to overcome positive recoil pressures to initiate airflow. The level of PEEPi and imposed work may be reduced by measures that prolong expiratory time. In addition, in certain circumstances, trigger sensitivity may be reduced by the application of external PEEP to levels not exceeding 85% of PEEPi (123). Gottfried (124) recently provided practical recommendations for the use of external PEEP in patients with PEEPi. These are outlined in Table 4.

2. *Adverse Consequences of Prolonged DIA Inactivity*

DIA inactivity induced by unilateral denervation, tetrodotoxin nerve blockade, or spinal isolation resulted in a significant reduction in DIA-specific force (i.e., force/unit cross-sectional area) begins as early as 3 days after denervation and persists for as long as 6 weeks (125–127). Denervation was associated with either hypertrophy (early) or preservation (late) of type I and IIa DIA fiber cross-sectional areas, while types IIb/x fibers atrophied (125,127). The addition of malnutrition resulted in further atrophy of type IIb/x fibers and atrophy of types I and IIa fibers (127). Thus, the force-generating capacity of the whole DIA was significantly reduced (decreased mass, decreased contractility). While the above models differ from controlled mechanical ventilation with or without neuromuscular blockage, the direction of change is similar. For example, Bourdellés et al. (128) reported reduced DIA contractility in rats following 48 h mechanical ventilation. In human neonates, significant DIA fiber atrophy was noted following prolonged mechanical ventilation, in autopsy studies (129). There are few data on the effects of other modes of mechanical ventilation on DIA structure and function. Significant patient work has been well-documented with ventilatory modes such as assist control, SIMV, etc. (130,131). It is therefore unlikely that "disuse" atrophy would occur in the absence of prolonged controlled ventilation.

Recently, adverse sequelae of prolonged administration of neuromuscular blocking agents have been highlighted (132). Two clinical scenarios have been reported. The first is prolonged neuromuscular blockade reported in patients in which the elimination of active metabolites is impaired (e.g., renal insufficiency) (132). The second, more serious complication is that of a neuromyopathy, the effects of which may be prolonged or irreversible. This has been most commonly documented in patients receiving concomitant corticosteroids and prolonged infusions (>48 h) of a neuromuscular blocking agent (133). While the pathophysiologic mechanisms are unknown, the combined influences of muscle inactivity and corticosteroid-induced fiber atrophy may be important factors. While most data relate to the use of pancuronium or vercuronium (133,134), adverse complications with newer agents have been reported (135).

B. Acid-Base Changes and Disorders of Gas Exchange

There is good evidence in animal models that respiratory acidosis significantly impairs DIA contractility (136,137) (Fig. 13). In addition, Esau (138) demonstrated that a combination of respiratory acidosis and hypoxia had a greater

Table 4 Criteria for Use of PEEP or CPAP in Mechanically Ventilated Patients with Intrinsic PEEP

Relative indications	Relative contraindications
1. Severe COPD	Airway obstruction not severe Other causes of airway obstruction (e.g., acute asthma) Dynamic hyperinflation without airway obstruction High minute ventilation Rapid, shallow breathing Small or kinked endotracheal tube High expiratory circuit resistance
2. Intrinsic PEEP > 5 cm H_2O	Intrinsic PEEP < 5 cm H_2O
3. Flow limitation present Peak airway pressure, total PEEP, and lung volume stable where low levels of PEEP or CPAP applied	Flow limitation absent Peak airway pressure, total PEEP, and lung volume increase when low levels of PEEP or CPAP applied Expiratory muscles actively recruited when PEEP or CPAP applied
4. Assisted mechanical ventilation Assist-control ventilation Intermittent mandatory ventilation Pressure support ventilation	Controlled mechanical ventilation
5. Excessive patient effort Ineffective triggering Extreme dyspnea Marked asynchrony with ventilator Prominent accessory muscle use	Patient comfortable Triggers ventilator easily No noticeable dyspnea No accessory muscle use

Source: Gottfried S. The role of PEEP or CPAP in the mechanically ventilated COPD patient. In: Roussos C, ed. The Thorax. 2nd ed. New York: Marcel Dekker; 1995:2471–2500 (with permission).

detrimental effect on DIA contractility than respiratory acidosis alone. In man, respiratory acidosis has been shown to reduce Pdi and limit endurance (139). In dogs, metabolic acidosis has been shown to reduce Pdi at all frequencies of stimulation, with a greater detrimental impact noted in the compensated state (140). However, a more recent study reported no adverse effects of lactic acidosis on DIA function. Severe hypoxia has been show to impair DIA contractility in dogs (142). Impaired endurance capacity of the respiratory muscles complicated hypoxia in man in one study, but was not confirmed in another (143,144).

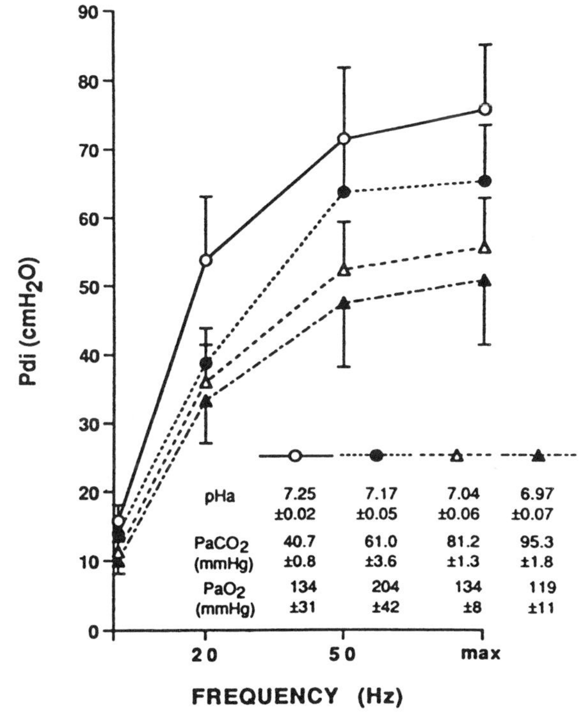

Figure 13 Relationship between frequency of stimulation and transdiaphragmatic pressure (Pdi) to increments of $PaCO_2$ in spontaneously breathing dogs. Note the progressive reduction in Pdi as the degree of respiratory acidosis increases. From: Schnader JY, Juan G, Howell S, Fitzgerald R, Roussos C. Arterial CO_2 partial pressure affects diaphragmatic function. J Appl Physiol 1985; 58:823–829, with permission.

C. Electrolyte Balance

Hypophosphatemia is prevalent in hospitalized and critically ill patients (145, 146). For example, hypophosphatemia was reported in 21.5% of 158 patients presenting with an acute exacerbation of COPD (145). Significant decrement in Pdi has been demonstrated in hypophosphatemic patients on mechanical ventilation for acute respiratory failure (147). Marked impairment of Pdi was noted following correction of the hypophosphatemia (147). Hypomagnesemia may also produce respiratory muscle weakness that is reversible with correction (148). It is of interest that serum levels of magnesium in ICU patients may not reflect muscle levels; in one study, serum levels of magnesium were reduced in 9.4% of patients, compared to reductions in muscle concentrations in 47% of patients (149). Hypocalcemia (150) and hypokalemia (151) may also cause respiratory muscle weakness.

D. Effects of Nutrition Deprivation on Respiratory Muscles

Prolonged nutrition deprivation (ND) results in significant atrophy of muscle fibers of the DIA and medial gastronemius muscles in rats (152–154) (Fig. 14). Of interest, atrophy is disproportionately greater in type II fibers, with the greatest impact on types IIx and IIb fibers (155). These latter fibers produce the high levels of force. Acute short-term ND may also produce DIA fiber atrophy, particularly in young growing animals that exhibit reduced "nutritional reserve" (156). In both acute and prolonged ND, DIA contractility is preserved (154,156). Thus, reduced DIA mass results in reduced total force-generating capacity. This may limit the functional force reserve and endurance capacity of the DIA, especially under loaded conditions. DIA reserve may be further compromised under conditions of stressed ND (e.g., sepsis) (157). In significantly undernourished patients without

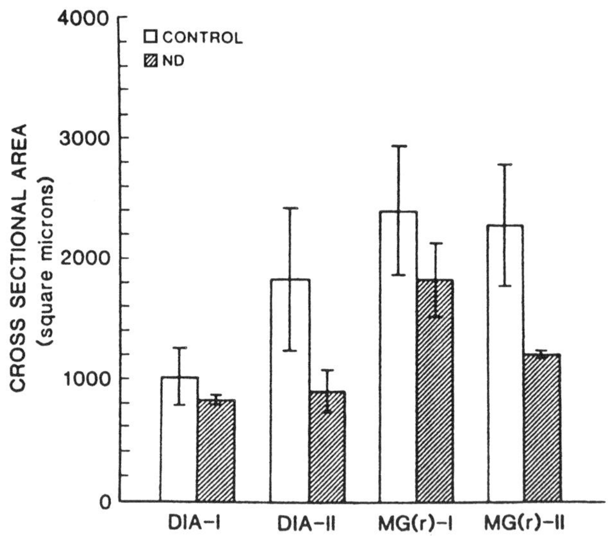

Figure 14 Bar graph depicting cross-sectional areas of type I and II muscle fibers in both diaphragm (DIA) and deep portion of medial gastrocnemius (Mg_r). Values are means ± SD. Note that although a significant reduction in cross-sectional area was noted for both fiber types in both muscles, a significantly ($P < .0001$) greater degree of atrophy was noted din type II fibers from both DIA and Mg_r. From: Sieck GC, Lewis MI, Blanco CE. Effects of undernutrition on diaphragm fiber size, SDH activity and fatigue resistance. J Appl Physiol 1989; 66:2196–2205, with permission.

lung disease (71% ideal body weight), Arora and Rochester reported that DIA mass was reduced by 43% compared to well-nourished controls (158). Recently, Murciano and colleagues (159) reported significantly reduced Pdi in patients with anorexia nervosa (63% ideal body weight) following phrenic stimulation or maximal sniff, which improved markedly following nutritional support.

1. Rationale for Nutritional Support

Nutritional support has become an integral component of critical care medicine (160). A number of studies suggest a relationship between nutritional status and outcome (161,162). For example, Bartlett et al. (161) reported a high rate of mortality in critically ill patients who had accrued an acute cumulative deficit of >10,000 calories compared to a control group in positive caloric balance. In addition, improved weaning success from mechanical ventilation has been reported in patients receiving adequate nutritional support compared to those in whom support was not provided (163,164). However, controversy regarding the role of nutritional supplementation in critically ill patients exists, as there are no randomized controlled trials providing high-grade evidence for reduced morbidity and mortality (165). As ND, particularly if accompanied by a hypermetabolic, hypercatabolic state, almost certainly impacts severely on the respiratory muscles (as well as pulmonary defense mechanisms, immune status, and respiratory drive), it seems prudent from the pathophysiological viewpoint to continue current treatment trends while awaiting better evidence. Indeed, Kelly et al. (166) demonstrated improved mouth pressures and increased body cell mass in critically ill patients receiving TPN.

2. Anabolic Steroids and Growth Factors

As nutritional supplementation may fail to augment lean body mass while expanding the fat component, measures aimed at augmenting somatic protein mass are being explored. We have recently demonstrated increased contractility, fiber hypertrophy, and increased maximum shortening velocity of the DIA in hamsters administered nandrolone (167). A recent study by Bhasin and co-workers (168) reported that supraphysiologic doses of testosterone increased muscle size and strength in normal men, while relatively low dose nandrolone improved mouth pressures and lean body weight in undernourished patients with COPD over and above nutritional supplementation measures (169). The possible role of anabolic steroids in critically ill patients awaits future trials.

Acute or prolonged ND is associated with reduced levels of insulinlike growth factor-1 (IGF-1) and resistance to the action of growth hormone (GH) (170). Indeed, serum levels of IGF-1 may be a sensitive marker of nutritional status. Partial (171) or complete (172) restoration of DIA fiber cross-sectional areas was demonstrated in adolescent rats subjected to severe or moderate degrees of acute ND, following the administration of IGF-1. There are limited studies in man regarding the impact of GH and/or IGF-1 on respiratory muscle function in critically ill patients. Most studies have examined the effects of these growth factors on improving nitrogen balance, wound healing, etc. (173,174). Improved mouth pressures and nitrogen balance was demonstrated in preliminary studies in patients with respiratory disease (175,176).

E. Pharmacologic Influences on Respiratory Muscles

Several different drugs have been demonstrated to influence respiratory muscle function in either a positive or an adverse manner. A summary of these pharmacologic effects follows.

1. Cardiac Glycosides

DIA strength (Pdi) was significantly increased 45 and 90 min following the administration of digoxin to patients with COPD in acute respiratory failure, with no increase in cardiac output observed (177). In dogs, the positive intropic effect on DIA produced by digoxin was not accompanied by an increase in DIA blood flow (178). In addition, deslanoside appeared to have some protective effect against DIA fatigue (179). The mechanism of action appears to be at the level of excitation-contraction coupling and may be linked to augmented calcium entry into the muscle cell.

2. Dopamine

Dopamine administered to patients with COPD during episodes of acute respiratory failure (10 μg/kg/min) resulted in a 30% increase in Pdi following supramaximal phrenic stimulation (180). The improved DIA strength was attributed to a 30% increase in DIA blood flow (60% increase in cardiac output) (Fig. 15) (180).

3. Milrinone

Preliminary in vitro studies of the phosphodiesterase inhibitor in rats demonstrated improved DIA force and fatigue resistance (181).

4. Methylxanthines

Intense interest in the use of aminophylline as a potential DIA inotrope followed Aubier and co-workers' (182) landmark report that aminophylline improved Pdi (15%) and reversed low-frequency fatigue induced by resistive breathing in normal subjects. Since then, the role of aminophylline as a therapeutic tool has undergone intense scrutiny, and its use remains a controversial topic. Early reports revealed positive inotropic effects of theophylline in vitro (using supratherapeutic levels) on the DIA. Likewise in dogs, supratherapeutic levels of aminophylline revealed positive influences in a dose-dependent fashion (see reviews for summary of early data and the origins of the controversy) (183,184). More recent animal data in vitro support the notion that supratherapeutic levels of theophylline are required to exert a positive impact (185,186). Prolonged infusion (2 weeks) of

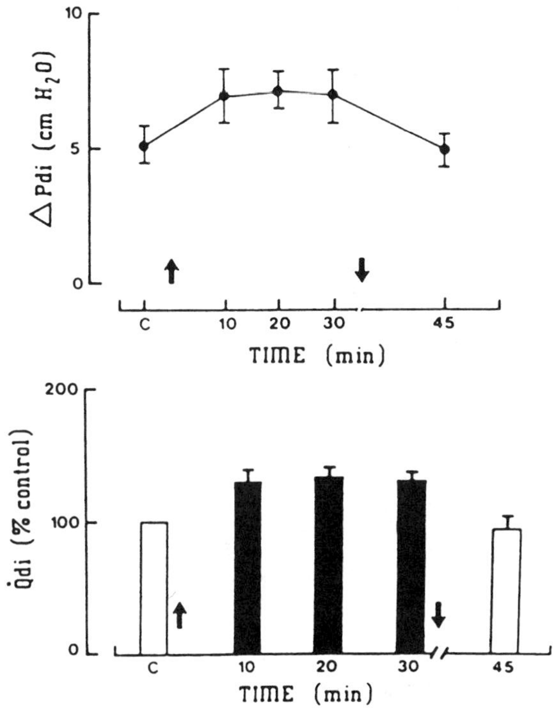

Figure 15 Graphs depicting increments in transdiaphragmatic pressures (Pdi; top panel) and diaphragm blood flow (Qdi; bottom panel) before, during, and after dopamine administration to patients in acute respiratory failure due to COPD exacerbation. From: Aubier M, Murciano D, Menu Y, Boczkowski J, Mal H, Pariente R. Dopamine effects on diaphragmatic strength during acute respiratory failure in chronic obstructive pulmonary disease. Ann Intern Med 1989; 110:17–23, with permission.

aminophylline in rats (blood levels 12.3 ± 2 mg/l) resulted in improved DIA contractility (187).

In man, the role of methylxanthines in improving DIA or accessory muscle contractility remains highly controversial (188–191), but important new insights have recently been reported. Gauthier et al. (192) evaluated the effects of aminophylline in normal subjects at different lung volumes (and therefore different DIA fiber lengths). Therapeutic levels of theophylline significantly increased twitch Pdi (following bilateral supramaximal phrenic stimulation) only at lung volumes above 75% of inspiratory capacity. The same results were observed in nonfatigued and fatigued states. Similar results were reported in dogs in which inotropic effects of theophylline in the foreshortened DIA was demonstrated (193). These studies have important clinical implications in states of hyperinflation, particularly dynamic hyperinflation in critically ill patients.

The mechanisms underlying the intrinsic action of theophylline in the DIA are not clear. Possibilities include enhanced transmembrane flux of calcium, as the inotropic effects are abolished by calcium channel blockers (194), or possibly improve T-tubular conduction (193).

5. *Sympathomimetic Amines*

Isoproternol, tebutaline, and albuterol (salbutamol) have no effect on the fresh DIA but appear to exhibit inotropic effects in the fatigued state (195–197). In man, albuterol was reported to have no effect on the fresh or fatigued DIA (198). Recent studies report that the new β_2 agonist broxaterol may enhance respiratory muscle endurance in patients with COPD (199).

6. *Cyclosporine*

Reduced exercise endurance time and skeletal muscle mitochemical respiration were reported in rats following 14 days of cyclosporine A administration (200). Whether these effects could explain in part the reduced exercise capacity and anaerobic threshold noted in transplant patients following active rehabilitation needs to be explored (201).

7. *Corticosteroids*

Corticosteroids have been reported in animal studies to induce atrophy of type IIb/x fibers (202–205). Fluorinated steroids appear to induce greater atrophy and myogenic changes (202,203,205). Short-term administration of either methylprednisone or triamcinolone to rats with dosage regimens used in the treatment of acute cellular rejection or status asthmaticus resulted in significant atrophy of type IIb/x diaphragm fibers (206). Studies in man suggest that steroid myopathy of respiratory muscles can ensue if large doses of corticosteroids are administered (e.g., dose equivalent to $\geqslant$ 40 mg/day prednisone) (207–209). Studies in patients with COPD with steroid-induced myopathy (average prednisone dosage, 14.2 $\pm$ 8.2 mg) revealed markedly reduced limb and respiratory muscle strength and evidence of myopathic changes affecting all fibers in quadriceps muscle biopsies (210). It should be emphasized, however, that steroid effects in critically ill patients may be compounded by a multitude of factors and/or drugs described throughout this review.

REFERENCES

1. De Troyer A, Estenne M. Functional anatomy of the respiratory muscles. Clin Chest Med 1988; 9:175–193.
2. Seick GC. Organization and recruitment of diaphragm motor units. In: Roussos C, ed. The Thorax. 2nd ed. New York: Marcel Dekker, 1995:783–820.

3. Grassino A, Clanton T. Respiratory muscle fatigue. Semin Resp Med 1991; 12: 305–321.
4. Aldrich TK. Central and transmission fatigue. Semin Resp Med 1991; 12:322–330.
5. Moxham J. Resp muscle fatigue: mechanisms, evaluation and therapy. Br J Anesthesiol 1990; 65:43–53.
6. Roussos C, Bellemare F, Moxham J. Respiratory muscle fatigue In: Roussos C, ed. The Thorax. 2nd ed. New York: Marcel Dekker, 1995:1405–1461.
7. Fitts RH. Cellular mechanisms of muscle fatigue. Physiol Rev 1994; 74:49–94.
8. NHLBI Workshop. Respiratory muscle fatigue: report of the respiratory muscle fatigue workshop group. Am Rev Respir Dis 1990; 142:474–480.
9. Laghi F, D'Alfonso N, Tobin J. Pattern of recovery from diaphragmatic fatigue over 4 hours. J Appl Physiol 1995; 79:539–546.
10. Drachman DB. Myasthenia gravis. N Engl J Med. 1994; 330:1797–1810.
11. Tobin MJ, Perez W, Guenther SM, et al. The pattern of breathing during successful and unsuccessful trials of weaning from mechanical ventilation. Am Rev Respir Dis 1986; 134:1111–1118.
12. Cohen C, Zagelbaum G, Gross D, Roussos C, Macklem PT. Clinical manifestations of inspiratory muscle fatigue. Am J Med 1982; 73:308–316.
13. Tobin JM, Perez W, Guenther SM, Lodado RF, Dantzker D. Does ribcage abdominal paradox signify respiratory muscle fatigue? J Appl Physiol 1987; 63:851–860.
14. Brochard L, Haarf A, Lorino H, Lemaire F. Inspiratory pressure support prevents diaphragmatic fatigue during weaning from mechanical ventilation. Am Rev Respir Dis 1989; 139:513–521.
15. Black LF, Hyatt RE. Maximal respiratory pressures: normal values and relationship to age and sex. Am Rev Respir Dis 1969; 99:698–702.
16. Wilson SH, Cooke NT, Edwards NT, Edwards RH, Spiro SG. Predicted normal values for maximum respiratory pressures in Caucasian adults and children. Thorax 1984; 39:535–538.
17. Multz A, Aldrich TK, Prezant DJ, Karpel JP, Hendler JM. Maximal inspiratory pressure is not a reliable test of inspiratory muscle strength in mechanically ventilated patients. Am Rev Respir Dis 1990; 142:529–532.
18. Laroche CM, Mier AK, Moxham J, Green M. Measurement of sniff esophageal pressures to assess global inspiratory muscle strength. Am Rev Respir Dis 1988; 138:598–603.
19. De Troyer A, Estenne M. Limitations of measurement of transdiaphragmatic pressure in detecting diaphragm weakness. Thorax 1981; 36:169–174.
20. Laporta D, Grassino A. Assessment of transdiaphragmatic pressure in humans. J Appl Physiol 1985; 58:1469–1476.
21. Miller JM, Moxham J, Green M. The maximal sniff in the assessment of diaphragm function in man. Clin Sci 1985; 69:91–96.
22. Bellemare F, Bigland-Ritchie B. Assessment of human diaphragm strength and activation using phrenic nerve stimulation. Respir Physiol 1984; 58:263–277.
23. Simolowski T, Fleury B, Launois S, Cathala, HP, Bouche P, Derenne J. Cervical magnetic stimulation: a painless method for bilateral phrenic nerve stimulation in conscious humans. J Appl Physiol 1989; 67:1311–1318.
24. Markand ON, Kincaid JC, Pourmand RA, et al. Electrophysiologic evaluation of

diaphragm by transcutaneous phrenic nerve stimulation. Neurology 1984; 34: 604–614.
25. Koulouris N, Vianna LG, Mulvey DA, Green M, Moxham J. Maximal relaxation rates of esophageal, nose and mouth pressures during a sniff reflect inspiratory muscle fatigue. Am Rev Resp Dis 1989; 139:1213–1217.
26. Goldstone J, Green M, Moxham J. Maximum relaxation rate of the diaphragm during weaning from mechanical ventilation. Thorax 1994; 49:54–60.
27. Roussos C, Macklem PT. Diaphragmatic fatigue in man. J Appl Physiol 1977; 43:189–197.
28. Bellemare F, Grassino A. Effect of pressure and timing of contraction on human diaphragm fatigue. J Appl Physiol 1982; 53:1190–1195.
29. Bellemare F, Wright D, Levine CM, Grassino A. Effect of tension and timing of contraction on the blood flow of the diaphragm. J Appl Physiol 1983; 54:1597–1606.
30. Field S, Sanci S, Grassino A. Respiratory oxygen consumption estimated by the diaphragm pressure-time index. J Appl Physiol 1984; 57:44–51.
31. Supinski G, DiMarco A, Dibner-Dunlap M. Alterations in diaphragm strength and fatiguability in congestive heart failure. J Appl Physiol 1994; 76:2707–2713.
32. Howell S, Maarek JM, Fournier M, Sullivan K, Zhan, WZ, Sieck GC. Congestive heart failure: differential adaptation of the diaphragm and latissimus dorsi. J Appl Physiol 1995; 79:389–397.
33. Aubier M, Trippenbach T, Roussos C. Respiratory muscle fatigue during cardiogenic shock. J Appl Physiol 1981; 51:499–508.
34. Viires N, Sillye G, Aubier M, Rassidakis A, Roussos C. Regional blood flow distribution in dogs during induced hypotension and low cardiac output. J Clin Invest 1983; 72:935–947.
35. McParland C, Krishnan B, Wang Y, Gallagher CG. Inspiratory muscle weakness and dyspnea in chronic heart failure. Am Rev Respir Dis 1992; 146:467–472.
36. Hammond MD, Bauer KA, Sharp JT, Rocha RD. Respiratory muscle strength in congestive heart failure. Chest 1990; 98:1091–1094.
37. Nishimura Y, Malda H, Tanaka K, Nakamura H, Hashimoto Y, Yokoyama M. Respiratory muscle strength and hemodynamics in chronic heart failure. Chest 1994; 105:355–359.
38. Evans SA, Watsonn L, Hawkins M, Cowzey AS, Johnston IDA, Kinnear WJM. Respiratory muscle strength in chronic heart failure. Thorax 1995; 50:625–628.
39. Mancini DM, Henson D, LaManca J, Levine S. Respiratory muscle function and dyspnea in patients with chronic congestive heart failure. Circulation 1992; 86:9009–9018.
40. Eddinger TJ, Moss RL. Mechanical properties of skinned single fibers of identified types from rat diaphragm. Am J Physiol 1987; 243:C210–C218.
41. Weiner DH, Fink LI, Maris J, Jones RA, Chance B, Wilson JR. Abnormal skeletal muscle bioenergetics during exercise in patients with heart failure: role of reduced muscle blood flow. Circulation 1986; 73:1127–1136.
42. Kassis E, Jacobsen TN, Mogensen F, Amtorp O. Sympathetic reflex control of skeletal muscle blood flow in patients with congestive heart failure: evidence for B-adrenergic circulatory control. Circulation 1986; 74:929–938.

43. Levine B, Kalman J, Mayer L, Fillit HM, Packer M. Elevated circulating levels of tumor necrosis factor in severe chronic heart failure. N Engl J Med 1990; 323: 236–241.
44. Carr JG, Stevenson LW, Walden JA, Heber D. Prevalence and hemodynamic correlates of malnutrition in severe congestive heart failure secondary to ischemic or idiopathic dilated cardiomyopathy. Am J Cardiol 1989; 63:709–713.
45. Gottlieb SS, Baruch L, Kukin ML, Bernstein JL, Fisher ML, Packer M. Prognostic implications of serum magnesium concentration in patients with congestive heart failure. J Am Coll Cardiol 1990; 16:827–831.
46. McParland C, Resch EF, Krishnan B, Wang Y, Cujec B, Gallagher CG. Inspiratory muscle weakness in chronic heart failure: role of nutrition and electrolyte status and systemic myopathy. Am J Respir Crit Care Med 1995; 151:1101–1107.
47. Bradley TD, Chartrand DA, Fitting JW, Killian KJ, Grassino A. The relation of inspiratory effort sensation to fatiguing patterns of the diaphragm. Am Rev Respir Dis 1986; 134:119–124.
48. Wilcox P, Baile EM, Hards J. Phrenic nerve function and its relationship to atelactasis after coronary artery bypass surgery. Chest 1988; 93:693–698.
49. Large SR, Haywood LJ, Flower CD, Cory-Pearce RR, Wallwork JJ, English TA. Incidence and etiology of raised hemidiaphragm after cardiopulmonary bypass. Thorax 1984; 40:444–447.
50. Esposito RA, Spencer FC. The effect of pericardial insulation on hypothermic phrenic nerve injury during open heart surgery. Ann Thorac Surg 1987; 43: 503–508.
51. De Vita JA, Robinson LR, Rehder J, Hattler B, Cohen C. Incidence and natural history of phrenic neuropathy occurring during open heart surgery. Chest 1993; 103: 850–856.
52. Efthimiou J, Butler J, Woodham C, Westaky S, Benson MK. Phrenic nerve and diaphragm function following open heart surgery: a prospective study with and without topical hypothermia. Q J Med 1992; 85:845–853.
53. Diehl JL, Lofaso F, Deleuze P, Similowski T, Lemaire F, Brochard L. Clinically relevant diaphragmatic dysfunction after cardiac operations. J Thorac Cardiovasc Surg 1994; 107:487–498.
54. Watanabe T, Trusler GA, Williams WG, Edmonds JF, Coles JG, Hosokawa Y. Phrenic nerve paralysis after pediatric cardiac surgery. J Thorac Cardiovasc Surg 1987; 94:383–388.
55. Russell RI, Mulvey D, Laroche C, Shinebourne EA, Green M. Bedside assessment of phrenic nerve function in infants and children. J Thorac Cardiovasc Surg 1991; 101:143–147.
56. Dureuil B, Viirés N, Pariente R, Desmonts JM, Aubier M. Effects of phrenic nerve cooling on diaphragmatic function. J Appl Physiol 1987; 63:1763–1769.
57. Curtis JJ, Nawarawong W, Walls JT, et al. Elevated hemidiaphragm after cardiac operations: incidence, prognosis and relationship to the use of typical ice slush. Ann Thorac Surg 1989; 48:764–768.
58. Chandler KW, Rozas CJ, Kory RC, Goldman AL. Bilateral diaphragmatic paralysis complicating local cardiac hypothermia during open heart surgery. Am J Med 1984; 77:243–249.

59. Raffa H, Kayali MT, Al-Ibrahim K, Mimish L. Fatal bilateral phrenic nerve injury following hypothermic open heart surgery. Chest 1994; 105:1268–1269.
60. Laroche CM, Carroll N, Moxham J, Green M. Clinical significance of severe isolated diaphragm weakness. Am Rev Respir Dis 1988; 138:862–866.
61. Lisboa C, Paré PD, Pertuzé J, Contreras G, Moreno R, Guillemi S, Cruz E. Inspiratory muscle function in unilateral diaphragmatic paralysis. Am Rev Respir Dis 1986; 134:488–492.
62. Gilbert R, Auchincloss JH, Peppi D. Relationship of rib cage and abdomen motion to diaphragm function during quiet breathing. Chest 1981; 80:607–612.
63. Russell RJ, Helps BA, Dicks-Mireaux CM, Helms PJ. Early assessment of diaphragmatic dysfunction in children in the ITU: chest radiology and phrenic nerve stimulation. Eur Respir J 1993; 6:1336–1339.
64. Chroni E, Patel RL, Taub N, Venn GE, Howard RS, Panayiotopoulos CP. A comprehensive electrophysiological evaluation of phrenic nerve injury related to open-heart surgery. Acta Neurol Scand 1995; 91:255–259.
65. Wilcox PG, Paré D, Pardy RL. Recovery after unilateral phrenic injury associated with coronary artery revascularization. Chest 1990; 98:661–666.
66. Driver AG, Blackburn BB, Marcuard SP, Austin EH. Bilateral diaphragm paralysis treated with cuirass ventilation. Chest 1987; 92:683–685.
67. Raine J, Samuels MP, Mok Q, Shinebourne EA, Southall DP. Negative extrathoracic pressure ventilation for phrenic nerve palsy after pediatric cardiac surgery. Br Heart J 1992; 67:3088–3011.
68. Abd AG, Braun NMT, Baskin MI, O'Sullivan MM, Alkaitis DA. Diaphragmatic dysfunction after open heart surgery treatment with a rocking bed. Ann Intern Med 1989; 111:881–886.
69. Graham DR, Kaplan D, Evans CC, Hind CR, Donelly RJ. Diaphragmatic plication for unilateral diaphragmatic paralysis: a 10-year experience. Ann Thorac Surg 1990; 49:248–252.
70. Ciccolella PE, Daly BD, Celli BR. Improved diaphragmatic function after surgical plication for unilateral diaphragmatic paralysis. Am Rev Respir Dis 1992; 146: 797–799.
71. Laub GW, Muralidharan S, Chen C, et al. Phrenic nerve injury: a prospective study. Chest 1991; 100:376–379.
72. Guinn GA, Beall AC, Lamki N, Heibig J, Thornby J. Phrenic nerve injury during coronary artery bypass. Texas Heart Inst J 1990; 17:48–50.
73. Maccherini M, Davoli G, Sani G, et al. Warm heart surgery eliminates diaphragmatic paralysis. J Cardiac Surg 1995; 10:257–261.
74. Bone R, Balk R, Cerra F, et al. Definitions for sepsis and organ failure and guidelines for the use of innovative therapies in sepsis. Chest 1992; 101:1644–1655.
75. Hussain S, Simkus G, Roussos C. Respiratory muscle fatigue: a cause of ventilatory muscle failure in septic shock. J Appl Physiol 1985; 59:1802–1808.
76. Hussain S, Roussos C. Distribution of respiratory muscle and organ blood flow during endotoxic shock in dogs. J Appl Physiol 1985; 59:1802–1808.
77. Hussain S, Graham R, Rutledge F, Roussos C. Respiratory muscle energetics during endotoxic shock in dogs. J Appl Physiol 1986; 60:486–493.

78. Kim WS, Ward ME, Hussain SNA. Pathological O_2 supply dependence of diaphragmatic and systemic O_2 uptake during endotoxemia. J Appl Physiol 1994; 77:1093–1100.
79. Boczkowski J, Vicaut E, Aubier M. In vivo effects of *Escherichia coli* endotoxemia on diaphragmatic microcirculation in rats. J Appl Physiol 1992; 72:2219–2224.
80. Harlan J. Leukocyte-endothelial interaction. Blood 1985; 65:513–525.
81. Hussain SNA, Rutledge F, Graham R, Magder S, Roussos C. Effects of norepinephrine and fluid administration on diaphragmatic O_2 consumption in septic shock. J Appl Physiol 1987; 62:1368–1376.
82. Supinski GS, DiMarco, AF, Gonzalez J, Altose MD. Effect of norepinephrine on diaphragm contractility and blood flow. J Appl Physiol 1990; 69:2019–2028.
83. Supinski GS, DiMarco, AF, Ketai L, Hussein F, Altose MD. Reversibility of diaphragm fatigue by mechanical hyperperfusion. Am Rev Respir Dis 1988; 138: 604–609.
84. Van Lambalgen AA, Van Kraats AA, Mulder MF, Van Den Box GC, Teerlink T, Thijs LG. Organ blood flow and distribution of cardiac output in dopexamine- or dobutamine-treated endotoxemic rats. J Crit Care 1993; 8:117–127.
85. Tang W, Pakula JL, Weil MH, Noc M, Fukui M, Bisera J. Adrenergic vasopressor agents and mechanical ventilation for the treatment of experimental septic shock. Crit Care Med 1996; 24:115–130.
86. Magder S, Erian R, Roussos C. Respiratory muscle blood flow in oleic acid-induced pulmonary edema. J Appl Physiol 1986; 60:1849–1856.
87. Murphy TD, Mayock DE, Standaert TA, Gibson RL, Woodrum DE. Group B *Streptococcus* has no effect on piglet diaphragmatic force generation. Am Rev Respir Dis 1992; 145:471–475.
88. Leon A, Boczkowski J, Dureuil B, Desmonts J, Aubier M. Effects of endotoxic shock on diaphragmatic function in mechanically ventilated rats. J Appl Physiol 1992; 72:1466–1472.
89. Boczkowski J, Dureuil B, Branger C, et al. Effects of sepsis on diaphragmatic function in rats. Am Rev Respir Dis 1988; 138:260–265.
90. Shindoh C, DiMarco A, Nethery D, Supinski G. Effect of PEG-superoxide dismutase on the diaphragmatic response to endotoxin. Am Rev Respir Dis 1992; 145: 1350–1354.
91. Mier A, Brophy C, Green M. Respiratory muscle weakness during upper respiratory tract infections. Am Rev Resp Dis 1988; 138:5–7.
92. Altose M. Viral infections and respiratory muscle contractility. Am Rev Respir Dis 1988; 138:1–2.
93. Anzueto A, Supinski GS, Levine SM, Jenkinson SG. Mechanisms of disease: are oxygen-derived free radicals involved in diaphragmatic dysfunction? Am J Resp Crit Care Med 1994; 149:1048–1052.
94. Supinski G, Nethery D, DiMarco A. Effect of free radical scavengers on endotoxin-induced respiratory muscle dysfunction. Am Rev Respir Dis 1993; 148:1318–1324.
95. Van Surell C, Boczkowski J, Pasquier C, Du Y, Franzini E, Aubier M. Effects of N-acetylcysteine on diaphragmatic function and malondialdehyde content in *Escherichia coli* endotoxemic rats. Am Rev Respir Dis 1992; 146:730–734.

96. Supinski G, Stofan D, DiMarco, A. Effect of ischemia-reperfusion on diaphragm strength and fatigability. J Appl Physiol 1993; 75:2180–2187.
97. Kobzik L, Reid MB, Bredt DS, Stamler JS. Nitric oxide in skeletal muscle. Nature 1994; 372:546–548.
98. Boczkowski J, Sambe A, Ungureanu-Longrois D, Viires N, Aubier M. Role of nitric oxide in diaphragmatic dysfunction in *E. coli* endotoxemic rats. Am J Respir Crit Care Med 1995; 151:A231.
99. Shindoh C, Kurosawa H, Wu D, Kikuchi Y, Hida W, Shirato K. Effects of L-NAME and L-arginine on diaphragm contraction after endotoxin administration. Am J Respir Crit Care Med 1995; 151:A231.
100. Hussain SNA. Role of nitric oxide in endotoxin-induced metabolic and vascular dysregulation of the canine diaphragm. Am J Respir Crit Care Med 1995; 152: 683–689.
101. Wilcox P, Osborne S, Bressler B. Monocyte inflammatory mediators impair in vitro hamster diaphragm contractility. Am Rev Respir Dis 1992; 146:462–466.
102. Diaz PT, Julian MW, Wewers MD, Clanton TL. Tumor necrosis factor and endotoxin do not directly affect in vitro diaphragm function. Am Rev Respir Dis 1993; 148: 281–287.
103. Wilcox PG, Bressler B. Effects of tumor necrosis factor α in vitro hamster diaphragm contractility. Am Rev Respir Dis 1992; 145:A457.
104. Wilcox PG, Wakai Y, Walley KR, Cooper DJ, Road J. Tumor necrosis factor α decreases in vivo diaphragm contractility in dogs. Am J Respir Crit Care Med 1994; 150:1368–1373.
105. Jiang TX, Wilcox PG. Effects of tumor necrosis factor-alpha (TNF-α) on hamster diaphragm contractility is mediated by nitric oxide. Am J Respir Crit Care Med 1996; 153:A439.
106. Boczkowski J, Dureuil B, Pariente R, Aubier M. Preventive effects of indomethacin on diaphragmatic contractile alterations in endotoxemic rats. Am Rev Respir Dis 1990; 142:193–198.
107. Ruff RL, Secrist D. Inhibitors of prostaglandin synthesis or cathepsin B prevent muscle wasting due to sepsis in the rat. J Clin Invest 1984; 73:1483–1486.
108. Rochester DF. Respiratory muscles and ventilatory failure: 1993 perspective. Am J Med Sci 1993; 305:394–402.
109. Rochester DF. Respiratory muscle failure and respiratory failure. Semin Resp Med 1992; 13:7–13.
110. Roussos C, Zakynthinos S. Ventilatory failure and respiratory muscles. In: Roussos C, ed. The Thorax. 2nd ed. New York: Marcel Dekker, 1995:2071–2099.
111. Tobin MJ, Chadha TS, Jenouri G, Birch SJ, Gazeroglu HB, Sackner MA. Breathing patterns 2. Disease subjects. Chest 1983; 84:286–294.
112. Bellemare F, Grassino A. Effect of pressure and timing of contraction on human diaphragm fatigue. J Appl Physiol 1982; 53:1190–1195.
113. Hlastala MP. Ventilation. In: Crystal RC, West JB, eds. The Lung, Scientific Foundations. New York: Raven Press, 1991:1209–1214.
114. Efthimiou J, Fleming J, Spiro S. Sternomastoid muscle function and fatigue in breathless patients with severe respiratory disease. Am Rev Respir Dis 1987; 136: 1099–1105.

115. Zakynthinos SG, Vassilakopoulos T, Roussos C. The load of inspiratory muscles in patients needing mechanical ventilation. Am J Respir Crit Care Med 1995; 152: 1248–1255.
116. Watchko JF, Johnson BD, Gosselin LE, Prakash YS, Sieck GC. Age-related differences in diaphragm muscle injury after lengthening activities. J Appl Physiol 1994; 77:2124–2133.
117. Martin JG, Habib M, Engel LA. Inspiratory muscle activity during induced hyperinflation. Respir Physiol 1980; 39:303–313.
118. Brochard L, Mancebo JJJ, Wysocki MM, et al. Noninvasive ventilation for acute exacerbations of chronic obstructive pulmonary disease. N Engl J Med 1995; 333: 817–822.
119. Kramer N, Meyer TJ, Meharg JJ, Cece RD, Hill NS. Randomized, prospective trial of non-invasive positive pressure ventilation in acute respiratory failure. Am J Respir Crit Care Med 1995; 151:1799–1806.
120. Bott J, Carroll MP, Conway JH, et al. Randomised controlled trial of nasal ventilation in acute ventilatory failure due to chronic obstructive airways disease. Lancet 1993; 341:1555–1557.
121. Meyer TJ, Hill NS. Noninvasive positive pressure ventilation to treat respiratory failure. Ann Intern Med 1994; 120:769–770.
122. Pepe PE, Marini JJ. Occult positive end-expiratory pressure in mechanically ventilated patients with airflow obstruction. The auto-PEEP effect. Am Rev Respir Dis 1982; 126:160–170.
123. Ranieri VM, Giuliana R, Cinnella G, et al. Physiologic effects of positive end-expiratory pressure in patients with chronic obstructive pulmonary disease during acute ventilatory failure and controlled mechanical ventilation. Am Rev Respir Dis 1993; 147:5–13.
124. Gottfried S. The role of PEEP on CPAP in the mechanically unilateral COPD patient. In: Roussos C, ed. The Thorax. New York: Marcel Dekker, 1995:2471–2500.
125. Zhan W-Z, Sieck GC. Adaptations of diaphragm and medial gastrocnemius muscles to inactivity. J Appl Physiol 1992; 72:1445–1453.
126. Miyata H, Zhan W-Z, Prakash YS, Sieck GC. Myoneural interactions affect diaphragm muscle adaptations to inactivity. J Appl Physiol 1995; 79:1640–1649.
127. Lewis M, LoRusso T, Zhan W-Z, Sieck G. The interactive effects of denervation and malnutrition on diaphragm structure and function. J Appl Physiol 1996; 81:2165–2172.
128. Le Bourdellés G, Viires N, Boczkowski J, Seta N, Pavlovic D, Aubier M. Effects of mechanical ventilation on diaphragm contractile properties in rats. Am J Resp Crit Care Med 1994; 149:1539–1544.
129. Knisely AS, Leal S, Singer DB. Abnormalities of diaphragmatic muscle in neonates with ventilated lungs. J Pediatr 1988; 113:1074–1077.
130. Marini JJ, Rodriguez RM, Lamb V. The inspiratory workload of patient-initiated mechanical ventilation. Am Rev Respir Dis 1986; 134:902–909.
131. Marini JJ, Smith TC, Lamb VJ. External work output and force generation during synchronized intermittent mechanical ventilation. Effect of machine assistance on breathing pattern. Am Rev Respir Dis 1988; 138:1169–1179.
132. Hansen-Flaschen J, Cowen J, Raps EC. Neuromuscular blockade in the intensive care unit: more than we bargained for. Am Rev Respir Dis 1993; 147:234–236.

133. Giostra E, Magistris MR, Pizzolato G, Cox J, Chevrolet JC. Neuromuscular disorder in intensive care unit patients treated with pancuronium bromide. Occurrence in a cluster group of seven patients and two sporadic cases, with electrophysiologic and histologic examination. Chest 1994; 106:210–220.
134. Barohn RJ, Jackson CE, Rogers SJ, Ridings LW, McVey A. Prolonged paralysis due to nondepolarizing neuromuscular blocking agents and corticosteroids. Muscle Nerve 1994; 17:647–654.
135. Manthous CA, Chatila W. Prolonged weakness after the withdrawal of atracurium. Am J Respir Crit Care Med 1994; 150:1441–1443.
136. Fitzgerald RS, Hauer MC, Bierkamper G, Raff H. Responses of in vitro rat diaphragm to changes in acid-base environment. J Appl Physiol 1984; 57:1202–1210.
137. Schnader JY, Juan G, Howell S, Fitzgerald R, Roussos C. Arterial CO_2 partial pressure affects diaphragmatic function. J Appl Physiol 1985; 58:823–829.
138. Esau SA. Hypoxic hypercapnic acidosis decreases tension and increases fatigue in hamster diaphragm muscle in vitro. Am Rev Respir Dis 1989; 139:1410–1417.
139. Juan G, Calverley P, Talamo C, Schnader JY, Roussos C. Carbon dioxide impairs diaphragm function in man. N Engl J Med 1984; 310:874–879.
140. Howell S, Fitzgerald RS, Roussos C. Effects of uncompensated and compensated metabolic acidosis on canine diaphragm. J Appl Physiol 1985; 59:1376–1382.
141. Yanos J, Wood LDH, Davis K, Keamy M III. The effect of respiratory and lactic acidosis on diaphragm function. Am Rev Respir Dis 1993; 147:616–619.
142. Bark H, Supinski G, Bundy R, Kelsen S. Effect of hypoxia on diaphragm blood flow, oxygen uptake, and contractility. Am Rev Respir Dis 1988; 138:1535–1541.
143. Jardim J, Farkas G, Prefault C, Thomas D, Macklem PT, Roussos C. The failing inspiratory muscles under normoxic and hypoxix conditions. Am Rev Respir Dis 1981; 124:274–279.
144. Ameredes BT, Clanton TL. Hyperoxia and moderate hypoxia fail to affect inspiratory muscle fatigue in humans. J Appl Physiol 1989; 22:894–900.
145. Fiaccadori E, Coffrini E, Ronda N, et al. Hypophosphatemia in the course of chronic obstructive pulmonary disease. Prevalence mechanisms, and relatiopnships with skeletal muscle phosphorus content. Chest 1990; 97:857–868.
146. Gravelyn TR, Brophy N, Siegert C, Peters-Golden M. Hypophosphatemia-associated respiratory muscle weakness in a general inpatient population. Am J Med 1988; 84:870–876.
147. Aubier M, Murciano D, Lecocgic Y, et al. Effect of hypophosphatemia on diaphragmatic contractility in patients with acute respiratory failure. N Engl J Med 1985; 313:420–442.
148. Malloy DW, Dhingra S, Solven FS. Hypomagnesemia and respiratory muscle power. Am Rev Respir Dis 1984; 129:497–498.
149. Fiaccadori E, Del Canale S, Coffrinii E, et al. Muscle and serum magnesium in pulmonary intensive care unit patients. Crit Care Med 1988; 16:751.
150. Aubier M, Viires N, Piquet J, et al. Effects of hypocalcemia on diaphragmatic strength generation. J Appl Physiol 1985; 58:2054–2061.
151. Bilbrey GL, Herbin L, Carter NW, Knochel JP. Skeletal muscle resting membrane potential in potassium deficiency. J Clin Invest 1973; 52:3011–3018.

152. Lewis MI, Sieck GC, Fournier M, Belman MJ. The effect of nutritional deprivation on diaphragm contractility and muscle fiber size. J Appl Physiol 1986; 60:596–603.
153. Sieck GC, Lewis MI, Blanco CE. Effects of undernutrition on diaphragm fiber size, SDH activity and fatigue resistance. J Appl Physiol 1989; 66:2196–2205.
154. Kelsen SG, Ference M, Kappor S. The effect of prolonged undernutrition on structure and function of the diaphragm. J Appl Physiol 1985; 58:1354–1359.
155. Lanz JK Jr, Donahoe M, Rogers RM, Ontell M. Effects of growth hormone on diaphragmatic recovery from malnutrition. J Appl Physiol 1992; 7:801–805.
156. Lewis M, Sieck G. Effect of acute nutritional deprivation on diaphragm structure and function in adolescent rats. J Appl Physiol 1992; 73:974–978.
157. Pingleton S, Boczkowski J, Viires N, Pavlovic D, Pariente R, Aubier M. Effect of combined starvation and sepsis upon diaphragmatic function. Am Rev Respir Dis 1990; 141:A549.
158. Arora NS, Rochester DF. Effect of body weight and muscularity on human diaphragm and muscle mass. J Appl Physiol 1982; 52:64–70.
159. Murciano D, Rigaud D, Pingleton S, Armengaud MH, Melchior JC, Aubier M. Diaphragmatic function in severely malnourished patients with anorexia nervosa: effects of renutrition. Am J Respir Crit Care Med 1994; 150:1569–1574.
160. Berger R, Adams L. Nutritional support in the critical care setting. Part 1. Chest 1989; 96:139–150.
161. Bartlett RH, Dechert RE, Mault JR, Ferguson SK, Kaiser AM, Erlandson EE. Measurements of metabolism in multiple organ failure. Surgery 1982; 92:771–779.
162. Mullen JL, Buzby GP, Mathews DC, Smale BF, Rosato EF. Reduction of operative morbidity by combined preoperative and post operative nutritional support. Ann Surg 1980; 192:604–613.
163. Larca L, Greenbaum DM. Effectiveness of intensive nutritional regimes in patients who fail to wean from mechanical ventilator. Crit Care Med 1982; 10:297–300.
164. Bassili HR, Deitel M. Effect of nutritional support on weaning patients off mechanical ventilators. JPEN 1985; 5:161–163.
165. Koretz, R. Nutritional Supplementation in the ICU. How critical is nutrition for the critically ill? Am J Respir Crit Care Med 1995; 151:570–573.
166. Kelly SM, Allan R, Field S, Coughlin M, Shizal H, Macklem P. Inspiratory muscle strength and body composition in patients receiving total parenteral nutrition therapy. Ann Rev Respir Dis 1984; 130:33–37.
167. Yeh AY, Fournier M, Micevych PE, Sieck GC, Lewis M. Impact of nandrolone treatment on hamster diaphragm structure and function. Am J Resp Crit Care Med 1996; 153:686A.
168. Bhasin S, Storer TW, Berman N, et al. The effects of supraphysiologic doses of testosterone on muscle size and strength in normal men. N Engl J Med 1996; 335: 1–7.
169. Schols AMWJ, Soeters PB, Mostert R, Pluymers RJ, Wouters EFM. Physiologic effects of nutritional support and anabolic steroids in patients with chronic obstructive pulmonary disease: a placebo-controlled randomized trial. Am J Respir Crit Care Med 1995; 152:1268–1274.
170. Thissen J, Ketelslegers J, Underwood LE. Nutritional regulation of insulin-like growth factors. Endocr Rev 1994; 15:80–101.

171. Lewis M, LoRusso T, Fournier M. Effect of growth hormone (GH) and insulin-like growth factor-I on diaphragm fiber size in malnourished adolescent rats. Am J Resp Crit Care Med 1995; 151:814A.
172. Feinberg AT, Fournier M, Lewis MI. The impact of growth factors on diaphragm fiber size with moderate nutritional deprivation. Am J Resp Crit Care Med 1996; 153:A686.
173. Bentham J, Rodriguez-Arnao J, Ross RJ. Acquired growth hormone resistence in patients with hypercatabolism. Horm Res 1993; 40:87–91.
174. Herndon DN, Barrow RE, Kunkel KR, Broemeling L, Rutan RL. Effects of recombinant human growth hormone on donor-site healing in severely burnt children. Ann Surg 1990; 212:424–429.
175. Suchner U, Rothkopf M, Stanislaus G, Elwyn D, Kvetan V, Askanazi J. Growth hormone and pulmonary disease: metabolic effects in patients receiving parental nutrition. Arch Intern Med 1990; 150:1225–1230.
176. Pape G, Friedman M, Underwood LE, Clemmons DR. The effect of growth hormone on weight-gain and pulmonary function in patients with chronic obstructive lung disease. Chest 1991; 99:1495–1500.
177. Aubier M, Murciano D, Viires N, et al. Effects of digoxin on diaphragmatic strength generation in patients with chronic obstructive pulmonary disease during acute respiratory failure. Am Rev Resp Dis 1987; 135:544–548.
178. Aubier MM, Viires N, Murciano D, Seta JP, Pariente R. Effects of digoxin on diaphragmatic strength generation. J Appl Physiol 1986; 61:1767–1774.
179. Kikuchi Y, Hida W, Shindoh C, et al. Effect of digitalis on the diaphragm in anesthetized dogs. J Appl Physiol 1987; 63:277–284.
180. Aubier M, Murciano D, Menu Y, Boczkowski J, Mal H, Pariente R. Dopamine effects on diaphragmatic strength during acute respiratory failure in chronic obstructive pulmonary disease. Ann Intern Med 1989; 110:17–23.
181. Rossing TH, Shannon K, Miller M. Effects of milrinone on contractility of the rat diaphragm in vitro. Am Rev Respir Dis 1987; 136:841–844.
182. Aubier M, De Troyer A, Sampson M, Macklem PT, Roussos C. Aminophylline improves diaphragmatic contractility. N Engl J Med 1981; 305:249–252.
183. Aubier M. Pharmacotherapy of respiratory muscles. Clin Chest Med 1988; 9: 325–336.
184. Moxham J. Aminophylline and the respiratory muscles: an alternative view. Clin Chest Med 1988; 9:325–336.
185. Reid MB, Miller MJ. Theophylline does not increase strength or endurance of diaphragm in vitro. J Appl Physiol 1989; 67:1655–1661.
186. Derom E, Janssens S, De Bock V, Decramer M. Theophylline minimally alters contractile properties of canine diaphragm in vitro. J Appl Physiol 1990; 69:1390–1396.
187. Kuei JH, Sieck GC. Chronic aminophylline administration. Effect on diaphragm contractility and fatigue resistance in vitro. Am Rev Respir Dis 1991; 144:121–125.
188. Levy RD, Nava S, Gibbons L, Bellemare F. Aminophylline and human diaphragm strength in vivo. J Appl Physiol 1990; 68:2591–2596.

189. Moxham J, Miller J, Wiles CM, Morris A Jr, Green M. Effect of aminophylline on the human diaphragm. Thorax 1985; 40:288–292.
190. Murciano D, Aubier M, Viirés, Mal H, Pariente R. Effects of theophylline and enprofylline on diaphragmatic contractility. J Appl Physiol 1987; 63:51–57.
191. Lewis M, Belman M, Sieck G. Aminophylline and fatigue of the sternomastoid muscle. Am Rev Respir Dis 1986; 133:672–675.
192. Gauthier AP, Yan S, Sliwinski P, Macklem PT. Effects of fatigue, fiber length, and aminophylline on human diaphragm contractility. Am J Respir Crit Care Med 1995; 152:204–210.
193. Gayan-Ramirez G, Decramer MM. Inotropic effects of theophylline on foreshortened canine diaphragm. Am J Respir Crit Care Med 1994; 149:920–924.
194. Kolbeck RC, Speir WA. Diltiazem, verapamil, and nifedipine inhibit theophylline-enhanced diaphragmatic contractility. Am Rev Respir Dis 1989; 139:139–145.
195. Howell S, Roussos C. Isoproterenol and aminophylline improve contractility of fatigued canine diaphragm. Am Rev Respir Dis 1984; 129:118–124.
196. Aubier M, Viires N, Murciano D, Medrano G, Lecocguic Y, Parient R. Effects and mechanism of action of terbutaline on diaphragmatic contractility and fatigue. J Appl Physiol 1984; 56:922–929.
197. Howell S, Fitzgerald RS, Roussos C. Effects of neostigmine and salbutamol on diaphragmatic fatigue. Resp Physiol 1985; 62:15–29.
198. Javaheri S, Smith JT, Thomas JP, Guilfoile TD, Donovan EF. Albuterol has no effect on diaphragmatic fatigue in humans. Am Rev Respir Dis 1988; 137:197–201.
199. Nava S, Crotti P, Gurrieri G, Fracchia C, Rampulla C. Effect of a B_2-agonist (Broxaterol) on respiratory muscle strength and endurance in patients with COPD with irreversible airway obstruction. Chest 1992; 101:133–140.
200. Mercier JG, Hokanson JF, Brooks GA. Effects of cyclosporine A on skeletal muscle mitochondrial respiration and endurance time in rats. Am J Respir Crit Care Med 1995; 151:1532–1536.
201. Ross DP, Waters P, Mohsenifar Z, Belman M, Kass R, Koerner S. Hemodynamic responses to exercise after lung transplantation. Chest 1993; 103:46–53.
202. Lewis M, Monn S, Sieck G. The effect of corticosteriods on diaphragm fatigue, SDH activity and muscle fiber size. J Appl Physiol 1992; 72:293–301.
203. Dekhuijzen PNR, Gayan-Ramirez G, Dom R, de Bock V, Decramer M. Triamcinolone and prednisolone affect contractile properties and histopathology of rat diaphragm differently. J Clin Invest 1993; 92:1534–1542.
204. Wilcox PG, Hards JM, Bockhold K, Bressler B, Pardy RL. Pathologic changes and contractile properties of the diaphragm in corticosteroid myopathy in hamsters: comparison to peripheral muscle. Am J Resp Cell Mol Biol 1989; 1:191–199.
205. Dekhuijzen PNR, Gayan-Ramirez G, Bisschop A, De Bock V, Dom R, Decramer M. Corticosteroid treatment and nutritional deprivation cause a different pattern of atrophy in rat diaphragm. J Appl Physiol 1995; 78:629–637.
206. Nava S, Gayan-Ramirez G, Rollier H, et al. Effects of acute steroid administration on ventilatory and peripheral muscles in rats. Am J Respir Crit Care Med 1996; 153: 1888–1896.

207. Decramer M, Stas K. Corticosteroid-induced myopathy involving respiratory muscles in patients with COPD or asthma. Am Rev Respir Dis 1992; 146:800–802.
208. Bowyer SI, LaMothe MP, Hollister JR. Steroid myopathy: incidence and detection in a population with asthma. J Allergy Clin Immunol 1985; 76:234–242.
209. Weiner P, Azgad Y, Sc M, Weiner MM. The effect of corticosteroids on inspiratory muscle performance in humans. Chest 1993; 104:1788–1791.
210. Decramer M, de Bock V, Dom R. Functional and histologic picture of steroid-induced myopathy in chronic obstructive pulmonary disease. Am J Respir Crit Care Med 1996; 153:1958–1964.

3

Ventilator Management and Weaning in the CCU

JAY UDANI

Cedars-Sinai Medical Center, Los Angeles, California

ZAB MOHSENIFAR

Cedars-Sinai Medical Center and University of California, Los Angeles, School of Medicine, Los Angeles, California

I. INDICATIONS FOR MECHANICAL VENTILATION IN THE CCU

There are many reasons and indications for mechanical ventilation in the CCU setting.

1. The most important indications for ventilation are to support pulmonary gas exchange, to reverse hypoxia, and to reverse acute respiratory acidosis, the goal being to normalize alveolar ventilation and to achieve and maintain a level of oxygen saturation which is acceptable for each clinical scenario (1).
2. Another clinical indication for ventilation is to increase lung volumes in order to prevent or treat atelectasis and maintain the functional residual capacity in settings such as adult respiratory distress syndrome (ARDS) and postoperative pain.
3. Mechanical ventilation can also decrease the work of breathing in order to unload the ventilatory muscles and to decrease cardiac demand.

Clinical settings in which mechanical ventilation may be helpful for management of patients include: adult respiratory distress syndrome, neuromuscular disease, obstructive airway disease, asthma, myocardial ischemia, and cardiogenic pulmonary edema.

II. CARDIOPULMONARY INTERACTIONS

The increased work of breathing in respiratory failure causes increased oxygen demand. This in turn can cause myocardial ischemia with a concomitant decrease in left ventricular compliance, an increase in pulmonary capillary pressure, a decrease in lung compliance, and an increase in the work of breathing. Positive pressure ventilation increases intrathoracic pressure and thus decreases venous return, increases lung volumes to increase the PaO_2, and decreases right to left shunting, all of which may increase the effective cardiac output by as much as 1 L (1), which can decrease the risk of myocardial ischemia and may even obviate the need for mechanical circulatory support (2) in extreme cases. There is, however, a great range of variability of response to positive pressure ventilation as the increasing lung volumes may increase the resistance of alveolar vessels while simultaneously decreasing the resistance of the extra-alveolar vessels. Therefore the change in cardiac output cannot always be predicted (1).

In pulmonary edema there is decreased elastic recoil secondary to alveolar flooding and increased airway resistance secondary to mucosal edema and bronchospasm. For spontaneous inspiration to achieve a fixed tidal volume, a significant increase in the transpulmonary pressure gradient must be generated by an exaggerated fall in intrathoracic pressure. This all generates increased work for the diaphragm resulting in increased O_2 consumption and then muscular fatigue. This then causes negative swings in the intrathoracic pressure and accelerates systemic venous blood flow, resulting in decreased left ventricular ejection fraction which then worsens the pulmonary edema. It may be necessary to treat with intubation and ventilation to decrease the intrathoracic blood volume, thereby decreasing the left ventricular afterload and the left ventricular O_2 demands (3).

III. MANAGEMENT OF MECHANICAL VENTILATION IN THE CCU

A. Assist Control

In assist control ventilation, every breath is supported by the ventilator, and there is a backup rate to ensure minimum ventilation. The programming may be volume-targeted or pressure-targeted, which is more physiologic and better tolerated. In general, this mode of ventilation is poorly tolerated in the nonsedated patient population. Other potential adverse effects include respiratory alkalosis and worsening of air trapping in patients with obstructive lung disease as the inspiratory and expiratory cycles of the patient and the ventilator may not be entirely in synch. This is best used as the initial mode of ventilation in patients who are well-sedated (1).

B. Synchronized Intermittent Mechanical Ventilation

In synchronized intermittent mechanical ventilation, there are a preset number of ventilator-delivered mandatory breaths of a predetermined tidal volume. The patient can take spontaneous breaths in addition to the mandatory breaths, and these breaths will not be ventilator-supported. The advantages are that the patient can vary the amount of respiratory work and, at the same time, have a backup (1). In addition, the patient is generally more comfortable and there is less need for sedation or paralytic agents (4). The potential risks of this method of ventilation include the possibility of hyperventilation or respiratory alkalosis if there is dyssynchrony between the patient and the ventilator. In addition, spontaneous efforts may increase the work of breathing in patients with obstructive airways diseases. This method of ventilation can be used for weaning, in which case the number of mechanically delivered mandatory breaths are systematically decreased with guidance from the patient's pH response (4).

C. Pressure Support

In pressure support ventilation, each breath must be patient-initiated and each spontaneous breath is augmented with a fixed amount of positive pressure. The patient can control the depth, length, and flow profile of each breath. This method of ventilation is generally regarded as very comfortable (1), but can only be used in patients with an intact respiratory drive. A low level of pressure support can be thought of as overcoming the resistance of the ETT and the demand valve. The disadvantage is that the tidal volume is not controlled (1). This is best used during periods of stable ventilatory support and as a method of weaning from ventilation. Weaning is accomplished by gradually decreasing the amount of pressure support as tolerated by the patient (4).

D. Flow-By or T-Tube

In T-tube or flow-by breathing mode, the patient is breathing unassisted by the ventilator, but is still intubated. The patient is responsible for all spontaneous breaths and is not given any positive airway pressure. The work of breathing with the T-tube apparatus may in fact be greater than spontaneous breathing without the T-tube, as the patient must overcome the dead space in the equipment and the resistance of the endotracheal tube, the inspiratory circuit, the humidifier, and the exhalation valve (4). When this method of ventilation is used for weaning from mechanical ventilation, it is advisable to add small amounts of pressure support to overcome the resistance as described above in order to make the patient more comfortable and increase the chance of successful weaning. The risks of this method of ventilation are that the patient must have an intact respiratory drive and should not be sedated, as there is no backup rate.

E. Noninvasive Ventilation

The purpose of noninvasive ventilation is to provide improved gas exchange while decreasing the risks associated with intubation. Noninvasive ventilation has also been shown to be able to reduce the length of the ICU stay (5). This system consists of a face mask through which pressure support is delivered at a constant, preset, positive airway pressure throughout the respiratory cycle. The respiratory rate, tidal volume, and inspiratory time are all regulated by the patient. The goal is to increase end-expiratory pressure to greater than atmospheric pressure to increase lung volume and oxygenation (1). The inspiratory pressure terminates when the inspiratory flow drops below 5 L/min or when airway pressure exceeds positive pressure setting by 1.5 cm H_2O (1). This procedure may help to recruit collapsed lung units.

A study of 17 patients showed that noninvasive ventilation was successful in 47% of the time regardless of underlying cause of respiratory failure, and was successful in 83% of the time in patients who had just failed extubation from invasive ventilatory support (6). In deciding who is eligible and most appropriate for noninvasive ventilatory support, CO_2 retention is a better indicator than severe hypoxia, and hyperventilation is a contraindication. This method of ventilation is similar to pressure support and flow-by ventilation in that it can only be used in patients who have an intact respiratory drive, as all breaths are initiated by the patient. In all cases, gas exchange will improve after the first hour regardless of whether or not the patient ultimately fails on noninvasive ventilation (7). The lack of significant improvement of PaO_2 on day 1 predicts the need for endotracheal intubation (7). Complications of noninvasive ventilation can include facial discomfort from the face mask and localized skin lesions (7). Other potential risks include hyperinflation and patient fatigue from excessive expiratory work.

F. Alternative Modes of Ventilation

There are three experimental modes of ventilation that can be used in special circumstances. In ARDS, only a small part of the lung parenchyma is accessible to the O_2 delivered from the ventilator. If the tidal volume from the ventilator is too high, it may overexpand and injure the small amount of functioning lung that is left. There are three modes of ventilation—high-frequency ventilation, inverse ratio ventilation, and airway pressure release ventilation—which are based on the principle of decreasing the end-inspiratory airway pressures and/or the tidal volumes delivered to the patient. There are currently no data suggesting that these methods are superior to the conventional methods of ventilation (1).

G. Complications of Ventilation

There are many potential complications of ventilatory support and positive pressure ventilation which the physician must be aware of when making the decision to place a patient on a ventilator. There is an increased risk of infection as the ETT allows the entry of pathogens and disrupts the cough and mucociliary clearance mechanisms, and secretions may enter around the balloon (1). Risks associated with the ETT itself include glottic injury, tracheal erosion, tracheal dilatation, and tracheomalacia. There is a risk of ETT misplacement and possible dislocation. The most common mislocation is into the right mainstem bronchus with the potential for overinflation of the right lung and atelectasis of the left lung. Through the use of oxygen and positive pressure ventilation, one can see oxygen toxicity and decreased cardiac output as described previously.

There can be renal dysfunction as the decreased cardiac output decreases renal perfusion, resulting in decreased free water clearance and then fluid retention leading to total body edema. These patients are also susceptible to GI hypomobility and obstipation secondary to immobility and medications. GI distress may be further worsened by aerophagia and mucosal irritation, ulceration, or bleeding. ICU patients, especially those on ventilators, are prone to develop mental and psychological distress secondary to sleep deprivation, loss of control of breathing, pain, fear, and the need for sedatives (1).

IV. WEANING

Weaning is the method of gradual discontinuation and withdrawal of ventilatory support and the return to spontaneous breathing by the patient. There are many methods of weaning, and there are many factors that contribute to the ultimate success or failure of a weaning trial. At the most basic level, the factors that predict successful weaning are adequacy of pulmonary gas exchange, performance of the respiratory muscles, and psychological factors (4). Oxygenation is usually not a factor in ventilator weaning, as hypoxia is a contraindication to the initiation of the weaning process. Inadequate respiratory muscle performance can be divided into decreased neuromuscular capacity, such as decreased respiratory center output, phrenic nerve dysfunction, neuromuscular disorders, and increased respiratory muscle pump load secondary to increased ventilatory requirements such as increased resistance, decreased compliance, auto-PEEP, increased CO_2 production, increased dead space ventilation, and an inappropriately increased respiratory drive (4). Other factors important for successful weaning include a resolution of the underlying cause of respiratory failure and resolution of any cardiac insufficiency.

A. Weaning Physiology

Weaning must be attempted only when cardiac insufficiency and risk of myocardial ischemia have been minimized. It is not recommended to wean patients who are hemodynamically unstable or who have pulmonary capillary leakage. Factors that increase the risk of myocardial ischemia when the patient is switched from positive pressure mechanical ventilation to spontaneous ventilation include atherosclerosis, mild oxygen desaturation, and increased LVEDP (8).

Weaning may cause hemodynamic deterioration, as the change from mechanical to spontaneous ventilation causes a decrease in pulmonary artery wedge pressure and a change from positive intrathoracic pressure to negative intrathoracic pressure generated by the muscles of respiration. This causes an increase in venous return which increases the left ventricular filling pressure, LVEDP, and left ventricular afterload. All of this increases myocardial work while increasing airway resistance via the narrowing of small airways and thus increasing respiratory work (3,8). These events may precipitate respiratory muscle failure and thus weaning failure. They may also cause myocardial ischemia, left ventricular failure, and pulmonary edema.

The change from assisted positive pressure ventilation to flow-by or T-piece is associated with significant increases in systolic and diastolic blood pressures and the heart rate (9). These same parameters are significantly increased during extubation and may place the susceptible patient at risk for myocardial ischemia. A recent study found that the use of β-blockers slightly but significantly decreased these physiologic responses in patients being weaned and extubated (9).

Two other studies examined the risk of myocardial ischemia during weaning. One study found evidence of ischemia on thallium scan in 47% of patients who were undergoing weaning after prolonged mechanical ventilation (10). The other study found evidence of silent ischemia in 14.3% of patients being weaned by flow-by, 9.1% of patients being weaned by CPAP, and 0% of patients being weaned by SIMV (11).

In general, pressure support may minimize the negative swings in intrathoracic pressure during spontaneous ventilation and may be a safer mode of weaning for patients at high myocardial risk (3).

B. Weaning Parameters

There are many weaning parameters thought to help predict successful weaning. Some are felt to be more accurate and have been validated better than others (12). Weaning parameters are doubly important because they can provide valuable information about the patient's underlying physiologic state. As the patient's state changes on a daily basis, the parameters should be assessed daily as well (1).

One parameter not often utilized is the presence of myocardial ischemia. Ischemia as documented by continuous ECG monitoring was found to be associated with an increased failure to wean in a study of 17 patients who had been on mechanical ventilation for $>$ 5 days (13). Other parameters used to predict successful weaning include respiratory rate, oxygen saturation, pH, maximal inspiratory pressure, and f/Vt (14).

C. Weaning Process

To prepare a patient for weaning from mechanical ventilation, he or she must first be medically stable. The following criteria should be used in deciding if the patient is stable for weaning. The most important criterion is that the underlying cause of the institution of mechanical ventilation has been resolved or markedly improved. Other specific medical parameters that should be followed include: temperature $< 38.5°C$ (101.3°F); hemoglobin > 8 g/dl or at least no significant change from baseline; no electrolyte disorders; and patient should be free of sedation. Cardiovascular parameters are no evidence of cardiac insufficiency, and no vasoactive drugs. Respiratory parameters to aid in the decision to wean include: PEEP of < 5; respiratory rate of < 35; $SpO_2 > 90\%$; and pH > 7.32 on FiO_2 of 40%. Once these parameters have been met, the f/Vt should be measured on room air flow-by for 60 sec (12), provided that the SpO_2 is $\geqslant 92$. If this is not the case, then the f/Vt should be done on the current O_2 setting. This parameter should be $\leqslant 100$. The ventilator is then returned to the previous setting, and 3 min later a maximum inspiratory pressure is measured and should be $\leqslant$ $(-)20$ (14).

D. Flow-by Trial

When the decision has been made to wean and all of the above parameters are met, all patients should undergo a flow-by trial (Fig. 1). The patient is placed on a flow-by circuit at the same FiO_2 as he or she was previously breathing. The trial should be aborted if any of the following occur:

1. Respiratory rate > 35 or increased by $> 50\%$
2. $SpO_2 < 90\%$ or $PaO_2 < 55$
3. pH < 7.32
4. Heart rate > 140 or there is a sustained change in heart rate which increases or decreases by $> 20\%$
5. Systolic blood pressure > 180 or < 90, or a sustained increase by $> 20\%$
6. Agitation, diaphoresis, anxiety, or worsening mental status

If the patient tolerates this flow-by circuit for 2 h, he or she is ready to extubate and will have a 75% chance of successful extubation. If the patient does not tolerate weaning, he or she should be placed back on assist control ventilation and rested until the following day (14).

For patients who fail the initial flow-by trial, there are two options—once-daily flow-by trials, or pressure support ventilation weaning (Fig. 1). In the two best studies available to date (15,16), these two methods and SIMV ventilation were compared. One study concluded flow-by had an increased success rate while the other found PSV to be superior. An ongoing study at Cedars-Sinai Medical Center is comparing flow-by and PSV weaning to determine if one of these two methods is faster or more successful.

Patient comfort during weaning is difficult to assess. A study of 21 patients randomly switched between weaning modes on a single day were surveyed to

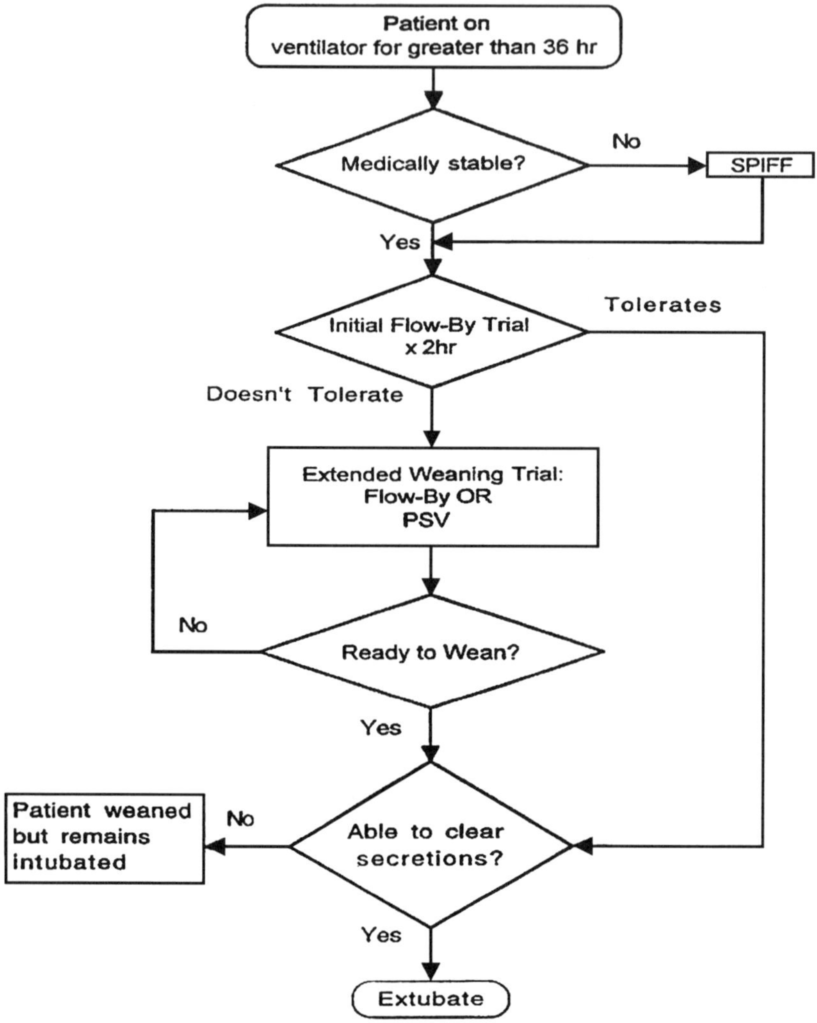

Figure 1 Ventilator weaning pathway.

measure dyspnea and anxiety. No significant difference between protocols was found (17).

E. Once-Daily Flow-by Trials

The patient is placed on the flow-by circuit using the same FiO_2 as previously used on the assist control ventilator setting and watched for signs of failure to wean as previously detailed. If the patient fails before 2 h, he or she is replaced on the previous method of ventilation and allowed to rest for 24 h before weaning again with a 2-h flow-by trial. When the patient tolerates the flow-by circuit for > 2 h, he or she is then ready to extubate.

F. Pressure Support Ventilation Weaning

With this method, the initial pressure support level is determined by adjusting the pressure support until the respiratory rate is between 20 and 30. Continuous positive airway pressure (CPAP) of up to 4 cm H_2O can be utilized to overcome the resistance of the circuit and to thus increase patient comfort. If the patient shows no signs of intolerance to the weaning trial, as described above for the flow-by trial, the level of pressure support can be decreased by 2 to 4 cm H_2O up to two times per day. If one or more signs of intolerance develop, return the pressure support to the previous level. The patient should be rested each night from 10 p.m. until 7 a.m. on Assist Control. If the patient tolerates PSV at a level of 5 cm H_2O for 2 h (the level of pressure support required to overcome the resistance of the endotracheal tube), he or she is then ready to extubate.

G. Other Considerations

Patients with coronary artery disease who are difficult to wean may benefit from diuresis. In a study of 15 ventilator-dependent COPD patients with coronary artery disease, nine of 15 were successfully weaned after 10 days of diuresis with a 5 kg weight loss each (9). It was felt that the diuresis caused a decrease in the circulating blood volume and thus decreased airway edema in the presence of left ventricular diastolic dysfunction, which allowed these patients to be successfully weaned.

H. Extubation

When the decision has been made that the patient is ready to breathe without the help of the ventilator, it must be determined if the patient is able to tolerate extubation. If the patient is unable to clear secretions on his or her own or unable to protect his or her airway to prevent aspiration, it is recommended that the patient remain intubated, but not ventilated. If these criteria are met, the patient is ready for extubation and should be extubated at the same level of FiO_2 that was used during weaning (14).

I. Postextubation Issues

After extubation, several problems may occur including laryngeal incompetence, aspiration, and, less commonly, laryngeal edema. Laryngeal edema is more common in patients who have been intubated for longer than 36 h, and studies utilizing dexamethasone did not show any decrease in the occurrence of edema (4). Extubation failure is defined as the need for reintubation within 7 days, and there is a 50% mortality associated with extubation failure (4).

REFERENCES

1. Slutsky AS. Mechanical ventilation. American College of Chest Physicians' Consensus Conference. Chest 1993; 104:1833–1859.
2. Goldenberg IF. Nonpharmacologic management of cardiac arrest and cardiogenic shock. Chest 1992; 102(5 suppl 2):596S–616S.
3. Pinsky MR. The effects of mechanical ventilation on the cardiovascular system. Crit Care Clin 1990; 6(3):663–678.
4. Tobin MJ, Alex CG. Principles and Practice of Mechanical Ventilation. New York: McGraw Hill, 1994:1177–1207.
5. Brochard L et al. Reversal of acute exacerbations of chronic obstructive lung disease by inspiratory assistance with a face mask. N Engl J Med 1990; 323.
6. Yang K, Tobin M. A prospective study of indexes predicting the outcome of trials of weaning from mechanical ventilation. N Engl J Med 1991; 324(21):1444–1450.
7. Wysocki M et al. Noninvasive pressure support ventilation in patients with acute respiratory failure. Chest 1993; 103:907–913.
8. Lemaire F et al. Acute left ventricular dysfunction during unsuccessful weaning from mechanical ventilation. Anesthesiology 1988; 69:171–179.
9. Dryden CM et al. The effect of preoperative beta-blocker therapy on cardiovascular responses to weaning from mechanical ventilation and extubation after coronary artery bypass grafting. J Cardiothorac Vasc Anesth 1993; 7(5):547–550.
10. Hurford WE et al. Myocardial perfusion as assessed by thallium-201 scintigraphy during the discontinuation of mechanical ventilation in ventilator dependent patients. Anesthesiology 1991; 74:1007–1016.
11. Abalos A et al. Myocardial ischemia during the weaning period. Am J Crit Care 1992; 1(3):32–36.
12. Sassoon C, Mahutte C. Airway occlusion pressure and breathing pattern as predictors of weaning outcome. Am Rev Respir Dis 1993; 148:860–866.
13. Hurford WE et al. Association of myocardial ischemia with failure to wean from mechanical ventilation. Crit Care Med 1995; 23:1475–1480.
14. Ventilator Weaning: Clinical Guideline. Cedars Sinai Medical Center Ventilator Weaning Guideline Committee, Los Angeles, 1995.

15. Brochard L et al. Comparison of three methods of gradual withdrawal from ventilatory support during weaning from mechanical ventilation. Am J Respir Crit Care Med 1994; 150:896–903.
16. Estcban A et al. A comparison of four methods of weaning patients from mechanical ventilation. N Engl J Med 1995; 332(6):345–350.
17. Knebel AR et al. Comparison of breathing comfort during weaning with two ventilator modes. Am J Respir Crit Care Med 1994; 149:14–18.

4

Detection of Sleep Apnea in the Cardiac Care Unit

VIAS MARKIDES and ADRIAN J. WILLIAMS

St. Thomas' Hospital, London, England

I. SLEEP-DISORDERED BREATHING AND SLEEP APNEA SYNDROME

Sleep-disordered breathing (SDB) is the broad term used to describe the endpoint of a number of conditions of diverse etiology that can disrupt breathing during sleep. *Apnea* is usually defined as the cessation of breathing for more than 10 sec. *Hypopnea* refers to a reduction in tidal volume without total cessation in respiration. Episodes of apnea and hypopnea often coexist in patients with sleep-disordered breathing, with apnea representing the more severe end of a spectrum of reduction in tidal volume.

Brief episodes of apnea or hypopnea are a feature of normal sleep, occurring most commonly during the transition from wakefulness to sleep, when the level of arterial carbon dioxide tension ($Paco_2$) in the body is reset to a level that is higher by approximately 5 mmHg. Such transitional apneas occur in most individuals but can be very pronounced in patients with frequent arousals during sleep.

In an attempt to differentiate between a normal and an abnormal frequency of apneic or hypopneic events, the apnea (AI) and apnea-hypopnea (AHI) indices are used. These refer, respectively, to the number of apneic or apneic and hypopneic events per hour of sleep. The upper limit of normal for AI has traditionally been considered to be 5 apneic events per hour, but some authors have suggested that the higher cutoff level of 10 events per hour should be used, especially in elderly individuals in whom the prevalence of mild and asymptomatic sleep-disordered breathing with AI of 5–10 per hour is extremely high and does not appear to be associated with worse outcome (1).

Sleep-disordered breathing is common and its prevalence increases with age. It is often accompanied by hypoxemia and hypercapnia, changes in heart rate and blood pressure, and arousals that may fragment sleep and lead to daytime fatigue and somnolence as well as cognitive changes. A significant proportion of patients, however, often those with mild disease, remain asymptomatic.

A. Sleep-Disordered Breathing

1. Prevalence

The exact prevalence of SDB in the general population is difficult to ascertain but a number of well-conducted epidemiological studies suggest that it is very common indeed.

The prevalence of SDB in men and women aged 30–60 years, defined as an apnea-hypopnea score of 5 or higher, was recently estimated as 9% for women and 24% for men (2). Another study found an overall prevalence of 18% for SDB in men and women of a similar age group using an AHI greater than 15 for the definition (3). It is quite possible, however, that this figure represents an overestimate of the prevalence of SDB, as subjects who had agreed to participate might have been more likely to have SDB than nonresponders.

A number of risk factors for sleep-disordered breathing have been identified in various studies (Table 1). Male sex and obesity appear to be among the strongest risk factors for SDB and have been found fairly consistently (2,3). Snoring is strongly associated with obstructive sleep apnea and therefore with SDB. Hypertension is associated with SDB for a number of reasons. First, risk factors such as obesity are shared between hypertensive patients and subjects with SDB. Second, hypertension may be exacerbated or even caused by SDB, at least in some patients (4,5). Current but not ex-smokers also appear to be at increased risk for SDB, after controlling for potential confounding factors (6).

Table 1 Risk Factors for Sleep-Disordered Breathing

Male sex	Snoring
Age	Hypertension
Obesity	Current smoking
Neck circumference	

B. Sleep Apnea Syndrome

The term *sleep apnea syndrome* (SAS) describes the presence of SDB accompanied by symptoms, in particular daytime hypersomnolence.

1. *Prevalence*

The prevalence of SAS has recently been found to be 2% for women and 4% for men aged 30–60 years (2). Another epidemiological study identified the lowest limit for prevalence of SAS in a group of middle-aged women as 2.5% (7).

The SAS is extremely common in the elderly and several studies have suggested that its prevalence in this age group may be as high as 18% or more. However, many of these patients may have satisfactory sleep, and the epidemiological link between SAS and cardiovascular disease and cognitive dysfunction in the elderly has not been confirmed. If, however, the diagnostic threshold is increased from 5 apneas to 10 apneas plus hypopneas per hour, elderly patients with SAS have more sleep disturbances, are more depressed, and have more cognitive deficits as compared to normal old persons. When an appropriate diagnostic index is used, SAS in the elderly resembles SAS in the middle-aged population. A high apnea-plus-hypopnea index is a predictor of mortality in the elderly population, and a very high level of SDB is a very significant risk factor for mortality during sleep phase in these patients (8–13).

2. *Clinical Significance*

Symptomatic sleep-disordered breathing is disabling for the sufferer. Sleep is disrupted at frequent intervals by arousals, which are a characteristic feature of both obstructive and central sleep apnea and contribute to the development of daytime hypersomnolence. Daytime somnolence, a hallmark of SAS, is a common subjective finding. It can be formally assessed using the multiple sleep latency test (MSLT) or one of its variants, such as the maintenance of wakefulness test (MWT) in which subjects are asked to remain awake in a quiet darkened room and then are monitored for electroencephalographic (EEG) evidence of sleep onset. Symptomatic sleep apnea patients have reduced sleep latency. The strongest nocturnal correlates of reduced sleep latency appear to be respiratory arousal index and, in the more severely affected patients, measures of nocturnal hypoxemia. These two factors contribute interactively to daytime dysfunction in patients with SAS (14).

Daytime hypersomnolence is also important in terms of safety at work and on the road, both for the patient and for others. An increased risk for road-traffic accidents as a result of falling asleep at the wheel has been well documented. Sleep-related vehicle accidents are believed to comprise up to 20% of road traffic accidents. However, hypersomnolence is often due to social and work-related reasons and not sleep-disordered breathing, especially in young subjects (15). Early-morning headache is another cardinal feature of severe SAS and is believed to be the result of nocturnal hypercapnia.

The SAS is also associated with cognitive impairment. Among a large cohort of middle-aged men and women, both habitual snoring and sleep apnea were associated with concentration problems but an association with memory problems has not been confirmed (16). There also appears to be an association between SAS and clinical depression.

Fatigue and loss of libido are also well described. Erectile dysfunction is common in male patients with SAS. In a large study of men with erectile dysfunction, more than 40% of participants had an apnea index equal to or greater than 5 per hour of sleep (17).

Snoring, often a feature of SDB, especially in patients with obstructive sleep apnea, may be disturbing for the bed partner and may even lead to marital disruption. Moreover, snoring is, in itself, a risk factor for hypertension, stroke, and ischemic heart disease (18).

Finally, SAS has important prognostic implications (19) (discussed below), which are of particular importance since SAS is an underrecognized but eminently treatable disorder.

The remainder of this discussion will focus on the different categories of disorders that result in sleep-disordered breathing, including obstructive and central sleep apnea, apnea that occurs in association with obstructive airways disease, and ischemic heart disease. Apnea in neuromuscular disease, which is also common and important, is beyond the scope of this chapter.

II. OBSTRUCTIVE SLEEP APNEA

A. Definition

Obstructive sleep apnea (OSA) is a disorder characterized by apneas or hypopneas in the presence of often greatly increased respiratory effort, which results from partial or complete collapse of the upper airway during inspiration. The term *obstructive sleep apnea syndrome* (OSAS) refers to symptomatic OSA. Partial upper airway obstruction, even without apnea or snoring, may be associated with frequent brief arousals that can disrupt sleep sufficiently to cause pathological daytime somnolence (99).

B. Prevalence

OSA is the commonest pattern of SDB. The exact prevalence of OSA in the general population remains unknown, in part because even some of the best studies on the prevalence of SDB have not classified it according to type. In one study, the minimum prevalence of OSA in a group of middle-aged men was estimated as 2.7% using an AHI equal to or greater than 10 as a cutoff point (20).

The prevalence of OSA may be even higher in cardiac patients, who share risk factors for ischemic heart disease and OSA such as obesity, hypertension, and smoking. OSA appears to be very common among patients with ischemic heart disease. In one small study, 50% of patients with angiographically proven ischemic heart disease had an apnea index of greater than 10 per hour. Approximately one-third of these patients were symptomatic. The findings of this study are particularly important since patients with ischemic heart disease may be particularly vulnerable to the adverse respiratory and hemodynamic effects of OSA such as hypoxemia and hypertension (21).

A higher-than-expected prevalence of obstructive apnea has been known to exist for some time among patients with hypertension. Two studies have suggested that the prevalence of sleep apnea and SAS in hypertensive patients may be as high as 30% and 9%, respectively (22,23). The prevalence of clinically significant OSA syndrome in patients with severe ventricular dysfunction awaiting transplantation appears to be similar to that of the general population, but as it may adversely affect cardiac function, it has been suggested that heart transplantation candidates be screened for symptoms suggestive of OSAS (24).

Of substantial significance both for the subjects themselves and for road safety were the somewhat disturbing results of a large study that examined the prevalence of SDB among commercial long-haul truck drivers. Not only did this study suggest a high prevalence of hypertension (16%) among these subjects, which had been most often previously undiagnosed, but almost 80% of drivers had an oxygen desaturation index (ODI) greater than 5 per hour and 10% had an ODI greater than 30 per hour. Both hypertension and ODI were associated with obesity. Drivers who had been with the company for longer than 1 year were more likely to be obese and hypertensive and have daytime fatigue and nonrefreshing sleep (25).

C. Predisposing Factors (Table 2)

Obesity has long been known to be an important risk factor for the development of OSA. A high body mass index (BMI) as well as more specific markers such as skin fold thickness and upper body obesity are associated with increased risk for OSA (99). In patients matched for BMI, neck circumference confers an increased risk for both snoring and sleep apnea (26).

Hypertension is certainly associated with OSA but may be at least in part a disease marker rather than a predisposing factor.

Hypothyroidism has traditionally been thought of as an important risk factor for the development of OSA but this has not been validated. In one study, the prevalence of hypothyroidism among patients with OSA was only 3.1%, which is not dissimilar from the prevalence in the general population. Conversely, the prevalence of moderate to severe OSA in hypothyroid patients was of the order of 10%, but the numbers in this group were too small for accurate conclusions to be drawn (27).

Table 2 Risk Factors for the Development of Obstructive Sleep Apnea

Age
Male sex
Obesity
High BMI
Skin fold thickness
Upper body obesity
Neck circumference
Shape of upper airway
"Congested" oropharynx
Macroglossia
Micrognathia
Increased upper airway or nasal resistance
Nasal obstruction in infants[(99)]
Increased upper airway resistance in patients with stroke
Congenital disorders
Marfan's syndrome[(28)]
Prader-Willi syndrome
Pierre Robin syndrome[(99)]
Endocrine disorders
Hypothyroidism
Acromegaly[(99)]

D. Pathogenesis

The pathogenesis of OSA is complex and incompletely understood. Upper airway narrowing due to abnormal bony morphology or deposition of fat in the neck and functional impairment of the upper airway dilating muscles appear to be important factors for its development (29,30).

Snoring, an important marker of increased upper airways resistance during sleep, is in part genetically determined (31). There also appears to be a strong genetic predisposition for SAS. In one study, almost half of the adult offspring of patients with SAS were also affected by the syndrome—this represented a highly significant difference in prevalence from that of the general population (32). Other studies have confirmed a significant genetic predisposition to sleep apnea (33).

In contrast to snoring as a marker of increased nocturnal upper airway resistance, a high nasal resistance has not been shown to increase the risk for OSA in adults, and reduction of nasal resistance by nasal surgery (septoplasty, turbinectomy, and/or polypectomy) does not appear to reduce the severity of OSA (34–36).

Upper airway muscle tone is often decreased in OSA but increases in the late apneic phase as a result of arousal. Electromyographic (EMG) studies have demonstrated that the activity of upper airway muscles such as genioglossus increases in the late apneic phase and, subsequently, decreases gradually. This increase in activity, which is normally responsible for apnea termination, is blunted during rapid-eye-movement (REM) sleep (37).

Other abnormalities have also been described in OSA patients including a reduction in the ventilatory response to hypercapnia but not hypoxia even when subjects are awake (38).

Regardless of the specific contributing factors in individual patients, the common end result is repetitive collapse of the upper airway leading to apneic episodes despite greatly increased inspiratory activity. Negative intrathoracic pressures of up to 60 mmHg produced by this inspiratory activity against a closed upper airway are not uncommon in OSA. This is of great importance for the cardiovascular system as huge swings are produced in the transmural pressures of all four cardiac chambers. Right ventricular preload increases dramatically as does left ventricular afterload. Bradycardia during the apneic period is rapidly succeeded, immediately after apnea termination, by sinus tachycardia. This, in association with an increase in stroke volume after apnea termination, leads to a dramatic increase in systemic blood pressure in the postapneic period.

Progressive hypoxemia and hypercapnia during the apneic period are corrected after a period of relative hyperventilation after arousal from sleep and restoration of upper airway patency in the postapneic period. Apnea termination in OSA, in contrast to central sleep apnea, appears to depend more on mechanoreceptor stimuli, especially from respiratory muscles, than on chemoreceptor stimuli (39).

The severity of OSA appears to change during the night. As the night progresses, the mean apnea duration increases both during non-REM and REM sleep. Moreover, the reduction in upper airway tone that is a characteristic of REM sleep becomes more significant as the night progresses as longer periods are spent in REM sleep (37,40).

Poor sleep quality and daytime sleepiness are probably largely the result of sleep fragmentation by repetitive arousals rather than nocturnal hypoxemia, although the latter may also have a role (14,41).

Obstructive sleep apnea is a progressive condition. This has been brought out by analysis of patients' symptoms over time as well as retrospective analysis of polysomnograms of patients followed up before the initiation of treatment. Increasing body weight appears to be an important marker of disease progression (42).

OSA is exacerbated by alcohol and perhaps by sedatives (1). Alcohol ingestion depresses the respiratory motor activity to upper airway muscles more than that to the diaphragm, a response pattern that favors upper airway obstruction during inspiration (43,44). It also induces vasodilatation and swelling of the respiratory mucosa and depresses respiratory centers resulting in hypotonia of oropharyngeal dilator muscles (45). Benzodiazepines may exacerbate sleep apnea only in a small subgroup of patients with OSA (46).

E. Recognized Adverse Cardiovascular Effects of OSA

A large number of important cardiovascular changes have been noted in patients with OSA, both acutely and in the long term. These occur against a background of repetitive and sometimes marked changes in the arterial tensions of oxygen and carbon dioxide, changes in intrathoracic pressure with consequent changes in left and right ventricular preload and afterload, as well as changes in pulmonary interstitial pressure. Arousals are linked to acute sympathetic activation, sleep disruption, and deprivation from beneficial effects of sleep.

Epidemiological surveys have indicated an increased risk of cardiovascular complications in patients with OSA. A survey of obese subjects in Sweden showed that high likelihood of OSA, as defined by self-reported loud snoring and observed breathing pauses, was associated with an increased risk of hypertension, severe dyspnea, hospital admissions with chest pain, and myocardial infarction after correction for body fat distribution and other potential confounding factors (47). Another study showed that the risk for hypertension, coronary, and peripheral vascular disease increased progressively and significantly between nonsnorers, snorers without SDB, and patients with SDB (48).

1. Changes in Heart Rate and Autonomic Imbalance

Cyclical changes in heart rate and systemic blood pressure accompany apneic events and are in part mediated by fluctuations in the activity of the autonomic nervous system. Increased vagal activity is largely responsible for the cyclical reductions in heart rate during apnea and is blocked by atropine but not by oxygen administration, although the latter does cause some blunting of the variability in heart rate (49). Cyclical elevations in systemic blood pressure result from recurrent peripheral vasoconstriction mediated by repetitive activation of the sympathetic nervous system, which coincides with arousals from sleep and termination of apnea at a time when stroke volume also increases (50).

Sympathetic activation appears to occur in many conditions associated with impaired alertness including OSA, narcolepsy, and idiopathic hypersomnolence as evidenced by increased urinary epinephrine plus norepinephrine levels (51). Whereas normal sleep is characterized by a fall in urinary epinephrine and norepinephrine levels, in patients with OSA only epinephrine levels fall during sleep. Short-term administration of nasal continuous positive airways pressure (nCPAP) allows nocturnal urinary epinephrine levels to fall (52).

Muscle nerve sympathetic activity (MSA) changes cyclically during apneic events. Mean MSA is higher even in awake patients with OSA than normal controls. Systolic blood pressure levels are positively correlated to MSA and it has been postulated that this may contribute to the development of systemic hypertension (53,54).

2. *Hypertension*

A well-documented association exists between OSA and systemic hypertension. Hypertension is present during wakefulness in approximately 50% of patients with OSA. Although age and obesity are important risk factors for diurnal hypertension in OSA, OSA almost certainly makes an independent contribution, especially in younger obese men (50). Cyclical elevations in blood pressure during sleep increase ventricular afterload and may thereby contribute to the development of left ventricular hypertrophy. Severe OSA is associated with daytime hypertension, failure of the BP to fall during sleep, and often a rise in BP as the night progresses (55). In some patients, hypertension related to OSA may prove refractory to standard medical therapy (56).

An exaggerated inspiratory fall in systolic blood pressure (BP) during obstructive apneas is followed by an increase in blood pressure during arousals. This may occur 30 or more times per hour. This pattern of exaggerated inspiratory fall followed by a rise in BP has been used in the diagnosis of OSA (56,57). The most important factor in the development of hypertension during sleep appears to be the presence of repetitive arousals, although hypoxemia may be a contributing factor (58). The average mean arterial pressure values are higher during obstructive apneas than during wakefulness in patients with OSA. This contributes to the disappearance of normal fall in blood pressure with sleep onset (59).

In many patients with OSA, even those without established hypertension, blood pressure may not fall and often rises during sleep. Autonomic cardiovascular reflexes including Valsalva ratio and baroreflex sensitivity index are suppressed. Moreover, plasma norepinephrine levels are often elevated (60).

It has, however, proved difficult to dissect out the effects of OSA from the effects of other potentially confounding factors, especially obesity. The high prevalence of OSA in patients with hypertension and of hypertension in patients with OSA is well documented but insufficient to establish a causal link between the two disorders. Several studies have been carried out in an attempt to establish or refute a causal link.

In one study, the effects of weight loss and nCPAP on systemic blood pressure were examined. Multivariate analysis revealed that weight loss but not nCPAP treatment contributed significantly to the course of hypertension (61). Another study indicated that both weight and minimum oxygen saturation during sleep in OSA were significantly correlated to diastolic blood pressure levels (62). In a large study of patients suspected to have OSA, patients with sleep apnea and nocturnal hypoxemia not only lost the normal morning dip in BP, but their BP was slightly higher in the morning than in the evening. The absolute morning BP was higher in patients with sleep apnea and hypoxemia than in nonapneic patients with normal oxygen levels, but this difference disappeared when the groups were matched for age and body mass index (63). These results stand in contradiction with the results of another well-conducted study in which ambulatory 24-hr blood pressure monitoring was performed in patients with OSAS. Stepwise multiple regression analysis revealed that diastolic, systolic, and mean BP values both during sleep and during wakefulness were significantly related to apnea/hypopnea index and age. Minimal arterial oxygen saturation also contributed to diastolic and mean BP values during sleep. Body mass index did not significantly contribute to any of the blood pressure values (64).

In a community-based study of BP during wakefulness and sleep in a healthy adult population, mean BP levels were found to be significantly higher in patients with sleep apnea than those without, both during wakefulness and during sleep. After controlling for factors including weight, age, and sex, sleep apnea was significantly associated with hypertension in a dose-response fashion, with odds ratios ranging from 2 to 5 for patients with apnea-hypopnea indices ranging from 5 to 25 (65).

Weight loss improves hypertension in patients with OSA. The degree to which weight loss directly contributes to the fall in BP in these patients, as opposed to the secondary effects of weight loss through improvement in sleep apnea, has been studied in patients participating in a hospital-based weight control program. Following weight loss, both BP and respiratory disturbance index (RDI) declined significantly. Soft palate width decreased and vital capacity increased. Regression analyses demonstrated that RDI rather than weight loss was the strongest independent predictor of fall in blood pressure, accounting for approximately 60% of the variability in this measurement (66).

Of substantial interest have been the results of studies of snorers with or without sleep apnea. Snoring in the absence of sleep apnea is probably not associated with hypertension. In one large study, age, male sex, apnea/hypopnea index, and body mass index but not snoring were significant determinants of early morning BP (67). In another, smaller study of male snorers with or without OSA, however, hypertension was not more common in the OSA group (68).

Perhaps the most compelling evidence in support of a causal link between OSA and hypertension comes from results of studies showing that long-term nCPAP administration significantly reduces BP in patients with OSA (131).

3. Pulmonary Hypertension and Cor Pulmonale; Polycythemia

As one might expect, there is a correlation between daytime hypercarbia and pulmonary hypertension as well as a negative correlation between daytime hypoxemia and FEV_1 and pulmonary hypertension. However, no correlation has been found between pulmonary hypertension and apnea or apnea-hypopnea indices or lowest saturation during sleep (69). Pulmonary hypertension is associated with COAD and severe obesity (with daytime hypoventilation) but not with OSA. It would appear that nocturnal desaturation in association with sleep apnea occurring in isolation is not enough to cause pulmonary hypertension. Sustained hypoxemia and/or hypercapnia over a 24-hr period is a necessary prerequisite for the development of cor pulmonale in patients with OSA, and diffuse airway obstruction (COAD) plays a major role in causing such hypoxemia (70). However, nocturnal desaturation may *contribute* toward the development of pulmonary hypertension and cor pulmonale (71).

Similarly, intermittent nocturnal hypoxemia associated with OSA is not associated with polycythemia but only with minor elevations in hematocrit values (72,73).

4. *Cardiac Arrhythmias*

Both nocturnal arrhythmias and nocturnal angina have been reported in patients with ischemic heart disease (IHD) and can be reversed with treatment of OSA with nasal CPAP (74).

Bradyarrhythmias (sinus arrest causing asystole, second- and third-degree atrioventricular block) as well as tachyarrhythmias (atrial flutter and fibrillation, ventricular tachycardia) have been reported and generally respond to treatment of the underlying sleep disorder (75,76). Bradyarrhythmias have been noted in patients with severe disease and poor compliance with treatment. This group of patients may also be at higher risk of death from myocardial infarction (77). Increased ventricular ectopy has been noted in patients with obstructive sleep apnea, especially when oxygen saturation falls below 60% (50). In one study, the incidence of serious ventricular arrhythmias during 24-hr electrocardiography in a group of patients with OSA was 26% (51). A controlled study, however, has not confirmed the observation that arrhythmias are more common in patients with OSA (78).

5. *Exacerbation of Ischemic Heart Disease*

Angina, and in particular nocturnal angina or angina out of proportion to the angiographic findings, has been reported in patients with OSA. Some evidence supports a link between myocardial ischemia and REM sleep in patients with OSA (50). In one small study, most patients presenting with nocturnal angina were found to have sleep apnea. In another study of patients with OSA without history of coronary heart disease, the vast majority of whom had negative exercise tests, almost one-third had ST-segment depression during sleep. Treatment with positive airway pressure appears to improve nocturnal angina and reduce nocturnal ST-segment depression (79–82).

An association between OSA and myocardial infarction has long been suspected. A retrospective study showed that, after adjustment for age, body mass index, hypertension, smoking, and cholesterol level, a high apnea index was associated with a greatly increased risk for myocardial infarction (83). Another study indicated that SDB was associated with poor LV function and coronary events (84).

6. *Left Ventricular Function*

It might be reasonable to assume that intermittent hypoxemia and increased ventricular afterload due to obstructed inspiration during sleep may cause chronic left ventricular (LV) hypertrophy or dysfunction. In a study of snorers with or without obstructive sleep apnea, echocardiographic measurements including end-diastolic LV and RV dimensions and wall thickness and indices of LV systolic and diastolic performance were within normal limits in OSA patients and not significantly different from those of nonapneic snorers (85). In another study of OSA in a pediatric population, RV function improved substantially after surgical relief of upper airway obstruction. In a minority of children, LV function also improved considerably (86). In another study, almost 30% of patients with OSA (but no patients with narcolepsy or idiopathic hypersomnolence) were found to have abnormal LV fractional shortening (51). In a controlled study of echocardiographic findings in patients with OSA, LV hypertrophy but not systolic dysfunction was found to occur significantly more frequently in the OSA syndrome group. The LV mass index was approximately 15% higher even among normotensive patients with OSA and no history of cardiac disease compared with the normotensive controls (87).

7. *Cerebral Perfusion and Stroke*

A number of small studies have focused on cerebral hemodynamics in patients with OSA and have produced conflicting results.

Two studies used transcranial Doppler to measure cerebral blood flow velocity during sleep in patients with OSA. In one study, cerebral blood flow velocity decreased during snoring but increased during apneas (88). In the other study, cerebral blood flow was found to be reduced in patients with SAS compared with controls, especially after controlling for their higher end-tidal $Paco_2$ (89).

Regardless of cerebral hemodynamics, the risk of stroke is increased both in habitual snorers and in patients with OSA (50,90). The extent to which hypertension associated with obstructive sleep apnea is responsible for the observed increase in risk remains uncertain.

8. *Mortality*

Several studies have shown that, untreated, OSA is associated with reduced survival (91,92). This mortality is predominantly cardiovascular and includes an increased risk of sudden death, often during sleep (50,90). Even habitual snorers appear to have a higher risk of sudden cardiovascular death during sleep, especially if they have other cardiovascular risk factors (50,93,94).

Severe disease, as measured by an apnea index greater than 20, is associated with a much worse prognosis, a difference that is particularly evident in relatively young patients in whom mortality from other causes is low. Treatment with either nCPAP or tracheostomy appears to be highly effective in preventing death or death from vascular causes in patients with OSA, but the results of treatment with uvulopalatopharyngoplasty or weight loss alone are disappointing (95,96).

Studies in elderly populations have yielded less impressive results. One study showed that RDI > 15 was not an independent predictor of mortality (97), whereas another showed that a RDI $\geqslant 5$ was strongly associated with mortality in women only and that patients with OSA had a tendency to die in their sleep (98).

F. Diagnosis

The initial evaluation of the patient with suspected OSAS is based on identification of disease markers by careful history taking and, to a lesser extent, physical examination. The physician may then choose to proceed with a relatively simple and inexpensive investigation such as overnight oximetry to confirm the presence of SDB before moving on to a definitive investigation, which is, without doubt, nocturnal polysomnography.

1. History

Although not every patient with OSA will be a middle-aged obese snorer with hypersomnolence, disease markers—which may be associations, risk factors, or disease effects—greatly contribute toward the diagnosis of OSAS.

As previously noted, it is well established that male sex and high body mass index are important risk factors for the development of OSA. The prevalence of the disease also increases with age. Snoring is common (70–95%) and, in some cases, it may even be the only symptom (99). Excessive daytime somnolence is highly correlated to the presence of OSAS (100). Sleep apnea, and obstructive apnea in particular, is extremely prevalent among hypersomnolent patients (101). It is, however, important to exclude other causes of hypersomnolence, especially sleep deprivation. Cognitive effects of sleep apnea such as memory loss have previously been described. A history of alcohol ingestion as well as a complete drug history should be obtained.

The interview should be extended to include questioning of the bed partner. This can yield invaluable information regarding important features of the disease of which the patient may be unaware, such as snoring, gasping, apnea, cyanosis, pathological somnolence, and changes in cognition.

Finally, it is important to note whether the patient has a history suggestive of other respiratory or cardiovascular disease that could be exacerbated by the presence of OSA.

2. Physical Examination

A thorough physical examination should be performed. The relationship between weight and height as well as neck size should be noted. The astute clinician will look for evidence of uncommon conditions associated with obstructive apnea such as Marfan's syndrome and acromegaly. General examination should include examination of thyroid status. One should also look for the presence of oropharyngeal crowding, micrognathism, or macroglossia.

A careful examination of the cardiovascular and respiratory systems should follow. It is particularly important to note the patient's BP, signs of right or left ventricular impairment, and evidence of associated obstructive or restrictive lung disease.

3. *Investigations*

Patients should have routine hematological and biochemical investigations. Thyroid function testing should also be part of the initial screen. A plain chest radiograph and electrocardiogram should be performed next. Lung function testing and assessment of daytime oxygen saturation and arterial blood gases should also be part of the initial evaluation. Transthoracic echocardiography provides useful information on baseline left and right ventricular function. Whenever possible, an assessment of pulmonary arterial pressure using Doppler echocardiography should be performed.

Overnight oximetry is a useful screening test for patients suspected of having OSA. It is highly sensitive and relatively inexpensive. It is simple to perform and totally noninvasive and can be performed reliably even in the community. It sensitivity has been reported to be as high as 98% although its specificity is closer to 50% and decreases in patients with coexistent obstructive lung disease (102,103).

A number of automated devices have been used in an attempt to improve the specificity of oximetry without resorting to polysomnography. These devices may include sound recorders for assessment of snoring, thermistors for detection of airflow, transducers for measurement of chest and abdominal wall movement with breathing, and accelerometers or other sensors for detecting limb movement. Several reports have confirmed that both sensitivity and specificity can be quite high, but these monitors tend to be expensive and generally inferior to full polysomnography.

Polysomnography remains the gold standard for the diagnosis of OSA, even though it requires expensive equipment in a dedicated sleep laboratory as well as highly trained personnel. During polysomnography, continuous and simultaneous recordings are made of: electrocardiogram (EKG); at least three electroencephalogram (EEG) channels; chin and leg electromyogram (EMG); electro-oculogram (EOG); oxygen saturation using finger or ear oximetry; airflow using a nasal thermistor; chest and abdominal wall movement using inductance bands or acceleration using piezo-electric crystals; and snoring using a microphone and sound recorder. The patient is ideally supervised throughout the study, and although unsupervised studies can be performed, the technician's observations often prove very useful. The recording is digitized and recorded on a computer before analysis. Using polysomnography, apneas and hypopneas can be recognized with relative ease and classified into obstructive, central, and mixed events. Changes in sleep stage and arousals are noted on the basis of EEG, EOG, and EMG features and are related to respiratory events. The severity of sleep apnea is indicated by the apnea and/or hypopnea index and indices of oxygen desaturation.

G. Treatment

1. *Weight Loss*

One of the most important aspects of treatment of OSA is patient education regarding the need for weight loss and provision of an appropriate weight reduction program. Many patients are obese and often hypertensive, and weight loss can improve sleep apnea as well as ameliorate hypertension, either directly or indirectly. However, weight reduction is often difficult in these patients, and in patients with severe disease in whom rapid improvement of clinical state is important, it may occur too slowly. Weight loss reduces apneas but it may not be curative in many patients (104). Furthermore, weight loss alone does not appear to reduce the mortality associated with OSA (96). Two studies have reported that weight reduction surgery, in addition to improving body mass index (BMI), also reduced apnea-hypopnea index. However, this effect was frequently lost within 7 years of surgery, an effect that was not totally explained by an associated increase in BMI (105,106). A combination of weight reduction, advice regarding the recommended sleep posture (patients are advised to sleep on their side), and use of a nasal decongestant in snorers has been reported to lead to minor improvement in apnea frequency (107).

2. *Avoidance of Alcohol and Sedatives*

Alcohol and sedatives are recognized as factors that can potentially exacerbate OSA. Avoidance of alcohol is therefore recommended for most patients. In rats, alcohol ingestion causes mismatching of hypoglossal and phrenic nerve activities, an effect reduced by pretreatment with medroxyprogesterone acetate (43). In patients with OSA whose disease is exacerbated by alcohol ingestion, medroxyprogesterone acetate appears to improve oxygenation during obstructive events but does not improve their number or duration (44).

3. *Oral Appliances*

A number of oral appliances that are worn at night have been designed in an attempt to improve the patency of the upper airway during sleep. Many of these appliances act either as semirigid splints that maintain oral airway patency or as mandibular advancement prostheses. Oral appliances are particularly useful in patients who have relatively mild disease or are unable to tolerate nasal CPAP. Temporomandibular joint discomfort is a common side effect (108,109).

4. *Oxygen Administration*

Administration of low-flow oxygen via nasal cannulae improves oxygen saturation but it prolongs apneas and therefore worsens hypercapnia during the apneic period (110). At least in the short term, oxygen administration does not have an effect on BP overall, or on BP variability during sleep (111). Moreover, pulmonary arterial pressure, which is usually maximal at the end of the apneic period, does not appear to be reduced by oxygen administration, perhaps reflecting concomitant hypercapnia (112). In patients with mixed apneas, oxygen reduces the frequency of central and mixed events but increases the frequency of obstructive events (113). Oxygen therapy can nonetheless be a valuable alternative to nasal CPAP in patients with mild or asymptomatic disease (114). Transtracheal administration of low-flow oxygen, which delivers oxygen below the level of upper airway obstruction, may be of benefit in patients in whom nasal oxygen is ineffective (115,116).

5. *Drugs*

The nonsedative tricyclic antidepressant protriptyline is one of the best-known pharmacological treatments for obstructive sleep apnea. However, its effects have only been studied in a handful of small studies. In two of the best studies, protriptyline was found to be beneficial but by no means curative. Protriptyline reduces the proportion of REM sleep, and as some of the most significant apneic events occur in this stage of sleep, it can improve oxygen desaturation and daytime hypersomnolence. Moreover, it may reduce actual apneic events during episodes of SDB. However, it is by no means effective in all patients and can only be used in patients with relatively mild disease that is not life-threatening. It can be associated with significant anticholinergic side effects including dryness of the mouth, constipation, hesitancy of micturition, and erectile dysfunction (117,118).

Methylxanthines have long been known to exert stimulant effects on both respiration and upper airway tone. In animal models, the former occur with relatively high doses of the drug whereas the latter may occur even with small doses (119). In a large study of patients with SAS, theophylline was found to provide long-term symptomatic improvement and to reduce the number of apneas. It was, however, most beneficial in patients with relatively mild disease (120). Theophylline can disrupt sleep architecture as well as sleep quality, at least in some patients (121,122). As it is not curative and its effects on mortality in obstructive apnea remain unknown at present, it is reasonable to consider this form of treatment only in patients with relatively mild disease.

6. *ENT Procedures*

Uvulopalatopharyngoplasty (UPPP) consists of surgical removal of the uvula, part of the muscular portion of the soft palate and redundant palatal mucosa, and the tonsils. It has been used for the treatment of OSA for 15 years. About half of the patients who undergo UPPP have a 50% or greater reduction in apnea index. Many studies have failed to identify preoperatively those patients most likely to benefit from UPPP, but dynamic nasopharyngoscopy may be helpful (123,124). Patients often report subjective improvement, but this may occur irrespective of postoperative polysomnographic findings. As retrospective follow-up data suggest that UPPP may not modify the increased mortality associated with moderate or severe obstructive apnea, and since recurrence of obstructive apnea is not uncommon, it is very important to ensure continuing and objective postoperative improvement in sleep apnea with follow-up polysomnography (125,126).

Nasal surgery, with a view to reduction of nasal resistance, may involve septoplasty, turbinectomy, and/or polypectomy. It may be of benefit in selected patients with OSA with normal cephalometry (36).

Tracheostomy, which was once standard treatment for OSA, is now used only in patients with disease refractory to other forms of treatment because of its invasive nature. Tracheostomy can normalize the apnea index and lead to symptomatic improvement and is known to reduce vascular morbidity and overall mortality in patients with OSA (95,96,127).

7. Continuous Positive Airway Pressure

Noninvasive CPAP is the mainstay of treatment for OSA. The application of positive pressure throughout the respiratory cycle creates a pneumatic splint that maintains upper airway patency. In general, nasal CPAP is more comfortable and better tolerated than the application of CPAP via face mask. A number of interfaces have been designed to deliver nasal CPAP (128). The interfaces most commonly used are nasal masks and nasal pillows. The level of CPAP required to relieve upper airway obstruction during sleep varies considerably. In general, high levels of CPAP are required in obese patients, especially those with a large neck circumference as well as patients with a collapsible pharynx or severe discasc (129).

In general, treatment with nasal CPAP is highly efficacious (169). The acute effects of CPAP in patients with OSA include a reduction in BP variability during sleep but not an overall reduction in BP (111). Nocturnal urinary epinenephrine levels fall (52). The apnea-hypopnea index falls and the number of oxygen desaturation events is reduced considerably.

With long-term administration of CPAP, symptomatic improvement occurs in the majority of patients. Sleep becomes more refreshing and patients often become free from morning headaches and daytime hypersomnolence. Patients are able to become more active, and quality of life improves. The administration of CPAP also appears to lead to an improvement in the underlying disease process. When patients with OSA are studied overnight off treatment after several months of regular nocturnal CPAP administration, sleep apnea is found to be substantially improved, even without an associated fall in BMI. Moreover, daytime Pao_2

increases and Pa_{CO_2} falls (130). Not only is nocturnal blood pressure variability reduced with long-term nCPAP, but diurnal systolic and diastolic blood pressure levels also fall significantly (131). CPAP treatment also reduces biochemical markers of sympathetic activation. Daytime plasma norepinephrine levels fall as do day- and nighttime vanillyl mandelic acid and metanephrine levels (132). LV function improves significantly after several months of treatment. The degree of improvement in LV systolic function is correlated with baseline function, with greater improvement noted in patients who have worse function before the initiation of treatment (133,134). Perhaps most significantly, nCPAP has been shown to improve the long-term prognosis in patients with OSA (95,96).

Even though nCPAP is highly efficacious in the treatment of OSA, several problems may arise. Acute LV failure as well as dysrhythmias occurring shortly after initiation of treatment have been reported (135,139). Moreover, not all patients find it reasonably comfortable or acceptable. With increasing CPAP levels, breathing often becomes less comfortable. Experience in finding the best possible interface is vital if delivery of CPAP is to be optimal, local pressure effects are to be avoided, and the patient is to find the treatment acceptable in the long term.

Compliance with treatment is a significant problem since around 25% of patients may not tolerate nCPAP (108). Self-reported compliance may not be a reliable indicator (136). Time counters are available on some machines and can be used to assess compliance (137). Compliance appears to be positively correlated with apnea severity, nocturnal hypoxemia, and daytime hypersomnolence before the initiation of treatment (137–139).

8. *Noninvasive Positive Pressure Ventilation (NIPPV)*

The administration of positive pressure ventilation (PPV) with positive end-expiratory pressure (PEEP) may become necessary in some patients with OSA and has been shown to be highly efficacious (140). These patients generally fall within two groups. The first group consists of patients, usually very obese, in whom the level of CPAP required to maintain upper airway patency is so high that breathing becomes difficult and uncomfortable. The second group consists of patients with OSA who have nocturnal hypoventilation and hypercapnia that are unresponsive to nCPAP. Many of these patients also have daytime hypercapnia and/or obstructive lung disease. Bilevel positive airway pressure (BiPAP) is widely used. It provides two different levels of positive pressure, one for inspiration and one for expiration, which can be easily adjusted according to patient needs (141).

9. *Other Devices*

A plastic nasal dilator is available for the treatment of OSA. Use of the nasal dilator is associated with a reduction in the frequency and severity of obstructed breathing and apnea index. Nocturnal oxygen saturation and snoring may improve substantially, but symptomatic improvement may not occur (142).

III. CENTRAL SLEEP APNEA

Unlike obstructive apnea, in which there is marked respiratory effort against a closed upper airway, patients with central sleep apnea (CSA) have repetitive cessation of airflow in the absence of respiratory effort.

A. Etiology and Pathogenesis

CSA is a heterogeneous disease entity. In general, patients can be classified into two broad groups based on awake levels of $Paco_2$ and their ventilatory response to carbon dioxide. The first group consists of patients who tend to hypoventilate and have high levels of $Paco_2$ in the absence of intrinsic lung disease and a blunted ventilatory response to carbon dioxide. They tend to have recurrent episodes of respiratory failure. Patients within this group often have disease with a clinical picture that merges into the spectrum of primary alveolar hypoventilation. Many of them are obese and have features of the obesity-hypoventilation syndrome. At the other end of the spectrum of CSA is the second group of patients that consists of subjects who either ventilate normally or hyperventilate and have normal or low awake $Paco_2$ levels and a normal or exaggerated ventilatory response to carbon dioxide. These patients often present with clinical features typical of sleep apnea. Many of them have Cheyne-Stokes respiration (CSR). Even though the clinical and physiological differences between the two groups are marked, the two groups may have similar nocturnal apneic events and sleep architecture (143,144).

CSR is characterized by alternating periods of hyperventilation and hypoventilation or apnea. It was first described by Hippocrates, but the classic descriptions by John Cheyne and William Stokes followed several centuries later (145). The etiology and pathogenesis of CSR have been argued since the description by John Cheyne in the 19th century of a patient with both enlarged cerebral ventricles and heart disease who had periodic breathing. Autopsy studies have shown that most subjects with CSR have structural abnormalities of the brain. The disease is, however, seen frequently in patients with cardiovascular disease and, in particular, heart failure. It is therefore hardly surprising that theories suggesting both neurological and cardiovascular mechanisms in the pathogenesis of the disease have been postulated. Proposed neurological abnormalities include cyclical medullary depression or medullary hyperexcitability alternating with periods of depression. Described cardiovascular abnormalities are centered around a circulatory delay related to heart failure (146).

It is now known that both neurological and cardiovascular factors contribute to the pathogenesis of the disease and that if the relationship between these cardiac and neurological components is altered, the stability of the respiratory control system is lost. Such disturbance in the control system may arise by prolongation of the circulation time, or by the system becoming more dependent on the arterial partial pressure of oxygen rather than carbon dioxide (147).

Patients with heart failure and CSR often hyperventilate. They have lower $Paco_2$ both when awake and during sleep than controls with heart failure but no CSR-CSA (148,149). Circulatory delay is a well-known feature of heart failure and animal models suggest that circulatory delay can indeed lead to periodic breathing. Whether the changes observed in animal models of CSR are also valid in humans with heart failure remains controversial as the magnitude of circulatory delay necessary to produce CSR in animals is rarely if ever seen in humans. Nonetheless, a strong correlation has been noted between circulation time and CSR-CSA cycle length in humans (148,150).

Arousal and apnea termination are associated with the hyperventilation stage of CSR. Termination of apnea in patients with periodic breathing appears to be related largely to chemoreceptor input, which is in contrast to the proposed mechanism for apnea termination in OSA in which mechanoreceptor input from the lungs is thought to be of primary importance. Arousals disrupt sleep and are associated with lack of slow-wave sleep and daytime hypersomnolence (151).

B. Prevalence

The exact prevalence of CSA remains unclear. It does, however, appear to be particularly high in patients with neurological disease, including structural brain stem and cerebrovascular disease, as well as in patients with cardiac dysfunction.

Several studies have shown that significant LV impairment is associated with SDB, CSA, and CSR. SDB has been reported to occur in up to 50% of patients with stable congestive heart failure, and LV systolic dysfunction may be an independent risk factor for sleep apnea in these patients (152). One small study showed that approximately 40% of patients on a heart transplant waiting list had periodic breathing and CSA (153). In another study, patients with LV impairment due to ischemic heart disease were found to have cyclical oxygen desaturations with a frequency 10 times higher than that observed in healthy controls (154). Similar results suggesting a very high prevalence of Cheyne-Stokes breathing and central apnea have been reported in patients with dilated cardiomyopathy (155).

C. Morbidity and Mortality

In one relatively small study designed to determine the impact of CSA with or without CSR on morbidity and mortality, CSR was found in 60% of patients with CSA. Patients with severe CSR had more central apneas, more, but shorter, desaturations, more awakenings, and spent more time awake during the night. Heart failure was associated with CSR. Even though patients with severe CSR were at almost twice the risk of dying compared with those with no apnea, CSR was not found to be an independent risk factor for increased mortality (156). Based on the limited information available, it appears that, even though CSA is associated with significant morbidity, the prognosis in patients with CSA is largely dependent on the underlying disease and not on the presence of sleep apnea per se.

D. Diagnosis

A history of cardiac dysfunction, cerebrovascular disease, or structural brain stem disease should alert the clinician to the possibility of CSA. Obese patients may have central apnea as part of the obesity-hypoventilation syndrome. Daytime hypercapnia in the absence of structural lung disease may be an indicator of worsening hypoventilation during sleep. Most patients with CSA, however, have normal or exaggerated ventilation during wakefulness. Most patients with cardiac failure fall within this group. They may have symptoms of nocturnal hypoventilation such as daytime hypersomnolence, early morning headache, and unrefreshing sleep, despite an adequate length of sleep. The bed partner may note apneic episodes in the absence of respiratory effort.

Screening tests such as overnight oximetry and some more sophisticated techniques are often useful, but their sensitivity and specificity in patients with CSA have not been established. Ultimately, the diagnosis relies on demonstration of repetitive apnea or hypopnea in the absence of respiratory effort during polysomnography.

E. Treatment

In patients with CSA, treatment of the underlying cause is of paramount importance, whenever possible. In patients with heart failure, ACE inhibition with captopril increases the proportion of sleep spent in slow-wave and REM sleep. Apneic episodes, arousals, and episodes of desaturation are also reduced (157). CSR in patients with advanced heart failure has been cured by heart transplantation (158,159).

1. Drugs

Even though respiratory stimulants such as methylxanthines would be a logical treatment for CSA, large controlled studies have not been performed. In two small studies, which included patients with heart failure, administration of theophylline resulted in a reduction in Cheyne-Stokes breathing and an improvement in oxygen desaturation events and sleep disruption (160,161). Aminophylline has also been reported to improve CSA due to structural brain stem disease (162). The tricyclic antidepressant imipramine may also reduce the number of apneas and improve both nocturnal and diurnal symptoms in patients with CSA (163).

Oxygen administration appears to be beneficial for patients with heart failure and CSA. Not only may oxygen relieve hypoxemia, but it may also reduce apneic episodes and arousals and improve sleep duration and quality (157,164). Oxygen may also be beneficial in patients with primary alveolar hypoventilation and CSA, again not only by relieving hypoxia and its cardiovascular complications but also by reducing the number and duration of apneic events (165,166).

2. *Noninvasive CPAP*

Use of nasal CPAP is a relatively well-described form of treatment for CSA. Its mechanism of action remains unclear, but CPAP administration may raise the level of $Paco_2$ above the apneic threshold in patients with CSA who have CSR (167).

The acute hemodynamic effects of nCPAP administration in patients with heart failure remain highly controversial, with a number of small studies reporting conflicting results. Some studies have reported adverse hemodynamic effects including a fall in cardiac index and a rise in systemic vascular resistance (168), and acute LV failure occurring shortly after initiation of treatment has been described (169). Conversely, other studies have reported that nCPAP either does not change or may improve the cardiac index in patients with LV dysfunction and elevated pulmonary arterial wedge pressure (170–172).

Regardless of these findings, long-term administration of nCPAP to patients with advanced cardiac failure and CSR appears to reduce the number of apneas and to improve symptoms of sleep apnea and oxygen saturation. LV function, daytime breathlessness, fatigue, and inspiratory muscle strength may also improve (167,173–177). Moreover, nCPAP is known to improve the imbalance between sympathetic and parasympathetic tone in heart failure as evidenced by a reduction in both nocturnal and daytime catecholamine levels and an increase in heart rate variability (178,179).

Nasal CPAP also appears to be effective in reducing hypoventilation and hypoxemia in patients with primary and central alveolar hypoventilation (180).

3. *Noninvasive and Invasive Positive Pressure Ventilation*

Although positive pressure ventilation, including nasal BiPAP, would seem a logical treatment for CSA and although it has been used fairly extensively, little evidence regarding its use is available from controlled studies. It has, nonetheless, been shown to be effective in patients with CSA, including primary alveolar hypoventilation, in whom apneas are reduced and hypercapnia and hypoxemia are corrected. It may be particularly useful in patients unresponsive to treatment with nCPAP or those who hypoventilate (141,181).

IV. SLEEP IN PATIENTS WITH CHRONIC OBSTRUCTIVE AIRWAYS DISEASE (COAD)

COAD is associated with specific patterns of SDB. Marked changes in oxygen saturation during sleep have been noted, especially during REM sleep (182).

Patients with obstructive lung disease rely on muscles other than the diaphragm—intercostal and accessory muscles—for their breathing, the diaphragm being in a position of mechanical disadvantage due to splinting related to hyperinflation. Paralysis of all respiratory muscles except for the diaphragm during REM sleep can thus bring about a substantial fall in ventilation, with a rise in $Paco_2$ and fall in Pao_2, although frank apneas are uncommon (183,184). Ventilation-perfusion mismatching may worsen. Exacerbation of hypoxemia and hypercapnia during sleep in patients with COAD may contribute to the development of pulmonary hypertension. Cardiac arrhythmias and ST-segment changes have also been described (185–187).

Ten to twenty percent of patients with sleep apnea syndrome have coexistent COAD. This "overlap" syndrome tends to occur mostly in male patients with SAS, and these patients tend to have lower Pao_2 and lower $Paco_2$ levels and a higher incidence of pulmonary hypertension. Episodes of nocturnal hypoxemia may be more marked, not only because of a lower baseline Pao_2, but also because of a steeper slope of desaturation due to reduced stores of oxygen in alveoli and blood as a result of obstructive lung disease. The reversible component of obstructive airways disease should be treated using conventional medical therapy. Elimination of the sleep apnea component by nCPAP or tracheostomy is of paramount importance as it can reduce nocturnal and even daytime hypoxemia and improve pulmonary hypertension and symptomatology. Patients left with REM-related desaturation can simply be treated with supplemental oxygen. Oxygen therapy alone should generally be avoided in patients with the overlap syndrome: oxygen saturation is improved, but apneas are prolonged, leading to a further rise in $Paco_2$ and a fall in pH (187–191).

Low-flow oxygen administration in patients with pure COAD appears much safer, even though the number of episodes of sleep-disordered breathing may remain unchanged or increase. The number and amplitude of oxygen desaturation events and time spent in desaturation are improved. Sleep quality improves and the ratio of REM sleep to total sleep increases (192–194). For patients with disease unresponsive to treatment with low-flow oxygen, nocturnal noninvasive positive pressure ventilation may be used.

Both triazolam and zolpidem can improve total sleep time and sleep efficiency in patients with mild to moderate COAD without a detrimental effect on oxygen saturation or apnea-hypopnea index (195). Conversely, ethanol ingestion in these patients increases the number and duration of apneic events, as well as ventricular ectopy, and reduces total sleep time (196).

V. SLEEP APNEA AFTER ACUTE MYOCARDIAL INFARCTION

Not only does sleep apnea appear to be an independent predictor of acute myocardial infarction (MI) (83), but nocturnal hypoxemia is very common in the first week after acute MI. Both episodic and sustained hypoxemia during this period, when the myocardium is particularly vulnerable to additional insults, are associated with worsening myocardial ischemia as evidenced by ST-segment changes and rhythm disturbances including atrioventricular block and supraventricular and ventricular arrhythmias. Based on the results of small studies, episodic desaturation occurs in 25–100% of patients during the first week after acute MI and may be severe (197–200).

Heart-rate-variability analyses suggest that MI leads to the loss of the physiological activation of the vagus during sleep. This results in relative sympathetic dominance even during sleep. Sleep apnea is also associated with sympathetic activation, large swings in blood pressure, hypoxemia, and hypercapnia. Although not proven, sympathetic overactivity in this setting and in combination with hypoxemia and myocardial irritability in the setting of AMI may well contribute toward the occurrence of nocturnal sudden death (201). It therefore seems prudent to recommend the routine administration of oxygen during sleep in the first few days after acute MI, even in the absence of daytime hypoxemia, preexisting lung disease, or pulmonary edema.

REFERENCES

1. Bresnitz EA, Goldberg R, Kosinski RM. Epidemiology of obstructive sleep apnea. Epidemiol Rev 1994; 16(2):210–227 (review).
2. Young T, Palta M, Dempsey J, Skatrud J, Weber S, Badr Safwan. The occurrence of sleep-disordered breathing among middle-aged adults. N Engl J Med 1993; 328(17): 1230–1235.
3. Olson LG, King MT, Hensley MJ, Saunders NA. A community study of snoring and sleep-disordered breathing. Prevalence. Am J Respir Crit Care Med 1995; 152(2): 711–716.
4. Engel S, Karoff M, Raschke F, Fischer J. Prevalence of sleep apnea syndrome with primary arterial hypertension in a cardiologic rehabilitation clinic. Pneumonologie 1995; 49(Suppl 1):145–147.
5. Fletcher EC. The relationship between systemic hypertension and obstructive sleep apnea: facts and theory. Am J Med 1995; 98(2):118–128 (review).
6. Wetter DW, Young TB, Bidwell TR, Badr MS, Palta M. Smoking as a risk factor for sleep-disordered breathing. Arch Intern Med 1994; 154(19):2219–2224.
7. Gislason T, Benediktsdottir B, Bjornsson JK, Kjartansson G, Kjeld M, Kristbjarnarson H. Snoring, hypertension, and sleep apnea syndrome. An epidemiologic survey of middle-aged women. Chest 1993; 103(4):1147–1151.
8. Fleury B. Sleep apnea syndrome in the elderly. Sleep 1992; 15(6 Suppl):S39–41 (review).
9. Knight H, Millman RP, Gur RC, Saykin AJ, Doherty JU, Pack AI. Clinical significance of sleep apnea in the elderly. Am Rev Respir Dis 1987; 136(4):845–850.

10. Ancoli-Israel S, Kripke DF, Mason W. Characteristics of obstructive and central sleep apnea in the elderly: an interim report. Biolog Psychiatry 1987; 22(6): 741–750.
11. Ancoli-Israel S, Kripke DF, Klauber MR, Mason WJ, Fell R, Kaplan O. Sleep-disordered breathing in community-dwelling elderly. Sleep 1991; 14(6):486–495.
12. Ancoli-Israeli S, Kripke DF. Prevalent sleep problems in the elderly. Biofeedback Self Regul 1991; 16(4):349–359.
13. Bliwise DL, Yesavage JA, Tinklenberg JR, Dement WC. Sleep apnea in Alzheimer's disease. Neurobiol Aging 1989; 10(4):343–346.
14. Poceta JS, Timms RM, Jeong DU, Ho SL, Erman MK, Mitler MM. Maintenance of wakefulness test in obstructive sleep apnea syndrome. Chest 1992; 101(4):893–897.
15. Horne JA, Reyner LA. Sleep related vehicle accidents. Br Med J 1995; 310 (6979): 565–567.
16. Jennum PJ, Sjol A. Cognitive symptoms with snoring and sleep apnea. An epidemiologic study of 1,504 women and men aged 30–60 years. Ugeskr Laeger 1995; 157(45):6252–6256.
17. Hirshkowitz M, Karacan I, Arcasoy MO, Acik G, Narter EM, Williams RL. Prevalence of sleep apnea in men with erectile dysfunction. Urology 1990; 36(3): 232–234.
18. Honsberg AE, Dodge RR, Cline MG, Quan SF. Incidence and remission of habitual snoring over a 5- to 6-year period. Chest 1995; 108(3):604–609.
19. Odens ML, Fox CH. Adult sleep apnea syndromes. Am Fam Phys 1995; 52(3):859–866, 871–872 (review).
20. Cirignotta F, D'Allessandro R, Partinen M, Zucconi M, Cristina E, Gerardi R, Cacciatore FM, Lugaresi E. Prevalence of every night snoring and obstructive sleep apneas among 30–69-year-old men in Bologna, Italy. Acta Neurol Scand 1989; 79(5):366–372.
21. Andreas S, Schulz R, Haro W, Werner GS, Kreuzer H. Sleep-related breathing disorders in patients with coronary heart disease. Dtsche Med Wochenschr 1995; 120(45):1533–1537.
22. Kales A, Bixler EO, Cadieux RJ, Schneck DW, Shaw LC 3d, Locke TW, Vela-Bueno A, Soldatos CR. Sleep apnoea in a hypertensive population. Lancet 1984; 2(8410): 1005–1008.
23. Vela-Bueno A, Fernandez Pinilla C, Espinar Sierra J, Recarte C, Dobladez B, Fernandez Cruz A, Martell Claros N, Luque Otero M. Sleep apnea in arterial hypertension. Med Clin 1993; 100(8):288–291.
24. Klink ME, Sethi GK, Copeland JG, Quan SF. Obstructive sleep apnea in heart transplant patients. A report of five cases. Chest 1993; 104(4):1090–1092.
25. Stoohs RA, Bingham LA, Itoi A, Guilleminault C, Dement WC. Sleep and sleep-disordered breathing in commercial long-haul truck drivers. Chest 1995; 107(5): 1275–1282.
26. Hoffstein V, Mateika SA. Differences in abdominal and neck circumferences in patients with and without obstructive sleep apnea. Eur Respir J 1992; 5(4):377–381.
27. Lin CC, Tsan KW, Chen PJ. The relationship between sleep apnea syndrome and hypothyroidism. Chest 1992; 102(6):1663–1667.

28. Cistulli PA, Sullivan CE. Sleep-disordered breathing in Marfan's syndrome. Am Rev Respir Dis 1993; 147(3):645–648.
29. Deegan PC, McNicholas WT. Pathophysiology of obstructive sleep apnoea. Eur Respir J 1995; 8(7):1161–1178 (review).
30. Leung AK, Robson WL. The ABZzzzs of snoring. Postgrad Med 1992; 92(3):217–222 (review).
31. Jennum P, Hein HO, Suadicani P, Sorensen H, Gyntelberg F. Snoring, family history, and genetic markers in man. The Copenhagen Male Study. Chest 1995; 107(5): 1289–1293.
32. Pillar G, Lavie P. Assessment of the role of inheritance in sleep apnea syndrome. Am J Respir Crit Care Med 1995; 151(3 Pt 1):688–691.
33. Redline S, Tishler PV, Tosteson TD, Williamson J, Kump K, Browner I, Ferrette V, Krejci P. The familial aggregation of obstructive sleep apnea. Am J Respir Crit Care Med 1995; 151(3 Pt 1):682–687.
34. Miljeteig H, Hoffstein V, Cole P. The effect of unilateral and bilateral nasal obstruction on snoring and sleep apnea. Laryngoscope 1992; 102(10):1150–1152.
35. Atkins M, Taskar V, Clayton N, Stone P, Woodcock A. Nasal resistance in obstructive sleep apnea. Chest 1994; 150(4):1133–1135.
36. Series F, St. Pierre S, Carrier G. Effects of surgical correction of nasal obstruction in the treatment of obstructive sleep apnea. Am Rev Respir Dis 1992; 146(5 Pt 1): 1261–1265.
37. Okabe S, Hida W, Kikuchi Y, Taguchi O, Takishima T, Shirato K. Upper airway muscle activity during REM and non-REM sleep of patients with obstructive sleep apnea. Chest 1994; 106(3):767–773.
38. Gold AR, Schwartz AR, Wise RA, Smith PL. Pulmonary function and respiratory chemosensitivity in moderately obese patients with sleep apnea. Chest 1993; 103(5): 1325–1329.
39. Kimoff RJ, Cheong TH, Olha AE, Charbonneau M, Levy RD, Cosio MG, Gottfried SB. Mechanisms of apnea termination in obstructive sleep apnea. Role of chemoreceptor and mechanoreceptor stimuli. Am J Respir Crit Care Med 1994; 149(3 Pt 1):707–714.
40. Charbonneau M, Marin JM, Olha A, Kimoff RJ, Levy RD, Cosio MG. Changes in obstructive sleep apnea characteristics through the night. Chest 1994; 106(6):1695–1701.
41. Colt HG, Haas H, Rich GB. Hypoxemia vs sleep fragmentation as cause of excessive daytime sleepiness in obstructive sleep apnea. Chest 1991; 100(6):1542–1548.
42. Svanborg E, Larsson H. Development of nocturnal respiratory disturbance in untreated patients with obstructive sleep apnea syndrome. Chest 1993; 104(2): 340–343.
43. St. John WM, Bartlett D Jr., Knuth KV, Knuth SL, Daubenspeck JA. Differential depression of hypoglossal nerve activity by alcohol. Protection by pretreatment with medroxyprogesterone acetate. Am Rev Respir Dis 1986; 133(1):46–48.
44. Collop NA. Medroxyprogesterone acetate and ethanol-induced exacerbation of obstructive sleep apnea. Chest 1994; 106(3):792–799.
45. Rains VS, Ditzler TF, Newsome RD, Lee-Gushi S, Morgan EJ. Alcohol and sleep apnea. Hawaii Med J 1991; 50(8):282–287.

46. Hoijer U, Hedner J, Ejnell H, Grunstein R, Odelberg E, Elam M. Nitrazepam in patients with sleep apnoea: a double-blind placebo-controlled study. Eur Respir J 1994; 7(11):2011–2015.
47. Grunstein RR, Stenlof K, Hedner J, Sjostrom L. Impact of obstructive sleep apnea and sleepiness on metabolic and cardiovascular risk factors in the Swedish Obese Subjects (SOS) Study. Int J Obes Related Metab Disord 1995; 19(6):410–418.
48. Olson LG, King MT, Hensley MJ, Saunders NA. A community study of snoring and sleep-disordered breathing. Health outcomes. Am J Respir Crit Care Med 1995; 152(2):717–720.
49. Guilleminault C, Connolly S, Winkle R, Melvin K, Tilkian A. Cyclical variation of the heart rate in sleep apnea syndrome. Mechanisms, and usefulness of 24 h electrocardiography as a screening technique. Lancet 1984; 1(8360):126–131.
50. Shepard JW Jr. Hypertension, cardiac arrhythmias, myocardial infarction, and stroke in relation to obstructive sleep apnea. Clin Chest Med 1992; 13(3):437–458 (review).
51. Boudoulas H, Schmidt HS, Clark RW, Geleris P, Schaal SF, Lewis RP. Anthropometric characteristics, cardiac abnormalities and adrenergic activity in patients with primary disorders of sleep. J Med 1983; 14(3):223–238.
52. Marrone O, Riccobono L, Salvaggio A, Mirabella A, Bonanno A, Bonsignore MR. Catecholamines and blood pressure in obstructive sleep apnea syndrome. Chest 1993; 103(3):722–727.
53. Carlson JT, Hedner J, Elam M, Ejnell H, Sellgren J, Wallin BG. Augmented resting sympathetic activity in awake patients with obstructive sleep apnea. Chest 1993; 103(6):1763–1768.
54. Hedner J, Ejnell H, Sellgren J, Hedner T, Wallin G. Is high and fluctuating muscle nerve sympathetic activity in the sleep apnoea syndrome of pathogenetic importance for the development of hypertension? J Hypertension 1988 (Suppl); 6(4): S529–531.
55. Noda A, Okada T, Hayashi H, Yasuma F, Yokota M. 24-hour ambulatory blood pressure variability in obstructive sleep apnea syndrome. Chest 1993; 103(5):1343–1347.
56. Isaksson H, Svanborg E. Obstructive sleep apnea syndrome in male hypertensives, refractory to drug therapy. Nocturnal automatic blood pressure measurements—an aid to diagnosis? Clin Exp Hypertension (A) 1991; 13(6–7):1195–1212.
57. Davies RJ, Vardi-Visy K, Clarke M, Stradling JR. Identification of sleep disruption and sleep disordered breathing from the systolic blood pressure profile. Thorax 1993; 48(12):1242–1247.
58. Okabe S, Hida W, Kikuchi Y, Taguchi O, Ogawa H, Mizusawa A, Miki H, Shirato K. Role of hypoxia on increased blood pressure in patients with obstructive sleep apnoea. Thorax 1995; 50(1):28–34.
59. Davies RJ, Crosby J, Vardi-Visy K, Clarke M, Stradling JR. Non-invasive beat to beat arterial blood pressure during non-REM sleep in obstructive sleep apnoea and snoring. Thorax 1994; 49(4):335–339.
60. Sforza E, Parchi P, Contin M, Cortelli P, Lugaresi E. Do autonomic cardiovascular reflexes predict the nocturnal rise in blood pressure in obstructive sleep apnea syndrome? Blood Pressure 1994; 3(5):295–302.

61. Rauscher H, Formanek D, Popp W, Zwick H. Nasal CPAP and weight loss in hypertensive patients with obstructive sleep apnoea. Thorax 1993; 48(5):529–533.
62. Mendelson WB. Sleepiness and hypertension in obstructive sleep apnea. Chest 1992; 101(4):903–909.
63. Hoffstein V, Mateika J. Evening-to-morning blood pressure variations in snoring patients with and without obstructive sleep apnea. Chest 1992; 101(2):379–384.
64. Lavie P, Yoffe N, Berger I, Peled R. The relationship between the severity of sleep apnea syndrome and 24-h blood pressure values in patients wtih obstructive sleep apnea. Chest 1993; 103(3):717–721.
65. Hia KM, Young TB, Bidwell T, Palta M, Skatrud JB, Dempsey J. Sleep apnea and hypertension. A population-based study. Ann Intern Med 1994; 120(5):382–388.
66. Kiselak J, Clark M, Pera V, Rosenberg C, Redline S. The association between hypertension and sleep apnea in obese patients. Chest 1993; 104(3):775–780.
67. Hoffstein V. Blood pressure, snoring, obesity, and nocturnal hypoxaemia. Lancet 1994; 344(8923):643–645.
68. Rauscher P, Popp W, Zwick H. Systemic hypertension in snorers with and without sleep apnea. Chest 1992; 102(2):367–371.
69. Apprill M, Weitzenblum E, Krieger J, Oswald M, Kurtz D. Frequency and mechanism of daytime pulmonary hypertension in patients with obstructive sleep apnoea syndrome. Cor Vasa 1991; 33(1):42–49.
70. Bradley TD, Rutherford R, Grossman RF, Lue F, Zamel N, Moldofsky H, Phillipson EA. Role of daytime hypoxemia in the pathogenesis of right heart failure in the obstructive sleep apnea syndrome. Am Rev Respir Dis 1985; 131(6):835–839.
71. Whyte KF, Douglas NJ. Peripheral edema in the sleep apnea/hypopnea syndrome. Sleep 1991; 14(4):354–356.
72. Hoffstein V, Herridge M, Mateika S, Redline S, Strohl KP. Hematocrit levels in sleep apnea. Chest 1994; 106(3):787–791.
73. Carlson JT, Hedner J, Fagerberg B, Ejnell H, Magnusson B, Fyhrquist F. Secondary polycythaemia associated with nocturnal apnoea—a relationship not mediated by erythropoietin? J Intern Med 1992; 231(4):381–387.
74. Liston R, Deegan PC, McCreery C, McNicholas WT. Role of respiratory sleep disorders in the pathogenesis of nocturnal angina and arrhythmias. Postgrad Med J 1994; 70(822):275–280.
75. Lazarus A, Py A, Guérin F, Valty J, Le Heuzey JY. [Arrhythmia and syndrome of obstructive sleep apnea in adults] translated: Arythmies et syndrome d'apnées obstructives du sommeil de l'adulte. Arch Mal Coeur Vaisseaux 1993; 86(12):1753–1759.
76. Rama PR, Sharma SC. Sleep apnea and complete heart block. Clin Cardiol 1994; 17(12):675–677.
77. Koehler U, Wetzig T, Peter JH, Ploch T, Schafer H, Stellwaag M. Morbidity and mortality in sleep apnea and nocturnal bradyarrhythmia. Dtsche Med Wochenschr 1994; 119(36):1187–1193.
78. Flemons WW, Remmers JE, Gillis AM. Sleep apnea and cardiac arrhythmias. Is there a relationship? Am Rev Respir Dis 1993; 148(3):618–621.
79. Loui WS, Blackshear JL, Fredrickson PA, Kaplan J. Obstructive sleep apnea manifesting as suspected angina: report of three cases. Mayo Clin Proc 1994; 69(3):244–248.

80. Abinader EG, Peled N, Sharif D, Lavie P. ST-segment depression during obstructive sleep apnea. Am J Cardiol 1994; 73(9):727 (letter).
81. Franklin KA, Nilsson JB, Sahlin C, Näslund U. Sleep apnoea and nocturnal angina. Lancet 1995; 345(8957):1085–1087.
82. Hanly P, Sasson Z, Zuberi N, Lunn K. ST-segment depression during sleep in obstructive sleep apnea. Am J Cardiol 1993; 71(15):1341–1345.
83. Hung J, Whitford EG, Parsons RW, Hillman DR. Association of sleep apnoea with myocardial infarction in men. Lancet 1990; 336(8710):261–264.
84. Tateishi O, Okamura T, Itou T, Murakami M, Suda T, Nishimuta I, Obata S, Nagata T. Observation of sleep-related breathing disorders in patients with coronary artery disease by ambulatory electrocardiogram-respiration monitoring system. Jpn Circ J 1994; 58(1):831–835.
85. Hanly P, Sasson Z, Zuberi N, Anderson M. Ventricular function in snorers and patients with obstructive sleep apnea. Chest 1992; 102(1):105–115.
86. Tal A, Leiberman A, Margulis G, Sofer G. Ventricular dysfunction in children with obstructive sleep apnea: radionuclide assessment. Pediatr Pulmonol 1988; 4(3): 139–143.
87. Hedner J, Ejnell H, Caidahl K. Left ventricular hypertrophy independent of hypertension in patients with obstructive sleep apnoea. J Hypertension 1990; 8(10): 941–946.
88. Siebler M, Nachtmann A. Cerebral hemodynamics in obstructive sleep apnea. Chest 1993; 103(4):1118–1119.
89. Fisher AQ, Chaudhary BA, Taormina MA, Akhtar B. Intracranial hemodynamics in sleep apnea. Chest 1992; 102(5):1402–1406.
90. Wiegand L, Zwillich CW. Obstructive sleep apnea. Disease-a-Month 1994; 40(4): 197–252 (review).
91. Westbrook PR. Sleep disorders and upper airway obstruction in adults. Otolaryngol Clin North Am 1990; 23(4):727–743 (review).
92. Lavie P, Herer P, Peled R, Berger I, Yoffe N, Zomer J, Rubin AH. Mortality in sleep apnea patients: a multivariate analysis of risk factors. Sleep 1995; 18(3):149–157.
93. Seppala T, Partinen M, Penttila A, Aspholm R, Tiainen E, Kaukianen A. Sudden death and sleeping history among Finnish men. J Intern Med 1991; 229(1):23–28.
94. Zaninelli A, Fariello R, Boni E, Corda L, Alicandri C, Grassi V. Snoring and risk of cardiovascular disease. Int J Cardiol 1991; 32(3):347–351.
95. He J, Kryger MH, Zorick FJ, Conway W, Roth T. Mortality and apnea index in obstructive sleep apnea. Experience in 385 male patients. Chest 1988; 94(1):9–14.
96. Partinen M, Jamieson A, Guilleminault C. Long-term outcome for obstructive sleep apnea syndrome patients. Mortality. Chest 1988; 94(6):1200–1204.
97. Mant A, King M, Saunders NA, Pond CD, Goode E, Hewitt H. Four-year follow-up of mortality and sleep-related respiratory disturbance in non-demented seniors. Sleep 1995; 18(6):433–438.
98. Ancoli-Israel S, Klauber MR, Kripke DF, Parker L, Cobarrubias M. Sleep apnea in female patients in a nursing home. Increased mortality. Chest 1989; 96(5):1054–1058.
99. Partinen M, Telakivi T, Epidemiology of obstructive sleep apnea syndrome. Sleep 1992; 15(Suppl):S1–4 (review).
100. De Benedetto M, Cuda D, Leante M. Diurnal hypersomnolence and chronic snoring: an epidemiologic study. Acta Otorhinolaryngol Ital 1991; 11(6):579–586.

101. Franceschi M, Zamproni P, Crippa D, Smirne S. Excessive daytime sleepiness: a 1-year study in an unselected inpatient population. Sleep 1982; 5(3):239–247.
102. Duchna HW, Rasche K, Orth M, Schultze-Werninghaus G. Sensitivity and specificity of pulse oximetry in diagnosis of sleep-related respiratory disorders. Pneumologie 1995; 49(Suppl 1):113–115.
103. Series F, Marc I, Cormier Y, La Forge J. Utility of nocturnal home oximetry for case finding in patients with suspected sleep apnea hypopnea syndrome. Ann Intern Med 1993; 119(6):449–453.
104. Grunstein RR, Wilcox I. Sleep-disordered breathing and obesity. Baillieres Clin Endocrinol Metab 1994; 8(3):601–628 (review).
105. Pillar G, Peled R, Lavie P. Recurrence of sleep apnea without concomitant weight increase 7.5 years after weight reduction surgery. Chest 1994; 106(6):1702–1704.
106. Charuzi I, Lavie P, Peiser J, Peled R. Bariatric surgery in morbidly obese sleep-apnea patients: short- and long-term follow-up. Am J Clin Nutr 1993; 55(2 Suppl):594S–596S.
107. Braver HM, Block AJ, Perri MG. Treatment for snoring. Combined weight loss, sleeping on side, and nasal spray. Chest 1995; 107(5):1283–1288.
108. Eveloff SE, Rosenberg CL, Carlisle CC, Millman RP. Efficacy of a Herbst mandibular advancement device in obstructive sleep apnea. Am J Respir Crit Care Med 1994; 149(4 Pt 1):905–909.
109. Clark GT, Arand D, Chung E, Tong D. Effect of anterior mandibular positioning on obstructive sleep apnea. Am Rev Respir Dis 1993; 147(3):624–629.
110. Block AJ, Hellard DW, Cicale MJ. Snoring, nocturnal hypoxemia, and the effect of oxygen inhalation. Chest 1987; 92(3):411–417.
111. Ali NJ, Davies RJ, Fleetham JA, Stradling JR. The acute effects of continuous positive airway pressure and oxygen administration on blood pressure during obstructive sleep apnea. Chest 1992; 101(6):1526–1532.
112. Marrone O, Bellia V, Pieri D, Salvaggio A, Bonsignore G. Acute effects of oxygen administration on transmural pulmonary artery pressure in obstructive sleep apnea. Chest 1992; 101(4):1023–1027.
113. Gold AR, Bleecker ER, Smith PL. A shift from central and mixed sleep apnea to obstructive sleep apnea resulting from low-flow oxygen. Am Rev Respir Dis 1985; 132(2):220–223.
114. Phillips BA, Schmitt FA, Berry DT, Lamb DG, Amin M, Cook YR. Treatment of obstructive sleep apnea. A preliminary report comparing nasal CPAP to nasal oxygen in patients with mild OSA. Chest 1990; 98(2):325–330.
115. Breitenbucher A, Keller-Wossildo H, Keller R. Transtracheal oxygen therapy in obstructive sleep apnea syndrome. Schweizerische Medizinische Wochenschrift. J Suisse Med 1989; 119(46):1638–1641.
116. Farney RJ, Walker JM, Elmer JC, Viscomi VA, Ord RJ. Transtracheal oxygen, nasal CPAP and nasal oxygen in five patients with obstructive sleep apnea. Chest 1992; 101(5):1228–1235.
117. Smith PL, Haponik EF, Allen RP, Bleecker ER. The effects of protriptyline in sleep-disordered breathing. Am Rev Respir Dis 1983; 127(1):8–13.
118. Brownell LG, West P, Sweatman P, Acres JC, Kryger MH. Protriptyline in obstructive sleep apnea: a double-blind trial. N Engl J Med 1982; 307(17):1037–1042.

119. Chiang CH, Tang YC, Wang SE, Hwang JC. Changes in phrenic, hypoglossal and recurrent laryngeal nerve activities after intravenous infusions of aminophylline in cats. Eur Respir J 1995; 8(4):632–636.
120. Meissner P, Dorow P, Thalhofer S, Heinemann S. Theophylline acceptance in long-term therapy of patients with obstructive sleep related respiratory disorder. Pneumologie 1995; 49(Suppl 1):187–189.
121. Espinoza H, Antic R, Thornton AT, McEvoy RD. The effects of aminophylline on sleep and sleep-disordered breathing in patients with obstructive sleep apnea syndrome. Am Rev Respir Dis 1987; 136(1):80–84.
122. Mulloy E, McNicholas WT. Theophylline in obstructive sleep apnea. A double-blind evaluation. Chest 1992; 101(3):753–757.
123. Aboussouan LS, Golish JA, Wood BG, Mehta AC, Wood DE, Dinner DS. Dynamic pharyngoscopy in predicting outcome of uvulopalatopharyngoplasty for moderate and severe obstructive sleep apnea. Chest 1995; 107(4):946–951.
124. Johnson NT, Chinn J. Uvulopalatopharyngoplasty and inferior sagittal mandibular osteotomy with genioglossus advancement for treatment of obstructive sleep apnea. Chest 1994; 105(1):278–283.
125. Rodenstein DO. Assessment of uvulopalatopharyngoplasty for the treatment of sleep apnea syndrome. Sleep 1992; 15(6 Suppl):S56–62 (review).
126. Keenan SP, Burt H, Ryan CF, Fleetham JA. Long-term survival of patients with obstructive sleep apnea treated by uvulopalatopharyngoplasty or nasal CPAP. Chest 1994; 105(1):155–159.
127. Partinen M, Guilleminault C. Daytime sleepiness and vascular morbidity at seven-year follow-up in obstructive sleep apnea patients. Chest 1990; 97(1):27–32.
128. Sanders MH, Kern NB, Stiller RA, Strollo PJ, Martin TJ, Atwood CW Jr. CPAP therapy via oronasal mask for obstructive sleep apnea. Chest 1994; 106(3):774–779.
129. Miljeteig H, Hoffstein V. Determinants of continuous positive airway pressure level for the treatment of obstructive sleep apnea. Am Rev Respir Dis 1993; 147(6 Pt 1):1526–1530.
130. Leech JA, Onal E, Lopata M. Nasal CPAP continues to improve sleep-disordered breathing and daytime oxygenation over long-term follow-up of occlusive sleep apnea syndrome. Chest 1992; 102(6):1651–1655.
131. Mayer J, Becker H, Brandenburg U, Penzel T, Peter JH, von Wichert P. Blood pressure and sleep apnea: results of long-term nasal continuous positive airway pressure therapy. Cardiology 1991; 79(2):84–92.
132. Hedner J, Darpo B, Ejnell H, Carlson J, Caidahl K. Reduction in sympathetic activity after long-term CPAP treatment in sleep apnoea: cardiovascular implications. Eur Respir J 1995; 8(2):222–229.
133. Krieger J, Grucker D, Sforza E, Chambron J, Kurtz D. Left ventricular ejection fraction in obstructive sleep apnea. Effects of long-term treatment with nasal continuous positive airway pressure. Chest 1991; 100(4):917–921.
134. Malone S, Liu PP, Holloway R, Rutherford R, Xie A, Bradley TD. Obstructive sleep apnea in patients with dilated cardiomyopathy: effects of continuous positive airway pressure. Lancet 1991; 338(8781):1480–1484.
135. Meurice JC, Mergy J, Rostykus C, Doré P, Paquereau J, Patte F. Atrial arrhythmia as a complication of nasal CPAP. Chest 1992; 102(2):640–642.

136. Rauscher H, Formanek D, Popp W, Zwick H. Self-reported vs measured compliance with nasal CPAP for obstructive sleep apnea. Chest 1993; 103(6):1675–1680.
137. Meurice JC, Dore P, Paquereau J, Neau JP, Ingrand P, Chavagnat JJ, Patte F. Predictive factors of long-term compliance with nasal continuous positive airway pressure treatment in sleep apnea syndrome. Chest 1994; 105(2):429–433.
138. Rolfe I, Olson LG, Saunders NA. Long-term acceptance of continuous positive airway pressure in obstructive sleep apnea. Am Rev Respir Dis 1991; 144(5):1130–1133.
139. Krieger J. Long-term compliance with nasal continuous positive airway pressure (CPAP) in obstructive sleep apnea patients and nonapneic snorers. Sleep 1992; 15(6 Suppl):S42–46.
140. Piper AJ, Sullivan CE. Effects of short-term NIPPV in the treatment of patients wtih severe obstructive sleep apnea and hypercapnia. Chest 1994; 105(2):434–440.
141. Becker H, Brandenburg U, Peter JH, Schneider H, Weber K, von Wichert P. Indications and application of BiPAP therapy. Pneumologie 1993; 47(Suppl 1):184–188.
142. Hoijer U, Ejnell H, Hedner J, Petruson B, Eng LB. The effects of nasal dilation on snoring and obstructive sleep apnea. Arch Otolaryngol Head Neck Surg 1992; 118(3):281–284.
143. Bradley TD, McNicholas WT, Rutherford R, Popkin J, Zamel N, Phillipson EA. Clinical and physiologic heterogeneity of central sleep apnea syndrome. Am Rev Respir Dis 1986; 134(2):217–221.
144. Hanly PJ. Mechanisms and management of central sleep apnea. Lung 1992; 170(1): 1–17 (review).
145. Dowell AR, Buckley CE, Cohen R, Whalen ER, Sieker HO. Cheyne-Stokes respiration. Arch Intern Med 1971; 127:712–726.
146. Brown HW, Plum F. The neurologic basis of Cheyne-Stokes respiration. Am J Med 1961; 30:849–860.
147. Tobin MJ, Snyder JV. Cheyne-Stokes respiration revisited: controversies and implications. Crit Care Med 1984; 12(10):882–887.
148. Naughton M, Benard D, Tam A, Rutherford R, Bradley TD. Role of hyperventilation in the pathogenesis of central sleep apneas in patients with congestive heart failure. Am Rev Respir Dis 1993; 148(2):330–338.
149. Hanly P, Zuberi N, Gray R. Pathogenesis of Cheyne-Stokes respiration in patients with congestive heart failure. Relationship to arterial Pco_2. Chest 1993; 104(4): 1079–1084.
150. Millar TW, Hanly PJ, Hunt B, Frais M, Kryger MH. The entrainment of low frequency breathing periodicity. Chest 1990; 98(5):1143–1148.
151. Hanly P, Zuberi-Khokhar N. Daytime sleepiness in patients with congestive cardiac failure and Cheyne-Stokes respiration. Chest 1995; 107(4):952–959.
152. Javaheri S, Parker TJ, Wexler L, Michaels SE, Stanberry E, Nishyama H, Roselle GA. Occult sleep-disordered breathing in stable congestive heart failure. Ann Intern Med 1995; 122(7):487– 492.
153. Lofaso F, Vershueren P, Rande JL, Harf A, Goldenberg F. Prevalence of sleep-disordered breathing in patients on a heart transplant list. Chest 1994; 106(6):1689–1694.
154. Rasche K, Hoffarth HP, Marek W, Reier W, von Dryander S. Nocturnal oxygen

saturation in patients with coronary heart disease—dependent on degree of left ventricular functional impairment. Pneumonologie 1991; 45(Suppl 1):261–264.
155. Thalhofer S, Dorow P, Schuler S, Hetzer R. Oxygen saturation and sleep structure in patients with dilated cardiomyopathy. Pneumonologie 1991; 45(Suppl 1):259–260.
156. Ancoli-Israel S, Engler RL, Friedman PJ, Klauber MR, Ross PA, Kripke DF. Comparison of patients with central sleep apnea. With and without Cheyne-Stokes respiration. Chest 1994; 106(3):780–786.
157. Walsh JT, Andrews R, Starling R, Cowley AJ, Johnston ID, Kinnear WJ. Effects of captopril and oxygen on sleep apnoea in patients with mild to moderate congestive cardiac failure. Br Heart J 1995; 73(3):237–241.
158. Andreas S, Mohr FW, Kreuzer H. Elimination of periodic respiration in heart failure by heart transplantation. Pneumonologie 1995; 49(7):428–430.
159. Collop NA. Cheyne-Stokes ventilation converting to obstructive sleep apnea following heart transplantation. Chest 1993; 104(4):1288–1289.
160. Dowdell WT, Javaheri S, McGinnis W. Cheyne-Stokes respiration presenting as sleep apnea syndrome. Am Rev Respir Dis 1990; 141:871–879.
161. Tomcsanyi J, Karlocai K. Effect of theophylline on periodic breathing in congestive heart failure measured by transcutaneous oxygen monitoring. Eur J Clin Pharmacol 1994; 46(2):173–174.
162. Raetzo MA, Junod AF, Kryger MH. Effect of aminophylline and relief from hypoxia on central sleep apnoea due to medullary damage. Bull Eur Physiopathol Resp 1987; 23(2):171–175.
163. Rubin AH, Alroy GG, Peled R, Lavie P. Preliminary clinical experience with imipramine HCl in the treatment of sleep apnea syndrome. Eur Neurol 1986; 25(2):81–85.
164. Hanly PJ, Millar TW, Steljes DG, Baert R, Frais MA, Kryger MH. The effect of oxygen on respiration and sleep in patients with congestive heart failure. Ann Intern Med 1989; 111(10):777–782.
165. McNicholas WT, Carter JL, Rutherford R, Zamel N, Phillipson EA. Beneficial effect of oxygen therapy in primary alveolar hypoventilation with central sleep apnea. Am Rev Respir Dis 1982; 125(5):773–775.
166. Barlow PB, Barlett D Jr, Hauri P, Hellekson C, Nattie EE, Remmers JE, Schmidt-Nowara WW. Idiopathic hypoventilation syndrome: importance of preventing nocturnal hypoxemia and hypercapnia. Am Rev Respir Dis 1980; 121(1):141–145.
167. Naughton MT, Benard DC, Rutherford R, Bradley TD. Effect of continuous positive airway pressure on central sleep apnea and nocturnal pco_2 in heart failure. Am J Respir Crit Care Med 1994; 150(6 Pt 1):1598–1604.
168. Liston R, Deegan PC, McCreery C, Costello R, Maurer B, McNicholas WT. Haemodynamic effects of nasal continuous positive airway pressure in severe congestive heart failure. Eur Respir J 1995; 8(3):430–435.
169. Becker H, Stammnitz A, Schneider H, Peter JH, von Wichert P. Nasal continuous positive airway pressure (nCPAP) therapy in obstructive sleep breathing disorders. Dtsche Med Wochenschr 1995; 120(22):783–789.
170. De Hoyos A, Liu PP, Benard DC, Bradley TD. Haemodynamic effects of continuous positive airway pressure in humans with normal and impaired left ventricular function. Clin Sci 1995; 88(2):173–178.
171. Naughton MT, Rahman MA, Hara K, Floras JS, Bradley TD. Effect of continuous

positive airway pressure on intrathoracic and left ventricular transmural pressures in patients with congestive cardiac failure. Circulation 1995; 91(6):1725–1731.
172. Bradley TD, Holloway RM, McLaughlin PR, Ross BL, Walters J, Liu PP. Cardiac output response to continuous positive airway pressure in congestive heart failure. Am Rev Respir Dis 145(2 Pt 1):377–382.
173. Takasaki Y, Orr D, Popkin J, Rutherford R, Liu P, Bradley TD. Effect of nasal continuous positive airway pressure on sleep apnea in congestive heart failure. Am Rev Respir Dis 1989; 140(6):1578–1584.
174. Naughton MT, Liu PP, Benard DC, Goldstein RS, Bradley TD. Treatment of congestive heart failure and Cheyne-Stokes respiration during sleep by continuous positive airways pressure. Am J Respir Crit Care Med 1995; 151(1):92–97.
175. Bradley TD, Takasaki Y, Orr D, Popkin J, Liu P, Rutherford R. Sleep apnea in patients with left ventricular dysfunction: beneficial effects of nasal CPAP. Prog Clin Biol Res 1990; 345:363–368.
176. Davies RJ, Harrington KJ, Ormerod OJ, Stradling JR. Nasal continuous positive airways pressure in chronic heart failure with sleep-disordered breathing. Am Rev Respir Dis 1993; 147(3):630–634.
177. Granton JT, Naughton MT, Benard DC, Liu PP, Goldstein RS, Bradley TD. CPAP improves inspiratory muscle strength in patients with heart failure and central sleep apnea. Am J Respir Crit Care Med 1996; 153(1):277–282.
178. Naughton MT, Benard DC, Liu PP, Rutherford R, Rankin F, Bradley TD. Effects of nasal CPAP on sympathetic activity in patients with heart failure and central sleep apnea. Am J Respir Crit Care Med 1995; 152(2):473–479.
179. Butler GC, Naughton MT, Rahman MA, Bradley TD, Floras JS. Continuous positive airway pressure increases heart rate variability in congestive heart failure. J Am Coll Cardiol 1995; 25(3):672–679.
180. Yu L, Huang XZ, Wu QY. Management of nocturnal nasal mask continuous positive airway pressure in central hypoventilation in patients with respiratory diseases. Chung-Hua Chieh Ho Ho Hu Hsi Tsa Chih Chinese J Tuberc Respir Dis 1994; 17(1): 38–40, 62–63.
181. Thalhofer S, Dorow P. Effect of n-BiPAP therapy on the hemodynamics in patients with central sleep apnea. Pneumologie 1995; 49(Suppl 1):165–166.
182. Douglas NJ. Nocturnal hypoxemia in patients with chronic obstructive pulmonary disease. Clin Chest Med 1992; 13(p3):523–532 (review).
183. Fleetham J, West P, Mezon B, Conway W, Roth T, Kryger M. Sleep, arousals, and oxygen desaturation in chronic obstructive pulmonary disease. The effect of oxygen therapy. Am Rev Respir Dis 1982; 126(3):429–433.
184. Littner MR, McGinty DJ, Arand DL. Determinants of oxygen desaturation in the course of ventilation during sleep in chronic obstructive pulmonary disease. Am Rev Respir Dis 1980; 122(6):849–857.
185. Levi-Valensi P, Weitzenblum E, Rida Z, Aubry P, Braghiroli A, Donner C, Aprill M, Zielinski J, Wurtemberger G. Sleep-related oxygen desaturation and daytime pulmonary haemodynamics in COPD patients. Eur Respir J 1992; 5(3):301–307.
186. Miyhara Y, Miyhara Y, Naito T, Ikeda S. Monitoring of nocturnal oxygen desaturation using pulse oximeter and apnomonitor in patients with chronic pulmonary disease. Respiration 1995; 62(6):348–352.

187. Flenley DC. Sleep in chronic obstructive lung disease. Clin Chest Med 1985; 6(4): 651–661.
188. Chaouat A, Weitzenblum E, Krieger J, Ifoundza T, Oswald M, Kessler R. Association of chronic obstructive pulmonary disease and sleep apnea syndrome. Am J Respir Crit Care Med 1995; 151(1):82–86.
189. Fletcher EC. Chronic lung disease in the sleep apnea syndrome. Lung 1990; 168 (Suppl):751–761 (review).
190. Goldstein RS, Ramcharan V, Bowes G, McNicholas WT, Bradley D, Phillipson EA. Effect of supplemental nocturnal oxygen on gas exchange in patients with severe obstructive lung disease. N Engl J Med 1984; 310(7):425–429.
191. Alford NJ, Fletcher EC, Nickeson D. Acute oxygen in patients with sleep apnea and COPD. Chest 1986; 89(1):30–38.
192. Muir JF, Rose D, Aubry P, Levi-Valensi P, Duron B. Ventilatory disorders and sleep abnormalities in severe chronic obstructive respiratory insufficiency. Effects of nocturnal oxygen therapy. Presse Med 1983; 12(27):1701–1706.
193. Weitzenblum E, Aprill M, Oswald M, Kurtz D. Drug therapy of sleep-related hypoxaemia. Lung 1990; 168(Suppl):948–954 (review).
194. Kearley R, Wynne JW, Block AJ, Boysen PG, Lindsey S, Martin C. The effect of low flow oxygen on sleep-disordered breathing and oxygen desaturation. A study of patients with chronic obstructive lung disease. Chest 1980; 78(5):682–685.
195. Steens RD, Pouliot Z, Millar TW, Kryger MH, George CF. Effects of zolpidem and triazolam on sleep and respiration in mild to moderate chronic obstructive pulmonary disease. Sleep 1993; 16(4):318–326.
196. Dolly FR, Block AJ. Increased ventricular ectopy and sleep apnea following ethanol ingestion in COPD patients. Chest 1983; 83(3):469–472.
197. Galatius-Jensen S, Hansen J, Rasmussen V, Bildsoe J, Therboe M, Rosenberg J. Nocturnal hypoxaemia after myocardial infarction: association with nocturnal myocardial ischaemia and arrhythmias. Br Heart J 1994; 72(1):23–30.
198. Galatius-Jensen S, Hansen JE, Jensen JB, Rasmussen V, Therbo-Pedersen M, Rosenberg J. Episodic hypoxemia and coinciding ECG changes after acute myocardial infarction. Ugerskr Laeger 1995; 157(14):1991–1995.
199. Saito T, Yoshikawa T, Sakamoto Y, Tanaka K, Inoue T, Ogawa R. Sleep apnea in patients with acute myocardial infarction. Crit Care Med 1991; 19(7):938–941.
200. Stark R, Kohler D. The value and consequences of nocturnal pulse oximetry in severe heart failure, suspected myocardial infarct and acute cerebral ischemia. Pneumologie 1989; 43(Suppl 1):596–599.
201. Vanoli E, Adamson PB, Ba-Lin Pinna GD, Lazzara R, Orr WC. Heart rate variability during specific sleep stages. A comparison of healthy subjects with patients after myocardial infarction. Circulation 1995; 91(7):1918–1922.

5

Nosocomial Pneumonia in the Critical Care Unit

A. REKHA K. MURTHY and ERIC S. DAAR

University of California, Los Angeles, School of Medicine, and Cedars-Sinai Medical Center, Los Angeles, California

MEHMET PEKEROL

Cedars-Sinai Medical Center, Los Angeles, California

I. INTRODUCTION

Studies in the United States report that hospital-acquired pneumonia, based on the Centers for Disease Control and Prevention (CDC) surveillance definition, accounts for 15% of all hospital-associated infections, with an estimated 250,000 cases per year (1–4). This nosocomial infection ranks second to urinary tract infections, with incidence rates of 0.6% to 1.1% (1,2,5), and occurs with a higher frequency in university-affiliated hospitals than in nonteaching hospitals (1,2). In addition, rates in intubated patients, a known risk factor for nosocomial pneumonia, are increased by fourfold to 21-fold over nonintubated patients (5,6). Intensive care unit (ICU) surveillance data collected by the CDC's National Nosocomial Infection Surveillance (NNIS) System reveals rates of ventilator-associated pneumonia to be highest in burn and neurosurgical ICUs, and higher in surgical ICUs than in medical ICUs (Table 1) (4).

Nosocomial pneumonia is associated with high mortality, with crude rates ranging from 20% to 50% (7–9). The mortality rate in ICU patients with nosocomial pneumonia is two to 10 times higher than in those without pneumonia (7,10); higher rates were also seen in older patients, those receiving mechanical ventilation, having underlying diseases, and organ failure (7,11,12). While bacteremia occurs in only 2% of subjects with nosocomial pneumonia, it is associated with a threefold increase in mortality (5,13). In addition, pneumonia due to gram-

Table 1 Rates of Ventilator-Associated Pneumonia by Intensive Care Unit Type

Type of ICU	Pooled mean (per 1000 ventilator days)
Burn	20.9
Neurosurgical	20.2
Trauma	16.9
Surgical	14.9
Medical/surgical	12.5
Coronary	9.9
Medical	9.4
Respiratory	6.4
Pediatric	5.9

NNIS Surveillance, Jan. 1990–Apr. 1995.
Source: Ref. 4.

negative bacilli is associated with a crude mortality rate of approximately 50%, compared to 10% to 20% in pneumonia due to gram-positive organisms (6,14–16).

Although the mortality in patients with nosocomial pneumonia is high, it is difficult to ascertain to what degree the pneumonia contributed to the ultimate demise of patients who often have severe comorbid disease. Several studies have attempted to determine the attributable mortality of nosocomial pneumonia, or the mortality directly due to the pneumonia itself. The attributable mortality of hospital-acquired pneumonia has been estimated to be approximately 7%, accounting for one-third of deaths in which pneumonia was diagnosed (8). Attributable mortality in intubated patients with pneumonia was even higher, estimated in one study to be 27%, representing 50% of all deaths (14). In addition to the direct contribution of nosocomial pneumonia to the mortality of hospitalized patients, those who survive experience increased morbidity, including increased length of hospitalization by an average of 7 days (8,17), increased duration of mechanical ventilation by 18 to 22 days (18,19), and increased cost. Since reimbursement by Medicare and other insurance providers is often based on the admitting diagnosis, much of the extra costs associated with nosocomial pneumonia represent a direct loss of hospital revenue. It has been estimated that nosocomial pneumonia could account for more than 1.75 million extra hospital days and nearly $1.5 billion in additional charges (20). In light of the increased morbidity, mortality, and cost associated with nosocomial pneumonia, it is critical that clinicians become aware of the diagnostic methods and treatment for this disease. More importantly, clinicians must understand the pathogenesis of this infection in order to apply methods for prevention of this complication of hospitalization.

II. PATHOGENESIS AND RISK FACTORS

Insights into the pathogenesis of nosocomial pneumonia improve our ability to define the microbiology of the disease and to prevent this common complication. Hospital-acquired pneumonia represents a complex interaction between host defenses and the invading pathogens. Host defense mechanisms include filtration and humidification of air in the upper airways, epiglottic and cough reflexes, ciliary transport by respiratory epithelium, phagocytes, and opsonins within the distal airways, and systemic cell-mediated immunity and humoral immunity. The development of nosocomial pneumonia requires that the pathogens reach the distal airways and then multiply to cause invasive disease, overcoming host defenses at each step.

Nosocomial pneumonia, not unlike other forms of pneumonia, typically occurs as a result of aspiration of bacteria colonizing the upper respiratory tract. It has been shown that approximately 45% of healthy individuals aspirate during sleep and that aspiration is markedly increased (up to 70%) in patients with impaired consciousness, abnormal swallowing, depressed gag reflexes, delayed gastric emptying, and decreased gastrointestinal motility (21).

The upper airway includes respiratory passages above the larynx which are known to be a reservoir for more than 200 microbial species. In fact, in healthy subjects, saliva contains approximately 10^8 to 10^9 bacteria per milliliter with a ratio of anaerobes to aerobes of nearly 10 to 1. Importantly, aerobic gram-negative bacilli are rarely present in this patient population (22,23). A major event that usually precedes hospital-acquired pneumonia is the alteration of the bacterial flora of the oropharyngeal airway (23–25). Although gram-negative bacilli, coliforms and *Pseudomonas aeruginosa* are not normal oropharyngeal constituents, their prevalence is increased in hospitalized patients, nursing home inhabitants, alcoholics, and diabetics (22,26). While one study showed that approximately 3% of inpatients with psychiatric disorders harbored aerobic gram-negative bacilli, oropharyngeal cultures from 16% of moderately ill and 57% of critically ill patients yielded such bacteria (22). In fact, patients admitted to an ICU become colonized during the first few days of admission (22). Johansen and Pierce showed that nosocomial pneumonia developed in 23% of patients who were colonized with gram-negative bacilli, compared to only 3% of uncolonized patients (22).

Bacterial adherence to respiratory epithelial cells is a major determinant, and is the initial event, in bacterial colonization of the airway (27,28). Adherence may be affected by multiple factors related to the bacteria (presence of pili, cilia, capsule, or production of elastase or mucinase), host cell (surface proteins and polysaccharides), and environment (pH and presence of mucin in respiratory secretions) (29–35). Alterations in the host appear to be necessary for airway colonization to occur. In fact, attempts to induce colonization in healthy individuals by direct inoculation of large numbers of aerobic gram-negative bacilli into the oropharyngeal airway have been unsuccessful (29). The stress of severe illness alters the surface of respiratory epithelial cells, permitting adhesive antigens on bacterial surfaces to attach to receptors on the surface of host epithelial cells, resulting in increased adherence of such organisms. In vitro studies suggest that adherence of gram-negative bacilli to buccal epithelial cells is facilitated by critical illness or surgical stress when cell-surface fibronectin is degenerated by increased levels of salivary proteases (32,35). Overall, enhanced binding of gram-negative bacilli to airway epithelial cells has been demonstrated in patients with life-threatening illnesses, following general surgery, and in the setting of malnutrition (28, 31,34,35). Further understanding of bacterial adherence may lead to a novel approach toward prevention of nosocomial pneumonia.

Gastric bacterial colonization is another potential source of pathogens in hospitalized patients. In healthy individuals, gastric colonization rarely occurs since gram-negative bacilli do not survive in the presence of a $pH < 2$ (36). In contrast, in patients with a gastric pH of $\geqslant 6$, bacterial colonization may reach up to 10^6 organisms per milliliter gastric fluid (37,38). Indeed, molecular typing studies in some subjects have demonstrated colonizing strains in gastric fluid to be identical to those subsequently isolated from infected lung (37). Increases in gastric colonization have been described in patients with advanced age, achlorhydria, administration of enteral feeding solutions, malnutrition, ileus, upper gastrointestinal disease, and treatment with antacids or antisecretory agents (36,39–42).

Bacteria can also be introduced into the lower respiratory tract of patients by contaminated respiratory therapy equipment. In addition, bacterial colonization of the hands of hospital personnel plays a major role in the spread of nosocomial pathogens from patient to patient. In fact, gram-negative bacilli are often present in high concentration in the hospital environment, and on the hands of hospital personnel (43,44). Less commonly, inhalation of fungi (such as *Aspergillus*) or hematogenous seeding and reactivation (tuberculosis or cytomegalovirus) can be the cause of pneumonia in hospitalized patients (1).

Aspiration often occurs after oropharyngeal colonization and can result in alteration of the normal flora to include more virulent and resistant nosocomial pathogens. While mucociliary clearance and alveolar macrophages are sufficient to remove small quantities of bacteria, containment of larger inocula depends on a normally functioning immune system. In patients with trauma or shock, clearance of aspirated bacteria is decreased by inflammation and lung injury as a consequence of cytokines released in the lung (45). In the absence of adequate host defenses, bacteria can proliferate and cause pneumonia.

Understanding the pathogenesis of nosocomial pneumonia makes it possible to identify specific risk factors for such infections. Many probable risk factors for hospital-acquired pneumonia have been examined (6–8,10,15,16,46–48). One of the difficulties in comparing these studies has been the inconsistency in the clinical definition of pneumonia used. Although specific risk factors may differ between study populations, general categories have been commonly described (Table 2). These include a myriad of host factors, as well as situations that can result in increased colonization with gram-negative bacteria, increased risk of aspiration, and hindered clearance of respiratory secretions (16,19,47,48).

Nosocomial pneumonia is more common in patients at increased risk of aspiration or reflux, such as those with endotracheal intubation, insertion of a nasogastric tube, or being maintained in the supine position. Other acute events that impair airway reflexes, as well as trauma to the head or chest, also increase the risk of pneumonia. Fagon et al. have reported that the risk of developing nosocomial pneumonia in mechanically ventilated patients is increased by 1%/day (16). This is probably a result of endotracheal intubation compromising the natural barrier between the oropharynx and trachea, facilitating the entry of bacteria into the lung. Moreover, endotracheal intubation not only impairs the cough reflex and mucociliary clearance, but also damages local tissue to which bacteria may then adhere (5–7). Leakage around the cuff of the endotracheal tube also allows subglottic secretions, which pool above the cuff, to enter the trachea (16,49). Finally, clearance of pulmonary secretions are inhibited in patients with chronic obstructive lung disease and surgery or trauma to the head, neck, chest, or upper abdomen (6,48). Of 520 thoracic and abdominal surgery patients followed by Garibaldi et al., 91 (17.5%) developed pneumonia (48). In this series, preoperative markers for severity of illness, such as low albumin and high-risk classification by anesthesiologists, were strongly associated with pneumonia.

Studies have shown that prior antibiotic treatment correlates with nosocomial pneumonia caused by antibiotic resistant organisms, including *P. aeruginosa*, as well as with higher mortality rates (15). Sprunt and Redman (50) have shown that patients receiving penicillin or streptomycin prior to cardiac surgery had a marked decrease in normal oral bacterial flora, with an increase in gram-negative bacteria.

Table 2 Risk Factors Associated with Nosocomial Pneumonia

Host factors	Enhanced colonization	Increased aspiration	Impaired pulmonary clearance
Extremes of age	Admission to ICU	Neuromuscular disease	Bedridden
Severe underlying disease	Antibiotic use	Altered consciousness	Chronic lung disease
Malnutrition	Antacids	Endotracheal intubation	Surgical procedure/trauma
Chronic lung disease	Antisecretory agents	Nasogastric tube	—Head or neck
Corticosteroid use	Severity of illness	Supine position	—Chest
Immunosuppression			—Upper abdomen

Source: Refs. 16, 19, 22, 28, 31, 34–38, 47–49.

When antibiotics were stopped, gram-negative bacilli disappeared within 10 days and the number of gram-positive bacteria returned to normal. Flynn et al. reported that *Enterobacter* species become important pathogens in cardiac surgery patients when carriage was amplified by the administration of a first-generation cephalosporin (51). These studies all highlight the importance of antibiotic prescribing practices in the development of nosocomial pneumonia.

III. MICROBIOLOGY

Pathogens responsible for most hospital-acquired pneumonias reflect the composition of the colonizing oropharyngeal flora immediately preceding the onset of symptoms. Table 3 summarizes recent NNIS bacteriologic data collected from 1990 to 1996 (52). Gram-negative bacilli caused more than 50% of all nosocomial pneumonias. *Staphylococcus aureus* was the most common organism overall (19%), followed by *P. aeruginosa* (17%) and *Enterobacter* species (11%) (52). Common community-acquired pathogens, such as *Streptococcus pneumoniae* or *Haemophilus influenzae* are uncommon causes of nosocomial pneumonia; how-

Table 3 Microbiology of Nosocomial Pneumonia

	Pathogen	Percent of 13,433 isolates
Gram-negative	*Pseudomonas aeruginosa*	17
	Enterobacter species	11
	Klebsiella pneumoniae	8
	Haemophilus influezae	5
	Escherichia coli	4
	Acinetobacter species	4
	Serratia marcescens	3
	Proteus mirabilis	2
	Citrobacter species	1
	Other *Klebsiella* species	1
Gram-positive	*Staphylococcus aureus*	19
	Coagulase-negative staphylococci	2
	Enterococci	2
	Streptococcus species	2
Fungi	*Candida albicans*[a]	5
	Other *Candida* species	1
	Other fungi	1
Viruses	*All*	1

National Nosocomial Infection Surveillance Summary Report, 1990–1996.
[a]Not all are confirmed by biopsy; some may represent colonization.
Source: Ref. 52.

ever, they may play a larger role in community hospitals, where they have been isolated in 51% of episodes, with gram-negative bacilli only accounting for 26% of such infections (53). In addition, polymicrobial infections are common, occurring in up to 25% to 46% of mechanically ventilated patients (14,16,18,39,54,55).

Although aerobic bacteria are the most commonly isolated pathogens, diagnostic studies for anaerobic bacteria, *Legionella* species, viruses, mycobacteria, and fungi are not routinely performed in many hospitals. Thus, the frequency of these pathogens is likely to be underestimated (1,56–62). In particular, nosocomial pneumonia caused by *Legionella* species may be endemic in hospitals with contaminated cooling towers or water supplies (1,63–66). *Legionella* infection also occurs at increased frequency in patients who are immunocompromised, critically ill, or taking corticosteroids. These factors probably account for the nearly 40% mortality rate associated with nosocomial *Legionella* pneumonia (67,68). Similarly, viral pneumonia must be considered in specific situations. For example, viral pneumonitis presents more commonly in pediatric wards, where it may account for up to 20% of cases of nosocomial pneumonia. The most common respiratory viruses in this patient population are influenza and respiratory syncytial virus (59,69,70). In addition, nosocomial outbreaks of influenza pneumonia have occurred in patients in nursing homes, chronic disease facilities, ICUs, and pediatric wards (1,69,70). Although influenza is primarily spread person to person by large droplet nuclei, transmission by hands or fomites may occur.

The predominance of gram-negative bacilli and *S. aureus* in hospital-acquired pneumonia is directly related to host and environmental factors described in the pathogenesis section of this chapter. Patients without substantial comorbidity or extensive antibiotic use who develop nosocomial pneumonia are usually infected by *S. aureus*, nonpseudomonal gram-negative organisms, such as *Klebsiella* species, *Enterobacter* species, *Escherichia coli*, *Proteus* species, *Serratia marcescens*, and in some settings *H. influenzae* or *S. pneumoniae*. In contrast, a variety of factors place hospitalized patients at increased risk for other pathogens (Table 4) (71,72). Patients with previous antibiotic use, immunosuppression, prolonged hospitalization, endotracheal intubation, malnutrition, and chronic lung disease are more likely to be infected by resistant gram-negative bacilli, such as *P. aeruginosa* (15,16). In addition, corticosteroids and cytotoxic chemotherapy increase the likelihood of infection by *Legionella* species and fungi, such as *Aspergillus* species (67,71,73).

Patients with a witnessed aspiration or recent abdominal surgery are predisposed to mixed infections with aerobic and anaerobic bacteria (56,57,71). Nevertheless, in the setting of a witnessed aspiration it is sometimes difficult to distinguish between a chemical (noninfectious) pneumonitis, caused by the aspiration of gastric acid, and true bacterial infection. The risk of *S. aureus* pneumonia is increased in hospitalized patients who are comatose, have sustained an injury or trauma, present after a recent episode of influenza, and have diabetic mellitus or

Table 4 Risk Factors for Specific Pathogens

Clinical situations	Specific pathogens
All hospitalized patients	*P. aeruginosa*
S. aureus	Previous antibiotics
Klebsiella species	Immunosuppression
Enterobacter species	Intubation
E. coli	Malnutrition
Proteus species	Chronic lung disease
S. marcescens	*S. aureus*
Aspiration/recent abdominal surgery	Comatose
Anaerobic bacteria	Injury or trauma
Pathogens described in all hospitalized patients	Diabetes mellitus
	Renal failure
	Recent influenza
	Legionella species
	Corticosteroids
	Cytotoxic therapy
	Aspergillus species
	Corticosteroids
	Cytotoxic therapy
	Neutropenia

Source: Refs. 15, 16, 52, 53, 56–76.

renal failure (74,75). Moreover, prior antibiotics may increase the risk for methicillin-resistant *S. aureus* (76). Understanding the clinical situations in which various pathogens occur assists in the diagnostic evaluation and selection of empiric antimicrobial therapy.

IV. DIAGNOSIS

Nosocomial pneumonia can be difficult to diagnose, as clinical, laboratory, and imaging findings are neither sensitive nor specific (22,77–83). Identifying which patients truly have pneumonia and then defining the pathogen(s) involved allows for optimal therapy. Commonly used clinical criteria for the diagnosis of hospital-acquired pneumonia include fever, cough, purulent sputum, and a new and persistent pulmonary infiltrate on chest radiograph, accompanied by a suggestive Gram strain of sputum, tracheal, or pleural aspirate (23). Although these criteria together with sputum or tracheal aspirate cultures are relatively sensitive, they are not specific for nosocomial pneumonia and often lead to overdiagnosis. This is particularly true in intubated subjects and those with congestive heart failure, pulmonary emboli, and adult respiratory distress syndrome (ARDS) (80). Fagon et al. (16) reported that an accurate diagnosis of pneumonia in mechanically ventilated patients was made by clinicians only 62% of the time, and appropriate antibiotic therapy was administered for only 33% of those patients, with another 16% of patients receiving antibiotics unnecessarily. This was further illustrated by Meduri et al. (84), who found that at autopsy, more than 70% of patients who died with ARDS had pneumonia. When clinicians were blinded to the autopsy results of these patients and asked to evaluate them for pneumonia by clinical criteria, 30% of cases without histologic evidence of pneumonia were diagnosed clinically as having pneumonia. General principles in the clinical diagnosis of nosocomial pneumonia, given the difficulties outlined, include a high index of suspicion for pneumonia in patients at risk.

Once the clinical diagnosis of pneumonia has been made, an effort should ensue to identify the causative pathogen(s). Gram stain of purulent sputum should be performed and if there is a preponderance of one type of bacteria in an area with many polymorphonuclear (PMN) cells and few squamous cells, a presumptive diagnosis can be made and antimicrobial therapy initiated. In a setting of a previously untreated patient where a purulent sputum Gram stain has a paucity of bacteria, consideration of pathogens not readily visualized by Gram stain, such as *Legionella*, anaerobes, *Mycoplasma*, mycobacteria, and viruses, should be considered. In contrast to sputum Gram stain, cultures are less helpful because of the high likelihood of contamination with oropharyngeal flora. While a positive culture may not necessarily reflect the offending pathogen, the lack of a positive culture for aerobic gram-negative bacilli or *S. aureus*, in untreated subjects, makes infection by these organisms unlikely. Blood cultures should also be obtained routinely, although in the majority of cases they are negative. If pleural fluid is present, an aspirate should be analyzed to assess for the presence of exudative fluid at risk for loculation, as well as for evidence of empyema. In either setting, immediate drainage will be required.

Sputum Gram stain analysis and culture is noninvasive, relatively inexpensive, and readily available in most institutions; however, its lack of specificity has led to studies of other methods of making a microbiologic diagnosis of pneumonia. Initial attempts to standardize sputum analysis have largely proven unrewarding. A report from the Mayo Clinic utilizing the criteria of more than 25 PMN cells and fewer than 10 epithelial cells per field as representative of an acceptable specimen of lower respiratory tract secretions resulted in discarding 74% of specimens (85). Patients who lack a productive cough present an additional problem; however, sputum production can often be facilitated by ultrasonic mobilization with hypertonic saline. Regardless, the collected specimen must transverse the oropharyngeal passage, allowing for potential contamination. Despite numerous attempts to improve specificity, routine sputum cultures as well as quantitative cultures have proven to be unreliable indicators of the organism(s) involved in nosocomial pneumonia (55,56,80).

Because of the limitation of induced sputum analysis, other methods have been evaluated for sensitivity and specificity (Table 5). One such example is endotracheal aspiration (EA), which is frequently utilized in intubated patients. Unfortunately, the proximity of the trachea to the upper airway allows for oropharyngeal bacteria to contaminate even these specimens. Studies of the utility of EA to predict pneumonia in intubated patients have used differing criteria to define pneumonia (81,86,87). Nevertheless, studies that used the most stringent of criteria, such as quantitative culture of EA with growth of 10^5 colony-forming units (cfu) per milliliter, detected 86% to 100% of infections but had a specificity of only 29% to 59% (81,86). This lack of specificity has led to the development of other methods which attempt to minimize oropharyngeal contamination.

One such method is transtracheal aspiration (TTA), which was originally described over 30 years ago and was commonly used in the 1970s. Despite studies showing the sensitivity and specificity of this method to be favorable, it has become unpopular because of concerns about risks to the patient due to its inherent invasiveness and the lack of personnel trained to perform this procedure (88). Alternative methods employed to identify the offending pathogen(s) include protected catheter aspiration (PCA), protected specimen brush (PSB), and quantitative bronchoalveolar lavage (BAL). The PCA procedure is performed by inserting a plugged catheter into the bronchial tree, either blindly or by bronchoscopic guidance; the plug is extruded and a relatively sterile sample of lower respiratory secretions is aspirated. The sample of 0.01 ml is then diluted 100-fold and plated for culture. Several studies evaluating this procedure have revealed that cultures growing at least 10^3 cfu/ml (representing 10^5 cfu/ml in the lung) usually indicate true infection. Although the specificity of this method has been estimated

Table 5 Sensitivity and Specificity of Various Diagnostic Methods for Nosocomial Pneumonia

Method (Reference)	Sensitivity (%)	Specificity (%)
Endotracheal aspirate (81,86,87)	44–100	29–100
Protected catheter aspirate (55,82,86,87)	61–100	84–100
Protected specimen brush (56,77,82,89,90)	65–100	59–100
Quantitative bronchoalveolar lavage (77,78,91,92)	80–100	65–100

Source: Refs. 55, 56, 77, 78, 81, 82, 86, 87, 89–92.

to be 84% to 100%, since both the sample size and the area sampled are small, the sensitivity of PCA has been reported to be as low as 60% (55,82,86,87).

PSB, a technique related to PCA, is performed by inserting a small sheathed brush bronchoscopically into the bronchial tree to collect a sample for quantitative cultures. This method also uses 10^3 cfu/ml as a threshold value to define a positive culture. PSB has been extensively studied and found to have a wide variation in sensitivity and specificity, 65% to 100% and 59% to 100%, respectively (56,77, 82,89,90). Not surprisingly, administration of antimicrobial therapy decreased both sensitivity and specificity of these techniques, while persistent contamination with colonizing organisms contributes to false-positive results (89,90).

A final method that has been utilized to determine the etiology of nosocomial pneumonia is quantitative BAL. This method sequentially instills and aspirates a physiologic solution into lung subsegments through a catheter. The procedure is performed by advancing a catheter into the bronchial tree, either by fiberoptic bronchoscopy or blindly, with a particular lung segment being isolated by inflating an occluding balloon. Sterile saline (from 50 to 150 ml) is instilled through the catheter, and samples are aspirated. Sampling is selected based on the location of the infiltrate on chest radiograph or by direct visualization of the subsegment containing purulent secretions. Complications from BAL are generally minor, including benign postbronchoscopy fever, abnormalities in chest radiography, short-lived declines in PaO_2, and, rarely, pneumothorax, hemoptysis, and exacerbation of respiratory failure. Quantitative BAL cultures have several potential advantages over PCA and PSB in the evaluation of patients with nosocomial pneumonia. BAL samples larger areas, increasing its sensitivity, and allows for larger sampling volume for simultaneous culture and direct microscopic examination. Generally, 10^4 cfu/ml has been used as the threshold for positive quantitative BAL cultures, resulting in relatively high sensitivity and specificity (Table 5) (77,78,91,92). In addition, microscopic identification of intracellular organisms recovered by bronchoalveolar lavage (BAL-ICO) may allow for early and accurate diagnosis of pneumonia in mechanically ventilated patients. Although limited data regarding this particular technique exist, the sensitivity of BAL-ICO has been reported to be 63% to 100%, with specificity as high as 100% (77,93).

More research is needed to improve diagnostic methods for defining the etiology of hospital-acquired pneumonia. Although the techniques described above are promising, data remain somewhat limited, standardization is poor, and sensitivity and specificity vary among institutions. In addition, bronchoscopic and TTA methods require special expertise, are invasive, and are expensive. At this time, most patients should be evaluated by sputum analysis, with more invasive methods reserved for those who fail to respond to empiric therapy. Clearly, there is also a need for future studies to determine the effect of these procedures on therapeutic decisions and patient outcomes.

V. ANTIMICROBIAL THERAPY

Several factors have been shown to be associated with poor outcome in nosocomial pneumonia (6,8,10,94). These include patients with severe pneumonia, as assessed by chest radiograph, high A-a gradient, signs of impending respiratory failure, or shock (6,10,95). Other poor prognosticators include advanced age, underlying neoplasm, and other severe underlying diseases (6,8,10,95). Poor outcomes can also be predicted by a delay in therapy or the initiation of inappropriate antimicrobials. Finally, there is a less favorable prognosis for those infected by resistant and/or virulent pathogens, such as *P. aeruginosa* (6,16,94). Consequently, once the clinical diagnosis of nosocomial pneumonia has been made, appropriate empiric therapy is imperative to minimize morbidity and mortality.

Efforts should be directed toward identifying an etiologic agent so that antimicrobial use can be guided by susceptibility studies. Appropriate empiric therapy should be primarily guided by host factors and sputum Gram stain. In severely ill patients who develop a hospital-acquired pulmonary infection, empiric therapy should be directed toward the most virulent aerobic gram-negative bacilli, such as *P. aeruginosa*. Depending on the clinical situation and initial Gram stain, consideration should also be given to treating aerobic streptococci and anaerobes, which normally colonize the oropharyngeal area, as well as *S. aureus*, the single most commonly isolated pathogen (52,56,57).

Several microbiologic and antimicrobial factors should be considered when choosing empiric therapy for patients with nosocomial pneumonia. First and foremost, the clinician must be cognizant of the antimicrobial resistance patterns of the specific hospital and unit. In addition, antimicrobials have unique properties that are often relevant to specific situations. Some agents used in combination are synergistic, while others can be antagonistic. β Lactams with aminoglycosides represent one combination where synergistic killing is consistently observed for *P. aeruginosa* and many other virulent gram-negative bacilli (96). In contrast, cephalosporin-penicillin combinations have been described to be antagonistic against such bacteria in vitro (97). In addition, some agents alone or in combination are more likely to promote the emergence of resistance than others. For example, cephalosporins have been shown to rapidly induce resistance when used to treat *Enterobacter* species (98).

Recent guidelines published by the American Thoracic Society (99) propose an approach to empiric therapy for nosocomial pneumonia based on three factors: the severity of the pneumonia, the timing of onset of the pneumonia (<5 d v >5 d of admission), and the presence of specific host or therapeutic factors predisposing to specific pathogens. In light of the virulence of pathogens implicated in severe hospital-acquired pneumonias, many recommend empiric therapy with an aminoglycoside and a β-lactam agent, such as an antipseudomonal penicillin (mezlocillin, piperacillin, azlocillin, or a β-lactam/β-lactamase inhibitor combination) or

Table 6 Approach to Empiric Therapy of Nosocomial Pneumonia

Mild to moderate pneumonia
  Treat nonpseudomonal gram-negative bacilli
    Options
      Nonpseudomonal third-generation cephalosporin (ceftriaxone, ceftizoxime, cefotaxime)
      β-lactam/β-lactamase inhibitor combination
      Fluoroquinolone (ciprofloxacin, ofloxacin)
      Imipenem/cilastatin[a]
      Clindamycin and Azthreonam
Severe pneumonia
(Includes moderate pneumonia in patients with prolonged hospitalization, previous antibiotics, intensive care unit)
  Treat nosocomial gram-negative bacilli, including *P. aeruginosa*
    Options
      Aminoglycosides[b] *PLUS*
      Antipseudomonal penicillin (piperacillin, azlocillin, mezlocillin)
      Ceftazidime
      Aztreonam
      Imipenem/cilastatin
      β-lactam/β-lactamase inhibitor combination
      Fluoroquinolone (ciprofloxacin)
Special considerations
  Corticosteroids—add treatment for *Legionella* species
    Erythromycin ± rifampin
  Diabetes mellitus, coma, trauma, renal failure, Gram stain with gram-positive cocci in clusters—add treatment for *S. aureus*
    Nafcillin, oxacillin, vancomycin (if risk for methicillin resistance[c])
  Witnessed aspiration or thoracoabdominal surgery—add treatment for anaerobes
    Clindamycin, metronidazole, β-lactam/β-lactamase inhibitor

[a]Imipenem/cilastatin is generally reserved for resistant pathogens.
[b]Synergy most reliable if aminoglycosides used with β-lactams; consider once-daily dosing.
[c]Methicillin-resistant *S. aureus* more common in subjects with prior antibiotic use, in intensive care unit, or nursing home-acquired.
Source: Refs. 53, 71, 96, 99–103.

ceftazidime (Table 6). Alternative agents to β-lactams would include imipenem-cilastatin, which has broad spectrum of activity for aerobic gram-negative bacilli, including *P. aeruginosa*; gram-positive bacteria, including methicillin-sensitive *S. aureus*; and essentially all anaerobes. Options in patients who have life-threatening allergic reactions to penicillins or known allergies to all β-lactams include aztreonam, a monobactam that does not cross-react with β-lactams, or fluoroquinolones. Although studies have shown that synergism is critical for the treatment of pseudomonal pneumonia, studies in less severely ill patients with less virulent pathogens have shown equivalent outcomes with monotherapy as that with combinations (53,100).

While aminoglycosides offer synergy, which may be important in treating particularly virulent organisms, there are genuine concerns in using this class of agents. First, they do not achieve high levels in pulmonary secretions and are inactivated by an acid environment, as is often seen in areas of infection. These limitations make this drug inappropriate as monotherapy for gram-negative pneumonia. In addition, many clinicians are reluctant to use aminoglycosides because of the potential for oto- and nephrotoxicity. This concern should only rarely be a problem for empiric therapy, pending identification of the offending pathogen. If the pneumonia is not severe or if virulent pathogens such as *P. aeruginosa* are not detected, the aminoglycoside may be discontinued and the patient may be treated with monotherapy (100). The dosing of aminoglycosides has also evolved from multiple daily infusions, with careful monitoring of peaks and troughs to ensure efficacy and limit toxicity, to once-daily dosing. Daily dosing of 5 to 7 mg/kg/day of drugs such as gentamicin or tobramycin in patients with normal renal function maximizes peak levels, which correlate with efficacy, and have been shown in several studies to result in less nephrotoxicity (101–103).

Reasonable guidelines for empiric therapy of nonneutropenic patients with severe nosocomial pneumonia, those in ICUs, or those with prior antibiotic use would include a once-daily aminoglycoside with an antipseudomonal β-lactam antibiotic. Patients with severe nosocomial pneumonia would include those admitted to an ICU, those who require mechanical ventilation, those who require $>40\%$ oxygen to maintain an arterial oxygen saturation of $>90\%$, and those with rapid radiographic progression, multilobar pneumonia, or evidence of sepsis with hypotension or end-organ dysfunction (71). Patients without these risk factors, or those who have experienced a good clinical response and found not to be infected with *P. aeurginosa* or other resistant pathogens, can then be changed to appropriate monotherapy. Other therapies that should be considered empirically, or based on additional microbiologic data, include treatment for *S. aureus* in those with diabetes mellitus, renal failure and/or a suggestive Gram stain or positive culture, and antianaerobic therapy for those with overt aspiration or negative cultures. In addition, failure to respond to β-lactam therapy, or patients at high risk, should be evaluated and treated for *Legionella* infection. Therapy in all patients should be modified based on subsequent microbiologic culture and susceptibility data, when available.

VI. PREVENTIVE MEASURES

Several interventions have been identified that can reduce the risk of acquiring nosocomial pneumonia. These include measures that delay colonization of reservoir sites, prevent inoculation into the distal lung, or aid host defenses. The CDC

Table 7 Prevention of Nosocomial Pneumonia

Education of health care workers
Surveilance of high-risk patients
Isolation of patients and multiply resistant respiratory pathogens
Aseptic technique for respiratory tract manipulation
Proper disinfection and maintenance of respiratory equipment
Ventilator circuit changes at intervals of ⩾48 h
Precautions to avoid drainage of ventilator tubing condensate toward patient
Hand washing
Use of barrier equipment and gloves
Elevation of head of bed for patients at risk for gastric aspiration
Preservation of gastric acidity
Optimization of nutritional status of severely ill patients
Vaccination—pneumococcal influenza

Source: Refs. 1, 37, 39, 104, 106, 109.

has recently published guidelines incorporating many of these measures (1). These include simple as well as more complex and controversial interventions (Table 7).

Maneuvers such as positioning and drainage of subglottic secretions may be beneficial. Positioning of patients can prevent pooling of secretions, stasis and hypoventilation in the lung, and aspiration. In fact, studies have shown that placing patients in a semirecumbent position, elevated to a 45° angle, decreased the incidence of aspirating a tracer when compared to the supine position (104). The role of subglottic drainage, such as through specially designed endotracheal tubes, although promising in two randomized studies, remains controversial and requires further study before being broadly recommended (105,106).

Since it has been shown that colonization of gastric secretions may act as a reservoir for bacteria, a great deal of interest has been focused on the detrimental effects of stress ulcer prophylaxis with antacids and antisecretory agents. Although controversy exists regarding the role of increased gastric pH and the development of nosocomial pneumonia, many studies support avoiding agents which decrease gastric acidity in hospitalized subjects (37,39). Other investigators have evaluated the use of selective digestive decontamination (SDD) as a way to decrease the reservoir of bacterial pathogens in the gastrointestinal tract. Studies have primarily utilized nonabsorbable antibiotics, such as polymyxin, aminoglycosides, amphotericin B, and sometimes fluoroquinolones or third-generation cephalosporins to lower bacterial colony counts (107). Although bacterial counts do appear to be reduced by such measures, consistent decreases in the rates of nosocomial pneumonia have not been shown (108). Because of the cost of such interventions and the concern of promoting resistance, SDD has not been endorsed pending more definitive outcome studies.

Universally accepted measures to prevent nosocomial pneumonia include adequate reprocessing of ventilation equipment and infection control measures in the patient care area. The CDC guidelines emphasize aseptic technique for respiratory tract manipulation, proper disinfection and maintenance of respiratory therapy equipment, and hand washing to prevent transmission of pathogenic microorganisms between patients (1). Other measures include changing ventilator circuits at intervals of 48 h or longer, precautions to prevent drainage of ventilator tubing condensate toward the patient, elevating the head of the bed by at least 30° for patients at risk for gastric aspiration, and optimizing the nutritional status of severely ill patients (1) (Table 7). Poor nutritional status has also been associated with nosocomial pneumonia, leading to the current trend of early nutritional supports for critically ill patients (109). Early enteral feeding may help maintain epithelial barriers and prevent pneumonia caused by translocation or migration of bacteria across the GI epithelial barrier (110).

VII. CONCLUSION

Nosocomial pneumonia represents a common complication of hospitalization which contributes to morbidity, mortality, cost of medical care, and the emergence of resistant pathogens. This problem persists despite the development of increasingly potent and broad-spectrum antimicrobials and substantial interest in preventing and managing nosocomial pneumonia. Major advances in this disease will require improving and standardizing the sensitivity and specificity of diagnostic criteria as well as the diagnostic tests utilized to identify the causative pathogen(s). Pending such advances, a high index of suspicion is required and early broad-spectrum antimicrobial therapy must be initiated based on the microbiologic and resistance patterns of the given institution. Empiric therapy should then be modified based on the individual clinical response and the results of microbiologic studies. Optimal management of patients with hospital-acquired pneumonia requires a close multidisciplinary collaboration between pulmonary and critical care specialists, infectious disease specialists, infection control practitioners and hospital microbiologists. This type of collaborative approach will result in early recognition and appropriate management of resistant pathogens and common source outbreaks. Prevention of nosocomial pneumonia is the most effective way to avoid disease-associated mortality, as well as the most cost-efficient approach. Preventive measures should be applied in all patients at risk.

REFERENCES

1. Tablan OC, Anderson LJ, Arden NH, Breiman RF, Butler JC, McNeil MM, Pearson ML. Guidelines for prevention of nosocomial pneumonia. Hospital Infection Control Practices Advisory Committee, Centers for Disease Control and Prevention. MMWR 1997; 46(No. RR-1):1–77.

2. Horan TC, White JW, Jarvis WR. Nosocomial infection surveillance, 1984. MMWR 1986; 35:17SS–29SS.
3. Haley RW, Culver DH, White JW, et al. The efficacy of infection surveillance and control programs in preventing nosocomial infections in US hospitals. Am J Epidemiol 1985; 121:182–205.
4. National Nosocomial Infections Surveillance (NNIS) Semiannual Report, May 1995. Am J Infect Control 1995; 23:373–385.
5. Haley RW, Hooton TM, Culver DH, et al. Nosocomial infections in US hospitals, 1975–1976: estimated frequency by selected characteristics of patients. Am J Med 1981; 70:947–959.
6. Celis R, Torres A, Gatell JM, Almela M, Rodriguez-Roisin R, Agusti-Vidal A. Nosocomial pneumonia: a multivariate analysis of risk and prognosis. Chest 1988; 93:318–324.
7. Craven DE, Kunches LM, Kilinsky V, Lichtenberg DA, Make BJ, McCabe WR. Risk factors for pneumonia and fatality in patients receiving continuous mechanical ventilation. Am Rev Respir Dis 1986; 16:128–140.
8. Leu HS, Kaiser DL, Mori M, Woolson RF, Wenzel RP. Hospital-acquired pneumonia: attributable mortality and morbidity. Am J Epidemiol 1989; 129:1258–1267.
9. Fagon JY, Novara A, Stephan F, Girou E, Safar M. Mortality attributable to nosocomial infections in the ICU. Infect Control Hosp Epidemiol 1994; 15(7):428–434.
10. Torres A, Aznar R, Gatell JM, et al. Incidence, risk, and prognosis factors of nosocomial pneumonia in mechanically ventilated patients. Am Rev Respir Dis 1990; 142:523–528.
11. Kollef MH. Ventilator-associated pneumonia. JAMA 1993; 270:1965–1970.
12. Emori TG, Banerjee SN, Culver DH, et al. Nosocomial infections in elderly patients in the United States, 1986–1990. Am J Med 1991; 91(suppl 3B):289S–293S.
13. Freeman J, Rosner BA, McGowan JE. Adverse effects of nosocomial infection. J Infect Dis 1979; 140:732–740.
14. Fagon J-Y, Chastre J, Hance AJ, Montravers P, Novara A, Gibert C. Nosocomial pneumonia in ventilated patients: a cohort study evaluating attributable mortality and hospital stay. Am J Med 1993; 94:281–288.
15. Rello J, Ausina V, Ricart M, Castella J, Prats G. Impact of previous antimicrobial therapy on the etiology and outcome of ventilator-associated pneumonia. Chest 1993; 104:1230–1235.
16. Fagon J-Y, Chastre J, Domart Y, et al. Nosocomial pneumonia in patients receiving continuous mechanical ventilation: prospective analysis of 52 episodes with use of a protected specimen brush and quantitative culture techniques. Am Rev Respir Dis 1989; 139:877–884.
17. Emori TG, Gaynes RP. An overview of nosocomial infections, including the role of the microbiology laboratory. Clin Microbiol Rev 1993; 6:428–442.
18. Jiminez P, Torres A, Rodriguez-Roisin R, et al. Incidence and etiology of pneumonia acquired during mechanical ventilation. Crit Care Med 1989; 17:882–885.
19. Rodriguez JL, Gibbons KJ, Bitzer LG, Dechert RE, Steinberg SM, Flint LM. Pneumonia: incidence, risk factors, and outcome in injured patients. J Trauma 1991; 31:907–912.
20. Wiblin RT, Wenzel RP. Hospital-acquired pneumonia. Curr Clin Top Infect Dis 1996; 16:195–214.

21. Huxley EJ, Viroslav J, Gray WR. Pharyngeal aspiration in normal adults and patients with suppressed consciousness. Am J Med 1978; 64:564–568.
22. Johanson WG, Pierce AK. Nosocomial respiratory infections with gram-negative bacilli: the significance of colonization of the respiratory tract. Ann Intern Med 1972; 77:701–706.
23. Johanson WG, Pierce AK, Sanford JP. Changing bacterial flora of hospitalized patients: emergence of gram-negative bacilli. N Engl J Med 1969; 281:1137–1140.
24. Rosenthal S, Tager IB. Prevalence of gram-negative rods in normal pharyngeal flora. Ann Intern Med 1975; 83:355–357.
25. Mackowiak PA, Martin RM, Jones SR, Smith JW. Pharyngeal colonization by gram-negative bacilli in aspiration-prone persons. Arch Intern Med 1978; 138:1224–1227.
26. Valenti WM, Trudell RG, Bentley DW. Factors predisposing to oropharyngeal colonization with gram-negative bacilli in the aged. N Engl J Med 1978; 298:1108–1111.
27. Niederman MS. Bacterial adherence as a mechanism of airway colonization. Eur J Clin Microbiol Infect Dis 1989; 8:15–20.
28. Johnason WG Jr, Higuchi JH, Chaudhuri TR. Bacterial adherence to epithelial cells in bacillary colonization of the respiratory tract. Am Rev Respir Dis 1980; 121: 55–63.
29. LaForce FM, Hopkins J, Trow R. Human oral defenses against gram-negative rods. Am Rev Respir Dis 1976; 114:929–935.
30. Johanson WG, Woods DE, Chaudhuri T. Association of respiratory tract colonization with adherence of gram-negative bacilli to epithelial cells. J Infect Dis 1979; 139:667–673.
31. Higuchi JH, Johanson WG. The relationship between adherence of *Pseudomonas aeruginosa* to upper respiratory cells in vitro and susceptibility to colonization in vivo. J Lab Clin Med 1980; 95:698–704.
32. Woods DE, Straus DC, Johanson WG Jr, Bass JA. Role of salivary protease activity in adherence of gram-negative bacilli to mammalian buccal epithelial cells in vivo. J Clin Invest 1981; 68:1435–1440.
33. Woods DE, Straus DC, Johanson WG Jr, Berry VK, Bass JA. Role of pili in adherence of *Pseudomonas aeruginosa* to mammalian buccal epithelial cells. Infect Immun 1980; 29:1146–1151.
34. Niederman MS, Merrill WW, Polomski LM, Reynolds HY, Gee JB. Influence of sputum IgA and elastase on tracheal cell bacterial adherence. Am Rev Respir Dis 1986; 133:255–260.
35. Woods DE, Straus DC, Johanson WG, Bass JA. Role of fibronectin in the prevention of adherence of *Pseudomonas aeruginosa* to buccal cells. J Infect Dis 1981; 143: 784–790.
36. Gianella RA, Broitman SA, Zamcheck N. Influence of gastric acidity on bacterial and parasitic enteric infections: a perspective. Ann Intern Med 1973; 78:271–276.
37. du Moulin GC, Paterson DG, Hedley-Whyte J, Libson A. Aspiration of gastric bacteria in antacid-treated patients: a frequent cause of postoperative colonisation of the airway. Lancet 1982; 1:242–245.
38. Atherton ST, White DJ. Stomach as source of bacteria colonizing respiratory tract during artificial ventilation. Lancet 1978; 2:968–969.

39. Prod'hom G, Leuenberger P, Koerfer J, et al. Nosocomial pneumonia in mechanically ventilated patients receiving antacid, ranitidine, or sucralfate as prophylaxis for stress ulcer: a randomized controlled trial. Ann Intern Med 1994; 120(8): 653–662.
40. Arnold I. The bacterial flora within the stomach and small intestine: the effect of experimental alterations of acid-base balance and the age of the subject. Am J Med Sci 1933; 186:471–481.
41. Drasar BS, Shiner M. Studies of the intestinal flora. II. Bacterial flora of the small intestine in patients with gastrointestinal disorders. Gut 1969.
42. Donowitz LG, Page MC, Mileur GL, Guenthner SH. Alteration of normal gastric flora in critical care patients receiving antacid and cimetidine therapy. Infect Control 1986; 7:23–26.
43. Maki DG. Control of colonization and transmission of pathogenic bacteria in the hospital. Ann Intern Med 1978; 89:777–780.
44. Albert RK, Condie F. Handwashing patterns in medical intensive care units. N Engl J Med 1981; 304:1465–1466.
45. Rodriguez JL. Hospital-acquired pneumonia in critically ill, injured patients. Am J Surg 1993; 165(2A suppl):34S–42S.
46. Mosconi P, Langer M, Cigada M, Mandelli M. Epidemiology and risk factors of pneumonia in critically ill patients. Intensive Care Unit Group for Infection Control. Eur J Epidemiol 1991; 7:320–327.
47. Chevret S, Hemmer M, Carlet J, Langer M. Incidence and risk factors of pneumonia acquired in intensive care units: results from a multicenter prospective study on 996 patients. European Cooperative Group of Nosocomial Pneumonia. Intens Care Med 1993; 19:256–264.
48. Garibaldi RA, Britt MR, Coleman ML, Reading JC, Pace NL. Risk factors for postoperative pneumonia. Am J Med 1981; 70:677–680.
49. Craven DE, Steger KA. Epidemiology of nosocomial pneumonia: new perspectives on an old disease. Chest 1995; 108(2)suppl:1S–6S.
50. Sprunt K, Redman W. Evidence suggesting importance of role of interbacterial inhibition in maintaining balance of normal flora. Ann Intern Med 1968; 68:579–590.
51. Flynn DM, Weinstein RA, Nathans C, Gaston MA, Kabins SA. Patients' endogenous flora as the source of "nosocomial" *Enterobacter* in cardiac surgery. J Infect Dis 1987; 156:363–368.
52. NNIS Semiannual Report, Centers for Disease Control and Prevention, May 1996.
53. Schleupner CJ, Cobb DK. A study of the etiologies and treatment of nosocomial pneumonia in a community-based teaching hospital. Infect Control Hosp Epidemiol 1992; 13:515–525.
54. Rello J, Quintana E, Ausina V, et al. Incidence, etiology, and outcome of nosocomial pneumonia in mechanically ventilated patients. Chest 1991; 100:439–444.
55. Torres A, de la Bellacasa JP, Xaubet A, et al. Diagnostic value of quantitative cultures of bronchoalveolar lavage and telescoping plugged catheters in mechanically ventilated patients with bacterial pneumonia. Am Rev Respir Dis 1989; 140: 306–310.
56. Bartlett JG, O'Keefe P, Tally F, Louie TJ, Gorbach SL. Bacteriology of hospital-acquired pneumonia. Arch Intern Med 1986; 146:868–871.

57. Lorber B, Swenson RM. Bacteriology of aspiration pneumonia: a prospective study of community- and hospital-acquired cases. Ann Intern Med 1974; 81:329–331.
58. Muder RR, Yu VL, McClure JK, Kroboth FJ, Kominos S, Lumish RM. Nosocomial Legionnaires' disease uncovered in a prospective pneumonia study: implications for underdiagnosis. JAMA 1983; 249:3184–3188.
59. Valenti WM, Hall CB, Douglas JR. Nosocomial viral infections I: epidemiology and significance. Infect Control 1980; 1:33–37.
60. Arnow PM, Anderson RL, Mainous PD, Smith EJ. Pulmonary aspergillosis during hospital renovation. Am Rev Respir Dis 1978; 118:49–53.
61. Hopkins CC, Weber DJ, Rubin RH. Invasive aspergillosis infection: possible non-ward common source within the hospital environment. J Hosp Infect 1989; 13: 19–25.
62. Fischl MA, Daikos GL, Uttamchandani RB, et al. Clinical presentation and outcome of patients with HIV infection and tuberculosis caused by multiple-drug-resistant bacilli. Ann Intern Med 1992; 117:184–190.
63. Kirby BD, Snyder KM, Meyer RD, Finegold SM. Legionnaires' disease: report of sixty-five nosocomially acquired cases and review of the literature. Medicine 1980; 59:188–205.
64. Marie TJ, MacDonald S, Clarke K. Nosocomial Legionnaires' disease: lessons from a four-year prospective study. Am J Infect Control 1991; 19:79–85.
65. Haley CE, Cohen ML, Halter J, Meyer RD. Nosocomial Legionnaires' disease: a continuing common-source epidemic at Wadsworth Medical Center. Ann Intern Med 1979; 90:583–586.
66. Yu VL, Beam TR Jr, Lumish RM, et al. Routine culturing for *Legionella* in the hospital environment may be a good idea: a three-hospital prospective study. Am J Med Sci 1987; 294:97–99.
67. Carratala J, Gudiol F, Pallares R, et al. Risk factors for nosocomial *Legionella pneumophila* pneumonia. Am J Respir Crit Care Med 1994; 149:625–629.
68. Roig J, Aguilar X, Ruiz J, et al. Comparative study of *Legionella pneumophila* and other nosocomial-acquired pneumonias. Chest 1991; 99:344–350.
69. Hall CB. Nosocomial viral respiratory infections: perennial weeks on pediatric wards. Am J Med 1981; 70:670–676.
70. Hall CB, Douglas RG, Geiman JM, Messner MK. Nosocomial respiratory syncytial virus infections. N Engl J Med 1975; 293:1343–1346.
71. Mandell LA, Marrie TJ, Niederman MS. Initial antimicrobial treatment of hospital acquired pneumonia in adults: a conference report. Can J Infect Dis 1993; 4: 317–321.
72. Skerrett SJ, Niederman MS, Fein AM. Respiratory infections and acute lung injury in systemic illness. Clin Chest Med 1989; 10:469–502.
73. Rodrigues J, Niederman MS, Fein AM, Pai PB. Nonresolving pneumonia in steroid-treated patients with obstructive lung disease. Am J Med 1992; 93:29–34.
74. Esperson F, Gabrielsen J. Pneumonia due to *Staphylococcus arueus* during mechanical ventilation. J Infect Dis 1981; 144:19–23.
75. Rello J, Quintana E, Ausina V, Puzo C, Net A, Prats G. Risk factors for *Staphylococcus aureus* nosocomial pneumonia in critically ill patients. Am Rev Respir Dis 1990; 142:1320–1324.

76. Rello J, Torres A, Ricart M, et al. Ventilator-associated pneumonia by *Staphylococcus aureus*: comparison of methicillin-resistant and methicillin-sensitive episodes. Am J Respir Crit Care Med 1994; 150:1545–1549.
77. Chastre J, Fagon J-Y, Soler P, et al. Diagnosis of nosocomial bacterial pneumonia in intubated patients undergoing ventilation: comparison of the usefulness of bronchoalveolar lavage and the protected specimen brush. Am J Med 1988; 85:499–506.
78. Griffin JJ, Meduri GU. New approaches in the diagnosis of nosocomial pneumonia. Med Clin North Am 1994; 78(5):1091–1121.
79. Davidson M, Tempest B, Palmer DL. Bacteriologic diagnosis of acute pneumonia. JAMA 1976; 235:158–163.
80. Andrews CP, Coalson JJ, Smith JD, Johanson WG. Diagnosis of nosocomial bacterial pneumonia in acute, diffuse lung injury. Chest 1981; 80:254–258.
81. Salata RA, Lederman MM, Shlaes DM, et al. Diagnosis of nosocomial pneumonia in intubated, intensive care unit patients. Am Rev Respir Dis 1987; 135: 426–432.
82. Pham LH, Brun-Buisson C, Legrand P, et al. Diagnosis of nosocomial pneumonia in mechanically ventilated patients: comparison of a plugged telescoping catheter with the protected specimen brush. Am Rev Respir Dis 1991; 143:1055–1061.
83. Meduri GU. Diagnosis and differential diagnosis of ventilator-associated pneumonia. Clin Chest Med 1995; 16(1):61–93.
84. Meduri GU. Diagnosis of ventilator-associated pneumonia. Infect Dis Clin North Am 1993; 7:295–329.
85. Murray PR, Washington JA. Microscopic and bacteriologic analysis of sputum. Mayo Clin Proc 1975; 50:339–344.
86. Torres A, de la Bellacasa JP, Rodriguez-Roisin R, de Anta MTJ, Agusti-Vidal A. Diagnostic value of telescoping plugged catheters in mechanically ventilated patients with bacterial pneumonia using the Metras catheter. Am Rev Respir Dis 1988; 138:117–120.
87. Jorda R, Parras F, Ibanez J, Reina J, Bergada J, Raurich JM. Diagnosis of nosocomial pneumonia in mechanically ventilated patients by the blind protected telescoping catheter. Intens Care Med 1993; 19:377–382.
88. Griffith DE, Mazurek GH. Pneumonia in chronic obstructive lung disease. Infect Dis Clin North Am 1991; 5:467–484.
89. Chastre J, Viau F, Brun P, et al. Prospective evaluation of the protected specimen brush for the diagnosis of pulmonary infections in ventilated patients. Am Rev Respir Dis 1984; 130:924–929.
90. Fagon J-Y, Chastre J, Hance AJ, et al. Detection of nosocomial lung infection in ventilated patients: use of a protected specimen brush and quantitative culture techniques in 147 patients. Am Rev Respir Dis 1988; 138:110–116.
91. Meduri GU, Beals DH, Maijub AG, Baselski V. Protected bronchoalveolar lavage: a new bronchoscopic technique to retrieve uncontaminated distal airway secretions. Am Rev Respir Dis 1991; 143:855–864.
92. Baselski VS, el-Torky M, Coalson JJ, Griffin JP. The standardization of criteria for processing and interpreting laboratory specimens in patients with suspected ventilator-associated pneumonia. Chest 1992; 102(suppl 1):571S–579S.
93. Sole-Violan J, Rodriguez de Castro F, Rey A, Martin-Gonzalez JC, Cabrera-Navarro

P. Usefulness of microscopic examination of intracellular organisms in lavage fluid in ventilator-associated pneumonia. Chest 1994; 106(3):889–894.

94. George D. Nosocomial pneumonia. In: Mayhall G, ed. Hospital Epidemiology and Infection Control. Baltimore: Williams Wilkins, 1996.
95. Kollef MH. Ventilator-associated pneumonia: a multivariate analysis. JAMA 1993; 270:1965–1970.
96. Hilf M, Yu VL, Sharp J, Zuravleff JJ, Korvick JA, Muder RR. Antibiotic therapy for *Pseudomonas aeruginosa* bacteremia: outcome correlations in a prospective study of 200 patients. Am J Med 1989; 87:540–546.
97. Sanders CC. Novel resistance selected by the new expanded spectrum cephalosporins: a concern. J Infect Dis 1983; 147:585.
98. Chow JW, Fine MJ, Shlaes DM, et al. *Enterobacter* bacteremia: clinical features and emergence of antibiotic resistance during therapy. Ann Intern Med 1991; 115: 585–590.
99. Campbell DG, Niederman MS, Broughton WA, Craven DE, Fein AM, Fink MP, Gleeson K, Hornick DB, Lynch JP, Mandell LA, Mason CM, Torres A, Wunderink RG. Hospital-acquired pneumonia in adults: diagnosis, assessment of severity, initial antimicrobial therapy, and prevention strategies. A Consensus Statement, American Thoracic Society. Am J Respir Crit Care Med 1996; 153;1711–1725.
100. Niederman MS. An approach to empiric therapy of nosocomial pneumonia. Med Clin North Am 1994; 78(5):1123–1141.
101. Miyagawa CI. Aminoglycosides in the intensive care unit. An old drug in a dynamic environment. New Horizons 1993; 1:172–180.
102. Prins JM, Buller HR, Lujper EF, Kuijper J, Tange RA, Speelman P. Once versus thrice daily gentamicin in patients with serious infections. Lancet 1993; 341:335–339.
103. Nicolau DP, Freeman CD, Belliveau PP, Nightingale CH, Ross JW, Quintiliani R. Experience with a once-daily aminoglycoside program administered to 2,184 adult patients. Antimicrob Agents Chemother 1995; 39:650–655.
104. Torres A, Serra-Batlles J, Ros E, et al. Pulmonary aspiration of gastric contents in patients receiving mechanical ventilation: the effect of body position. Ann Intern Med 1992; 116:540–543.
105. Valles J, Artigas A, Rello J, et al. Continuous aspiration of subglottic secretions in preventing ventilator-associated pneumonia. Ann Intern Med 1995; 122(3): 179–186.
106. Mahul PH, Auboyer C, Jospe R, et al. Prevention of nosocomial pneumonia (NP) in intubated patients: respective role of mechanical subglottic secretions drainage and stress ulcer prophylaxis. Intens Care Med 1992; 18:20–25.
107. Duncan RA, Steger KA, Craven DE. Selective decontamination of the digestive tract: risks outweigh benefits for intensive care unit patients. Semin Respir Infect 1993; 8:308–324.
108. Ferrer M, Torres A, Gonzalez J, et al. Utility of selective digestive decontamination in mechanically ventilated patients. Ann Intern Med 1994; 120:389–395.
109. Gorse GJ, Messner RL, Stephens ND. Association of malnutrition with nosocomial infection. Infect Control Hosp Epidemiol 1989; 10:194–203.
110. Deitch EA, Berg R. Bacterial translocation from the gut: a mechanism of infection. J Burn Care Rehab 1987; 8:475–482.

6

Cardiac Infections

STEFAN SCHNEIDER

Cedars-Sinai Medical Center, Los Angeles, California

PAULA L. GAUT

Cedars-Sinai Medical Center and University of California, Los Angeles, School of Medicine, Los Angeles, California

I. VIRAL MYOCARDITIS

A. Introduction

Myocarditis, an inflammatory process of the myocardium, continues to present clinicians with considerable diagnostic difficulties and limited therapeutic options (1). The diagnosis is suggested by typical clinical features and confirmed pathologically by transvenous endomyocardial biopsy (TEB) if indicated (2,3). A wide variety of viruses have been implicated as causes of myocarditis (Table 1). Most prominent are the enteroviruses, specifically of the Coxsackie B group, causing up to 40% of myocarditis (4–7). The chronological association of cardiac disease to a viral syndrome, viral cultures of pharyngeal secretions or stool, and a fourfold rise in neutralizing antibody titers to candidate viruses are commonly used as supportive evidence for a viral etiology (6). However, the isolation of a virus from myocardial tissue or pericardial fluid is extremely rare, particularly in adults (7–10).

The current working model for the pathogenesis of viral myocarditis proposes two phases:

1. An acute phase with direct myocyte infection and cytolysis concluding with viral clearance by lymphocytes, macrophages, and specific antibodies
2. A chronic late phase characterized by immune-mediated injury via inflammatory cells and cardiotropic antibodies (6,11).

Table 1 Viral Causes of Myocarditis

Coxsackie A and B	Rubella
Echo	Vaccinia
Influenza A and B	Coronaviruses
Polio	Rabies
Herpes simplex	Hepatitis B
Varicella zoster	Arboviruses
Epstein-Barr	Juninvirus
Cytomegalovirus	HIV
Mumps	

Source: Ref. 11.

Microvascular spasm has recently been suggested as an important mechanism in the pathogenesis of myocarditis (12).

Myocarditis is of particular interest as the inciting event of a pathologic process ultimately leading to the development of idiopathic dilative cardiomyopathy (IDC). This hypothesis is supported by animal models, increased viral antibody titers in patients with IDC compared to controls, identification of viral genome sequences in myocardial tissue by recombinant DNA technology, and the presence of cardiac symptoms and electrocardiographic abnormalities in an increased number (19% in one study) of patients within 6 years after a positive throat culture for Coxsackie virus (13–16). In addition, the incidence of IDC after clinically suspected myocarditis may be as high as 12%, compared to seven cases per 100,000 in the general population (17).

The majority of cases of viral myocarditis are clinically inapparent, and the true incidence and natural history remain unknown (1). A great majority of patients are believed to recover completely (18). Nevertheless, some patients go on to develop IDC and congestive failure. An analysis of TEB findings in patients with congestive heart failure revealed a rate of active myocarditis of approximately 10% (19). Estimates of the prevalence of myocarditis derived from autopsy series may vary from 2.5% to 5% in unselected cases to 21% when victims of sudden death are included (6). The establishment of the so-called Dallas criteria requiring nonsequential myofiber necrosis, either patchy or diffuse together with an inflammatory infiltrate, has been an important step toward standardizing the pathological diagnosis of myocarditis (20–23). Based on these criteria, a recent autopsy series has revealed an incidence of 1.06% for histologically proven myocarditis in adults (20). An unusually high incidence of myocarditis, 35% to 52%, has been reported from autopsy series of patients with acquired immunodeficiency syndrome (AIDS) (24,25). Moreover, a prospective study of echocardiographic findings in hospitalized patients with AIDS showed persistent tachycardia associated with decreased left ventricular fractional shortening and wall thickness in 54%, suggestive of a high frequency of underlying myocardial damage (26).

B. Clinical Manifestations

The clinical manifestations of myocarditis and pericarditis overlap widely. Fever may be present in over 50% of patients. A prodrome of malaise, aches, and sore throat often precedes the onset of myocarditis by approximately 2 weeks (7,27). Chest pain, often atypical or pericardial in character, is present in 35% (28). Of note, myocardial infarction has been described as a rare complication of myocarditis (29). Death in the acute phase is uncommon but can occur due to arrhythmias or heart failure (6,30).

C. Diagnosis

1. *Laboratory Findings*

An elevated erythrocyte sedimentation rate may be present in 60% of patients, with leukocytosis in 24% and a raised creatine kinase MB in 12% of patients (28). The latter may be abnormal in 70% of patients with ST segment elevation and remain elevated for approximately 4 days after myocardial injury (31). Troponin T may persist longer than the creatine kinase MB after myocardial necrosis (32).

2. *Electrocardiographic Findings*

Typical electrocardiographic changes evolve over approximately the first 10 days and resolve by 2 months (32). ST segment elevation, the first electrocardiographic sign of myocardial injury, usually develops on day 1 and is persistent. On days 3 to 5, T-wave inversion is noted. After 1 week, the electrocardiogram (ECG) may regain its normal morphology. At 2 weeks, T-wave inversions will again be seen, followed by a return of the ECG to baseline at 2 months (32,33). Due to the patchy nature of the myocardial lesions, R-wave depression or Q-waves are rarely seen. Right or left bundle branch block may occur in 13% and 18% of patients, respectively; abnormal P-waves in 42%, and atrioventricular (AV) block in 20% of patients (34). Fifteen percent of patients may show T-wave changes only; in these patients, the use of β blockers might aid in distinguishing these changes from functional, nonspecific T-wave alterations (33,34). One study showed abnormal ECGs in 96% of patients fulfilling the Dallas criteria for myocarditis (34).

3. *Echocardiographic Findings*

Up to 69% of patients with histologically proven myocarditis show echocardiographic evidence of left ventricular dysfunction (35). The most common findings are segmental wall motion abnormalities in 64% of patients, end-diastolic diameter above 3.3 cm/m^2 in 50%, decreased ejection fraction in 56%, altered myocardial texture in 23%, right ventricular dysfunction in 23%, abnormal ventricular filling in 20%, and ventricular wall thrombus in 15% of patients (35). Transient ventricular hypertrophy has been described as well (36).

ECG and echocardiographic abnormalities in histologically proven myocarditis may have prognostic significance. In the study by Morgera et al, a left bundle branch block, abnormal QRS complex, and depressed left ventricular ejection fraction were predictive of a worse prognosis (34). Death due to arrhythmia or congestive heart failure was significantly more common when these abnormalities were present, and survival during the 5 years of follow up fell from approximately 90% to 50%.

4. *Nuclear Imaging Studies*

Gallium-67 and indium-111 scanning can be used for the diagnosis of myocarditis since the respective tracers will enhance in areas of mononuclear infiltrate (Ga^{67}) and myocyte necrosis (In^{111}), the two obligate histologic features of viral myocarditis. Indium-111 antimyocyte imaging is 83% to 100% sensitive and 53% to 58% specific when compared to the yield from endomyocardial biopsy. A normal scan had a negative predictive value of 92% (37,38). For Ga^{67} scanning, a sensitivity of 83% and specificity of 86% have been reported (39). These methods may be useful screening tools in the identification of patients most likely to benefit from an endomyocardial biopsy.

5. *Transvenous Endomyocardial Biopsy (TEB)*

Introduced in the 1960s, this technique can provide a histological diagnosis of myocarditis in vivo without surgery, and permits an evaluation of extent and severity of disease (40). Due to the patchy nature of myocarditis, a minimum of four to six specimens needs to be obtained. When TEB is performed in this fashion, sampling error may be $< 5\%$ (41). In suspected myocarditis, TEB needs to be performed soon after onset of symptoms since resolution of active infiltrates has been shown within 4 days of the initial biopsy (42). At present, the only universally accepted diagnoses that warrant TEB are suspected transplant rejection and anthracycline toxicity (3). However, the role of traditional virus isolation as well as newer molecular biologic techniques such as polymerase chain reaction methods in endomyocardial biopsy is currently being evaluated.

D. Treatment

Symptomatic interventions remain the mainstay of treatment for viral myocarditis. Admission for electrocardiographic monitoring is advised to detect and treat associated arrythmias and to exclude myocardial infarction (4,34). Bed rest is recommended based on the increased mortality in mice when exercised early in infection (13). In a mouse model of myocarditis, nonsteroidal anti-inflammatory drugs (NSAIDS) were found to increase viral replication and myocardial necrosis in early but not late disease (43–46). These agents should therefore not be used during the first 2 weeks of viral myocarditis (47). Although ribavirin has been promising in acute myocarditis in animal models, no human data are available to support its clinical use (48).

The use of immunosuppression for the treatment of patients with myocarditis is controversial. Several case reports and uncontrolled trials have both supported and refuted this concept, which is based on the evidence for an autoimmune processes propagating the inflammation in the later stages of myocarditis (49–52). The Myocarditis Treatment Trial was designed to clarify this issue (19). In this randomized controlled study, 111 patients with myocarditis diagnosed by TEB employing the Dallas criteria and a left ventricular ejection fraction (LVEF) of less than 0.45 received either conventional treatment for congestive heart failure alone or immunosuppression for 24 weeks. No difference was demonstrated between the treatment assignments in LVEF, the primary outcome measure, or survival at 24 weeks and 1 year. Therefore, immunosuppressive therapy for the treatment of patients with myocarditis cannot be recommended at this time. Further study may identify certain subgroups of patients who may benefit from this form of therapy (19,53).

Finally, cardiac transplantation is available for patients with terminal heart failure due to viral myocarditis. Because of the high rate of spontaneous recovery from myocarditis, even in the face of severe hemodynamic abnormalities, patients should receive a prolonged trial of drug treatment and, if needed, mechanical support prior to transplantation (11). Furthermore, 1-year patient survival after transplantation for myocarditis is only 58%, compared with 82% when transplanted for other causes, and graft survival is also diminished (54).

E. Complications

1. Arrythmias

Myocarditis may involve the conduction system and is commonly complicated by rhythm disturbances (4). Complex premature ventricular beats have been documented in 27% of patients in one series (55). The potential for arrhythmias may be particularly high during the early phase of myocarditis (55). In the study by Morgera et al, complete AV block was observed in 31% of patients with disease of less than 1 month's duration (34). Bundle branch blocks are common; however, pacing is only rarely required (56). The true incidence of sudden death in myocarditis is unknown. Severe and fatal arrhythmias have been documented (57). When victims of cardiac arrest are examined, histological evidence of myocarditis may be found in 20% to 33% of patients (58,59).

If antiarrhythmic treatment is needed, negative inotrope agents, including β blockers, are best avoided (46,47). Given that a significant proportion of adult patients improve spontaneously, the use of amiodarone and automatic implantable cardioverter defibrillator (AICD) devices should be reserved for life-threatening arrhythmias (11,60,61).

2. Congestive Heart Failure

The true incidence of heart failure in acute myocarditis remains unknown. In general, this complication more commonly occurs in neonates, and is rare in adults

(62). When patients with unexplained heart failure related to dilated cardiomyopathy are examined by TEB, the incidence of myocarditis has ranged from 0% to 67% (63,64). Recent series employing the Dallas criteria have found histologic evidence of myocarditis in such patients in 4% to 12% of patients with unexplained heart failure (19,65,66).

The treatment of cardiac failure in such patients may include rest, salt restriction, diuretics, digitalis glycosides, angiotensin-converting enzyme (ACE) inhibitors, and anticoagulants (11). Digitalis glycosides should be used with caution, since patients with myocarditis may be particularly sensitive to their toxicity. Patients with IDC experience improved survival when ACE inhibitors are administered (67,68). The use of ACE inhibitors has therefore been recommended in patients with myocarditis and systolic dysfunction who are able to tolerate these agents. For patients intolerant of ACE inhibitors, combination therapy with hydralazine and isosorbide dinitrate may be an alternative. Anticoagulation should be considered even when ventricular dysfunction is mild, since active myocarditis appears to be associated with an increased risk of mural thrombus formation (69,70).

II. PERICARDITIS

A. Introduction

All major categories of microbes have been reported as causes of infectious pericarditis, including viruses, bacteria, mycobacteria, fungi, and parasites (71). Infectious pericarditis represents a distinct minority of acute pericarditides in recent series, accounting for as few as 7% of cases, whereas the idiopathic form has been described in up to 86% of cases (72). While the idiopathic form is commonly suspected to be of viral origin, support for this etiology can be found only in 15% to 20% of cases. Virus isolation from pericardial fluid is the exception (73,74).

The purulent form of pericarditis, caused chiefly by bacterial or fungal pathogens, was a common cause of pericarditis in the preantibiotic era (75). With the advent of antibiotics, the incidence of purulent pericarditis has declined and the spectrum of causative bacteria has shifted. *Staphylococcus aureus* and aerobic gram-negative bacilli have replaced *Streptococcus pneumoniae* as the leading pathogens (76,77). Purulent pericarditis may result from direct extension of infection from the lung, a myocardial or subdiaphragmatic abscess, as well as from hematogenous spread and direct inoculation by trauma or surgery (77). In a recent review of purulent pericarditis, the relative frequency of bacteria as etiologic agents was *S. pneumoniae* in 33%, *S. aureus* in 23%, streptococci in 11%, and aerobic gram-negative bacilli including *Haemophilus influenzae* and *Neisseria meningitidis* in 26% (78). In children, *S. aureus*, *H. influenzae*, and *N. menin-*

gitidis are most common (79). In a series from the U.S., tuberculous pericarditis occurs in 1% of patients with tuberculosis (80). Although less common in industrialized nations, tuberculous pericarditis remains an important cause of heart disease worldwide (72,81–83). Overall fungi are a rare cause of pericarditis, most commonly observed in the setting of *Histoplasma capsulatum* outbreaks, where it may occur in up to 6% of cases (84). Pericarditis due to *Candida* sp. and *Aspergillus* sp. occurs as a rare complication in immunocompromised patients, those with prolonged antibiotic use, or subsequent to thoracic surgery (85,86).

B. Clinical Manifestations

Symptoms of infectious pericarditis vary with etiology. The cardinal symptom of viral pericarditis is chest pain, typically retrosternal, exacerbated by inspiration on lying flat, and alleviated by leaning forward. These features assist in distinguishing it from ischemic pain. Pain referred to the trapezius muscle is considered highly characteristic of pericarditis (87). Pain was noted in 67% to 80%, fever in 59% to 85%, and an influenzalike prodrome in 36% to 65% of patients, the last preceding hospital admission for pericarditis by an average of 12 days (7,27). In distinction to the rather insidious onset of viral pericarditis, purulent pericarditis presents abruptly with fever, rigors, and toxicity, often during the course of a systemic illness (86,88). Fever is present in 96% to 100% of patients, with chest pain occurring in only one-third of patients (86,88). Tuberculous disease is characterized by an insidious onset with fever in over 90% of patients as well as weight loss, cough, chest pain, and night sweats (81,89).

The pathognomonic physical finding in pericarditis is the triphasic friction rub, a sound reminiscent of the squeaking of leather. The three phases parallel atrial systole, ventricular systole, and the diastole of the ventricle (90). Repeated sequential auscultation is important since the rub is frequently evanescent and may be incomplete, with only one or two phases, and difficult to distinguish from Hammond's crunch, mitral or tricuspid regurgitation, and other murmurs or artifacts (87). In viral pericarditis the rub is present in 70% to 80% of cases, but only in 32% to 46% of those with purulent pericarditis (27,86,91). In cases with a significant effusion or tamponade, there will be jugular venous distension, distant heart sounds, tachycardia, pulsus paradoxus, and hypotension.

C. Diagnosis

1. Laboratory Findings

Leucocytosis and elevated erythrocyte sedimentation rate are common but nonspecific findings in all forms of infectious pericarditis and are present in virtually all cases of purulent pericarditis. Neutrophilic leukocytosis $> 20{,}000/mm^3$ is seen more commonly in purulent pericarditis than in cases of viral etiology (27,92,93). In contrast, lymphopenia is suggestive of other etiologies, such as systemic lupus erythematosus (87). In cases of viral myopericarditis, cardiac enzymes may be elevated (27,94).

2. *Electrocardiographic Findings*

Acute pericarditis is characterized by relatively specific ECG changes which evolve over time. ST segment elevations are present in most leads except aVR and V1, where depression is usually present (Fig. 1). In contrast to what is seen with myocardial infarction, Q waves are never present with pericarditis alone, and T-wave inversion does not accompany ST segment elevation (87,95). Other ECG findings associated with pericarditis include low voltage, electrical alternans, and a downwardly concave ST segment. The progression of ECG changes with ST elevation reverting transiently to baseline, followed by T-wave inversion may be an important clue to the diagnosis. Although pericarditis has the potential to induce atrial fibrillation, most patients remain in sinus rhythm, and serious arrhythmias do not occur (96,97).

3. *Chest Radiographic Findings*

Although chest radiography may first reveal a pleural effusion (water bottle configuration, fat pad sign), pericardial fluid amounts below 250 cc are routinely undetectable, and even large amounts of fluid may be indistinguishable from four-chamber dilatation (98,99). In contrast, an enlarged cardiac silhouette from rapid accumulation of pericardial fluid in association with clear lung fields is very suggestive (98).

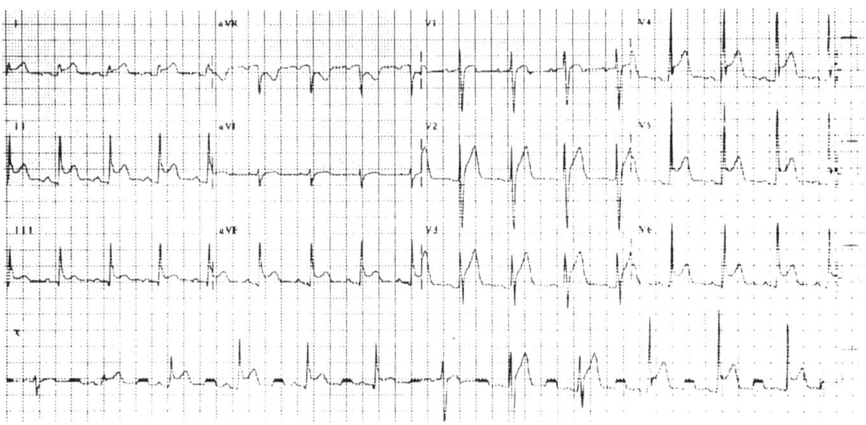

Figure 1 Electrocardiographic recording of a young patient presenting with pleuritic chest pain, showing generalized ST segment elevation in both the limb and precordial leads.

4. *Echocardiographic Findings*

Echocardiography has become the method of choice for the detection and follow-up of pericardial effusions (98). Sensitivity approaches 100% and specificity is excellent for effusions of more than 15 to 20 ml (100). Two-dimensional mode is now the standard because of its superior spatial resolution as well as its ability to detect fibrinous strands or a pericardial peel within an effusion (101,102). Echocardiographic signs of cardiac tamponade have been described, including early diastolic right ventricular collapse, late diastolic right atrial collapse, reciprocal respiratory variation in left and right ventricular dimension, reduced inspiratory inferior vena cava collapse, swinging heart with mitral pseudoprolapse, and exaggerated inspiratory flow across the tricuspid and pulmonic valve. Nevertheless, clinical correlation along with echocardiographic findings are necessary to properly evaluate those presenting with pericarditis (103,104).

5. *Diagnostic Approach*

Soler-Soler et al described a systematic, three-step diagnostic approach to acute pericarditis that is directed at infectious as well as noninfectious etiologies, such as collagen-vascular disease (72). As a first step routine laboratory studies, echocardiogram, antistreptolysin titer, rheumatoid factor, tuberculin skin test, antitoxoplasma antibodies, and selected viral studies are performed. Antinuclear antibodies as well as sputum or gastric aspirate analysis for mycobacteria are added if the illness lasts longer than 1 week. Thoracentesis is performed whenever a pleural effusion is present. In a second step, a diagnostic or therapeutic pericardiocentesis is performed in cases of tamponade or suspected purulence. Pericardial fluid stains and cultures for bacteria, mycobacteria, fungi, and viral agents are obtained. The addition of a adenosine deaminase determination to the conventional studies of pericardial fluid may serve as a useful predictor of pericardial tuberculosis (105). If clinical activity persists beyond 3 weeks, no etiologic diagnosis has been made, or tamponade persists or recurs after pericardiocentesis, a pericardial biopsy should be performed.

D. Treatment

1. *General Principles*

The treatment of viral pericarditis is generally supportive. Bed rest is recommended because physical activity aggravates symptoms and, in cases of viral perimyocarditis, may worsen outcome based on animal experiments (13). Control of pain with NSAIDS is a central component in the management of viral pericarditis. This commonly includes indomethacin at a dosage of 25 to 75 mg four times daily; however, other drugs of this group, including aspirin at a dosage of 650 mg every 4 hours, may also be employed (106).

2. *Directed Therapy*

a. Bacterial Pericarditis. Surgical drainage and appropriate antibiotic therapy are the cornerstones of the treatment for most cases of bacterial pericarditis (76,86,107). Intrapericardial administration of antibiotics is unnecessary because many important agents including penicillin, methicillin, gentamicin, cefazolin, and vancomycin penetrate well into the pericardial space (108–110). Because large-scale, controlled clinical trials are lacking, treatment recommendations in many instances are based on anecdotal reports and clinical experience.

S. aureus is now the most common organism causing bacterial pericarditis in the antibiotic era, accounting for approximately 25% to 50% of cases (78). Staphylococci, both coagulase-positive and coagulase-negative strains, are of particular concern after cardiac surgery and in pericarditis due to endocarditis in intravenous drug users (78). Staphylococcal pericarditis may also have to be considered in HIV-infected patients, even in the absence of the above risk factors (111). Staphylococcal disease tends to be serious and requires vigorous therapy, including the removal of suspected sources such as indwelling catheters, and surgical drainage, since pericardiocentesis alone is usually insufficient (112). In patients who are not surgical candidates, catheter drainage with intrapericardial instillation of streptokinase and streptodornase has been described (113). For methicillin-sensitive staphylococci, a penicillinase-resistant penicillin or first-generation cephalosporin is the treatment of choice. Alternatively, vancomycin can be used in cases with methicillin-resistant organisms or severe β-lactam allergy (78,114). Given the severity of staphylococcal disease, a total of 4 weeks of treatment has been suggested by some (114,115).

With the advent of antibiotics, *S. pneumoniae* has become a less prominent cause of bacterial pericarditis (77,92). In the preantibiotic era, mortalities of 100% had been reported, whereas cure is now achievable with complete drainage and parenteral antibiotics. Penicillin G in high doses is the drug of choice for the treatment of penicillin-sensitive strains (92). Because of the emergence of penicillin resistance, sensitivity testing must be performed on all isolates. Vancomycin or, depending on the minimal inhibitory concentration (MIC) of the organism, high-dose cefotaxime are used to treat resistant strains (78).

N. meningitidis can infect the pericardium during meningococcemia with or without coexistent meningitis (116–118). It accounts for 9% of cases in children and is less common in adults (79,119). Penicillin is highly effective and has been recommended at high doses (114). Although catheter drainage has been reported, surgical drainage or pericardiectomy is still frequently needed, even emergently in cases with acute constriction (91,120,121). Sterile pericardial fluid has been described in patients with pericarditis due to *N. meningitidis*. This phenomenon may result from prior antibiotic use, but also from an immune-mediated process which is exudative but not purulent and can be managed with corticosteroids or NSAIDs rather than antibiotics (117,122).

In the past, *H. influenzae* pericarditis was frequently a cause of purulent pericarditis in children (91). Although a decrease in incidence after the introduction of the *H. influenzae* type b vaccine can be expected, unvaccinated populations remain at risk (123). Ampicillin is recommended for the treatment of β-lactamase-negative strains, while third-generation cephalosporins may be used to treat β-lactamase-producing strains (124). The high viscosity of effusions caused by *H. influenzae* usually necessitate surgical drainage and often early pericardiectomy. This combined approach has led to survival rates > 90% (125,126). Alternatively, several reports have shown success using tube drainage with or without streptokinase irrigation (127,128).

Aerobic gram-negative bacilli, such as *Klebsiella pneumoniae*, *Escherichia coli*, *Pseudomonas aeruginosa*, and *Proteus*, have been reported with increasing frequency in hospitalized patients and those who are severely ill or immunocompromised (77,78,119). *Mycoplasma pneumoniae* has only infrequently been isolated from the pericardium, but may be more common than previously recognized. Good outcomes have been achieved in patients with pericarditis due to *M. pneumoniae* who have been treated with surgical drainage followed by 1 to 3 months of antibiotic therapy with either erythromycin or doxycycline (129).

Although anaerobes are a rare cause of pericarditis, appropriate antimicrobial therapy and drainage achieve a reasonably good outcome (130).

b. Tuberculous Pericarditis. Pericardial involvement in tuberculosis is typically the result of spread from adjacent nodes (131). While symptoms may vary, tuberculous pericarditis is characterized by an insidious onset, dyspnea, tachycardia, absence of murmurs, and bloody pericardial fluid which readily reaccumulates after pericardiocentesis (114). Although the optimal therapy for tuberculous pericarditis is controversial, it is clear that antituberculous drugs have significantly reduced mortality (132). In addition, many experts favor the use of adjuvant corticosteroids to reduce inflammation and prevent late constriction (71). Recent studies in which prednisone was added to the standard antituberculous therapy show more rapid resolution of pericardial effusions, within 48 to 72 h, resulting in a lower incidence of constriction requiring pericardectomy and decreased mortality (82,89). In general, the role of pericardiectomy in this setting is controversial, with early pericardiectomy being recommended by some to avoid the future necessity of operating on fibrotic, adherent pericardium (133). Others have suggested surgery only in selected patients, such as those with evidence of tamponade (81,82,134).

c. Fungal Pericarditis. Fungi are a less frequent cause of pericarditis. The most common pathogen is *H. capsulatum*, with *Candida* sp. and *Aspergillus* sp.

being seen less frequently. Uncommon causes include *Cryptococcus neoformans*, *Blastomyces dermatitides*, and *Coccidioides immitis*.

Pericarditis due to *Candida* sp. has been described most frequently in patients with severe illness (85). The diagnosis is often obscured by the underlying condition and the lack of specific clinical signs (85,86). The reported case fatality rate has been as high as 54% (85). Usual therapy includes the combination of pericardiectomy and intravenous amphotericin B. The role of 5-flucytosine and fluconazole has not been clearly defined (135).

Pericarditis due to *H. capsulatum* may develop from nonspecific inflammation during acute disease or as the result of progressive dissemination (84,136–138). While the former does not usually require antifungal therapy, the latter will, particularly in the immunocompromised host. High-dose amphotericin B is generally recommended in this setting (139).

E. Complications

1. Cardiac Tamponade

Cardiac tamponade is a life-threatening complication of pericarditis. The amount necessary to produce tamponade varies from 150 ml to 1 L or more, depending on the rapidity of accumulation (140). Dyspnea, tachypnea, tachycardia, hypotension, jugular venous distension, and pulsus paradoxus (inspiratory fall of sytolic blood pressure $>$ 10 mm Hg) in association with enlargement of the cardiac silhouette and clear lung fields on chest radiograph are highly suggestive (140). Unless the patient is moribund and in circulatory collapse, tamponade should always be confirmed by echocardiography prior to pericardiocentesis. This will localize and quantify the effusion and help to prevent inappropriate and potentially fatal attempts at pericardiocentesis (141). Furthermore, it may show a pericardial peel or fibrinous strands of a purulent effusion (102). Pericardiocentesis should be performed with electrocardiographic monitoring in a setting equipped to handle complications. Moreover, echocardiographic guidance reduces the risk and increases the diagnostic yield of the procedure (142–144). If the etiology is unclear and tuberculous or purulent pericarditis is considered, surgical drainage with biopsy of the pericardium and creation of a pericardial window is preferable to pericardiocentesis alone (71,145).

2. Constrictive Pericarditis

Pericardial constriction is a severe and late complication of pericarditis. Treatment usually requires pericardiectomy, which in this setting is associated with an operative mortality of 6% to 25% (146). Constriction is rare after bacterial pericarditis and is largely avoidable if complete drainage and needed pericardiectomy are employed (76,123). Although the frequency of tuberculous pericarditis has declined in Western nations, constriction develops in approximately 50% of patients and usually requires pericardectomy (81,147,148). In contrast, idiopathic pericarditis results in transient, self-limiting constriction in 20% of patients, and pericardectomy is not usually needed.

III. INFECTIVE ENDOCARDITIS

A. Introduction

Infective endocarditis (IE), an infection of the endothelial surface of the heart, is a highly dangerous form of endovascular infection, posing significant risk to the patient of life-threatening cardiac and extracardiac complications. With an estimated incidence of 1.7 to 4 cases per 100,000 of the general population, it currently accounts for 10,000 to 15,000 new cases per year in the United States (149–152). In the past, two classic presentations of infective endocarditis have been recognized: the acute form, a rapidly fatal disease where virulent organisms such as *S. aureus* and *S. pneumoniae* infect normal valves, causing early valvular destruction and embolic complications; and the subacute form, a more indolent process where less virulent organisms such as viridans streptococci and enterococci infect structurally abnormal valves and classic IE stigmata may be evident. Currently, a more useful approach is the categorization of endocarditis as native valve endocarditis, endocarditis in intravenous drug abusers, and prosthetic valve endocarditis (152). These entities have implications for etiologic agent and likelihood of preexisting heart disease, and serve as a basis for treatment and prognosis.

B. Epidemiology

1. Native Valve Endocarditis

Although native valve IE may occur in healthy persons with normal valves, predisposing factors are usually present. Underlying structural diseases of the heart increase susceptibility to IE, as 70% to 75% of patients have preexisting cardiac abnormalities (152–157). In most recent series, the predominant valvular process has shifted from rheumatic valvulitis to mitral valve prolapse and calcific atherosclerotic valvular heart disease in the elderly (158,159). Congenital heart disease is the underlying lesion in 10% to 20% of patients. Patients with debilitating diseases such as diabetes, alcoholism, or malignancy, and those on immunosuppressive therapy are also at increased risk for IE (160,161). Lastly, native valve IE remains predominantly a disease of men, with an approximate male:female ratio of 3:1 (162,163).

Bacteria are the leading causative agents of native valve IE. Streptococci account for 50% to 70%; viridans streptococci are the predominant pathogens (164,165). *Streptococcus bovis*, associated with the presence of colonic polyps or colonic malignancy, and enterococci, associated with genitourinary procedures or disease in older men, represent 10% of cases (166–169). Staphylococci account for 25% of cases, 90% of which are *S. aureus* infections (170). Although more commonly causing infection of prosthetic valves, coagulase-negative staphylococci have been reported to infect native valves in patients with underlying heart disease (171–173). Less than 10% of infections are caused by aerobic gram-negative bacilli (174,175). Fungi rarely cause native valve endocarditis in the absence of intravenous drug abuse; predisposing factors include severe underlying disease, corticosteroid therapy, prolonged administration of broad-spectrum antibiotics, and presence of intravascular catheters (176–178). Culture-negative endocarditis, accounting for 5% to 10% of cases, may occur in the setting of prior antibiotic use as well as infection due to fastidious organisms such as nutritionally deficient streptococci, HACEK organisms (*Haemophilus aphrophilus* and *H. parainfluenzae*, *Actinobacillus actinomycetemcomitans*, *Cardiobacterium hominis*, *Eikenella corrodens*, and *Kingella kingae*), *Brucella*, *Coxiella burnetii*, and *Chlamydia* (179,180). Current trends in the etiology of native valve IE show an increasing frequency of staphylococcal infections and a declining frequency of streptococal infections, an observation that may be more indicative of a referral or reporting bias in the literature than of a true epidemiologic phenomenon (151,163).

2. *Endocarditis in Intravenous Drug Abusers*

The incidence of IE in intravenous drug abusers is 2% to 5% per year, varying according to the type and frequency of drug use as well as the mode of preparation (181,182). A male predominance is recognized, and 20% have underlying structural heart disease, primarily congenital cardiac lesions or residua of previous infective endocarditis. In contrast to endocarditis in nonaddicts, *S. aureus* is the etiologic agent in over 50% of patients and accounts for 80% of cases with tricuspid infection (183,184). Streptococci and enterococci are found in 20%, largely affecting the aortic and mitral valves. Other common pathogens include aerobic gram-negative bacilli, predominantly *Pseudomonas* and *Serratia*, in 10%, and fungi in 5%. More than one organism is isolated from the blood in 5% of patients, either initially or during the course of therapy. *E. corrodens*, a common isolate from skin abscesses in addicts using methylphenidate or metamphetamine, may also be the causative agent of IE in these patients (185).

3. *Prosthetic Valve Endocarditis*

Prosthetic valve infections account for 10% to 20% of cases of IE, with an overall incidence of 1% to 4% per year (186,187). Current trends show an increasing number of cases, resulting from the expanded reservoir of elderly patients with prosthetic valves who have benefited from recent advances in cardiovascular surgery (151). Increased risk is associated with black race, male sex, and longer cardiopulmonary bypass time (188). The aortic prosthetic valve is more prone to infection, and the frequency of infection is also higher with multiple valve replacement. No difference in infectivity is recognized between mechanical and heterograft valves (189). Prosthetic valve IE is classified into two categories:

1. Early-onset infection, within 60 days of valve insertion, resulting from perioperative contamination, in which *S. epidermidis* is the predominant organism, followed by *S. aureus*, aerobic gram-negative bacilli, fungi, and diphtheroids
2. Late-onset disease, more than 60 days after valve insertion, in which the source of infection and microbiology closely resembles that of native valve IE, except for a 30% incidence of *S. epidermidis* infections (190,191).

However, two studies have suggested that the spectrum of infecting organisms of early-onset prosthetic valve IE extend over the first 12 months postsurgery, not merely during the first 2 months (189,192).

4. Nocosomial Endocarditis

Nocosomial endocarditis now comprises 13% to 14% of endocarditis cases in recent series (193,194). Over 50% of patients are elderly, and the majority have underlying valvular heart disease with left-sided involvement. A recent series reported a 45% incidence of endocarditis in patients with prosthetic valves who developed nocosomial bacteremia (195). Risk factors include the use of intravenous catheters, such as central venous and pulmonary artery catheters, and postsurgical procedures. Etiologic agents include *S. aureus* (50%), coagulase-negative staphylococci (30%), streptococci and enterococci (20%), and diphtheroids (10%).

C. Clinical Manifestations

The wide array of clinical signs and symptoms of IE reflect the underlying infectious process and its complications. Bacteremia produces nonspecific constitutional symptoms, such as fever, chills, malaise, loss of appetite, anorexia, and vomiting (153,154). Infection of the valve and local invasion may result in valvular regurgitation, congestive heart failure, rupture of the chordae tendineae or papillary muscles, fistular formation, and pericarditis with cardiac tamponade (196). Embolization from the infected cardiac valve or immune complex deposition may produce inflammation, abscess, or infarction of the organ involved, with the presenting signs and symptoms localized to that area.

Fever is found in 80% to 90% of patients but may be absent in association with advanced age, congestive heart failure, uremia, intracerebral hemorrhage, and immunosuppressive therapy (153). Cardiac murmurs due to either underlying valvular pathology or IE itself are present in 90% of patients (197). Frequent auscultation is important to detect changing murmurs, which have been reported in up to 36% to 52% of patients with IE (164,197). Pallor and anemia are noted in 75% to 80% of patients; splenomegaly may be found in 25% to 30% (164,198). Cutaneous manifestations, although more specific, are present in only approximately 50% of patients. Petechiae may occur in 30% of patients, particularly with longer courses of disease (153,198). Splinter hemorrhages, linear red-brown vertical streaks under the nail, are found in 10% to 28% of patients (164,198,199). Osler's nodes, tender, 2 to 15 mm, subcutaneous nodules on the digits and thenar, and Janeway lesions, small, nontender, hemorrhagic, erythematous macules, are present in 10% to 25% and 5% of patients, respectively, most typically in staphylococcal endocarditis (199). Roth spots, retinal hemorrhages, often oval with a pale center, usually found in the vicinity of the optic disc, are noted in less than 5% of patients (200).

D. Diagnosis

A normochromic normocytic anemia is found in 75% to 80% of patients, with leukocytosis in 20% to 30% (201). The erythrocyte sedimentation rate, although nonspecific, is elevated in 90% (154,201). Proteinuria, hematuria, or red cell casts on urinalysis parallel the degree of renal involvement. Chest radiograph may show evidence of congestive heart failure associated with valvular dysfunction, as well as pulmonary emboli, infiltrates, or cavitation complicating tricuspid valve IE. Electrocardiogram may show progressive conduction delay resulting from intraventricular septal abscess.

Blood culture is the most important laboratory test for the diagnosis of IE, allowing for the identification of the infecting microorganism and hence the institution of the most appropriate antimicrobial therapy. Two sets of blood cultures have a reported sensitivity of over 90% (202,203). Three or four sets of blood cultures should be obtained over a 2- to 4-hour period prior to the initiation of antibiotics (204–206). Cultures may be negative in 10% to 15% of patients, in association with prior antibiotic use, infection by fastidious pathogens or fungi, and mural or subvalvular location of infection (201). In all cases of suspected IE, BC should be held for 4 weeks to allow optimal time for the identification of slow-growing or fastidious microorganisms such as HACEK bacteria, *Brucella*, some anaerobes, or mycobacteria. In cases of suspected fungal or mycobacterial endocarditis, lysis centrifugation cultures have highest yield for isolation (206).

An echocardiogram should be performed in all patients with suspected endocarditis (207). It plays a vital role in the diagnosis of IE by identifying valvular vegetations, valve leaflet perforations, and valve ring abscesses while also assessing the hemodynamic complications of infection (208,209) (Fig. 2). Transthoracic echocardiography with Doppler evaluation is performed first, as it is noninvasive and less costly. If negative or equivocal results are obtained, the more sensitive transesophageal echocardiogram should be performed (151,207,210,211). It is particularly superior for the evaluation of prosthetic valves, for the detection of

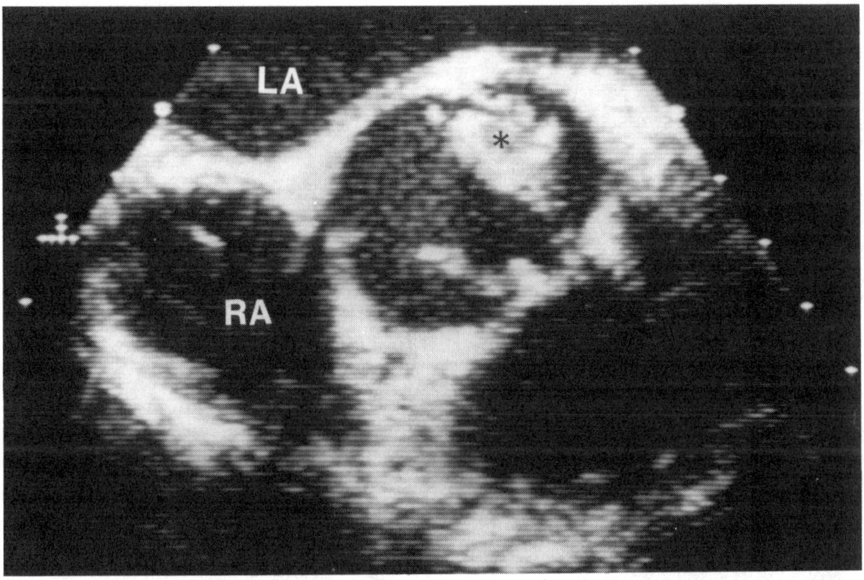

Figure 2 Transesophageal echocardiogram short-axis view of the aortic valve showing a 1.4×1.0 cm vegetation of the left coronary cusp of the aortic valve in a patient with endocarditis due to *C. hominis*. (RA = right atrium; LA = left atrium.)

smaller vegetations of the mitral valve, and for the delineation of abscesses and valve perforations (212–218) (Fig. 3).

In the past, the diagnosis of IE has rested upon the presence of four cardinal Oslerian manifestations: persistent bacteremia or fungemia, active valvulitis, large-vessel embolic complications, and immunologic vascular phenomena (219). With the current shift in the microbiologic spectrum of IE in favor of staphylococci and the rising incidence of IE in elderly patients, intravenous drug abusers, and prosthetic valve recipients, fewer patients meet all four of these criteria (220). This has prompted the development of a diagnostic system based on carefully defined major and minor clinical, microbiologic, and echocardiographic criteria similar to the Jones' criteria for rheumatic fever (209) (Table 2). In contrast to previous definitions, the new system incorporates echocardiographic findings, the positive predictive value of bacteremia due to typical IE organisms, and the risk factors of a predisposing heart condition or intravenous drug abuse. It has been shown to be more sensitive for clinically diagnosing IE in several prospective and retrospective studies, and is particularly useful in the setting of *S. aureus* bacteremia, right-sided valvulitis, and negative blood cultures (209,220–224). Moreover, two recent studies have reported a high degree of specificity as well,

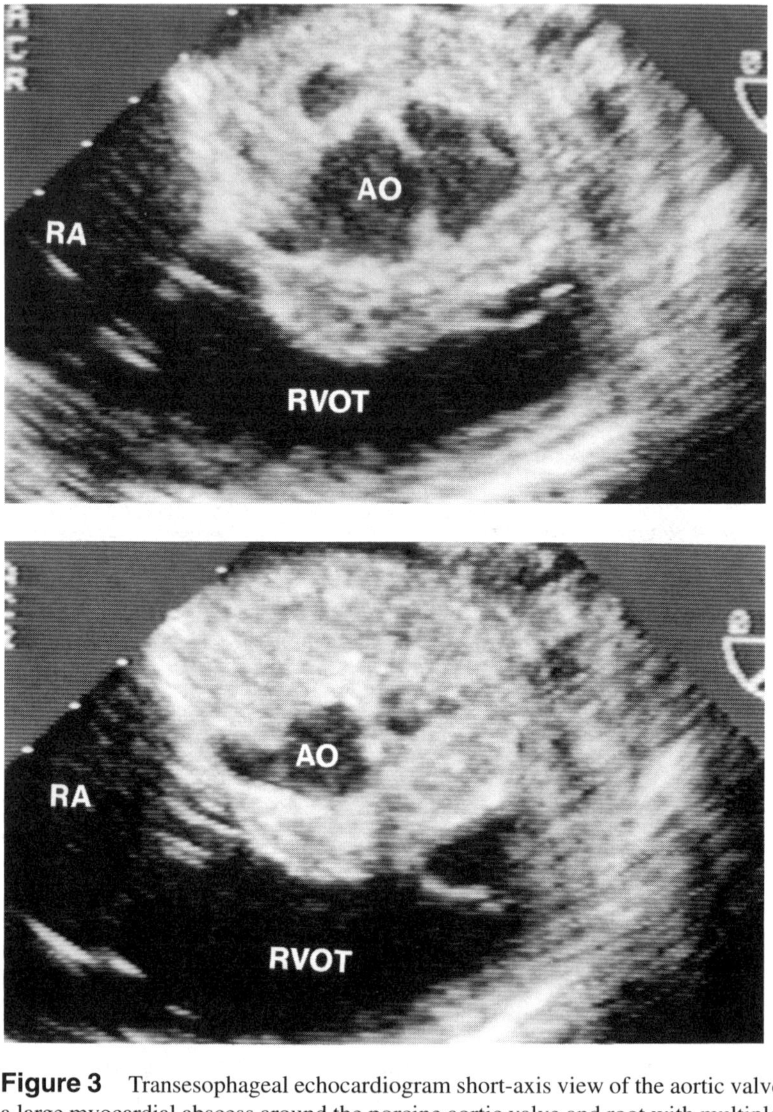

Figure 3 Transesophageal echocardiogram short-axis view of the aortic valve showing a large myocardial abscess around the porcine aortic valve and root with multiple fenestrations in a patient with prosthetic valve endocarditis due to viridans streptococci. Aortic root abscess, valve in systole (top). Aortic root abscess, valve in diastole (bottom). (RA = right atrium; RVOT = right ventricular outflow tract; AO = aortic valve.)

Table 2 Criteria for Infective Endocarditis

Major criteria
Positive blood culture
Bacteremia with typical microorganism (viridans streptococci, *S. bovis*, HACEK group; community-acquired *S. aureus* or enterococcus in absence of primary focus)
Persistent bacteremia[a]
Echocardiographic findings (oscillating intracardiac mass, abscess, new dehiscence of prosthetic valve)
Minor criteria
Predisposing heart condition or intravenous drug use
Fever >38°C (100.4°F)
Vascular phenomena (major arterial emboli, septic pulmonary infarcts, mycotic aneurysm, intracranial hemorrhage, conjunctival hemorrhages, Janeway lesions)
Immunologic phenomena (glomerulonephritis, Osler's nodes, Roth spots, rheumatoid factor)
Microbiologic findings not meeting major criterion[b]
Echocardiographic findings consistent with IE but not meeting major criterion
Definite diagnosis by clinical criteria
2 major criteria, or
1 major and 3 minor criteria, or
5 minor criteria

[a]Positive blood cultures drawn more than 12 h apart, or all of three or a majority of four positive blood cultures with first and last drawn at least 1 h apart.
[b]Positive blood culture not meeting major criteria or serologic evidence of active infection with organism consistent with IE.
Source: Reprinted by permission of the publisher from Ref. 209. Copyright 1994 by Excerpta Medica, Inc.

although the findings await confirmation in higher-risk patient groups (225,226). Despite this, some authorities find aspects of the criteria too imprecise to warrant inclusion in a strict case definition for IE (219,227). Further study and wider application of the new definition will provide a greater understanding of its role as a diagnostic tool for the management of patients with suspected IE.

E. Treatment

1. General Principles

Several general principles of therapy for IE are recognized:

1. Antimicrobial therapy should be bactericidal and administered intravenously of sufficient dose and duration.
2. The offending organism should be isolated in pure culture with determination of MIC and MBC.

3. Patients with associated myocarditis, arrhythmias, or congestive heart failure should be monitored in an intensive care unit setting.
4. Surveillance blood cultures should be obtained in the first 3 or 4 days of therapy and weekly thereafter.
5. Anticoagulation is discouraged due to risk of severe hemorrhage.
6. Surgical intervention should be promptly instituted when appropriate.

While blood culture results are pending, empiric antimicrobial therapy should be initiated and directed at the likely pathogen or pathogens for the clinical setting (228). For patients with native valve endocarditis and a subacute presentation, therapy with activity against streptococci and enterococci is indicated; penicillin or ampicillin plus gentamicin is reasonable. In the patient presenting with a rapidly progressive acute illness and in the intravenous drug abuser, an anti-staphylococcal agent should be added to the regimen. In areas with high endemicity of methicillin-resistant *S. aureus* (MRSA) among the addict population, vancomycin is the preferred drug. Patients with suspected prosthetic valve IE should receive vancomycin in combination with rifampin and gentamicin because of the relatively high frequency of isolation of *S. epidermidis* or MRSA in this setting.

When culture results reveal the offending agent, therapy should be narrowed to the most effective and least costly regimen. If cultures remain negative, the patient clinically responds, and the suspicion for endocarditis remains high, the initial regimen should be continued for a full course. If no pathogen is recovered and no clinical response is observed in 7 to 10 days, then special studies for unusual organisms such as *Brucella*, *Rickettsia*, and *Chlamydia* may be indicated (228). Empiric therapy for the fastidious HACEK microorganisms may be added. In the intravenous drug abuser and the patient with a prosthetic valve, the possibility of a fungal etiology should be strongly considered, particularly in the setting of a large vegetation or embolus.

2. *Directed Therapy*

The following review of directed therapy is adapted from the recently published updated recommendations from the American Heart Association for the antibiotic treatment of adults with IE due to streptococci, enterococci, staphylococci, and HACEK microorganisms (229) (Table 3). Treatment for viridans streptococcal IE varies with the penicillin susceptibility of the isolate. For highly penicillin-susceptible organisms (MIC < 0.1 μg/ml), a 4-week course of either parenteral penicillin G or ceftriaxone is appropriate (230–232). A short-course (2-week) regimen of combination therapy with penicillin plus gentamicin is appropriate for patients who are *not* HIV-infected and who have *no* evidence for intracardiac or extracardiac complications (233). For relative penicillin resistance (MIC > 0.1 μg/ml and < 0.5 μg/ml), IV gentamicin should be given for the first 2 weeks of

Table 3 Suggested Regimens for Therapy of Native Valve Endocarditis

Organism	Drug and daily dosage
Viridans streptococci, *Streptococcus bovis* (penicillin MIC < 0.1 μg/ml)	Penicillin G 12–18 million U/24 h IV either continuously or in 6 divided doses or Ceftriaxone 2 g once daily IV or IM
Viridans streptococci, *Streptococcus bovis* (penicillin MIC > 0.1 μg/ml and < 0.5 μg/ml)	Penicillin G 12–18 million U/24 h IV either continuously or in 6 divided doses *plus* gentamicin 1 mg/kg IV every 8 h
Enterococci	Penicillin G 18–30 million U/24 h IV (or ampicillin 12 g/24 h) either continuously or in 6 divided doses *plus* gentamicin 1 mg/kg IV every 8 h
Staphylococcus aureus, coagulase-negative staphylococci (methicillin-sensitive)[a]	Nafcillin (or oxacillin) 12 g/24 h IV in 6 divided doses[b]
Staphylococcus aureus, coagulase-negative staphylococci (methicillin-resistant)	Vancomycin 30 mg/kg/24 h in 2 divided doses (not to exceed 2 g/24 h unless serum levels are monitored)[b]
HACEK organisms	Ceftriaxone 2 g/24 h IV or IM[c]

[a]Susceptibility must be conclusively demonstrated.
[b]Gentamicin 1 mg/kg/8 h IV is added the first 3–5 days. For prosthetic valve endocarditis, gentamicin 1 mg/kg/8 h IV is added the first 2 weeks plus rifampin 300 mg orally every 8 h for the full treatment course.
[c]Cefotaxime may be substituted.
Source: Ref. 229.

the 4-week course of penicillin therapy. For highly resistant isolates (MIC > 0.5 μg/ml), for nutritionally deficient streptococci, and for prosthetic valve infection with viridans streptococci or *S. bovis*, the standard regimen for enterococcal endocarditis is recommended as described below. Vancomycin is an effective alternative for patients with immediate hypersensitivity to penicillin.

Enterococci are inhibited but not killed by clinically relevant concentrations of penicillins or vancomycin; however, the addition of an aminoglycoside exerts a synergistic bactericidal effect on these organisms (169,234). Therefore, standard therapy for enterococcal endocarditis entails a minimum 4-week course of combination therapy with parenteral penicillin or ampicillin plus gentamicin. A 6-week course of therapy is recommended for patients whose symptoms have existed > 3 months, and for patients with prosthetic valve IE (235). Therapy may be complicated by rising resistance patterns among enterococci. In many areas, a substantial proportion of enterococcal strains exhibit resistance to penicillins, vancomycin, or both, but high-level aminoglycoside resistance is the most common and serious impediment to successful therapy (236). Prolonged therapy with high-dose penicillin or ampicillin will cure approximately one-half of patients infected by strains with high-level gentamicin and streptomycin resistance; those failing therapy should be under strong consideration for valve replacement. Because of the greater experience with penicillin or ampicillin in treating life-threatening enterococcal infections, the physician might entertain cautious penicillin administration or desensitization per standard protocols and subsequent use of penicillin rather than the use of vancomycin as alternative therapy.

Patients with native valve endocarditis due to methicillin-sensitive *S. aureus* should receive a 4- to 6-week course of parenteral oxacillin or nafcillin, with the optional addition of gentamicin for the initial 3 to 5 days of therapy. Although synergistic in animal models and associated with more rapid bloodstream sterilization, the addition of gentamicin to nafcillin in *S. aureus* native valve endocarditis failed to improve cure rates while increasing nephrotoxicity (237,238). Cefazolin is alternative therapy for patients with delayed-type penicillin hypersensitivity. Patients with immediate-type penicillin hypersensitivity, and those with methicillin-resistant strains, should receive vancomycin. Caution is advised when choosing vancomycin for convenience in dosing, as suboptimal therapeutic response has been reported (151,239). Rifampin may be added to the therapeutic regimen for patients who are not responding adequately.

For patients with prosthetic valve endocarditis due to methicillin-sensitive *S. aureus*, use of combination therapy with oxacillin or nafcillin plus rifampin for 6 weeks, with the addition of gentamicin for the first 2 weeks, is recommended. Vancomycin should replace the oxacillin or nafcillin component for patients with prosthetic valve IE due to methicillin-resistant *S. aureus* or coagulase-negative staphylococci, and for those with penicillin allergy. Because of the potential occurrence of heteroresistance, coagulase-negative staphylococci should be assumed to be methicillin-resistant unless in vitro susceptibility has been conclusively demonstrated (240).

Treatment recommendations for endocarditis due to the HACEK microorganisms have been modified. Formerly, these bacteria were almost uniformly susceptible to ampicillin, and standard therapy consisted of ampicillin plus gentamicin for 4 to 6 weeks. Currently, penicillinase-producing strains resistant to ampicillin have emerged (241). These strains as well as ampicillin-sensitive strains are susceptible to third-generation cephalosporins; limited clinical data support their efficacy (232). Because antimicrobial susceptibility testing may be difficult to perform, all HACEK microorganisms should be considered ampicillin-resistant, and either cefotaxime or ceftriaxone therapy is recommended. Duration of therapy should be 4 weeks for native valve IE, and 6 weeks for prosthetic valve IE.

A 6-week course of combination therapy with an extended-spectrum penicillin plus aminoglycoside is indicated for the treatment of endocarditis due to *Pseudomonas* and *Serratia*. Published experience with third-generation cephalosporins is not extensive, but cures have been reported when used in combination with aminoglycosides (242). Medical therapy alone rarely cures left-sided *P. aeruginosa* IE, and many favor prompt valve replacement. Limited data exist regarding treatment of other Enterobacteriaceae (*E. coli*, *Enterobacter*, *Klebsiella*), but combination therapy with aminoglycoside plus either a third-generation cephalosporin or imipenem is reasonable. Imipenem is not a first-line agent due to its broad spectrum of activity, potential to cause seizures, and cost. Resistance to β-lactam agents may emerge during therapy for *Enterobacter*, *Citrobacter*, and *Serratia* and result in reactivation of disease.

Because of the threat of major emboli from bulky, friable vegetations and the high incidence of myocardial abscesses, early surgical intervention coupled with a prolonged postoperative course of amphotericin B is the treatment of choice for fungal endocarditis (176–178). This approach more than doubles overall survival in both native valve and prosthetic valve endocarditis (243).

F. Complications

1. Congestive Heart Failure

Congestive heart failure due to valvular dysfunction is the most common and most serious complication of IE (244). The risk is especially great in the acute form of the disease produced by such microorganisms as *S. aureus*, *S. pneumoniae*, *H. influenzae*, *N. meningitidis*, and *Neisseria gonorrheae* (196). It is reported in 15% to 65% of patients, and may occur as early as 1 month or as late as 1 year after the onset of IE. Eighty percent of patients develop insufficiency of the aortic valve, an often rapidly progressive process requiring urgent valve replacement. Destructive intracardiac lesions, such as fenestration of valve leaflets, rupture of chordae tendinae or papillary muscles, or aneurysms of the sinus of Valsalva, may be responsible for intractable heart failure in some cases. In patients with prosthetic valves, cardiac failure may result from disruption of the prosthesis or by valvular outflow obstruction by a vegetation, most often seen with fungal and staphylococcal IE. Echocardiography is an extremely useful modality to monitor the hemodynamic status of the patient; however, the presence and size of a visualized vegetation are not primary determinants of risk of severe heart failure and need for valve replacement (151). Intensive medical therapy is indicated as a first approach. Early surgical intervention is warranted in patients with progressive or severe heart failure who fail to respond rapidly and completely to medical therapy. The presence of an active infection is never a contraindication to the removal of an infected valve or to any procedure involving the heart (196). The risk of PVE after valve replacement may be minimized by careful and thorough debridement of friable necrotic material at the time of surgery (245,246).

2. *Myocardial Abscess*

Myocardial abscess may develop in up to 20% of patients with acute IE due to virulent microorganisms, most commonly affecting the aortic valve and also prosthetic valves (247,248). Localized abscesses may occur at any intracardiac site, but most commonly involve the perivalvular area (249,250). More serious complications include intracardiac fistulae, suppurative pericarditis, and myocarditis (250). Clinically, abscesses are difficult to recognize, but suggestive features include infection of the aortic valve, valvular regurgitation of recent development, presence of pericarditis, and a high degree of AV block (250,251). Intraventricular septal abscesses are of particular note in light of the corresponding ECG findings. Septal abscesses arising from contiguous spread from the mitral valve involve the lower aspect of the intraventricular septum and may present with gradual increase in conduction time progressing to left bundle branch block on ECG (252,253). With aortic valve IE and involvement of the upper septum, the ECG is less specific. Transesophageal echocardiography is highly sensitive for the detection of myocardial abscesses (213–217). Surgical therapy for drainage of the abscess is indicated in nearly all cases.

3. *Pericarditis*

Pericarditis may develop in a minority of patients, most often in the setting of staphylococcal IE, as the result of bacteremic seeding of the pericardium or via rupture of a myocardial or septal abscess or aneurysm of sinus of Valsalva. Echocardiography is the mainstay for diagnosis. Aggressive prompt pericardiocentesis and surgical drainage of the purulent material are essential. Pericardiectomy may be required for some patients. Pericarditis in association with less virulent organisms is rarely infectious in origin, more likely due to immune complex deposition.

4. *Myocardial Infarction*

Myocardial infarction may occur as the result of coronary artery embolization, or secondary to local inflammation and thrombus formation from an adjacent suppurative focus of infection (254). Reported incidence ranges from 3% to 25% (255,256). Management is similar to that for patients with myocardial infection secondary to atherosclerotic coronary artery disease.

5. *Arterial Embolization*

Next to intracardiac complications, arterial embolization is the second most common life-threatening event in patients with IE (196,257). The risk of clinically significant emboli, estimated at 22% to 43%, is highest in association with infections that produce large, bulky vegetations, such as those caused by *Haemophilus parainfluenzae* and other fastidious gram-negative HACEK organisms, fungi (especially *Aspergillus*), nutritionally deficient streptococci, and group B streptococci (177–179,245). Emboli originating from the left side of the heart most commonly involve the brain, spleen, kidney, and coronary arteries, and the presenting symptoms correlate with the site of enlodgment (258). Of the 30% of patients with IE who suffer neurologic complications, embolic stroke is the most common neurologic syndrome and occurs most often in association with *S. aureus* infection (259–264). The middle cerebral artery is most often embolized, and hemiplegia is the most frequent manifestation (259,260). Emboli originating from the tricuspid valve, as seen with staphylococcal IE in the intravenous drug abuser, may result in pulmonary emboli, infiltrates, or cavitation. In the setting of culture-negative IE, patients with major peripheral embolization should undergo embolectomy with histologic examination and culture when feasible; *Aspergillus* is most often diagnosed in this manner.

6. Mycotic Aneurysms

Mycotic aneurysms develop in about 25% of patients with IE and constitute 2.5% to 6% of all aneurysms of the brain (196). Most authorities believe that septic embolization from vegetations to the vasa vasorum is the most common cause (259,260). Mycotic aneurysms may involve any artery, usually at points of bifurcation, most often in association with organisms of low virulence such as viridans streptococci (260,265). In descending order of frequency, the vessels affected are the aorta, cerebral arteries, visceral arteries, and arteries of the upper and lower extremities. Those involving the cerebral circulation, coronary arteries, superior mesenteric and splenic arteries, and ligated ductus arteriosus pose the greatest threat to life (196). Mycotic aneurysms may be clinically silent until rupture occurs. A severe, localized headache is highly suggestive of intracerebral mycotic aneurysm; prompt evaluation with cerebral angiography may provide an early diagnosis before a sudden, massive, often fatal subarachnoid or intracerebral hemorrhage occurs (260,261,265,266). A tender, pulsatile mass, pressure on adjacent structures, or unexplained blood loss is indicative of intrathoracic or intraabdominal mycotic aneurysm (267–269). It may be detected on computerized tomography (CT) or magnetic resonance imaging (MRI) in a patient with unexplained fever, abdominal mass, or back pain (268–270). Hematemesis, hematobilia, and jaundice suggest mycotic aneurysm of the hepatic artery (245). Patients with rupture of a mycotic aneurysm into the small or large bowel experience sudden onset of gastrointestinal hemorrhage and massive diarrhea.

When suspected, angiography is the best method for establishing the presence and location of an aneurysm, assessing the condition of the involved vessel, noting the presence of other aneurysms, and guiding surgical therapy. Because of the risk for rupture and hemorrhage, prompt surgical intervention is generally recommended (245). For intrathoracic and intra-abdominal mycotic aneurysms, excision of infected material is not feasible in most cases (271,272). Revascularization carries a high risk of reinfection and rupture, and mortality is high.

Peripheral mycotic aneurysms may be ligated and excised without sacrifice of the extremity.

The management of patients with intracranial mycotic aneurysms is controversial. With an overall mortality of 60%, which increases to 80% if rupture ensues, many favor prompt excision or ligation whenever feasible anatomically (265,273). The very low frequency of rupture and anecdotal reports of aneurysm resolution with antibiotic therapy alone lead others to advocate a more conservative approach (266,274–276). Patients with a single, peripheral aneurysm or those less amenable to surgical excision may be followed with serial CT and angiographic studies. If one or more aneurysms enlarge or bleed, prompt surgical excision should be attempted (273). Multiple aneurysms and those proximal to the first bifurcation present especially complex surgical dilemmas. Highest risk of rupture and death has been observed in patients with staphylococcal IE (196).

G. Indications for Surgery

When medical therapy fails to control native valve or prosthetic valve IE, surgery is indicated. Table 4 summarizes the generally accepted recommendations for surgery, stratified according to absolute and relative indications. Moderate to severe or progressive heart failure that does not respond rapidly and completely to medical therapy is the most common indication for surgery, usually resulting from infection-related aortic and/or mitral insufficiency (277,278). The aortic valve is most often involved and is notable for its atypical clinical features and rapidly progressive cardiac decompensation that may be heralded by the finding of premature closure of the mitral valve on echocardiography (279,280). Severe

Table 4 Indications for Surgery in Native Valve Endocarditis

Absolute
Congestive heart failure
Valvular incompetence
Valvular stenosis
Uncontrolled infection
Persistent bacteremia
Suppurative intracardiac disease
Fungal endocarditis
Relative
Systemic emboli
Echocardiographically demonstrable vegetations
Virulent microorganisms (*S. aureus*, aerobic gram-negative bacilli)
Relapse

Source: Ref. 278, reprinted by permission of Lippincott-Raven Publishers, Copyright 1992.

congestive heart failure associated with mitral insufficiency is less common and easily recognized clinically. Occasional patients with mitral insufficiency develop congestive heart failure as the result of valvular stenosis caused by large, obstructing vegetations, often in the setting of staphylococcal or fungal IE (281). Mortality in patients who develop moderate to severe heart failure during IE is 50% to 90%, and several reports have demonstrated survival benefit with surgical intervention (279,282,283). Although timing of surgery should be dictated by the hemodynamic status of the patient, early aggressive surgical intervention is recommended to optimize outcome (284–286).

Another generally accepted indication for surgery in IE is uncontrollable infection, which may occur in 7% of patients with native valve IE and a greater percentage of those with prosthetic valve IE (287). Persistent bacteremia after more than 1 week of appropriate antimicrobial therapy, in absence of a metastatic focus of infection, is associated with a substantially higher mortality rate when treated with medical therapy alone versus a combined medical-surgical approach (282). Evaluation to exclude metastatic extracardiac sites of infection, such as septic pulmonary emboli, splenic abscess, or osteomyelitis, should be performed prior to consideration of an operative procedure in these patients. Suppurative intracardiac disease, such as perivalvular or myocardial abscess as well as fistulae and aneurysms of the sinus of Valsalva, is associated with an increased mortality and generally requires drainage (278). While no large trials have demonstrated the efficacy of surgical intervention for fungal IE, medical therapy alone is nearly universally fatal due to the associated large-vessel emboli, invasion of periannular structures, and limited efficacy of available antifungal agents (176–178,243,277, 278,284,288).

Because embolic events complicating IE may result in irreversible organ dysfunction, with a particularly high mortality in the setting of an embolic stroke, the presence of recurrent systemic emboli is a relative indication for surgery. The exact parameters are not clearly defined. One approach recommends surgical therapy if a *second* major emboli event occurs, particularly in association with staphylococcal or fungal IE (196,277). Another approach, based on the observation that the incidence of embolic events decreases 10-fold over the first 2 weeks of medical therapy, suggests surgical intervention for patients with recurrent emboli who have had at least 2 weeks of appropriate antibiotic therapy for infection by microorganisms with a high frequency of embolization (245,289). A related factor is the presence of echocardiographically demonstrable vegetations. The finding by some investigators that large (>10 mm), mobile vegetations on TTE increase the risk of embolization has led to the recommendation that elective cardiac valve replacement be strongly considered for these patients (290,291). However, more recent studies have failed to find an association between vegetation size and risk of embolization (263,289,292). Most authorities do not recommend valvular replacement surgery solely on the basis of echocardiographically demonstrable vegetations (278).

Infecting organisms which are difficult to treat are a relative indication for surgery in IE. Because of the increased mortality and high frequency of complications such as congestive heart failure and perivalvular abscess, patients with left-sided staphylococcal IE should be strongly considered for valve replacement. Patients who demonstrate clearing of bacteremia or who lack evidence of suppurative intracardiac disease or significant hemodynamic compromise are appropriately managed initially with medical therapy (278). Intravenous drug abusers with tricuspid valve IE due to *S. aureus* are usually cured with medical therapy alone and require surgery only if an absolute indication develops (164,283,293). A combined medical and surgical approach is highly desirable for the treatment of left-sided IE due to selected bacteria such as *P. aeruginosa* in the setting of antibiotic resistance or relapsing disease (242,294). Relapsing disease in itself, in the absence of a metastatic focus of infection, is a relative indication for surgery in IE (278). Recommendations vary according to type of infecting organism and number of relapses. First relapse in patients with IE due to *S. aureus*, aerobic gram-negative bacilli, or *C. burnetii*, should be strongly considered for valve replacement (266). First relapses in patients with IE due to enterococci or nutritionally deficient streptococci are usually cured with retreatment, and a surgical approach is entertained if a second relapse ensues.

Valve dehiscence and obstruction are absolute indications for surgery in patients with prosthetic valve IE, due to the grave hemodynamic consequences of valvular dysfunction (277). Relative indications include:

1. Early prosthetic valve IE, commonly caused by *S. aureus*, coagulase-negative staphylococci, or aerobic gram-negative bacilli and associated with a high mortality
2. Nonstreptococcal late prosthetic valve IE
3. Periprosthetic leak

Table 5 High-Risk Procedures for Which Chemoprophylaxis Is Advised[a]

Dental procedures known to induce gingival or mucosal bleeding
Tonsillectomy and/or adenoidectomy
Incision and drainage of infected tissue
Upper respiratory tract procedures (bronchoscopy with rigid bronchoscope, surgical operations that involve respiratory mucosa)
Gastrointestinal procedures (esophageal dilation, sclerotherapy for esophageal varices, endoscopic retrograde cholangiography with biliary obstruction, gallbladder surgery, surgical operations that involve gastrointestinal mucosa)
Genitourinary procedures (cystoscopy, ureteral dilation, prostatic surgery)

[a]Optional for high-risk patients: bronchoscopy with flexible bronchoscope +/− biopsy, transesophageal echocardiography, endoscopy +/− biopsy, vaginal delivery, vaginal hysterectomy.
Source: Adapted from Ref. 296.

4. Recurrent systemic emboli
5. Relapse of infection (277).

H. Prevention

Antibiotic prophylaxis is currently recommended for selected patients at risk for endocarditis when undergoing health care procedures that result in bacteremia (295,296). Because no adequate, controlled clinical trials of antibiotic regimens for the prevention of endocarditis exist, guidelines are based on animal models, in vitro susceptibility data, retrospective analyses, and organisms likely to produce bacteremia at a given site (295). When both the underlying cardiac condition and the procedure involve substantial risk, antibiotic prophylaxis is advised (296). A recent review provides a listing of high risk and intermediate risk cardiac disorders based on the frequency of association with endocarditis (296). Table 5 summarizes the high-risk procedures for which preventative therapy is recommended (295–297). Standard chemoprophylactic regimens are listed in Table 6, based upon recently updated guidelines by the American Heart Association (295). These new

Table 6 Recommended Standard Prophylactic Regimens for Endocarditis

	Preprocedure	Postprocedure
Dental, oral, respiratory, or esophageal		
Standard	Amoxicillin[a] 2.0 g orally 1 h before	
Unable to take oral medications	Ampicillin 2.0 gm IM/IV 30 min before	
Genitourinary/ gastrointestinal		
High-risk patients	Ampicillin[b] 2.0 g IV or IM plus gentamicin 1.5 mg/kg IV or IM (not to exceed 80 mg) 30 min before	Amoxicillin 1 g orally 6 h after OR Ampicillin 1 g IM/IV
Moderate-risk patients	Amoxicillin 2.0 g orally 1 h before OR Ampicillin[b] 2.0 g IM/IV 30 min before	

[a]Alternative oral regimens for penicillin-allergic patients include: clindamycin 600 mg or azithromycin/clarithromycin 500 mg. Also cephalexin or cefadroxil 2.0 g if no immediate-type hypersensitivity (urticaria, angioedema, or anaphylaxis).
[b]For penicillin-allergic patients, vancomycin 20 mg/kg IV over 1–2 h may be substituted.
Source: Adapted from Ref. 295. Copyright 1997 by the American Medical Association.

recommendations more clearly define the indications for antibiotic prophylaxis and simplify previous prophylactic regimens. As further research and clinical experience are gathered, guidelines for the prevention of endocarditis may continue to undergo modification in the future (297).

REFERENCES

1. Peters NS, Poole-Wilson PA. Myocarditis—continuing clinical and pathologic confusion. Am Heart J 1991; 121:942–947.
2. Weinstein C, Fenoglio JJ. Myocarditis. Hum Pathol 1987; 18:613–618.
3. Mason JW, O'Connell JB. Clinical merit of endomyocardial biopsy. Circulation 1989; 79:971–979.
4. Reyes MP, Lerner AM. Coxsackievirus myocarditis—with special reference to acute and chronic effects. Prog Cardiovasc Dis 1985; 27:373–394.
5. Grist NR, Bell EJ. A six year study of Coxsackie B infection in heart disease. J Hyg (Camb) 1974; 73:165–172.
6. Woodruff JF. Viral myocarditis. Am J Pathol 1980; 101:427–479.
7. Koontz CH, Ray CG. The role of Coxsackie Group B virus infections in sporadic myopericarditis. Am Heart J 1971; 82:750–758.
8. Sutton GC, Harding HB, Truehart LRP, Clarke HP. Coxsackie B4 myocarditis in an adult: successful isolation of virus from ventricular myocardium. Aerospace Med 1967; 38:66–69.
9. Van Creveld S, De Jager H. Myocarditis in newborns, caused by Coxsackie virus: clinical and pathological data. Ann Pediatr 1956; 187:100–112.
10. Monif GRG, Lee CW, Hsiung GD. Isolated myocarditis with recovery of ECHO type 9 virus from the myocardium. N Engl J Med 1967; 277:1353–1355.
11. Brown CA, O'Connell JB. Myocarditis and idiopathic dilated cardiomyopathy. Am J Med 1995; 99:309–314.
12. Sole MJ, Liu P. Viral myocarditis: a paradigm for understanding the pathogenesis and treatment of dilated cardiomyopathy. J Am Coll Cardiol 1993; 22(suppl A):99–105.
13. Reyes MP, Ho KL, Smith F, Lerner AM. A mouse model of dilated-type cardiomyopathy due to Coxsackie virus B3. J Infect Dis 1981; 144:232–236.
14. Cambridge G, McArthur CGC, Waterson AP, Goodwin JF, Oakley CM. Antibodies to Coxsackie B viruses in congestive cardiomyopathy. Br Heart J 1979; 41:692–696.
15. Bowles NE, Richardson PJ, Olsen EG, Archard LC. Detection of Coxsackie-B virus-specific RNA sequences in myocardial biopsy samples from patients with myocarditis and dilated cardiomyopathy. Lancet 1986; 1:1120–1123.
16. Orinius E. The late cardiac prognosis after Coxsackie B infection. Acta Med Scand 1968; 183:235–237.
17. O'Connell JB, Mason JW. Diagnosing and treating active myocarditis. West J Med 1989; 150:431–435.
18. Friman G, Fohlman J. The epidemiology of viral heart disease. Scand J Infect Dis 1993; 88(suppl):7–10.
19. Mason JW, O'Connell JB, Herskowitz A, et al. A clinical trial of immunosuppressive therapy for myocarditis. N Engl J Med 1995; 333:269–275.

20. Gravanis MB, Sternby NH. Incidence of myocarditis. A 10-year autopsy study from Malmo, Sweden. Arch Pathol Lab Med 1991; 115:390–392.
21. Gore I, Saphir O. Myocarditis: a classification of 1402 cases. Am Heart J 1947; 34:827–830.
22. Okuni M, Yamada T, Mochizuki S, Sakurai I. Studies on myocarditis in childhood, with special reference to the possible immunological process and the thymus in the chronicity of the disease. Jpn Circ J 1975; 39:463–470.
23. Aretz HT, Fallon JT, Billingham ME, et al. Myocarditis—a histopathologic definition and classification. Am J Cardiovasc Pathol 1986; 1:3–14.
24. Anderson DW, Virmani R, Reilly JM, et al. Prevalent myocarditis at necropsy in the acquired immunodeficiency syndrome. J Am Coll Cardiol 1988; 11:792–799.
25. Baroldi G, Corallo S, Moroni M, et al. Focal lymphocytic myocarditis in acquired immunodeficiency syndrome (AIDS): a correlative morphologic and clinical study in 26 consecutive fatal cases. J Am Coll Cardiol 1988; 12:463–469.
26. Corallo S, Mutinelli MR, Moroni M, et al. Echocardiography detects myocardial damage in AIDS: prospective study in 102 patients. Eur Heart J 1988; 9:887–892.
27. Smith WG. Coxsackie B myopericarditis in adults. Am Heart J 1970; 80:34–46.
28. Myocarditis Treatment Trial investigators. Incidence and clinical characteristics of myocarditis. Circulation 1991; 84(suppl 2):11–12.
29. Costanzo-Nordin MR, O'Connell JB, Subramanian R, Robinson JA, Scanlon PJ. Myocarditis confirmed by biopsy presenting as acute myocardial infarction. Br Heart J 1985; 53:25–29.
30. Sainani GS, Krompotic E, Slodki SJ. Adult heart disease due to Coxsackie virus B infection. Medicine 1968; 47:133–147.
31. Heikkila J, Karjalainen J. Evaluation of mild acute infectious myocarditis. Br Heart J 1982; 47:381–391.
32. Karjalainen J. Clinical diagnosis of myocarditis and dilated cardiomyopathy. Scand J Infect Dis 1993; 88(suppl):33–43.
33. Karjalainen J. Functional and myocarditis-induced T-wave abnormalities. Chest 1983; 83:868–874.
34. Morgera T, DiLenarda A, Dreas L, et al. Electrocardiography of myocarditis revisited: clinical and prognostic significance of electrocardiographic changes. Am Heart J 1992; 124:455–467.
35. Pinamonti B, Alberti E, Cigalotto A, et al. Echocardiographic findings in myocarditis. Am J Cardiol 1988; 62:285–291.
36. Hauser AM, Gordon S, Cieszkowski J, Timmis GC. Severe transient left ventricular "hypertrophy" occurring during acute myocarditis. Chest 1983; 83:275–277.
37. Dec GW, Palacios I, Yasuda T, et al. Antimyosin antibody cardiac imaging: its role in the diagnosis of myocarditis. J Am Coll Cardiol 1990; 16:97–104.
38. Yasuda T, Palacios IF, Dec GW, et al. Indium-111 monoclonal antimyosin antibody imaging in the diagnosis of acute myocarditis. Circulation 1987; 76:306–311.
39. O'Connell JB, Henkin RE, Robinson JA, Subramanian R, Scanlon PJ, Gunnar RM. Gallium-67 imaging in patients with dilated cardiomyopathy and biopsy-proven myocarditis. Circulation 1984; 70:58–62.
40. Konno S, Sekiguchi M, Sakakibara S. Catheter biopsy of the heart. Radiol Clin North Am 1971; 9:491–510.

41. Spiegelhalter DJ, Stovin PGI. An analysis of repeated biopsies following cardiac transplantation. Stat Med 1985; 2:33–40.
42. Keogh AM, Billingham ME, Schroeder JS. Rapid histological changes in endomyocardial biopsy specimens after myocarditis. Br Heart J 1990; 64:406–408.
43. Costanzo-Nordin MR, Reap EA, O'Connell JB, Robinson JA, Scanlon PJ. A nonsteroid antiinflammatory drug exacerbates Coxsackie B3 murine myocarditis. J Am Coll Cardiol 1985; 6:1078–1082.
44. Rezkalla S, Khatib G, Khatib R. Coxsackievirus B3 murine myocarditis: deleterious effects of nonsteroidal anti-inflammatory agents. J Lab Clin Med 1986; 107: 393–395.
45. Rezkalla S, Khatib R, Khatib G, et al. Effect of indomethacin in the late phase of Coxsackievirus myocarditis in a murine model. J Lab Clin Med 1988; 112: 118–121.
46. Rezkalla S, Kloner RA, Khatib G, Smith FE, Khatib R. Effect of metoprolol in acute Coxsackie virus B3 murine myocarditis. J Am Coll Cardiol 1988; 12:412–414.
47. Rezkalla SH, Kloner RA. Management strategies in viral myocarditis. Am Heart J 1989; 117:706–708.
48. Matsumori A, Wang H, Abelmann WH, Crumpacker CS. Treatment of viral myocarditis with ribavirin in an animal preparation. Circulation 1985; 71:834–839.
49. Mason JW, Billingham ME, Ricci DR. Treatment of acute inflammatory myocarditis assisted by endomyocardial biopsy. Am J Cardiol 1980; 45:1037–1044.
50. Vignola PA, Kazutaka A, Swayze PS, et al. Lymphocytic myocarditis presenting as unexplained ventricular arrythmias: diagnosis with endomyocardial biopsy and response to immunosuppression. J Am Coll Cardiol 1984; 4:812–819.
51. Hosenpud JD, McAnulty JH, Niles NR. Lack of objective improvement in ventricular systolic function in patients with myocarditis treated with azathioprine and prednisone. J Am Coll Cardiol 1985; 6:797–801.
52. Hobbs RE, Pelegrin D, Ratliff NB, et al. Lymphocytic myocarditis and dilated cardiomyopathy—treatment with immunosupressive agents. Cleve Clin J Med 1989; 56:628–635.
53. McKenna WJ, Davies MJ. Immunosuppression for myocarditis. N Engl J Med 1995; 333:312–313.
54. O'Connell JB, Dec GW, Goldenberg IF, et al. Results of heart transplantation for active lymphocytic myocarditis. J Heart Transplant 1990; 9:351–356.
55. Karjalainen J, Viitasalo M, Kala R, Heikkila J. 24-Hour electrocardiographic recordings in mild acute infectious myocarditis. Ann Clin Res 1984; 16:34–39.
56. Granath A, Kimby AG, Sodermark T, Volpe U, Zetterquist S. Stokes-Adams attacks requiring pacemaker treatment in three patients with acute nonspecific myocarditis. Acta Med Scand 1980; 207:177–181.
57. Tai YT, Lau CP, Fong PC, Li JP, Lee KL. Incessant automatic ventricular tachycardia complicating acute Coxsackie B myocarditis. Cardiology 1992; 80:339–344.
58. Phillips M, Robinowitz M, Higgins JR, Boran KJ, Reed T, Virmani R. Sudden cardiac death in Air Force recruits—a 20-year review. JAMA 1986; 256:2696–2699.
59. Hosenpud JD, McAnulty JH, Niles NR. Unexpected myocardial disease in patients with life threatening arrhythmias. Br Heart J 1986; 56:55–61.

60. Bengtsson E, Lamberger B. Five-year follow-up study of cases suggestive of acute myocarditis. Am Heart J 1966; 72:751–763.
61. Kopecky SL, Gersh BJ. Dilated cardiomyopathy and myocarditis: natural history, etiology, clinical manifestations and management. Curr Prob Cardiol 1987; 12: 569–647.
62. Grist NR. Viral myocarditis: a frequently misdiagnosed problem. Pract Cardiol 1984; 10:193–202.
63. Rose AG, Fraser RC, Beck W. Absence of evidence of myocarditis in endomyocardial biopsy specimens from patients with dilated (congestive) cardiomyopathy. S Afr Med J 1984; 66:871–874.
64. Dec GW Jr, Palacios IF, Fallon JT, et al. Active myocarditis in the spectrum of acute dilated cardiomyopathies: clinical features, histologic correlates, and clinical outcome. N Engl J Med 1985; 312:885–890.
65. Chow LC, Dittrich HC, Shabetai R. Endomyocardial biopsy in patients with unexplained congestive heart failure. Ann Intern Med 1988; 109:535–539.
66. Vasiljevic JD, Kanjuh V, Seferovic P, Sesto M, Stojsic D, Olsen EGJ. The incidence of myocarditis in endomyocardial biopsy samples from patients with congestive heart failure. Am Heart J 1990; 120:1370–1377.
67. CONSENSUS Trial Study Group. Effects of enalapril on mortality in severe congestive heart failure. Results of the Cooperative North Scandinavian Enalapril Study. N Engl J Med 1987; 316:1429–1435.
68. SOLVD Investigators. Effect of enalapril on survival in patients with reduced left ventricular ejection fractions and congestive heart failure. N Engl J Med 1991; 325:293–302.
69. Tomioka N, Kishimoto C, Matsumori A, Kawai C. Mural thrombus in experimental viral myocarditis in mice: relation between thrombosis and congestive heart failure. Cardiovasc Res 1986; 20:665–671.
70. Kojima J, Miyazaki S, Fujiwara H, Kumada T, Kawai C. Recurrent left ventricular mural thrombi in a patient with acute myocarditis. Heart Vessel 1988; 4:120–122.
71. Savoia MC, Oxman MN. Myocarditis and pericarditis. In: Mandell GL, Bennett JE, Dolin R, eds. Principles and Practice of Infectious Diseases. 4th ed. New York: Churchill Livingstone, 1995:799–812.
72. Soler-Soler J, Permanyer-Miralda G, Sagrista-Sauleda J. A systematic diagnostic approach to primary acute pericardial disease. The Barcelona experience. Cardiol Clin 1990; 8:609–620.
73. Fowler NO. Pericardial disease. Heart Dis Stroke 1992; 1:85–94.
74. Brodie HR, Marchessault V. Acute benign pericarditis caused by Coxsackie virus group b. N Engl J Med 1960; 262:1278–1280.
75. Flory WD. Pericarditis: report of seven cases. Minn Med 1962; 45:502–510.
76. Boyle JD, Pierce ML, Guze LB. Purulent pericarditis: review of literature and report of eleven cases. Medicine 1961; 40:119–144.
77. Klacsmann PG, Bulkley BH, Hutchins GM. The changed spectrum of purulent pericarditis. Am J Med 1977; 63:666–673.
78. Park S, Bayer AS. Purulent pericarditis. Curr Clin Top Infect Dis 1992; 12:56–83.
79. Feldman WE. Bacterial etiology and mortality of purulent pericarditis in pediatric patients. Review of 162 patients. Am J Dis Child 1979; 133:641–644.

80. Larrieu AJ, Tyers GFO, Williams EH, Derrick JR. Recent experience with tuberculous pericarditis. Ann Thorac Surg 1980; 29:464–468.
81. Sagrista-Sauleda J, Permanyer-Miralda G, Soler-Soler J. Tuberculous pericarditis: ten year experience with a prospective protocol for diagnosis and treatment. J Am Coll Cardiol 1988; 11:724–728.
82. Strang JIG, Kakaza HH, Gibson DG, et al. Controlled clinical trial of complete open surgical drainage and of prednisolone in treatment of tuberculous pericardial effusion in Transkei. Lancet 1988; 2(8614):759–764.
83. Hugo-Hamman CT, Scher H, DeMoor MM. Tuberculous pericarditis in children: a review of 44 cases. Pediatr Infect Dis J 1994; 13:13–18.
84. Wheat LJ, Stein L, Corya BC, et al. Pericarditis as a manifestation of histoplasmosis during two large urban outbreaks. Medicine 1983; 62:110–119.
85. Schrank JH, Dooley DP. Purulent pericarditis caused by *Candida* species: case report and review. Clin Infect Dis 1995; 21:182–187.
86. Rubin RH, Moellering RC. Clinical, microbiologic and therapeutic aspects of purulent pericarditis. Am J Med 1975; 59:68–78.
87. Shabetai R. Acute pericarditis. Cardiol Clin 1990; 8:639–644.
88. Sagrista-Sauleda J, Barrabes JA, Permanyer-Miralda G, Soler-Soler J. Purulent pericarditis: review of a 20-year experience in a general hospital. J Am Coll Cardiol 1993; 22:1661–1665.
89. Rooney JJ, Crocco JA, Lyons HA. Tuberculous pericarditis. Ann Intern Med 1970; 72:73–78.
90. Spodick DH. Acoustic phenomena in pericardial disease. Am Heart J 1971; 81: 114–124.
91. Okorama EO, Perry LW, Scott LP. Acute bacterial pericarditis in children: report of 25 cases. Am Heart J 1975; 90:709–713.
92. Kauffmann CA, Watanakunnakorn C, Phair JP. Purulent pneumococcal pericarditis. Am J Med 1973; 54:743–750.
93. Helin M, Savola J, Lapinleimu K. Cardiac manifestations during a Coxsackie B5 epidemic. Br Med J 1968; 3:97–99.
94. Proby CM, Hackett D, Gupta S, Cox TM. Acute myopericarditis in influenza A infection. Q J Med 1986; 60:887–892.
95. Spodick DH. Electrocardiogram in acute pericarditis. Am J Cardiol 1974; 33: 470–474.
96. Spodick DH. Arrhythmias during acute pericarditis: a prospective study of 100 cases. JAMA 1976; 235:39–41.
97. Spodick DH. Frequency of arrhythmias in acute pericarditis determined by holter monitoring. Am J Cardiol 1984; 53:842–845.
98. Hoitt BD. Imaging the pericardium. Cardiol Clin 1990; 8:587–600.
99. Lorell BH, Braunwald E. Pericardial disease. In: Braunwald E, ed. Heart Disease. A Textbook of Cardiovascular Medicine. 4th ed. Philadelphia: WB Saunders, 1992:1465–1516.
100. Horowitz MS, Schultz CS, Stinson EB, Harrison DC, Popp RL. Sensitivity and specificity of echocardiographic diagnosis of pericardial effusion. Circulation 1974; 50:239–247.
101. Friedman MJ, Sahn DJ, Haber K. Two-dimensional echocardiography and B-mode

ultrasound for the diagnosis of loculated pericardial effusion. Circulation 1979; 60:1644–1649.

102. Wolf WJ. Echocardiographic features of a purulent pericardial peel. Am Heart J 1986; 111:990–992.
103. Ameli S, Shah PK. Cardiac tamponade: pathophysiology, diagnosis, management. Cardiol Clin 1991; 9:665–674.
104. Fowler NO. Cardiac tamponade: a clinical or an echocardiographic diagnosis? Circulation 1993; 87:1738–1741.
105. Niwa Y, Kishimoto H, Shimokata K. Carcinomatous and tuberculous pleural effusions. Comparison of tumor markers. Chest 1985; 87:351–355.
106. Sternbach GL. Pericarditis. Ann Emerg Med 1988; 17:214–220.
107. Sinzobahamvya N, Ikeogu MO. Purulent pericarditis. Arch Dis Child 1987; 62: 696–699.
108. Geraci JE, Heilman FR, Nichols DR, Wellman WE, Ross GT. Some laboratory and clinical experiences with a new antibiotic, vancomycin. Antibiot Ann 1956–1957: 90–106.
109. Tan JS, Holmes JC, Fowler NO, Manitsas GT, Phair JP. Antibiotic levels in pericardial fluid. J Clin Invest 1974; 53:7–12.
110. Dudley MN, Nightingale CH, Drezner AD, Low HB, Quintiliani R. Comparative penetration of cefonicid and cefazolin into the atrial appendage and pericardial fluid of patients undergoing open-heart surgery. Antimicrob Agents Chemother 1984; 26:347–350.
111. Decker CF, Tuazon CU. *Staphylococcus aureus* pericarditis in HIV-infected patients. Chest 1994; 105:615–616.
112. Yoshikawa TT. Bacterial pericarditis. West J Med 1975; 122:305–307.
113. Mann-Segal DDM, Shanahan EA, Jones B, Ramasamy D. Purulent pericarditis: rediscovery of an old remedy. J Thorac Cardiovasc Surg 1996; 111:487–488.
114. Gleckman RA. Nonviral infectious pericarditis. Cardiovasc Clin 1976; 7:159–175.
115. Wise RI. Modern management of severe staphylococcal disease. Medicine 1973; 52:295–304.
116. Roberts KB, Neff JM. Meningococcal pericarditis without meningitis in a child. Am J Dis Child 1972; 124:440–441.
117. Pierce HI, Cooper EB. Meningococcal pericarditis. Clinical features and therapy in five cases. Arch Intern Med 1972; 129:918–922.
118. Naraqi S, Kabins SA. Acute meningococcal pericarditis without meningitis. Arch Intern Med 1975; 135:314–316.
119. Gould K, Barnett JA, Sanford JP. Purulent pericarditis in the antibiotic era. Arch Intern Med 1974; 134:923–927.
120. Scott LP, Knox D, Perry LW, Pineros-Torres FJ. Meningococcal pericarditis: report of 2 cases, 1 complicated by acute constrictive pericarditis. Am J Cardiol 1972; 29:104–108.
121. Biancaniello TM, Anagnostopoulos CE, Bernstein HE, Proctor C. Purulent meningococcal pericarditis: chronic percutaneous drainage with a modified catheter aided by echocardiography. Clin Cardiol 1985; 8:542–544.
122. Chow AW, Culver B, Yoshikawa TT, Guze LB. Primary meningococcal pericarditis presenting with tamponade. Chest 1975; 67:611–613.

123. Dupuis C, Pascale G, Kachaner J, et al. Bacterial pericarditis in infancy and childhood. Am J Cardiol 1994; 74:807–809.
124. Weingarten S, Weinberg H, Fang M, Meyer R. *Haemophilus influenzae* pericarditis in two adults. West J Med 1986; 145:690–694.
125. Morgan RJ, Stephenson LW, Woolf PK, et al. Surgical treatment of purulent pericarditis in children. J Thorac Cardiovasc Surg 1983; 85:527–531.
126. Cheatham JE, Grantham RN, Peyton MD, et al. *Haemophilus influenzae* purulent pericarditis in children. J Thorac Cardiovasc Surg 1980; 79:933–936.
127. Houghton JL, Becherer PR. *Haemophilus influenzae* pericarditis successfully treated by catheter drainage. South Med J 1987; 80:766–768.
128. Bennett EV. Purulent pericarditis. J Thorac Cardiovasc Surg 1984; 87:641–642. Letter.
129. Kenney RT, Li JS, Clyde WA Jr, et al. Myocardial pericarditis: evidence of invasive disease. Clin Infect Dis 1993; 17(suppl 1):58–62.
130. Skiest DJ, Steiner D, Werner M, Garner JG. Anaerobic pericarditis: case report and review. Clin Infect Dis 1994; 19:435–440.
131. Bellet S, McMillan TM, Gonley BA. Tuberculous pericarditis: a clinical and pathologic study based upon a series of seventeen cases. Med Clin North Am 1934; 18: 201–218.
132. Quale JM, Lipschik GY, Heurich AE. Management of tuberculous pericarditis. Ann Thorac Surg 1987; 43:653–655.
133. Carson TJ, Murray GF, Wilcox BR, Starek PJK. The role of surgery in tuberculosis pericarditis. Ann Thorac Surg 1974; 17:163–167.
134. Suwan PK, Potjalongsilp S. Predictors of constrictive pericarditis after tuberculous pericarditis. Br Heart J 1995; 73:187–189.
135. Geisler C, Ernst P, Vejlsgaard R. *Candida* pericarditis in a patient with leukaemia. Scand J Haematol 1981; 27:75–78.
136. Young EJ, Vainrub B, Musher DM. Pericarditis due to histoplasmosis. JAMA 1978; 240:1750–1751.
137. Prager RL, Burney DP, Waterhouse G, Bender HW. Pulmonary, mediastinal and cardiac presentations of histoplasmosis. Ann Thorac Surg 1980; 30:385–390.
138. Smith JW, Utz JP. Progressive disseminated histoplasmosis. Ann Intern Med 1972; 76:557–565.
139. Sarosi GA, Voth DW, Dahl BA, Doto IL, Tosh FE. Disseminated histoplasmosis: results of long-term follow-up. A Center for Disease Control cooperative mycoses study. Ann Intern Med 1971; 75:511–516.
140. Kuhn LA. Acute and chronic cardiac tamponade. Cardiovasc Clin 1976; 7:177–195.
141. Mazurek B, Jehle D, Martin M. Emergency department echocardiography in the diagnosis and therapy of cardiac tamponade. J Emerg Med 1991; 9:27–31.
142. Taatvitsainen M, Bondestam S, Mankinen P, Pitkaranta P, Tierala E. Ultrasound guidance for pericardiocentesis. Acta Radiol 1991; 32:9–11.
143. Callahan JA, Seward JB, Nishimura RA, et al. Two-dimensional echocardiography-guided pericardiocentesis: experience in 117 consecutive patients. Am J Cardiol 1985; 55:476–479.
144. Clarke DP, Cosgrove DO. Real-time ultrasound scanning in the planning and guidance of pericardiocentesis. Clin Radiol 1987; 38:119–122.

145. Kirkorian JG, Hancock EW. Pericardiocentesis. Am J Med 1978; 65:808–814.
146. Culliford AT, Lipton M, Spencer FC. Operation for chronic constrictive pericarditis. Do the surgical approach and degree of pericardial resection influence the outcome significantly? Ann Thorac Surg 1980; 29:146–152.
147. Paul O, Castleman B, White PD. Chronic constrictive pericarditis: a study of 53 cases. Am J Med Sci 1948; 216:361–377.
148. Cameron J, Oesterle SN, Baldwin JC, Hancock EW. The etiologic spectrum of constrictive pericarditis. Am Heart J 1987; 113:354–360.
149. King JW, Nguyen VQ, Conrad SA. Results of a prospective statewide reporting system for infective endocarditis. Am J Med Sci 1988; 295:517–527.
150. Griffen MR, Wilson WR, Edwards WD, O'Fallon WM, Kurland LT. Infective endocarditis, Olsted County, Minnesota, 1950 through 1981. JAMA 1985; 254: 1199–1202.
151. Bayer AS. Infective endocarditis. Clin Infect Dis 1993; 17:313–322.
152. Harris SL. Definitions and demographic characteristics. In: Kaye D, ed. Infective Endocarditis. 2d ed. New York: Raven Press, 1992:1–18.
153. Lerner PI, Weinstein L. Infective endocarditis in the antibiotic era. N Engl J Med 1966; 274:199–206.
154. Weinstein L, Rubin RH. Infective endocarditis—1973. Prog Cardiovasc Dis 1973; 16:239–274.
155. Kaye D. Changes in the spectrum, diagnosis, and management of bacterial and fungal endocarditis. Med Clin North Am 1973; 57:941–957.
156. Weinberger I, Rotenberg Z, Zacharovitch D, et al. Native valve infective endocarditis in the 1970's versus the 1980's: underlying cardiac lesions and infecting organisms. Clin Cardiol 1990; 13:94–98.
157. Steckelberg JM, Wilson WR. Risk factors for infective endocarditis. Infect Dis Clin North Am 1993; 7:9–19.
158. Nagger CZ, Forgacs P. Infective endocarditis: a challenging disease. Med Clin North Am 1986; 70:1279–1294.
159. McKinsey DS, Ratts TE, Bisno AL. Underlying cardiac lesions in adults with infective endocarditis. Am J Med 1987; 82:681–688.
160. Pantely GA, Rahimtoola S. Infective endocarditis. In: Eliot RS, ed. Cardiac Emergencies. 2d ed. New York: Futura Publishing Co., 1982:451–467.
161. Buchbinder NA, Roberts WC. Alcoholism, an important but unemphasized factor predisposing to infective endocarditis. Arch Intern Med 1973; 132:689–692.
162. Watanakunaknorn C. Changing epidemiology and newer aspects of infective endocarditis. Adv Intern Med 1977; 22:21–47.
163. Steckelberg JM, Melton LJ III, Ilstrup DM, Rouse MS, Wilson WF. Influence of referral bias on the apparent clinical spectrum of infective endocarditis. Am J Med 1990; 88:582–588.
164. Von Reyn CF, Levy BS, Arbeit RD, Friedland G, Crumpacker CS. Infective endocarditis: an analysis based on strict case definitions. Ann Intern Med 1981; 94:505–518.
165. Kaye D. Changing pattern of infective endocarditis. Am J Med 1985; 78(suppl 6B): 157–162.
166. Klein RS, Catalano MT, Edberg SC, Casey JI, Steibigel NH. *Streptococcus bovis* septicemia and carcinoma of the colon. Ann Intern Med 1979; 91:560–562.

167. Leport C, Bure A, Leport J, Vilde JL. Incidence of colonic lesions in *Streptococcus bovis* and enterococcal endocarditis. Lancet 1987; 1(8535):748. Letter.
168. Emiliani VJ, Chodos JE, Comer GM, Holness LG, Schwartz AJ. *Streptococcus bovis* brain abscess associated with an occult colonic villous adenoma. Am J Gastroenterol 1990; 85:78–80.
169. Megran DW. Enterococcal endocarditis. Clin Infect Dis 1992; 15:63–71.
170. Mortara LA, Bayer AS. *Staphylococcus aureus* bacteremia and endocarditis. Infect Dis Clin North Am 1993; 7:53–68.
171. Caputo GM, Archer GL, Calderwood SB, DiNubile MJ, Karchmer AW. Native valve endocarditis due to coagulase-negative staphylococci: clinical and microbiologic features. Am J Med 1987; 83:619–625.
172. Arber N, Militianu A, Ben-Yehuda A, Krivoy N, Pinkhas J, Sidi Y. Native valve *Staphylococcus epidermidis* endocarditis: report of seven cases and review of the literature. Am J Med 1991; 90:758–762.
173. Whitener C, Caputo GM, Weitekamp MR, Karchmer AW. Endocarditis due to coagulase-negative staphylcocci: microbiologic, epidemiologic, and clinical considerations. Infect Dis Clin North Am 1993; 7:81–96.
174. Cohen PS, Maguire JH, Weinstein L. Infective endocarditis caused by gram-negative bacteria: a review of the literature, 1945–1977. Prog Cardiovasc Dis 1980; 22:205–242.
175. Geraci JE, Wilson WR. Endocarditis due to gram-negative bacteria: report of 56 cases. Mayo Clin Proc 1982; 57:145–148.
176. Rubinstein E, Noriega ER, Simberkoff MS, Holzman R, Rahal JJ Jr. Fungal endocarditis: analysis of 24 cases and review of the literature. Medicine 1975; 54: 331–344.
177. Moyer DV, Edwards JE Jr. Fungal endocarditis. In: Kaye D, ed. Infective Endocarditis. 2nd ed. New York: Raven Press, 1992:299–312.
178. Rubinstein E, Lang R. Fungal endocarditis. Eur Heart J 1995; 16(suppl B):84–89.
179. Ellner JJ, Rosenthal MS, Lerner PI, McHenry MC. Infective endocarditis caused by slow-growing, fastidious, gram-negative bacteria. Medicine 1979; 58:145–158.
180. Van Scoy RE. Culture-negative endocarditis. Mayo Clin Proc 1982; 57:149–154.
181. Banks T, Fletcher R, Nayab A. Infective endocarditis in heroin addicts. Am J Med 1973; 55:444–451.
182. Chambers HF, Morris DL, Tauber MG, Modin G. Cocaine use and the risk for endocarditis in intravenous drug users. Ann Intern Med 1987; 106:833–836.
183. Sande MA, Lee BL, Mills J, Chambers HF III. Endocarditis in intravenous drug users. In: Kaye D, ed. Infective Endocarditis. 2d ed. New York: Raven Press, 1992:345–359.
184. Mathew J, Addai T, Anand A, Morrobel A, Maheshwari P, Freels S. Clinical features, site of involvement, bacteriologic findings, and outcome of infective endocarditis in intravenous drug users. Arch Intern Med 1995; 155:1641–1648.
185. Brooks GF, O'Donoghue JM, Rissing JP, Soapes K, Smith JW. *Eikenella corrodens*, a recently recognized pathogen: infections in medical-surgical patients and in methylphenidate abuse. Medicine 1974; 53:325–342.
186. Wilson WR, Danielson GK, Giuliani ER, Geraci JE. Prosthetic valve endocarditis. Mayo Clin Proc 1982; 57:155–161.

187. Heimberger TS, Duma RJ. Infections of prosthetic heart valves and cardiac pacemakers. Infect Dis Clin North Am 1989; 3:221–245.
188. Ivert TA, Dismukes WE, Cobbs CG, Blackstone EH, Kirklin JW, Bergdahl LA. Prosthetic valve endocarditis. Circulation 1984; 69:223–232.
189. Calderwood SB, Swinski LA, Waternaux CM, Karchmer AW, Buckley MJ. Risk factors for the development of prosthetic valve endocarditis. Circulation 1985; 72: 31–37.
190. Chastre J, Trouillet JL. Early infective endocarditis on prosthetic valves. Eur Heart J 1995; 16(suppl B):32–38.
191. Horstkotte D, Piper C, Niehues R, Wiemer M, Schultheiss HP. Late prosthetic valve endocarditis. Eur Heart J 1995; 16(suppl B):39–47.
192. Karchmer AW, Archer GL, Dismukes WE. *Staphylococcus epidermidis* causing prosthetic valve endocarditis: microbiologic and clinical observations as guides to therapy. Ann Intern Med 1983; 98:447–455.
193. Friedland G, VonReyn CF, Levy B, Arbeit R, Dasse P, Crumpacker C. Nosocomial endocarditis. Infect Control 1984; 5:284–288.
194. Terpenning MS, Buggy BP, Kauffman CA. Hospital-acquired infective endocarditis. Arch Intern Med 1988; 148:1601–1603.
195. Fang G, Keys TF, Gentry LO, et al. Prosthetic valve endocarditis resulting from nosocomial bacteremia. Ann Intern Med 1993; 119:560–567.
196. Weinstein L. Life-threatening complications of infective endocarditis. Arch Intern Med 1986; 146:953–957.
197. Garvey GJ, Neu HC. Infective endocarditis—an evolving disease: a review of endocarditis at the Columbia-Presbyterian Medical Center, 1968–1973. Medicine 1978; 57:105–127.
198. Terpenning MS, Buggy BP, Kauffman CA. Infective endocarditis: clinical features in young and elderly patients. Am J Med 1987; 83:626–634.
199. Pelletier LL, Petersdorf RG. Infective endocarditis: a review of 125 cases from the University of Washington Hospitals, 1963–1972. Medicine 1977; 56:287–313.
200. Silverberg HH. Roth spots. Mt Sinai J Med 1970; 37:77–79.
201. Kaye KM, Kaye D. Laboratory findings including blood cultures. In: Kaye D, ed. Infective Endocarditis. 2nd ed. New York: Raven Press, 1992:117–124.
202. Werner AS, Cobbs CG, Kaye D, Hook EW. Studies on the bacteremia of bacterial endocarditis. JAMA 1967; 202:199–203.
203. Washington JA. The role of the microbiology laboratory in the diagnosis and antimicrobial treatment of infective endocarditis. Mayo Clin Proc 1982; 57:22–32.
204. Dismukes WE. Management of infective endocarditis. In: Rackley CE, ed. Critical Care Cardiology. Philadelphia: F. A. Davis Company, 1981:189–208.
205. Washington JA, Ilstrup DM. Blood cultures: issues and controversies. Rev Infect Dis 1986; 8:792–802.
206. Aronson MD, Bor DH. Blood cultures. Ann Intern Med 1987; 106:246–253.
207. Khanderia BK. Suspected bacterial endocarditis: to TEE or not to TEE. J Am Coll Cardiol 1993; 21:222–224. Editorial.
208. Murphy JG, Foster-Smith K. Management of complications of infective endocarditis with emphasis on echocardiographic findings. Infect Dis Clin North Am 1993; 7: 153–165.

209. Durack DT, Lukes AS, Bright DK. New criteria for diagnosis of infective endocarditis: utilization of specific echocardiographic findings. Am J Med 1994; 96: 200–209.
210. Daniel WG, Schroeder E, Nonnast-Daniel B, Lichtlen PR. Conventional and transesophageal echocardiography in the diagnosis of infective endocarditis. Eur Heart J 1987; 8:287–292.
211. Daniel WG, Schroeder E, Mugge A, Lichtlen PR. Transesophageal echocardiography in infective endocarditis. Am J Cardiac Imagery 1988; 2:78–85.
212. Taams MA, Gussenhoven EJ, Bos E, et al. Enhanced morphological diagnosis in infective endocarditis by transoesophageal echocardiography. Br Heart J 1990; 63: 109–113.
213. Daniel WG, Mugge A, Martin RP, et al. Improvement in the diagnosis of abscesses associated with endocarditis by transesophageal echocardiography. N Engl J Med 1991; 324:795–800.
214. Birmingham GD, Rahko PS, Ballantyne R. Improved detection of infective endocarditis with transesophageal echocardiogram. Am Heart J 1992; 123:774–781.
215. Karalis DG, Bansal RC, Hauck AJ, et al. Transesophageal echocardiographic recognition of subaortic complications in aortic valve endocarditis: clinical and surgical implications. Circulation 1992; 86:353–362.
216. Aguado JM, Gonsalez-Vilchez F, Martin-Duran R, Arjona R, Vasquez de Prada JA. Perivalvular abscesses associated with endocarditis: clinical features and diagnostic accuracy of two-dimensional echocardiography. Chest 1993; 104:88–93.
217. Shapiro SM, Young E, DeGuzman S, et al. Transesophageal echocardiography in diagnosis of infective endocarditis. Chest 1994; 105:377–382.
218. Vered Z, Mossinson D, Peleg E, Kaplinsky E, Motro M, Beker B. Echocardiographic assessment of prosthetic valve endocarditis. Eur Heart J 1995; 16(suppl B):63–67.
219. von Reyn CF, Arbeit RD. Case definitions for endocarditis. Am J Med 1994; 96: 220–222. Editorial.
220. Bayer AS. Diagnostic criteria for identifying cases of endocarditis—revisiting the Duke criteria two years later. Clin Infect Dis 1996; 23:303–304. Editorial.
221. Bayer AS, Ward JI, Ginzton LE, Shapiro SM. Evaluation of new clinical criteria for the diagnosis of infective endocarditis. Am J Med 1994; 96:211–219.
222. Hoen B, Selton-Suty C, Danchin N, et al. Evaluation of the Duke criteria versus the Beth Israel criteria for the diagnosis of infective endocarditis. Clin Infect Dis 1995; 21:905–909.
223. Del Pont JM, De Cicco LT, Vartalitis C, et al. Infective endocarditis in children: clinical analyses and evaluation of two diagnostic criteria. Pediatr Infect Dis J 1995; 14:1079–1086.
224. Bayer AS. Revised diagnostic criteria for infective endocarditis. Cardiol Clin North Am 1996; 14:345–350.
225. Dodds GA III, Sexton DJ, Durack DT, Bashore TM, Corey GR, Kisslo J. Negative predictive value of the Duke criteria for diagnosis of infective endocarditis. Am J Cardiol 1996; 77:403–407.
226. Hoen B, Beguinot I, Rabaud C, et al. The Duke criteria for diagnosing infective endocarditis are specific: analysis of 100 patients with acute fever or fever of unknown origin. Clin Infect Dis 1996; 23:298–302.

227. von Reyn CF, Arbeit RD, Freidland GH, Crumpacker CS III. Criteria for the diagnosis of infective endocarditis. Clin Infect Dis 1994; 19:368–370. Letter.
228. Baldassarre JS, Kaye D. Principles and overview of antibiotic therapy., In: Kaye D, ed. Infective Endocarditis. 2d ed. New York: Raven Press, 1992:169–190.
229. Wilson WR, Karchmer AW, Dajani AS, et al. Antibiotic treatment of adults with infective endocarditis due to streptococci, enterococci, staphylococci, and HACEK microorganisms. JAMA 1995; 274:1706–1713.
230. Stamboulian D, Bonvehi P, Arevalo C, et al. Antibiotic management of outpatients with endocarditis due to penicillin-susceptible streptococci. Rev Infect Dis 1991; 13(suppl 2):160–163.
231. Francioli P, Etienne J, Hoigne R, Thys JP, Gerber A. Treatment of streptococcal endocarditis with a single daily dose of ceftriaxone sodium for 4 weeks: efficacy and outpatient treatment feasibility. JAMA 1992; 267:264–267. Comment.
232. Francioli PB. Ceftriaxone and outpatient treatment of infective endocarditis. Infect Dis Clin North Am 1993; 7:95–115.
233. Wilson WR, Thompson RL, Wilkowske CJ, Washington JA II, Giuliani ER, Geraci JE. Short-term therapy for streptococcal infective endocarditis: combined intramuscular administration of penicillin and streptomycin. JAMA 1981; 245:360–363.
234. Eliopoulos GM. Enterococcal endocarditis. In: Kaye D, ed. Infective Endocarditis. 2nd ed. New York: Raven Press, 1992:209–223.
235. Rice LB, Calderwood SB, Eliopoulos GM, Farber BF, Karchmer AW. Enterococcal endocarditis: a comparison of prosthetic and native valve disease. Rev Infect Dis 1991; 13:1–7.
236. Eliopoulos GM. Aminoglycoside resistant enterococcal endocarditis. Med Clin North Am 1993; 17:117–133.
237. Sande MA, Courtney KB. Nafcillin-gentamicin synergism in experimental staphylococcal endocarditis. J Lab Clin Med 1976; 88:118–124.
238. Korzeniowski O, Sande MA. Combination antimicrobial therapy for *Staphylococcus aureus* endocarditis in patients addicted to parenteral drugs and in non-addicts: a prospective study. Ann Intern Med 1982; 97:496–503.
239. Karchmer AW. *Staphylococcus aureus* and vancomycin: the sequel. Ann Intern Med 1991; 115:739–741.
240. Deighton M, Pearson S, Capstick J, Spelman D, Borland R. Phenotypic variation of *Staphylococcus epidermidis* isolated from a patient with native valve endocarditis. J Clin Microbiol 1992; 30:2385–2390.
241. LeQuellec A, Bessis D, Perez C, Ciurana AJ. Endocarditis due to B-lactamase-producing *Cardiobacterium hominis*. Clin Infect Dis 1994; 19:994–995. Letter.
242. Hessen MT, Abrutyn E. Gram-negative bacterial endocarditis. In: Kaye D, ed. Infective Endocarditis. 2nd ed. New York: Raven Press, 1992:251–264.
243. Denning DW, Stevens DA. Antifungal and surgical treatment of invasive aspergillosis: review of 2,121 published cases. Rev Infect Dis 1990; 12:1147–1201.
244. Mansur AJ, Grinberg M, Lemos da Luz P, Bellotti G. The complications of infective endocarditis: a reappraisal in the 1980s. Arch Intern Med 1992; 152:2428–2432.
245. Steckelberg JM, Murphy JG, Wilson WR. Management of complications of infective endocarditis. In: Kaye D, ed. Infective Endocarditis. 2nd ed. New York: Raven Press, 1992:435–453.

246. Lytle BW, Priest BP, Taylor PC, et al. Surgical treatment of prosthetic valve endocarditis. J Thorac Cardiovasc Surg 1996; 111:198–207.
247. Rose RI Jr, Higgins LS, Helgason AH. Bacterial endocarditis, pericarditis, and tamponade. Am J Cardiol 1967; 19:447–451.
248. Kim HS, Weilbaecher DG, Lie JT, Titus JL. Myocardial abscesses. Am J Clin Pathol 1978; 70:18–23.
249. Ryon DS, Pastor BH, Meyerson RM. Abscesses of the myocardium. Am J Med Sci 1966; 251:698–705.
250. Arnett EN, Roberts WC. Valve ring abscess in active infective endocarditis. Circulation 1976; 54:140–145.
251. Blumberg EA, Karalis DA, Chandrasekaran K, et al. Endocarditis-associated paravalvular abscesses. Chest 1995; 107:898–903.
252. DiNubile MJ, Calderwood SB, Steinhaus DM, Karchmer AW. Cardiac conduction abnormalities complicating native valve active infective endocarditis. Am J Cardiol 1986; 58:1213–1217.
253. Weisse AB, Khan MY. The relationship between new cardiac conduction defects and extension of valve infection in native valve endocarditis. Clin Cardiol 1990; 13: 337–345.
254. Schlaifer JD, Martin TD, Hill JA, Kerensky RA. Coronary artery obstruction caused by perivalvular abscess in aortic valve endocarditis. Am Heart J 1996; 131:413–416.
255. Wenger NK, Bauer S. Coronary embolism: review of the literature and presentation of fifteen cases. Am J Med 1958; 25:549–557.
256. Buchbinder NA, Roberts WC. Left-sided valvular active infective endocarditis: a study of forty-five necropsy patients. Am J Med 1972; 53:20–35.
257. Woo KS, Lam YM, Kwok HT, Tse LKK, Vallance-Owen J. Prognostic index in prediction of mortality from infective endocarditis. Int J Cardiol 1988; 24:47–54.
258. Erbel R, Liu F, Ge J, Rohmann S, Kupferwasser I. Identification of high-risk subgroups in infective endocarditis and the role of echocardiography. Eur Heart J 1995; 16(suppl B):588–602.
259. Pruitt AA, Rubin RH, Karchmer AW, Duncan GW. Neurologic complications of bacterial endocarditis. Medicine 1978; 57:329–343.
260. Lerner PI. Neurologic complications of infective endocarditis. Med Clin North Am 1985; 69:385–398.
261. Jones HR Jr, Siekert RG. Neurologic manifestations of infective endocarditis. Brain 1989; 112:1295–1315.
262. Salgado AV, Furlan AJ, Keys TF, Nichols TR, Beck GJ. Neurologic complications of endocarditis: a 12-year experience. Neurology 1989; 39:173–178.
263. Hart RG, Foster JW, Luther MF, Kanter MC. Stroke in infective endocarditis. Stroke 1990; 21:695–700.
264. Kanter MC, Hart RG. Neurologic complications of infective endocarditis. Neurology 1991; 41:1015–1020.
265. Brust JCM, Dickinson PCT, Hughes JEO, Holtzman RNN. The diagnosis and treatment of cerebral mycotic aneurysms. Ann Neurol 1990; 27:238–246.
266. Wilson WR, Giuliani ER, Danielson GK, Geraci JE. Management of complications of infective endocarditis. Mayo Clin Proc 1982; 57:162–170.

267. Kaufman SL, White RI, Harrington DP, Barth KH, Siegelman SS. Protean manifestations of mycotic aneurysms. AJR 1978; 131:1019–1025.
268. Mansur AJ, Grinberg M, Leao PP, Chung CV, Stolf NAG, Pileggi F. Extracranial mycotic aneurysms in infective endocarditis. Clin Cardiol 1986; 9:65–72.
269. Gonda RL Jr, Gutierrez OH, Azodo MVU. Mycotic aneurysms of the aorta: radiologic features. Radiology 1988; 168:343–346.
270. McCuskey WH, Loehr SP, Smidebush GC, Link KM. Detection of mycotic pseudoaneurysm of the ascending aorta using MRI. Magn Reson Imag 1993; 11:1223–1226.
271. Anderson CB, Butcher HR, Ballinger WF. Mycotic aneurysms. Arch Surg 1974; 109:712–716.
272. Johansen KJ, Devin J. Mycotic aortic aneurysms: a reappraisal. Arch Surg 1983; 118:583–588.
273. Bohmfalk GL, Story JL, Wissinger JP, Brown WE Jr. Bacterial intracranial aneurysm. J Neurosurg 1978; 48:369–382.
274. Bingham WF. Treatment of mycotic intracranial aneurysms. J Neurosurg 1977; 46: 428–437.
275. Moskowitz MA, Rosenbaum AE, Tyler HR. Angiographically monitored resolution of cerebral mycotic aneurysms. Neurology 1974; 24:1103–1108.
276. Morawetz RB, Karp RB. Evolution and resolution of intracranial bacterial (mycotic) aneurysms. Neurosurgery 1984; 15:43–49.
277. Alsip SG, Blackstone EH, Kirklin JW, Cobbs CG. Indications for cardiac surgery in patients with active infective endocarditis. Am J Med 1985; 78(suppl 6B):138–148.
278. Douglas JL, Dismukes WE. Surgical therapy of infective endocarditis on natural valves. In: Kaye D, ed. Infective Endocarditis. 2nd ed. New York: Raven Press, 1992:397–411.
279. Mills J, Utley J, Abbott J. Heart failure in infective endocarditis: predisposing factors, course, and treatment. Chest 1974; 66:151–157.
280. Mann T, McLaurin L, Grossman W, Craige E. Assessing the hemodynamic severity of acute aortic regurgitation due to infective endocarditis. N Engl J Med 1975; 293:108–113.
281. Karchmer AW, Stinson EB. The role of surgery in infective endocarditis. In: Remington JS, Swartz MS, eds. Curr Clin Top Infect Dis. New York: McGraw Hill, 1980:124–157.
282. Croft CH, Woodward W, Elliott A, Commerford PJ, Barnard CN, Berk W. Analysis of surgical versus medical therapy in active complicated native valve infective endocarditis. Am J Cardiol 1983; 51:1650–1655.
283. Richardson JD, Karp RB, Kirklin JW, Dismukes WE. Treatment of infective endocarditis: a ten year comparative analysis. Circulation 1978; 58:589–597.
284. Larbalestier RI, Kinchla NM, Aranki SF, Couper GS, Collins JJ Jr, Cohn LH. Acute bacterial endocarditis: optimizing surgical results. Circulation 1992; 86(suppl II):68–74.
285. Mullany CJ, Chua YL, Schaff HV, et al. Early and late survival after surgical treatment of culture-positive active endocarditis. Mayo Clin Proc 1995; 70:517–525.
286. Jamieson SW. Surgical therapy for infective endocarditis. Mayo Clin Proc 1995; 70:598–600. Editorial.

287. Black S, O'Rourke RA, Karliner JS. Role of surgery in the treatment of primary infective endocarditis. Am J Med 1974; 56:357–369.
288. Turnier E, Kay JH, Bernstein S, Mendez AM, Zubiate P. Surgical treatment of *Candida* endocarditis. Chest 1975; 67:262–268.
289. Steckelberg JM, Murphy JG, Ballard D, et al. Emboli in infective endocarditis—the prognostic value of echocardiography. Ann Intern Med 1991; 114:635–640.
290. O'Brien JT, Geiser EA. Infective endocarditis and echocardiography. Am Heart J 1984; 108:386–394.
291. Mugge A, Daniel WG, Gunter F, Lichtlen PR. Echocardiography in infective endocarditis: reassessment of prognostic implications of vegetation size determined by the transthoracic and the transesophageal approach. J Am Coll Cardiol 1989; 14:631–638.
292. Heinle S, Wilderman N, Harrison JK, et al. Value of transthoracic echocardiography in predicting embolic events in active infective endocarditis. Am J Cardiol 1994; 74:799–801.
293. Hecht SR, Berger M. Right-sided endocarditis in intravenous drug users. Ann Intern Med 1992; 117:560–566.
294. Levitsky S, Mammana RB, Silverman NA, Weber F, Hiro S, Wright RN. Acute endocarditis in drug addicts: surgical treatment for gram-negative sepsis. Circulation 1982; 66(suppl 2):1135–1138.
295. Dajani AS, Taubert KA, Wilson W, et al. Prevention of bacterial endocarditis: recommendations by the American Heart Association. JAMA 1997; 277:1794–1801.
296. Durack DT. Prevention of infective endocarditis. N Engl J Med 1995; 332:38–44.
297. Terpenning MS. Infective endocarditis. Clin Geriatr Med 1992; 8:903–912.

7

Management of the Postoperative Cardiac Surgery Patient

STEVEN S. KHAN

Cedars-Sinai Medical Center and University of California, Los Angeles, School of Medicine, Los Angeles, California

I. INTRODUCTION

Each year, about 250,000 coronary bypass surgery procedures and 50,000 valve replacements are performed in the United States. About 20% of coronary bypass surgery procedures each year are reoperations. With the advent of percutaneous coronary angioplasty and other catheter-based procedures in the 1980s, many predicted the impending end of cardiac surgery. However, this has not come to pass. Instead, the last several years have seen an explosion of new procedures in all aspects of cardiac surgery including coronary revascularization, valve replacement, arrhythmia surgery, and, perhaps most exciting, surgical treatment of end-stage heart failure. The advent of these procedures suggests that the role of cardiac surgery may expand considerably in the future. Therefore, a working knowledge of the management of the postcardiac surgical patient is crucial to the well-trained intensivist.

It is important to note at the outset that the care of the open heart surgery patient differs from the care of either general surgery or cardiology patients. The etiology and treatment of arrhythmias, low output states, and bleeding are frequently different from other critical care populations, primarily because of the use of cardiopulmonary bypass (CPB) and systemic hypothermia in most patients. Therefore, we will briefly review the intraoperative course of patients undergoing heart surgery.

II. INTRAOPERATIVE COURSE

In most centers, routine coronary artery bypass and valve surgery are performed using hypothermic cardiopulmonary bypass with cross-clamping of the aorta. After the chest is opened, a cannula is placed in the right atrium and connected to the heart lung machine. A cannula is also inserted in the ascending aorta to return blood from the heart lung machine to the aorta. A second aortic cannula is placed proximal to the first for infusion of cardioplegia.

Once these cannulae are placed, a portion of the venous blood returning to the heart is drained off through the atrial cannual and oxygenated by the heart lung machine. This phase of surgery is called partial cardiopulmonary bypass. During this phase, the patient's blood temperature is gradually lowered by using a heat exchanger in the heart lung machine to cool the blood. At a temperature of about 25°C, the patient usually develops ventricular fibrillation and the aorta is cross-clamped. At this point the patient is on complete cardiopulmonary bypass. After the cross-clamping of the aorta, cardioplegia is infused into the proximal aortic root cannula to perfuse the coronary arteries. However, if the aortic valve is not competent, cardioplegia may instead flow into the left ventricle instead of the coronary arteries. Topical hypothermia is then administered by packing the heart in ice slush.

A. Pump Oxygenators

Pump oxygenators can be either bubble oxygenators or membrane oxygenators. Bubble oxygenators place blood in direct contact with fine oxygen bubbles to allow diffusion of oxygen in and carbon dioxide out. Membrane oxygenators use a semipermeable membrane to separate the blood and oxygen during the diffusion process.

Pump oxygenators may damage the red blood cells, platelets, and white blood cells. For short pump runs (<3 h), there is no difference between the two types of oxygenators in the amount of trauma to the formed elements of blood. Membrane oxygenators may be superior for longer pump times and are currently in exclusive use by many institutions.

B. Heparin-Protamine Administration

Clotting of blood in the CPB machine is reduced by routine use of heparin. After bypass is completed, the heparin is reversed using protamine (about 1.3 mg protamine for each 1 mg heparin given). If the ACT remains elevated, more protamine is usually administered.

C. Alternative CPB Techniques

Although most centers use the method of myocardial preservation described above, other techniques are also used. Major interest in avoiding hypothermia has led to the use of warm blood cardioplegia in the last 5 years. The potential benefits were felt to include fewer pulmonary complications, less myocardial depression, decreased ICU stays, and less diaphragmatic paralysis. These benefits of warm cardioplegia are anecdotal and not proven. In onc randomized clinical trial of warm vs. cold cardioplegia, the only significant difference seen was an increase in the incidence of perioperative stroke in the patients receiving warm cardioplegia (1). In a randomized trial of 1732 patients, the Warm Heart Investigators (2) found no differences in stroke between warm and cold methods. Although, CK-MB release was less in warm patients, Q-wave MI, mortality, and reoperation for bleeding were similar.

Cardiac surgery can also be performed without cardioplegia by either performing surgery on the beating heart or by intermittently cross-clamping the aorta during surgery. Although few surgeons use the technique of intermittent cross-clamping, the current interest in minimally invasive cardiac surgery has prompted the development of a new generation of devices to facilitate surgery on the beating heart. Generally, these procedures are most easily done on anterior vessels such as the left anterior descending and diagonals, and, with somewhat greater difficulty, the right coronary artery. Surgery on the circumflex artery with this approach remains difficult.

D. Total Circulatory Arrest

Total circulatory arrest with profound hypothermia is a technique used in surgery on the aortic arch and in other procedures where it is difficult to continue to provide blood flow to the brain with standard bypass techniques. Ice packs are used to cool the head and body and after the core temperature is lowered to approximately 15°C, perfusion is stopped and the surgery proceeds. Following surgery, the patient is rewarmed and the remaining phases of surgery are completed. Although rare, there is a small risk of inadequate cooling of the brain and anoxic brain damage.

E. Discontinuation of Cardiopulmonary Bypass

Cardiopulmonary bypass is discontinued once the procedures requiring it are completed (for example, when the distal anastomoses are performed in coronary bypass surgery) and air is removed from the heart. Development of ST elevation on the ECG during this phase is suggestive of coronary air embolism.

III. NORMAL POSTOPERATIVE COURSE

A. Normal Findings

Patients may be slightly thrombocytopenic, but platelet transfusions are unnecessary unless the patient is actively bleeding. Patients with mechanical prosthetic valves may have an elevated LDH due to low-grade hemolysis, although the LDH is usually less than twice the upper limit of normal.

On arrival in the cardiac surgery intensive care unit patients are frequently still hypothermic, and their hemodynamics reflect this (3). Thus, patients may have a low cardiac index with a high systemic vascular resistance (SVR) due to reduced metabolic needs and vasoconstriction. The cardiac output should increase as the patient warms with a reduction in SVR. In most cases, patients with an initially low cardiac output after surgery need only simple rewarming.

B. Clinical Exam

Patients will typically have two mediastinal tubes, one in the anterior and one in the posterior mediastinum. Patients who have had a left or right mammary bypass may also have a pleural tube on the same side. Some surgeons place atrial and/or ventricular pacing wires which exit the chest just below the rib cage. Wires to the right of midline are usually atrial, and on the left, ventricular, although this should be confirmed with the surgeon or by pacing. Most patients will have an arterial line and at least a central venous line. Pulmonary artery catheters are not placed in all patients, and many elective coronary bypass procedures can be performed without hemodynamic monitoring.

Auscultation of the heart will frequently reveal a two- or three-component pericardial rub or mediastinal crunch early after surgery due to the mediastinal chest tubes. These rubs normally do not require treatment and disappear after the tubes are removed. Patients with prosthetic heart valves may have muffled prosthetic sounds for the first day or two after surgery. Nearly all patients with aortic prostheses will have a systolic murmur. No patient should have a regurgitant murmur from any heart valve prosthesis, however.

C. Electrocardiographic and Chest X Ray Findings

Patients may have nonspecific ST and T-wave changes after cardiac surgery. Diffuse ST elevation is usually due to pericarditis while focal ST segment elevation, if new, may be due to coronary air embolism or rarely graft occlusion. Epicardial pacing wires occasionally can't be seen on an AP portable chest film and a lateral chest x-ray may need to be done to visualize them. The postoperative chest x-ray should be examined for the presence of a significant pneumothorax. Some patients have air below the diaphragms, but this is of little practical consequence and may be due to perforation of the diaphragm during placement of the atrial pacing wires. Pneumopericardium is occasionally seen and is usually of no clinical significance. Atelectasis is a common pulmonary finding as well as pleural effusions. Pleural effusions can ordinarily be managed conservatively with diuresis if there is associated volume overload or heart failure. Effusions occupying more than about half of the lung field on the PA film or those causing respiratory compromise should be removed by thoracentesis.

D. Normal Postoperative Care

Patients are normally extubated within 6 to 7 hours after surgery. Some institutions are extubating selected low-risk coronary bypass patients on the operating table before transfer to the ICU. Early extubation is felt to be important in speeding transfer from the ICU on post operative day 1 and early discharge from the hospital. The chest tubes are generally removed 8–12 hours after surgery or when the drainage has been less than 40 cc/h for 4 h or more.

Many patients are atrially paced on return to the ICU, primarily because of hypothermia-induced bradycardia. Pacing can usually be discontinued when the patient has warmed and the pacemaker converted to a standby mode. In addition to pacing for bradycardia and heart block, atrial pacemaker leads can also be used for diagnosis of arrhythmias and for rapid pacing to convert atrial flutter.

E. Prophylactic Drug Therapy

1. *Atrial Fibrillation*

The use of prophylactic drug therapy to prevent a variety of complications after heart surgery has gained widespread acceptance. Prophylaxis for atrial fibrillation is now used by most institutions after both coronary bypass and valve surgery. The most convincing evidence for a beneficial effect of treatment is with β blockers. A number of randomized trials have shown a reduction in the incidence of atrial fibrillation of about 50% with routine postoperative β blocker therapy. The newest β blocker to be used for postoperative prophylaxis of atrial fibrillation is sotalol (4), but use of low doses of standard β blockers such as atenolol 25 mg PO BID or propranolol 10 to 20 mg PO TID is well accepted and effective. There is no convincing evidence that digoxin prevents atrial fibrillation although it is still occasionally given after surgery in patients with frequent premature atrial contractions so that the heart rate is controlled if the patient develops atrial fibrillation. Calcium blockers can also be used for rate control in atrial fibrillation. Recent data suggest that procainamide, given as a bolus of 12 mg/kg followed by a 2 mg/min drip, may also be beneficial in reducing atrial fibrillation after coronary bypass surgery (5).

2. *Bleeding*

There has been considerable recent interest in prophylactic therapy to reduce perioperative bleeding after heart surgery. The antifibrinolytic drugs, ϵ amino caproic acid (EACA), tranexamic acid, and aprotinin have been most studied and many centers are now routinely administering one of these agents to patients at increased risk for bleeding, such as patients undergoing a reoperation. A recent meta-analysis suggested that these agents all reduce bleeding compared to placebo. Administration of either EACA or aprotinin was associated with a 30% and 36% reduction in bleeding, respectively (both $P < .0001$) and with a reduction in the volume of red cell transfusions ($P < .0001$ for both agents). Reoperation for bleeding was also reduced although this was of borderline significance (both $P = .07$). The percentage of patients requiring transfusions was only lowered in the aprotinin groups, however. EACA has been shown to reduce bleeding in low-risk patients undergoing a first-time CABG in a randomized placebo-controlled trial (6). Bleeding was reduced by about 200 cc in the first 12 h ($P = .002$) with EACA compared to placebo.

Aprotinin may also be associated with an increased incidence of coronary bypass graft closure. In a very small, placebo-controlled study of 32 patients, although bleeding was significantly reduced in aprotinin patients, 31% had at least one graft closed compared to none of the placebo patients (7). In contrast, other studies have demonstrated no increase in graft occlusion with aprotinin (8). Another randomized trial of aprotinin demonstrated a significant reduction in blood product exposure with aprotinin compared to placebo, the greatest difference being seen in patients who were undergoing reoperation (0.3 exposures per patient for aprotinin, 10.7 exposures per patient for placebo). However, with aprotinin, the mortality was no better (5.6% aprotinin, 3.7% placebo), the graft patency was slightly worse (92% aprotinin vs. 95.1% placebo), and myocardial infarctions were slightly more common in the aprotinin group (8.9% aprotinin vs. 5.6% placebo).

Another reported potential complication of aprotinin is the development of renal insufficiency. A large randomized trial recently studied this in 216 patients undergoing CABG. Creatinine levels rose more often in aprotinin patients (19% vs. 12%), although the differences were not statistically significant. There was no difference in the number of patients developing clinically significant renal dysfunction. In practical terms, it appears that aprotinin may have a slight edge over EACA in efficacy but at a significantly higher monetary cost and a small increase in the risk of thrombotic complications compared to placebo. The benefit of aprotinin and EACA seems to be greatest in patients at risk for bleeding such as those undergoing reoperation and those on aspirin preoperatively (8).

DDAVP (desmopressin) is another agent that has been investigated for prevention of bleeding. Current data suggest that DDAVP has little effect in reducing bleeding when given routinely (9) although it does appear to be effective when given to patients who are actively bleeding (10).

3. *Antithrombotic Therapy*

Antithrombotic therapy can also be considered a form of prophylactic therapy after heart surgery. Early postoperatively, patients are placed on subcutaneous heparin for prophylaxis against deep venous thrombosis and pulmonary embolism. This complication appears to be more common in CABG patients than valve patients (see below).

In addition, patients undergoing coronary artery bypass surgery should generally receive preoperative dipyrridamole 75 mg followed by aspirin 160 to 325 mg

6 or 7 h after surgery. All patients should then be placed on long-term aspirin at a dose of at least 160 mg/day (80 mg BID or 160 mg once a day). There are data that low doses of 55 mg may not be as effective in preventing graft occlusion unless given with a supplemental antiplatelet agent (11); the only definitive randomized clinical trial data are for an aspirin dose of 325 mg QD. This has led to the American College of Chest Physicians recommending a standard dose of 325 mg for all CABG patients (12). The duration of therapy should be for at least 2 years for graft patency; however, therapy should be continued past 2 years since aspirin is also indicated indefinitely in patients with coronary artery disease.

Patients undergoing valve replacement should be placed on warfarin long term as outlined in Table 1. Anticoagulation is optional in patients undergoing valve repair, but many centers anticoagulate patients receiving an artificial ring for 3 months after surgery with a target INR of 2 to 3. Anticoagulation for patients receiving aortic tissue valves is optional and at our institution is generally not used for the very elderly (age >80) or patients felt to be at major risk for bleeding complications. However, most younger aortic valve recipients do receive warfarin for three months.

4. *Arterial Graft Spasm*

Younger patients undergoing coronary bypass surgery may receive one of the newer arterial conduits such as the gastroepiploic artery or the radial artery in addition to one or two internal mammary arteries (IMA). However, it is important to recall that these conduits are different from the IMA in that they have a well-developed muscularis layer. This makes them prone to spasm in the postoperative

Table 1 Anticoagulation Regimen for Patients After Open Heart Surgery

Indication	Therapy	Target
Mechanical prosthetic heart valves[a]	Warfarin	INR = 2.5–3.5
Bioprosthetic heart valves[a]		
Mitral valves	Warfarin × 3 months	INR = 2.0–3.0
Aortic valves	Warfarin optional but encouraged	INR = 2.0–3.0
Coronary artery bypass surgery[b]	ASA 325 mg qd (begun 6 h postop)	
Valve repair	ASA 325 mg qd	

[a]Stein PD, Alpert JS, Copeland J, et al. Antithrombotic therapy in patients with mechanical and biological prosthetic heart valves. Chest 1995; 108:371S–379S.
[b]Stein PD, Dalen JE, Goldman S, et al. Antithrombotic therapy in patiets with saphenous vein and internal mammary artery bypass grafts. Chest 1995; 108:424S–430S.

period; patients receiving alternative arterial conduits should therefore routinely receive calcium channel blockers to prevent or reduce the development of spasm.

IV. PERIOPERATIVE COMPLICATIONS

A. Complications of Cardiopulmonary Bypass

Discontinuation of bypass may be difficult in patients with significant ventricular dysfunction. Difficulty weaning patients from bypass may be due to occlusion of vein grafts, inadequate graft flow, myocardial infarction or stunning, hypovolemia, bradycardia, and arrhythmias, as well as acidosis, hypoxemia, and other metabolic problems.

Platelet dysfunction and thrombocytopenia are common after cardiopulmonary bypass. Platelet dysfunction may be due to platelet activation as blood passes through the tubing of the bypass machine. Thrombocytopenia occurs due to sequestration of platelets in the CPB tubing and filters as well as sequestration in the liver and spleen.

Another potential problem after cardiopulmonary bypass is a protamine reaction. When patients receive protamine to reverse heparin at the end of CPB, they may develop an allergic or anaphylactoid reaction to protamine. Affected patients typically have a low blood pressure and low SVR and may require pressors for circulatory support. Insulin-dependent diabetic patients, patients with a history of fish allergy, and patients who have undergone prior heart surgery are at increased risk for this reaction. If a protamine reaction is suspected, patients should be treated with steroids, antihistamines, and, if appropriate, vasopressors and volume infusion. If a patient has a prior history of protamine reactions, hexadimethrine bromide (Polybrene) can be used instead of protamine.

Cross-clamping of the aorta may be a major source of postoperative neurologic events. Clamping a diseased or calcified aorta can cause systemic emboliztion and significant neurologic damage. One approach to try to reduce this risk is routine preoperative echocardiographic scanning of the aorta. In a study of surface ultrasound scanning of the aorta, the rate of diagnosis of aortic pathology was increased from 2% to 10% with a significant reduction in stroke compared to historical control data (13). The aorta can also be evaluated using transesophageal echocardiography. Aortic pathology is treated by prophylactic aortic root replacement if necessary.

V. POSTOPERATIVE COMPLICATIONS

A. Low-Output State and Hypotension

There are many possibilities in the differential diagnosis of low-output state after heart surgery. Hypovolemia is probably the commonest cause, and in the absence of evidence to the contrary, many patients are empirically treated with fluids to increase blood pressure and cardiac output. However, it is wise to use fluid replacement judiciously to avoid excessive edema and pleural effusions postoperatively. Other entities to consider include cardiac tamponade, typically due to right atrial compression from a hematoma, myocardial infarction or ischemia, arrhythmias (usually evident on the monitor), tension pneumothorax, and failure of a valve repair or replacement. Empiric support of blood pressure is frequently done with catecholeamines such as dopamine and occasionally with epinephrine drips. However, therapy of the low-output state or hypotensive episode should be appropriate to the precipitating cause. Patients with a refractory low output can be supported using a mechanical assist device. Generally, intra-aortic balloon pumps are insufficient for this, their primary role is in relieving ischemia and afterload reduction of the left ventricle. Left ventricular assist devices are much more effective at providing adequate cardiac output.

B. Perioperative MI

Perioperative myocardial infarction (MI) occurs in about 5% of stable patients and 10% of unstable angina patients after coronary bypass surgery when defined by both enzyme and ECG criteria (14). In the recent Bypass Angioplasty Revascularization Investigation (BARI) study, the incidence of Q-wave infarction was 4.6% after bypass surgery (15). There are a wide variety of potential causes including preoperative myocardial ischemia; intraoperative hemodynamic stress, particularly during intubation; intraoperative coronary air embolism; and technical problems with graft anastomoses. The diagnosis of perioperative MI is usually made by observing the appearance of new Q waves on the ECG after surgery. The presence of new ST or T-wave abnormalities is not a specific indicator of perioperative myocardial infarction. CPK isoenzymes are limited in usefulness for diagnosis of perioperative infarction since CPK-MB is frequently elevated above normal levels after surgery (16). This is felt to be related to the atriotomy made for cannulation since the atria have high amounts of CPK-MB in them. However, some authors have suggested that markedly elevated CPK-MB levels (>80 mg/dl) are helpful in the diagnosis of perioperative myocardial infarction (17,18). In general, patients with small perioperative myocardial infarction do well and require no special care or specific extension of their hospital stay. However, the long-term prognosis of patients with Q-wave infarctions may be reduced (19,20).

C. Postoperative Hypertension

Hypertension occurs in 30–60% of patients in the postoperative period, usually within 1–2 hours after surgery (21) and is probably caused by high catecholamine levels (22). Control of blood pressure is important to minimize the risk of graft occlusion as well as reduce the risk of bleeding. Although many agents are available, we have favored the use of short acting angiotensin converting enzyme inhibitors such as captopril. Other choices include calcium channel blockers such as nifedipine and beta blockers such as atenolol or propranolol. The latter drugs have the additional advantage of reducing perioperative atrial fibrillation.

D. Arrhythmias

1. Atrial Arrhythmias

Atrial arrhythmias are extremely common after open heart surgery. Between 30% and 50% of patients develop supraventricular arrhythmias after surgery (23,24). Atrial fibrillation and atrial flutter are the commonest clinically significant arrhythmias. In a recent multicenter study by the McSPIE investigators of patients undergoing coronary bypass surgery (25), the incidence of postoperative atrial fibrillation was 27%. The most consistent risk factor for atrial fibrillation in both the McSPIE and multiple prior studies has been advanced patient age. Other risk factors in the McSPIE study included male sex, history of CHF, history of atrial fibrillation, and preoperative sinus tachycardia. Intraoperative pulmonary vein venting and bicaval venous cannulation also increased the risk of atrial fibrillation. There appear to be two peaks in the incidence of atrial fibrillation after heart surgery, one occurring 2 to 3 days after surgery and the other 5 to 7 days after. The occurrence of atrial fibrillation extends hospital stay by an average of about 2.5 days and the ICU stay by about 12 h.

Most cases of postoperative atrial fibrillation will convert back to sinus rhythm spontaneously within 24 to 48 h; however, a few require drug therapy or cardioversion. The first goal of therapy is to control the heart rate using either digoxin or β blockers. In the setting of acute, paroxysmal atrial fibrillation, β blockers may be more effective than digoxin at rate control. Patients can be loaded with digoxin intravenously, typically by giving 0.25 mg IV for four doses until a total of 1 mg has been reached. The patient is then kept on maintenance digoxin for about 4 to 6 weeks. β Blockers can also be used, either propranolol or a longer acting β blocker such as atenolol. If the patient does not convert spontaneously to sinus rhythm, chemical conversion can be attempted with either quinidine, procainamide, or ibutilide. Our practice has generally been to use an intravenous procainamide bolus of 500 to 1000 mg followed by an infusion of 1 to 2 mg/min. However, ibutilide offers a good alternative to procainamide with the possibility of more rapid conversion back to sinus rhythm.

Rapid atrial pacing can also be used to convert atrial flutter to sinus rhythm (26). Atrial pacing cannot be used to convert atrial fibrillation, however. To convert atrial flutter one must have access to an atrial pacing box capable of pacing at rates of 350 to 800 beats/min. The method used is to connect the two atrial wires to the pacemaker and set the output at its highest setting. Pacing is then begun at a slow rate to ensure that the leads are not connected to the wrong chamber. When satisfied, the pacemaker rate is then increased slowly to 10% above the atrial flutter rate, and pacing is continued for at least 30 sec. The pacemaker can then be turned off or slowly lowered to the patients intrinsic rate. Patients who fail drug therapy and rapid pacing should be cardioverted, particularly if compromised in any way by their arrhythmia.

2. *Ventricular Arrhythmias*

Short runs of PVCs and nonsustained ventricular tachycardia are not uncommon. The use of type 1 antiarrhythmic agents may precipitate these arrhythmias. Runs of 6 to 7 PVCs in a row are more serious and should be observed. Sustained VT/VF occurs less commonly (about 2% of patients) and is associated with a high mortality (27). These patients should be referred for electrophysiology testing and potentially for placement of an AICD (implantable defibrillator).

3. *Heart Block*

Mobitz 1 and Mobitz 2 second-degree blocks are more common after heart surgery than complete heart block. Conduction disturbances are more common after valve replacement surgery than after bypass surgery. Risk factors for complete heart block after CABG include presence of a preoperative LBBB, concomitant left ventricular aneurysmectomy, and age >64 years (28). The first step in management is to ensure that the patient has an adequate heart rate and, if not, to institute ventricular pacing using the epicardial wires or a transvenous wire. Any concomitant medications which could precipitate heart block should be discontinued including digoxin or β blockers. The medication sheet should be searched for other potential causes of heart block, particularly β-blocking eye drops. Patients with prolonged pauses (>3 sec) or persistent symptomatic bradyarrhythmias are referred for permanent pacemaker placement.

4. *Bundle Branch Block*

Bundle branch block is a not uncommon complication after cardiac surgery. Right bundle branch block is generally considered to be a benign occurrence and may be related to mechanical trauma from the Swann-Ganz catheter. Left bundle branch block may be a more serious event if it indicates the occurrence of a new perioperative myocardial infarction. However, in the absence of perioperative myocardial infarction, LBBB does not carry an adverse prognosis.

E. Postpericardiotomy Syndrome

Symptoms of postpericardiotomy syndrome typically develop 2 to 8 weeks after open heart surgery and include fever, tachycardia, chest pain, and atrial arrhythmias. Treatment consists of oral therapy with nonsteroidal antiinflammatory agents such as ibuprofen, indomethacin, or naprosyn. Refractory cases should be given a trial of steroids. A few patients with postpericardiectomy syndrome will go on to develop constrictive pericarditis (29). A major concern with constrictive pericarditis after coronary artery bypass surgery is that the inflammatory process may extend to involve one of the bypass grafts leading to its closure (30,31).

F. Tamponade

Cardiac tamponade after open heart surgery is usually quite different from cardiac tamponade in the CCU or medical intensive care unit. In many cases the tamponade is caused by a leak at the site of the right atrial cannulation. The hematoma that accumulates selectively compresses the vena cava (32) or right atrium and tends to cause a focal right atrial tamponade. Thus, equilibration of pressures in the right and left heart is not a universal diagnostic criteria for postoperative tamponade (33). It is more characteristic to see a progressive elevation in right atrial pressures with a corresponding drop in the cardiac output.

Echocardiography is also helpful in the diagnosis of postoperative tamponade. In an echocardiographic study of 29 patients with postoperative tamponade (34), the majority of patients (66%) had a localized posterior effusion while only 34% had a generalized effusion. RA diastolic collapse was evident in 34%, RV diastolic collapse in 27%, and LV diastolic collapse in 65%. Treatment is surgical relief of tamponade.

It is important to realize that pericardial effusions are common after open heart surgery. In a study of 803 patients, 64% had pericardial effusions on echocardiography at 8 days after surgery with 30% being moderate in size and 1.6% large in size (35). Most effusions were loculated rather than diffuse. Tamponade occurred in 1.9% and was more common after valve replacement than CABG. The most reliable diagnostic finding for postoperative tamponade in this study was an inspiratory decrease in aortic and mitral flow velocities.

G. Perioperative Bleeding

Some bleeding in the postoperative period is common and normally stops without therapy. However, a minority of patients will develop more severe bleeding, requiring therapy. There are a number of potential causes of postoperative bleeding including both quantitative and qualitative platelet abnormalities, heparin administration, abnormalities of coagulation factors, and mechanical reasons such as disruption of a graft anastomosis.

Platelet counts may drop due to sequestration of platelets in the liver or spleen or in the cardiopulmonary bypass tubing (36), and qualitative platelet disorders may also occur (37). Activation of the coagulation cascade by the cardiopulmonary bypass system may lead to a systemic fibrinolytic state (38).

In a large recent series (39) reoperation for bleeding was required in 3.8% of 2221 patients. Reoperation was three times more likely in valve cases (OR = 3.4) An identifiable source of bleeding was identified in 67% of patients, and 53% had an associated coagulopathy. Reoperation for bleeding was associated with a longer ICU stay, greater need for an intra-aortic balloon pump, and greater risk of death.

Perioperative bleeding can usually be managed medically with therapy directed to the specific cause of the bleeding. In most cases, the bleeding is associated with abnormal coagulation parameters, and the initial approach should be to correct the coagulation abnormalities. Therefore, the PT, PTT, platelet count, and template bleeding time should be evaluated. Patients with a prolonged prothrombin time should receive fresh frozen plasma. Patients with a prolonged PTT may have heparin rebound and can be reversed with further protamine infusion. However, excessive protamine may also be a risk factor for postoperative bleeding (40). Patients with low platelet counts are given platelets; those with normal platelet counts and prolonged bleeding times are given DDAVP (10). Patients who continue to bleed after correction of coagulation abnormalities or who have massive acute bleeding should be reexplored surgically.

VI. RESPIRATORY COMPLICATIONS

A subset of patients develop diaphragmatic dysfunction after cardiac surgery, and these patients may develop significant long-term complications. Diaphragmatic dysfunction is usually caused by cold injury to the phrenic nerve from ice slush used for topical cooling of the heart (41,42). In a study by Diehl (43) 2.1% of patients undergoing surgery with topical hypothermia developed postoperative diaphragmatic dysfunction. Of these, 11/13 patients developed nosocomial pneumonia, five had cardiorespiratory arrest after extubation, and three died. The incidence of diaphragmatic dysfunction was only 0.5% in patients who did not receive topical cooling. In general, postoperative diaphragmatic dysfunction resolves spontaneously although resolution may take 2 or 3 months. Diagnosis may be done quickly using the sniff test where diaphragmatic movement is observed under fluoroscopy while the patient sniffs (44), or by more extensive transdiaphragmatic pressure measurements. In patients with normal pulmonary function preoperatively, unilateral diaphragmatic function does not usually cause clinical problems. However, significant respiratory problems may occur in patients with prior lung disease who develop unilateral dysfunction and in normal patients who develop bilateral diaphragmatic paralysis (45,46). Resolution of paralysis may take 3 or 4 months, but intervals up to 27 months have been reported (47). Rocking bed ventilation appears to be an effective method of support for severely affected patients (47) but may not be well tolerated by some patients.

Patients who are taking the antiarrhythmic drug amiodarone before surgery are at risk for the development of adult respiratory distress syndrome (ARDS) after cardiac surgery (48). The pathogenesis of this is not clear but may be related to potentiation of oxygen toxicity by amiodarone in patients exposed to high oxygen concentrations during surgery. These patients typically have a normal chest x-ray and blood gases for the first 24 to 48 h and then develop progressive hypoxia and diffuse pulmonary infiltrates. Patients are treated supportively, but the mortality rate remains high.

A. Neurologic Events

Neurologic complications after heart surgery may be due to preexisting cerebrovascular disease, perioperative embolism, hemodynamic changes, medications, or peripheral nerve injury (49). Intraoperative embolism may be due to air, atheroma, or thrombus. Air embolism may occur at the end of cardiopulmonary bypass and is usually prevented by venting of the left ventricle. Atheromatous embolism can occur at the time of cross-clamping of the aorta, as discussed previously, or from native carotid disease. Thombotic embolism may occur from an intracardiac source such as a left atrial or left ventricular thrombus. Thomboembolism can also occur in the early postoperative period from prosthetic heart valves and atrial fibrillation. Neurologic events can be devastating and in many instances markedly prolong the length of hospital stay. Studies to prevent neurologic sequelae have been performed with a variety of agents. Pilot studies of GM1 ganglioside have failed to show a benefit (50). The calcium channel blocker nimodopine has similarly shown no benefit (51) and was associated with an increase in deaths (10.7% vs. 1.3%, $P = .02$) and an increase in major bleeding (13.3% vs. 4.1%, $P = .04$).

B. Renal Failure

Postoperative renal dysfunction occurs in about 10% of patients. However, frank renal failure is less common. In a recent study of 775 patients (52), renal dysfunction defined as a creatinine between 1.5 and 2.5 mg/dl developed in 11.4%. Renal failure, defined as creatinine over 2.5 mg/dl, occurred in 3.7%. Risk factors for renal impairment included use of an intra-aortic balloon pump, deep hypothermic circulatory arrest, low-output syndrome, advanced age, emergency operation, and low urine output during cardiopulmonary bypass. In other series, the risk of postoperative renal failure ranges from 1.5% to 5% depending on the patient population and definition of renal failure (53–55).

C. Pulmonary Embolism

Pulmonary embolism is uncommon after valve replacement surgery but does occur after coronary artery bypass surgery. In one series, pulmonary embolism developed in 3.2% of 1033 cardiac surgery patients (56) and occurred exclusively in CABG patients, not in isolated valve surgery patients ($P < .05$). Diagnosis was made by pulmonary angiography in the majority and by ventilation/perfusion scanning in a minority. The mortality rate was 19% in patients with a documented pulmonary embolism. Risk factors for pulmonary embolism included prolonged postoperative recovery, obesity, and hyperlipidemia. In summary, although pulmonary embolism is a rare complication of valve replacement surgery, it is not uncommon in CABG patients.

D. Gastrointestinal Complications

Gastrointestinal complications occur 0.5% to 1.5% of patients undergoing cardiac surgery (57,58). Gastrointestinal bleeding is the commonest GI complication after open heart surgery, and most patients should receive prophylactic therapy with H_2 antagonists, antacids, or sucralfate.

Other potential complications that appear to have a specific relationship to cardiac surgery include acute cholecystitis, paralytic ileus, and pancreatitis. The etiology of the cholecystitis, paralytic ileus, and possibly pancreatitis may be related to postoperative visceral hypotension (59).

Hyperbilirubinemia can occur early (1 to 10 days after surgery) or late (10 to 90 days postoperatively). Early hyperbilirubinemia with normal liver enzymes is usually due to red cell damage during cardiopulmonary bypass and is usually seen within 24 to 48 h after surgery. Early hyperbilirubinemia with elevated liver enzymes is usually due to liver damage from low cardiac output and hypoxemia. In patients with late elevation of bilirubin and elevation of liver enzymes, one must rule out infectious hepatitis.

Acute acalculous cholecystitis may present as either early or late hyperbilirubinemia and develops in about 0.3% of patients. It generally occurs within the first week after surgery (60). Patients typically present with right upper quadrant pain and nonspecific changes in liver enzymes. The diagnosis can be made by either ultrasound or technetium cholescintography. In the series by Sessions (60), 20 patients underwent cholecystectomy and nine (41%) were found to have gangrenous gallbladders, two with perforation. The overall mortality rate for these patients was 32%, highlighting the serious nature of this complication and that cholecystecomy should not be delayed due to the recent cardiac surgery. Acute cholecystitis may be the second commonest reason for gastrointestinal consultation in patients after heart surgery and may account for 20% of consults (61).

Pancreatitis is an uncommon but serious complication of cardiac surgery. Intraoperative administration of large doses of calcium has also been postulated as a possible cause of pancreatitis (62) as well as the visceral hypotension, as mentioned above. The diagnosis cannot be made from an elevated amylase alone since 30% to 50% of patients undergoing cardiopulmonary bypass develop asymptomatic hyperamylasemia that is generally not of pancreatic origin (63).

E. Valve-Related Complications

After valve replacement, many patients will have low-grade hemolysis caused by mechanical damage to the red cells from the new heart valve. This is reflected in an elevated LDH after surgery; however, the LDH should not be more than twice normal. Greater degrees of hemolysis are of concern and may be due to a paravalvular leak (leakage of blood around the sewing ring of the valve) or thrombosis of the valve. LDH levels typically decline 2 to 3 weeks after surgery. Thrombosis of mechanical valves is uncommon early after surgery but may be diagnosed with transesophageal echocardiography or by cinefluoroscopy. Thrombosed valves can be treated either surgically or with thrombolytic therapy (64,65). A dreaded complication of mitral valve replacement is rupture of the posterior left ventricular wall, most common in patients with a large posterior infarct (66).

VII. HIGH-RISK PATIENT GROUPS

A. Chronic Obstructive Pulmonary Disease

A recent study of patients with chronic obstructive lung disease (COPD) undergoing CABG (67) demonstrates the expected greater ICU stay (1.4 days), longer hospital stay (1.5 days), and greater need for prolonged ventilation. However, COPD patients also had more significant postoperative arrhythmias (73% vs. 24%, $P < .0001$), and 80% of the deaths in the COPD patients over the ensuing 16 months were due to arrhythmias. These findings suggest that arrhythmias are an important source of morbidity and mortality in COPD patients undergoing coronary bypass surgery.

B. Dialysis Patients

Dialysis-dependent patients are at significantly increased risk for morbidity and mortality after cardiac surgery. Perhaps as importantly, the long-term prognosis is poor in these patients. In a study of 21 dialysis-dependent patients 48% developed perioperative complications and two died (68). Although actuarial survival was 94% at 1 year, at 2 years it was only 45%, however. In another study of 25 patients with chronic renal failure (21 on hemodialysis, three on peritoneal dialysis), all patients were managed with dialysis within 24 h before surgery (69). Following surgery, 22 of the patients underwent immediate peritoneal dialysis through a Technoff catheter placed during surgery (18 patients) or inserted previously (four patients). Patients were then switched to hemodialysis when stable hemodynamically. The overall operative mortality was 16% although all of the deaths were in the 11 patients having nonelective surgery. This subgroup had a 36% mortality. The median lengths of stay in the ICU, telemetry unit, and total postoperative hospitalization were 3 days, 8 days, and 16 days, respectively. In a review of the 296 cases reported in the literature, these authors reported an overall mortality of 9% for dialysis patients (69).

C. Patients with Prior Stroke

Patients with a prior completed stroke may be at increased risk of neurologic complications after open heart surgery. In some cases this is manifest as a worsening of the prior deficit. In many cases, this is transient and reverses partially or completely over time. However, it seems prudent to evaluate these patients for carotid disease prior to their open heart procedure. It is still not clear whether these patients are at risk for new permanent neurologic deficits postoperatively. In a study of 43 patients with prior stroke and no extracranial carotid disease undergoing open heart surgery, only one patient (2.3%) developed new neurological symptoms (70). It is important to run these patients at higher mean pressures while on pump, typically at pressures of 90 to 100 mm Hg to minimize the risks of watershed ischemic events.

REFERENCES

1. Martin TD, Craver JM, Gott JP, et al. Prospective, randomized trial of retrograde warm blood cardioplegia: myocardial benefit and neurologic threat. Ann Thorac Surg 1994; 57: 298–302.
2. Warm Heart Investigators. Randomised trial of normothermic versus hypothermic coronary bypass surgery. Lancet 1994; 343:559–563.
3. Czer L, Hamer A, Murphy F, et al. Transient hemodynamic dysfunction after myocardial revascularization: temperature dependence. J Thorac Cardiovasc Surg 1983; 86: 226–234.
4. Nystrom U, Edvardsson N. Berggren H, Pizzarelli GP, Radegran K. Oral sotalol reduces the incidence of atrial fibrillation after coronary artery bypass surgery. Thorac Cardiovasc Sur 1993; 41: 34–37.
5. Laub GW, Janeira L, Muralidharan S, et al. Prophylactic procainamide for prevention of atrial fibrillation after coronary artery bypass grafting: a prospective, double–blind, randomized placebo–controlled pilot study. Crit Care Med 1993; 21:1471–1478.
6. Daily PO, Lamphere JA, Dembitsky WP, et al. Effect of prophylactic epsilon–aminocaproic acid on blood loss and transfusion requirements in patients undergoing first–time coronary artery bypass grafting. J Thorac Cardiovas Surg 1994; 108:99–108.
7. Laub GW, Riebman JB, Chen C, et al. The impact of aprotinin on coronary artery bypass graft patency. Chest 1994; 106:1370–1375.
8. Murkin JM, Lux J, Shannon NA, et al. Aprotinin significantly decreases bleeding and transfusion requirements in patients receiving aspirin and undergoing cardiac operations. J Thorac Cardiovasc Surg 1994; 107:554–561.
9. Fremes SE, Wong BI, Lee E, et al. Metaanalysis of prophylactic drug treatment in the prevention of postoperative bleeding. Ann Thorac Surg 1994; 58:1580–1588.
10. Czer L, Bateman T, Gray R, et al. Treatment of severe platelet dysfunction and

hemorrhage after cardiopulmonary bypass: reduction in blood product usage with desmopressin. J Am Coll Cardiol 1987; 9:1139–1147.

11. Sanz G, Pajaron A, Alegria E, et al. Prevention of early aortocoronary bypass occlusion by low–dose aspirin and dipyridamole. Circulation 1990; 82:765–773.
12. Stein PD, Dalen JE, Goldman S, et al. Antithrombotic therapy in patients with saphenous vein and internal mammary artery bypass grafts. Chest 1995; 108:424S–430S.
13. Duda AM, Letwin LB, Sutter FP, Goldman SM. Does routine use of aortic ultrasonography decrease the stroke rate in coronary bypass surgery? J Vasc Surg 1995; 21:98–107.
14. National Institutes of Health. Consensus development conference statement. Coronary artery bypass surgery: scientific and clinical aspects. N Engl J Med 1981; 304: 680–684.
15. BARI Investigators. Comparison of coronary bypass surgery with angioplasty in patients with multivessel disease. N Engl J Med 1996; 335:217–225.
16. Lee ME, Sethna DH, Conklin CM, et al. MB–K release following coronary artery bypass grafting in the absence of myocardial infarction. Ann Thorac Surg 1983; 35:277–279.
17. Gray RJ, Shell W, Conklin C, et al. Quantification of myocardial injury during coronary artery bypass graft surgery. Circulation 1978; 58(suppl I):I38–I42.
18. Gray RJ, Matloff JM, Conklin CM, et al. Perioperative myocardial infarction: late clinical course after coronary bypass surgery. Circulation 1982; 66:1185–1189.
19. Schaff HV, Gersh BJ, Fisher LD, et al. Detrimental effect of perioperative myocardial infarction on late survival after coronary artery bypass. Report from the Coronary Artery Surgery Study—CASS. J Thorac Cardiovasc Surg 1984; 88:972–981.
20. Chaitman BR, Alderman EL, Sheffield LT, et al. Use of survival analysis to determine the clinical significance of new Q waves after coronary bypass surgery. Circulation 1983; 67:302–309.
21. Hoar P, Hickey R, Ullyot D. Systemic hypertension following myocardial revascularization. J Thorac Cardiovasc Surg 1976; 71:859–864.
22. Roberts A, Niarchos A, Subramanian V, et al. Systemic hypertension associated with coronary artery bypass surgery. Predisposing factors, hemodynamic characteristics, humoral profile, and treatment. J Thorac Cardiovasc Surg 1977; 74:846–859.
23. Lauer MS, Eagle KA, Buckley MJ, DeSanctis RW. Atrial fibrillation following coronary artery bypass surgery. Prog Cardiovasc Dis 1989; 31:367–378.
24. Rubin DA, Nieminski KE, Reed GE, Herman MV. Predictors, prevention, and long–term prognosis of atrial fibrillation after coronary artery bypass graft operations. J Thorac Cardiovasc Surg 1987; 94:331–335.
25. Mathew JP, Parks R, Savino JS, et al. Atrial fibrillation following coronary artery bypass graft surgery. JAMA 1996; 276:300–306.
26. Waldo AL, MacLeen WA, Cooper TB, et al. Use of temporarily placed epicardial atrial wire electrodes for the diagnosis and treatment of arrhythmias following open heart surgery. J Thorac Cardiovasc Surg 1978; 76:500–505.
27. Pires LA, Wagshal AB, Lancey R, Huang SK. Arrhythmias and conduction disturbances after coronary artery bypass graft surgery: epidemiology, management, and prognosis. Am Heart J 1995; 129: 799–808.

28. Emlein G, Huang SK, Pires LA, et al. Prolonged bradyarrhythmias after isolated coronary artery bypass graft surgery. Am Heart J 1993; 126:1084–1090.
29. Killian DM, Furiasse JG, Scanlon J, Loeb HS, Sullivan JH. Constrictive pericarditis after cardiac surgery. Am Heart J 1989; 118:563–568.
30. Urschl HC, Razzuk MA, Gardner M. Coronary artery bypass occlusion secondary to postcardiotomy syndrome. Ann Thorac Surg 1972; 22:528–531.
31. Kabbani SS, Bashow T, Ellertson G, et al. Constrictive pericarditis following myocardial revascularization: a possible cause of graft occlusion. Am Heart J 1985; 110:493–495.
32. Weiss M, Bateman TM, Kass RM, et al. Extravascular obstruction of the superior vena cava after open–heart surgery by hematoma and diagnosis by scintigraphy. Am J Cardiol 1983; 51:1229–1231.
33. Bateman T, Gray R, Chaux A, et al. Right atrial tamponade complicating cardiac surgery: clinical, hemodynamic, and scintigraphic correlates. J Thorac Cardiovasc Surg 1982; 84:413–419.
34. Chitin K. Tischler MD, Pandian NG, Lee RT, Mohanty PK. Diagnosis of cardiac tamponade after cardiac surgery: relative value of clinical, echocardiograhic, and hemodynamic signs. Am Heart J 1994; 127(4 pt 1):913–918.
35. Pepi M, Muratori M, Barbier P, et al. Pericardial effusion after cardiac surgery: incidence, site, size, and haemodynamic consequences. Br Heart J 1994; 72:327–331.
36. Salzman E. Blood, platelets, and extracorporeal circulation. Transfusion 1963; 3: 274–277.
37. Friedenberg W, Myers W, Plotka E, et al. Platelet dysfunction associated with cardiopulmonary bypass. Ann Thorac Surg 1978; 25:298–305.
38. Boyd A, Engelman R, Beadet R, Lackner H. Disseminated intravascular coagulation following extracorporeal circulation. J Thorac Cardiovasc Surg 1972; 64:685–693.
39. Unsworth-White MJ, Herriot A, Valencia O, et al. Resternotomy for bleeding after cardiac operation: a marker for increased morbidity and mortality. Ann Thorac Surg 1995; 59:664–667.
40. Delaria GA, Tyner JJ, Hayes CL, Armstrong BW. Heparin–protamine mismatch. A controllable factor in bleeding after open heart surgery. Arch Surg 1994; 129: 944–950.
41. Rousou JA, Parker T, Engelman RM, Breyer RH. Phrenic nerve paresis associated with the use of iced slush and the cooling jacket for topical hypothermia. J. Thor Card Surg 1985; 89:921–923.
42. Curtis JJ, Nawarawong W, Walls JT, et al. Elevated hemidiaphragm after cardiac operations: incidence, prognosis, and relationship to the use of topical ice slush. Ann Thorac Surg 1989; 48:764–768.
43. Diehl JL, Lofaso F, Deleuze P, Similowski T, Lemaire F, Brochard L. Clinically relevant diaphragmatic dysfunction after cardiac operations. J Thorac Cardiovasc Surg 1994; 107:487–498.
44. Oh KS, Newman B, Bender T, Bowen A. Radiologic evaluation of the diaphragm. Radiol Clin North Am 1988; 26:355–364.
45. Chandler KW, Rozas CJ, Kory RC, Goldman A. Bilateral diaphragmatic paralysis complicating local cardiac hypothermia during open heart surgery. Am J Med 1984; 77:243–249.

46. Kohorst WR, Schonfeld SA, Altman M. Bilateral diaphragmatic paralysis following topical cardiac hypothermia. Chest 1984; 85:65–68.
47. Abd AG, Braun N, Baskin M, et al. Diaphragmatic dysfunction after open heart surgery: treatment with a rocking bed. Ann Intern Med 1989; 111:881–886.
48. Nalos P, Kass R, Gang E, et al. Life–threatening postoperative pulmonary complications in patients with previous amiodarone pulmonary toxicity undergoing cardiothoracic operations. J Thorac Cardiovasc Surg 1987; 93:904–912.
49. Brillman J. Central nervous system complications in coronary artery bypass graft surgery. Neurol Clin 1993; 11:475–495.
50. Grieco G, dHolosy M, Culliford AT, Jonas S. Evaluating neuroprotective agents for clinical anti–ischemic benefit using neurological and neuropsychological changes after cardiac surgery under cardiopulmonary bypass. Methodological strategies and results of a double-blind, placebo-controlled trial of GM1 ganglioside. Stroke 1996; 27:858–874.
51. Legault C, Furberg CD, Wagenknecht LE, et al. Nimodipine neuroprotection in cardiac valve replacement: report of an early terminated trial. Stroke 1996; 27:593–598.
52. Zanardo G, Michielon P, Paccagnella A, et al. Acute renal failure in the patient undergoing cardiac operation. Prevalence, mortality rate, and main risk factors. J Thorac Cardiovasc Surg 1994; 107:1489–1495.
53. Yeboah E, Petrie A, Pead J. Acute renal failure and open heart surgery. Br Med J 1972; 1:415–418.
54. Abel R, Buckley M, Austen W, et al. Etiology, incidence and prognosis of renal failure following operations. J Thorac Cardiovasc Surg 1976; 71:323–333.
55. Gailunas P, Chawla R, Lazarus J, et al. Acute renal failure following cardiac operations. J Thorac Cardiovasc Surg 1980; 79:241–243.
56. Josa M, Siouffi SY, Silverman AB, Barsamian EM, Khuri SF, Sharma GV. Pulmonary embolism after cardiac surgery. J Am Coll Cardiol 1993; 21:990–996.
57. Ohri SK, Desai JB, Gaer JAR, et al. Intraabdomonal complications after cardiopulmonary bypass. Ann Thorac Surg 1991; 52:826–831.
58. Johnston G, Vitikainen K, Knight R, Annest L, Garcia C. Changing perspective on gastrointestinal complications in patients undergoing cardiac surgery. Am J Surg 1992; 163:525–529.
59. Christenson JT, Schmuziger M, Maurice J, Simonet F, Velebit V. Postoperative visceral hypotension the common cause for gastrointestinal complications after cardiac surgery. Thorac Cardiovasc Surg 1994; 42:152–157.
60. Sessions SC, Scoma RS, Sheikh FA, McGeehin WH, Smink RD. Acute acalculous cholecystitis following open heart surgery. Am Surg 1993; 59:74–77.
61. Aranha G, Picklenan J, Pifarre R, et al. The reasons for gastrointestinal consultation after cardiac surgery. Am Surg 1984; 50:301–304.
62. Fernandez–Del Castillo C, Haringer W, Warshaw A, et al. Risk factors for pancreatic cellular injury after cardiopulmonary bypass. N Engl J Med 1991; 325:382–387.
63. Missavage A, Weaver D, Bouwnan D, et al. Hyperamylasemia after cardiopulmonary bypass. Am Surg 1984; 50:297–300.
64. Ledain LD, Ohayon JP, Colle JP, et al. Acute thrombotic obstruction with disc valve prostheses: diagnostic considerations and fibrinolytic treatment. J Am Coll Cardiol 1986; 7:743–751.

65. Silber H, Khan S, Matloff J, et al. The St. Jude valve: thrombolysis as the first line of therapy for cardiac valve thrombosis. Circulation 1993; 87:30–37.
66. Harold J, Bateman T, Czer L, et al. Left ventricular rupture complicating mitral valve replacement: relationship to recent infarction. J Am Coll Cardiol 1987; 9:277–282.
67. Cohen A, Katz M, Katz R, Hauptman E, Schachner A. Chronic obstructive pulmonary disease in patients undergoing coronary artery bypass grafting. J. Thorac Cardiovasc Surg 1995; 109:574–591.
68. Owen CH, Cummings RG, Sell TL, et al. Coronary artery bypass grafting in patients with dialysis–dependent renal failure. Ann Thorac Surg 1994; 58:1729–1733.
69. Ko W, Kreiger KH, Isom OW. Cardiopulmonary bypass procedures in dialysis patients. Ann Thorac Surg 1993; 55:677–684.
70. Beall AC, Jones JW, Guinn GA, Svensson LG, Nahas C. Cardiopulmonary bypass in patients with previously completed stroke. Ann Thorac Surg 1993; 55:1383–1384.

8

Hypercoagulable States in the Coronary Care Unit

SANJAY KAUL

Cedars-Sinai Medical Center, Los Angeles, California

I. INTRODUCTION

Intravascular thrombosis is one of the most frequent pathological events to occur in humans, accounting ultimately for more than 50% of deaths and a variety of clinical syndromes. Current evidence suggests that fissuring and disruption of an atherosclerotic plaque with resultant platelet deposition and thrombus formation and associated platelet-mediated vasoconstriction play a fundamental role in the pathogenesis of acute ischemic syndromes, including unstable angina, myocardial infarction, transient ischemic attack and stroke (1,2). The thrombotic process also complicates intravascular interventions such as coronary angioplasty, atherectomy, endovascular stents, endarterectomy, and bypass graft surgery, resulting in significant morbidity and mortality (3). The cardiologist is very familiar with the management of these acute thrombotic manifestations of atherosclerotic vascular disease. However, thrombosis is also an important complication of several inherited and acquired conditions, referred to generically as the thrombophilias or hypercoagulable states, which frequently present diagnostic and therapeutic challenges in the coronary care setting. The purpose of this chapter is to review the major pathophysiologic mechanisms underlying inherited and secondary hypercoagulable states and to evaluate the frequency, natural history, diagnosis, and management of these clinical disorders.

II. HYPERCOAGULABLE STATES AND THE CLOTTING CASCADE

Hypercoagulable states are those conditions in which the balance between prothrombotic and antithrombotic factors is distorted such that the individual is predisposed to thrombosis or recurrent thrombosis. To understand which elements of the clotting system, when defective, may lead to hypercoagulable states, a brief review of the normal hemostatic response is necessary and is described below.

The clotting cascade is initiated when endothelial injury occurs, exposing circulating platelets to thrombogenic substances in the subendothelium such as collagen, fibronectin, and laminin. Platelets adhere to the endothelial surface and become activated to release additional thrombogenic substances such as von Willebrand factor (VWF), fibrinogen, thrombospondin, and adenosine diphosphate (ADP), causing further aggregation of platelets (4). While this is occurring, the coagulation cascade is stimulated through either the intrinsic (contact factor, factor XII) or extrinsic pathways (tissue factor), culminating in a common pathway in which activated factor X, with factor V as a cofactor, converts prothrombin to thrombin. Thrombin then acts on fibrinogen to form fibrin, which secures the aggregated platelets in an insoluble clot (4).

Several physiologic anticoagulant systems act under normal circumstances to prevent excessive clot formation (4,5). These include antithrombin III, which binds to and neutralizes thrombin and several other clotting factors. Protein C, a vitamin K-dependent zymogen, is activated by thrombin, a process greatly amplified by the interaction of thrombin with thrombomodulin (5). Protein C exerts its anticoagulant activity by inactivating activated factors V and VIII, which are required as cofactors in the coagulation cascade. In conjunction with protein S, it may also promote fibrinolysis by inactivating plasminogen activator inhibitor-1 (PAI-1) (6). Protein S, also a vitamin K-dependent plasma protein, is required as a cofactor for the anticoagulant activity of protein C. Tissue factor pathway inhibitor (TFPI), also known as lipoprotein-associated coagulation factor (LACI), is a natural inhibitor of the extrinsic pathway of coagulation that neutralizes the factor VII/tissue factor complexes (4). Following clot formation, several types of plasminogen activators produce plasmin from plasminogen. Plasmin then dissolves clots by cleaving fibrin into fibrin degradation products.

Thus, normal hemostasis is closely regulated by a constant dynamic struggle between the prothrombotic and the opposing antithrombotic forces which under normal circumstances approximates a state of equilibrium. Why a particular individual develops thrombosis spontaneously, while others need a precipitating acquired factor, and in addition many others who never develop thrombosis no matter under which circumstances, may perhaps be explained by difference in intrinsic prothrombotic tendency, differences of resting and induced antithrombotic capacity, and nature and strength of the precipitating attack.

III. ETIOLOGY OF HYPERCOAGULABLE STATES

Conditions recognized as hypercoagulable states are usually divided into two categories–inherited or primary thrombotic disorders, and acquired or secondary thrombotic disorders (Table 1). Defects in any of the physiologic anticoagulant and fibrinolytic mechanisms result in primary hypercoagulable states. The primary hypercoagulable states are for the most part congenital deficiencies, generally inherited in an autosomal-dominant pattern. Patients with a variety of other conditions such as malignancies, nephrotic syndrome, sickle cell anemia, pregnancy, trauma, oral contraceptive use, and acute infections may demonstrate a predisposition to thromboembolic events; these patients are described as having secondary hypercoagulable states. Secondary hypercoagulability syndromes are classified into abnormalities of platelets, coagulation, and fibrinolysis, and blood vessels and rheology (Table 2).

A. Primary Disorders

1. Antithrombin III Deficiency

First described in 1965 by Egeberg in a Norwegian family, antithrombin-III (AT-III) deficiency impairs inactivation of the activated procoagulant factors Xa and IIa (thrombin), which leads to augmented thrombosis. AT-III deficiency may be either congenital or acquired. Congenital AT-III deficiency is inherited as an autosomal-dominant trait with incomplete penetrance, occurs with a frequency of 1:2000 to 1:5000, and results in either quantitative or qualitative deficiency of enzymatic activity (7–10). The risk of developing a thrombotic event in affected individuals during their lives is 50% to 70%, with most initial episodes occurring by the age of 30 (8,10,11). The tendency to thrombosis increases with advancing age, so that by age 50, 90% of affected patients have had thrombotic events. Acquired AT-III deficiency usually results from prolonged heparin therapy, estrogen administration (12,13), urinary losses of the protein in the nephrotic syndrome (14,15), hepatic insufficiency (16), DIC, and, rarely, excessive protein catabolism in malnourished individuals (17) and after asparaginase therapy (18).

Patients with this disorder are characterized by increased incidence of venous thrombosis, usually triggered by a prothrombotic stimulus, such as pregnancy, use of oral contraceptives, surgery, infection, or trauma (11,19,20). There is usually a family history of recurrent thrombosis, generally beginning in youth and often associated with surgery or trauma. Patents frequently present with deep vein thrombosis of the lower extremities, pulmonary embolism, and, occasionally, mesenteric and cerebral vein thrombosis. In rare cases, arterial thrombosis may occur, particularly in patients with atherosclerotic disease (17). Homozygous deficiency of AT-III has not been reported, presumably because this condition is incompatible with life.

Table 1 Hypercoagulable States

Inherited disorders	Acquired disorders
1. AT-III deficiency	1. Platelets
2. Protein C and S deficiency	a. Antiphospholipid syndrome
3. Activated protein C resistance (factor V Leiden type)	b. Heparin-induced thrombocytopenia
4. Fibrinolytic abnormalities	c. Myeloproliferative disorders
a. Plasminogen deficiency	d. Hypercholesterolemia
b. Decreased plasminogen activator activity	e. Dyslipidema
c. Increased plasminogen activator inhibitor-1	f. Diabetes mellitus
5. Dysfibrinogenemia	2. Coagulation and fibrinolysis
6. Heparin cofactor II deficiency	a. Malignancy (Trousseau's syndrome)
	b. Pregnancy
	c. Oral contraceptive use
	d. Nephrotic syndrome
	e. Warfarin-induced thrombosis
	f. Postoperative reduction in fibrinolytic activity
	3. Endothelium and rheology
	a. Homocystinuria/hyperhomocysteinemia
	b. Venous stasis
	c. Hyperviscosity
	d. Thrombotic thrombocytopenic purpura
	e. Arteritis

Table 2 Clinical Manifestations of Hypercoagulable States

1. Family history of thrombosis
2. Thrombosis at a young age
3. Idiopathic thrombosis
4. Recurrent thrombosis
5. Thrombosis at unusual sites (mesenteric, axillary, cerebral, renal, hepatic, inferior vena cava)
6. Thrombosis following minimal provocation (long car ride, airplane flight)
7. Progressive thrombosis despite anticoagulation
8. Resistance to anticoagulation with heparin (AT-III deficiency)
9. Coumarin necrosis (protein C and S deficiency)
10. Premature and accelerated atherosclerosis

Diagnosis of this disorder is usually made by the typical clinical presentation as described above and confirmed by both bioassay (functional activity) and immunoassay (antigenic) using RIA and ELISA. Patients generally have AT-III levels 25% to 60% of normal (140 μg/ml in pooled plasma) levels. Because the deficiency of AT-III may render heparin relatively ineffective, some patients will present with heparin resistance that is manifested by minimal prolongation of the PTT following therapeutic doses of heparin.

In asymptomatic carriers of AT-III deficiency, anticoagulant prophylaxis is not warranted unless exposed to prothrombotic stimuli such as major abdominal surgery. Following a thrombotic episode, patients should receive lifelong therapy with oral warfarin-type anticoagulants. Acute thrombotic episodes must be treated with heparin. If heparin resistance is encountered, AT-III should be administered along with heparin either in the form of fresh-frozen plasma or purified AT-III concentrates. AT-III has a half-life of about 60 h, and administration of 1 U/kg body weight of AT-III raises plasma activity by about 2%. The average dose of AT-III is usually 20 to 50 U/kg bolus, depending on the baseline levels. Danazol, an anabolic steroid, has also been tried with some benefit.

2. *Protein C and S Deficiency*

Protein C and S deficiencies are inherited in an autosomal-dominant manner with partial penetrance and variable expressivity (21–24). Protein C deficiency may also develop occasionally in patients with severe liver dysfunction and DIC (21). Heterozygous deficiency of protein C occurs with a prevalence of 1 in 200 to 1 in 300. A recent report demonstrated protein C and S deficiency in 4% and 5%, respectively, in 141 patients under the age of 45 who had venous thromboembolic disease (25).

The clinical manifestations are similar to the AT-III deficiency, except for two unique manifestations. Homozygous protein C deficiency causes lethal thrombosis in infancy (pupura fulminans) (26), and heterozygotes have an increased risk of developing warfarin-induced skin necrosis due to the half-life of this protein being shorter than other vitamin K-dependent, warfarin-suppressible zymogens (27). A few cases of arterial thrombosis have also been reported, especially in protein S deficiency (22,24,28,29).

Diagnosis is confirmed by functional and antigenic assays which are available in most coagulation laboratories. Laboratory evaluation of affected heterozygotes reveals depressed levels of protein C (40% to 60% of normal; 4 μg/ml) or protein S (15% to 50% of normal, 23 μg/ml). Anticoagulant therapy with oral warfarin is the treatment of choice for preventing thrombosis. A period of enhanced hypercoagulability follows initiation of warfarin therapy in patients with protein C deficiency because the half-life of protein C is only 6 to 7 h, much shorter than that of factor II, X, or IX. Heparin should therefore be given along with warfarin during the initiation of anticoagulation of such patients, and the heparin can subsequently be withdrawn. Purified protein C concentrates are also available for treatment. Anabolic steroids such as stanozolol and danazol have also been reported to be effective in protein C, but not protein S, deficiency.

3. *Abnormal Resistance to Activated Protein C, Factor V Leiden type*

A new inherited cause of thrombophilia (first described in 1993) is activated protein C (APC) resistance (28,30–32). Up to 90% of APC resistance is due to a single mutation of the factor V gene (factor V Leiden) (31). The factor V Leiden mutation is transmitted as an autosomal-dominant trait, has a prevalence of 3% to 7% in the general population, and is by far the most common inherited cause of a thrombotic tendency. APC resistance due to factor V Leiden is been observed in 50% of patients with familial thrombophilia and 40% of patients younger than age 45 with a first deep vein thrombosis (33). Thus, APC resistance is five to 10 times more common than a deficiency of AT-III, protein C, or protein S, which account for about 5% each in this population (30–33). Patients with the factor V Leiden mutation have up to a sevenfold increase in risk of venous thrombosis over normals, which may rise to as high as a 30-fold increase in smokers (34), obese individuals (34), and women on oral contraceptives (35).

The factor V Leiden mutation produces a factor V protein that has normal procoagulant activity but is resistant to degradation by activated protein C (APC). The defect in factor V Leiden is due to a single base mutation (G1691A) involving replacement of a G with an A in exon 10 of the factor V gene (31). This change results in replacement of arginine at position 506 by glutamine. Most patients with APC resistance are heterozygous for the factor V Leiden mutation. Patients who are homozygous for the mutation have severe, early onset of thrombosis. The absence of the factor V Leiden mutation does not exclude the possibility of activated protein C (APC) resistance due to other less common mutations in factor V.

Patients with APC resistance usually present with deep vein thrombosis or pulmonary embolism. No strong association has been found in patients with strokes or myocardial infarction. Among 14,916 apparently healthy men in the Physicians' Health Study, 374 of whom had myocardial infarctions, 209 had strokes, and 121 had deep venous thrombosis, pulmonary embolism, or both, during a mean follow-up of 8.6 years. Ridker et al. (36) found that the arg506-to-gln mutation of the factor V gene was present in 25.8% of men over the age of 60 in whom primary venous thrombosis developed. The presence of the mutation was not associated with an increased risk of myocardial infarction or stroke. They found that this factor was associated with four- to five-fold increased risk of recurrent thrombosis. The data raised the possibility that patients with idiopathic venous thromboembolism and factor V Leiden may require more prolonged anticoagulation to prevent recurrent disease compared to those without the mutation.

The initial diagnosis of this condition is made by a coagulation study in which aPTT and clotting time are measured in the presence or absence of exogenous APC. APC degrades factor Va and VIIIa and prolongs the aPTT in normal plasma by >40 sec. The ratio of aPTT in the presence and absence of exogenous APC is normally >2.0 to 2.2; a ratio of <2.0 is highly suggestive of abnormal resistance to APC (30,35). The coagulation test is useful for screening patients who have had thrombosis, but cannot be used when a patient is anticoagulated or has coexisting antiphospholipid antibodies. The identification of the specific mutation has led to more precise and specific DNA-based tests such as PCR amplification that allow the diagnosis to be made even if a patient is anticoagulated with heparin or warfarin or has coexisting antiphospholipid antibodies.

Current management of these patients is similar to the management of patients with AT-III, protein C, or protein S deficiencies—i.e., prophylactic anticoagulation therapy in situations that provoke thrombosis (surgery) and long-term anticoagulation in patients with recurrent thrombosis.

4. *Abnormalities of Fibrinolysis*

Patients with hypercoagulability syndromes have been identified with dysplasminogenemia (abnormal plasminogen) (37), hypoplasminogenemia (low levels of functionally normal plasminogen (38), impaired release of tissue plasminogen activator (tPA) from the endothelial cells (39), increased levels of inhibitor of plasminogen activator (PAI-1) (38), and factor XII (Hageman) deficiency (40). Recent studies have suggested that defective release of tPA and increased levels of PAI-1 may be important pathogenetic factors in as many as one-third of patients with documented venous thromboembolism (41). Moreover, reduced fibrinolytic activity caused by increased PAI-1 levels, which correlate strongly with elevated triglyceride levels, has also been found in young survivors of MI (42).

Lipoprotein (a) has been suggested as a link between atherogenesis and thrombosis (43–46). Lp(a) has a striking homology with plasminogen and has been shown in experimental models to compete with plasminogen for binding sites on fibrin and endothelial cells (45). Thus Lp(a) has the potential to inhibit fibrinolytic activity at the endothelial surface and contribute to the enhanced thrombogenicity of the endothelium (45).

Although aPTT is greatly prolonged in factor XII deficiency, it does not produce a hemorrhagic disorder, but, paradoxically, patients are prone to develop thromboembolic episodes (40). Factor XII has been implicated in the contact activation of fibrinolysis, and this process may be defective in factor XII-deficient patients. Impaired fibrinolysis may also contribute to the hypercoagulability state associated with postoperative states. Assays for plasminogen, tPA, PAI-1, and factor XII are currently only available in special diagnostic and research laboratories. Management of these patients entails routine therapy for the thromboembolic disorder.

5. *Dysfibrinogenemia*

Dysfibrinogenemias are a heterogeneous group of clinical disorders that present with a bleeding diathesis or recurrent venous or arterial thromboembolism or no clinical symptoms. They are inherited in an autosomal-dominant manner, and the defects can be detected by prolonged thrombin and reptilase time in presence of normal fibrinogen levels. Defects in the release of fibrinopetides A and B during conversion of fibrinogen to fibrin, abnormalities in fibrin polymerization, and abnormal resistance to plasmin-induced lysis have been reported (47). Therapy with warfarin appears to be beneficial.

6. *Heparin Cofactor II Deficiency*

Even though AT-III accounts for the majority of the antithrombin activity of plasma, another anticoagulant, called heparin cofactor II, interacts with heparin to inactivate thrombin with no effects on other serine proteases (factors IXa, Xa, and XIa) (48). Hereditary heterozygous deficiency of heparin cofactor II is associated with venous as well as arterial thromboses (48).

B. Secondary Disorders

1. *Antiphospholipid Syndrome*

The antiphospholipid syndrome (APS) is characterized by recurrent venous or arterial thrombosis, recurrent fetal loss, and thrombocytopenia in the presence of an autoantibody to the phospholipids such as anticardiolipin and lupus anticoagulant (49–52). The lupus anticoagulant, first described by Feinstein and Rapaport, is a misnomer because most patients with systemic lupus erythematosus (SLE) do not have the antibody, and in vivo it is thrombogenic even though the activated PTT is prolonged in vitro. Cardiolipin was first discovered as part of the VDRL test for syphilis, and subsequently a radioimmunoassay for the antibodies against this phospholipid was developed. The idea of APS came from the observation that patients with SLE and these antibodies seemed to suffer from more frequent thrombotic events than those without the antibodies.

The pathophysiology of the APS lies in the fact that these antibodies are directed against phospholipids that belong to the coagulation pathway, usually platelet membranes (49,52). The pathophysiology of the lupus anticoagulant is poorly understood, but it is directed against prothrombin, factor X, factor XII, and proteins C and S. As described above, the lupus anticoagulant acts as an anticoagulant in vitro, but in vivo it is thrombogenic. The anticardiolipin antibody is more specific and is directed against cardiolipin, but it actually recognizes and binds to an antigenic site residing in the plasma protein cofactor β_2-glycoprotein I (49), which is known to be involved in a variety of in vivo pathways including inhibition of platelet activation.

APS is the most common acquired defect associated with thrombosis with venous thromboses being more common than arterial (49,53–57). About 50% of patients with high antibody titers will develop thrombotic complications (55,56). Patients with anticardiolipin antibody titers above the 95th percentile have a fivefold increased risk of developing deep venous thrombosis or pulmonary embolism (54) and also have an increased risk of recurrent thromboses compared to controls. The most frequently seen arterial thrombotic manifestation is in the cerebral and extremity circulation, although thrombotic complications have been reported in the aortic, visceral, and coronary arteries (53,54). Cardiac abnormalities include verrucous endocarditis (Libman-Sacks endocarditis), particularly involving the mitral valve, and mitral valve thickening often with associated regurgitation (58). In addition, intracardiac thrombi and diffuse cardiomyopathy have also been reported in patients with APS. All of these can be a source of cardiac emboli. For this reason screening echocardiography should be considered in patients with APS and arterial thrombosis, especially with involvement of the cerebral and ocular circulation. Other clinical manifestation of APS are enumerated in Table 3.

Diagnosis is usually made by a history of either venous thrombosis, arterial thrombosis, recurrent fetal loss, or thrombocytopenia plus a persistently high titer of lupus anticoagulant or anticardiolipin antibody. To detect an antibody of the lupus anticoagulant type, several criteria have now been established by the subcommittee of the International Society of Thrombosis and Hemostasis. These include:

Table 3 Clinical Manifestations of Antiphospholipid Syndrome

1. Thromboembolic disease
   a. Venous: most common site is lower-extremity DVT
   b. Arterial: cerebral ischemia, TIAs, and embolic CVAs
2. Hematologic disorder
   a. Thrombocytopenia, hemolytic anemia, leukopenia, DIC
3. Neurologic associations
   a. CVA, TIA, severe migraine, multi-infarct dementia, myasthenia gravis
4. Cardiac abnormalities
   a. 25–35% of patients with APS have valvular abnormalities; Libman-Sacks endocarditis
   b. Left heart more commonly affected than right heart
5. Dermatologic
   a. Livedo reticularis, leg ulcers, necrotizing purpura, distal cutaneous ischemia
6. Obstetric
   a. Fetal loss, pre-eclampsia, premature delivery, chorea gravidorum

1. Prolongation of a phospholipid-dependent clotting test using two different test mechanisms—i.e., activated partial thromboplastin time (aPTT) and dilute Russell viper venom time (DRVVT);
2. Proof that the prolongation is not due to other causes—i.e., factor deficiencies or other inhibitors (mixing studies);
3. Confirmation of the phospholipid concentration dependence of the inhibitor—i.e., platelet neutralization procedure (PNP) and DRVVT confirmation;
4. Specific immunologic testing (ELISA) for anticardiolipin antibodies, particularly the IgG subtype;
5. Screening and confirmatory test systems must match; i.e., a positive DRVVT screening test must be confirmed by a DRVVT confirmatory test, and a prolonged lupus-sensitive aPTT must be confirmed by a PNP.

Treatment of these patients remains controversial, but usually consists of anticoagulation with warfarin with the possibility of using high-dose steroids for immunosuppression. The treatment of pregnant women with antiphospholipid antibodies to prevent a possible miscarriage is not well understood at the current time. Some women are helped by combinations of aspirin, prednisone, and/or subcutaneous heparin, whereas other women continue to have miscarriages even when they are taking these medications. Subcutaneous heparin is less likely than prednisone to cause diabetes and an increase in blood pressure during pregnancy. Other treatments, including plasmapheresis or intravenous gammaglobulin, may be considered in individual cases.

2. *Drug-Related Hypercoagulable States*

Certain drugs have an increased tendency for causing thrombosis. High-dose chemotherapy in cancer patients is associated with endothelial damage, which may contribute to thromboembolic events including pulmonary veno-occlusive disease (vincrystine and vinblastine), hepatic veno-occlusive disease, deep vein thrombosis, and myocardial infarction. Acquired deficiencies of protein C, protein S, and AT-III (L-asparaginase) (18) have also been reported in patients receiving chemotherapy (59). Oral estrogen-containing contraceptives have also been implicated in increased risk of thromboembolic disease (59). The exact etiology is unknown, but low levels of AT-III and protein S found in women taking these agents may be contributory (59,60). Cyclosporine and mitomycin are also associated with increased risk of venous thromboembolism, perhaps related to the development of thrombotic thrombocytopenic purpura secondary to these drugs. The two most widely used anticoagulants, heparin and warfarin, are rarely complicated by devastating thrombotic episodes described below.

3. *Heparin-Induced Thrombocytopenia*

Thrombocytopenia is a well-recognized complication of heparin therapy, occurring in about 1% of patients receiving porcine gut-derived heparin and in about

5% of patients receiving bovine lung-derived heparin (61–63). Thrombocytopenia usually begins between 3 and 15 days (median 10 days) after initiation of therapy but can occur earlier in patients who have been sensitized earlier, and can occur with high-dose therapy as well as with minimal exposure, as in intravenous line flushes. Heparin-induced thrombocytopenia (HIT) is generally mild with platelet counts usually >50,000/μl, and platelet counts promptly return to baseline within 4 days of stopping heparin. Thus one should monitor the platelet count daily and act if there is a sudden drop in the count. Another sign is heparin resistance (the sudden increase in the dose of heparin required to maintain therapeutic anticoagulation) secondary to the decrease in AT-III levels which is thought to reflect generalized activation of the coagulation system associated with this phenomenon.

Heparin-associated thrombosis, also called "white clot syndrome," is a rare but devastating complication of therapy that is usually associated with severe thrombocytopenia (HITT, heparin-induced thrombocytopenia with thrombosis) and occurs with an incidence of 0.5% in patients receiving bovine lung heparin and 0.4% in patients receiving porcine gut heparin. These thrombotic complications are often arterial, including stroke and myocardial infarction as well as peripheral arterial occlusion, skin necrosis, and purpura fulminans, and they result in major morbidity (20% limb loss) and mortality (30%). Venous thromboses have also been described, but it is unclear whether this is due to HIT or a manifestation of decreased levels of AT-III, which has also been described with this condition.

The pathophysiologic mechanism responsible for this disorder is believed to be a heparin-dependent IgG antibody directed against a heparin-binding protein, platelet factor 4 (PF4), found in the platelet α granules (64). The ternary complex of IgG bound to heparin-linked PF4 on platelet surface combines with platelet Fc receptors and activates the platelets leading to their consumption and removal with resultant thrombocytopenia. PF4 released from activated platelets binds to heparin and heparan sulfate on endothelial surface. The IgG antibody then reacts with the PF4-heparin/heparan antigen complex, producing endothelial injury, which, if extensive, leads to thrombosis and DIC. HIT is diagnosed by demonstrating the presence of antibodies in the plasma that aggregates platelets when heparin is added (the HAT assay).

The goal in the treatment of this disorder is prevention of thromboembolic complication by early detection. Platelet counts should be monitored daily, and evidence for heparin resistance should be carefully analyzed. Therapy consists of stopping all heparin drips and flushes and removing heparin-coated intravenous lines. Heparin can be safely stopped in patients on warfarin therapy for 4 or 5 days. Antiplatelet agents aspirin, dipyridamole and low-molecular-weight dextran, and the prostacyclin analogue iloprost, have been used as effective agents in patients not on warfarin. Patients with HIT and active thrombosis are extremely difficult to manage. Innovative therapy with such drugs as the and low-molecular-weight heparinoids, danaparoid Org 10172 (not approved by the FDA) or ancrod, a snake venom-derived defibrinogenating agent, is required. The ideal agents for use in HIT are the direct-acting antithrombins hirudin, bivalirudin (hirulog), and argatroban, which are totally unrelated to heparin and PF4. However, they have not been approved by the FDA and must be obtained by compassionate protocol. Use of low-molecular-weight heparins is risky because cross-reactivity with unfractionated heparin may occur. Platelet transfusion is contraindicated in HIT.

4. *Coumarin Skin Necrosis*

This is an extremely rare (one in 1 million) but very devastating complication of warfarin therapy. Classically it starts 4 days after initiation of therapy, with pain and skin discoloration. Then frank necrosis occurs in the affected area. Most common sites are the breasts and buttocks in women and the penis in men. Most reported cases that have occurred in patients with venous thrombosis were postsurgical or postpartum. Many but not all patients when tested had protein C or protein S deficiencies. The etiology of the skin necrosis is still debated, but it appears that protein C or S deficiency and an inflammatory state are prerequisites for occurrence. It has been postulated that a period of enhanced hypercoagulability follows initiation of warfarin therapy in patients with protein C deficiency because protein C (a vitamin K-dependent anticoagulant) levels fall rapidly due to the half-life of protein C (6 to 7 h) being much shorter than that of other vitamin K-dependent coagulation factors, II, X, or IX. The entity has not been described in patients anticoagulated for arterial events. A prudent approach would be to overlap warfarin therapy with heparin whenever anticoagulating patients with venous thrombotic events. In starting warfarin for arterial events or prophylaxis in atrial fibrillation, heparin coverage is probably not required if the patient does not have a personal or family history of venous thrombosis or evidence of antiphospholipid antibodies. Warfarin should be started at low doses (2 to 2.5 mg/day) and increased gradually over several weeks in these patients. This approach should avoid an abrupt fall in protein C levels before there is a reduction in factor II, X, or IX. Rarely, surgical debridement or skin grafting may be necessary.

Another complication of warfarin therapy is the "purple toes syndrome," which presents as bilateral painful peripheral discoloration of the plantar or the lateral aspects of the toes. Originally thought to represent a rare allergic manifestation to warfarin, it is now thought to be due to "multiple cholesterol emboli" arising from extensive aortic atherosclerosis.

5. *Homocystinuria/Hyperhomocysteinemia*

Homocystinuria is a rare hereditary disorder transmitted in an autosomal-recessive manner which is characterized by severe hyperhomocysteinemia and passage of homocysteine in the urine (65). It is most commonly caused by a deficiency in the enzyme cystathionine β-synthase leading to inability to metabolize homocysteine utilizing the transsulfuration pathway (65,66). Recently, remethylation abnormalities in homocysteine metabolism, including abnormal methylenetetrahydofolate reductase (absent or thermolabile variant) and abnormal methionine synthase, have also been reported to result in hyperhomocysteinemia (67). Elevated homocysteine levels may also result from low levels of folic acid, vitamin B_6, or vitamin B_{12}, all of which are cofactors in homocysteine metabolism (65). Normal circulating levels of total plasma homocysteine vary between laboratories but usually lie in the range of 5 to 15 μmol/L in the fasting state (65). A methionine-loading test may pick up some patients with latent abnormality but normal circulating plasma homocysteine levels (65).

Hyperhomocysteinemia is an established risk factor for atherosclerosis and vascular disease with a strong association reported with cerebrovascular, coronary artery, and peripheral artery disease in person younger than 55 years (65,66). Recent studies suggest that it may also be a risk factor for deep vein thrombosis in the general population (68). Several hypotheses have been proposed to explain the increased risk for thrombosis and atherosclerosis. Homocysteine is a highly reactive amino acid and may be toxic to vascular endothelium (69,70). It inhibits thrombomodulin expression and protein C activation (71,72) and suppresses endothelial heparan sulfate expression (73); both of these effects lead to hypercoagulability. In addition, reduced antithrombin-III activity and enhanced platelet activation in hyperhomocysteinemia may also provide a possible mechanism for increased risk of thrombosis. Binding of lipoprotein (a), an atherogenic lipoprotein, to fibrin is enhanced by homocysteine, providing a link among hyperhomocysteinemia, thrombosis, and premature atherosclerosis (74).

Patients with severe hyperhomocysteinemia should be treated with 1 mg of folic acid, 5 mg vitamin B_6, or 1 mg vitamin B_{12} daily. The optimal dose and vitamin combination to produce maximal reduction of homocysteine and the effect of lowering homocysteine levels on cardiovascular risk remain to be established.

6. *Trousseau's Syndrome*

Increased propensity to develop recurrent migratory thromboembolism in malignancy was first observed by Trousseau during the last century. This syndrome is usually associated with solid tumors of the pancreas, colon, lung, or breast that release tissue factor which initiates the extrinsic pathway of coagulation (75). The underlying pathophysiologic event is a chronic subclinical form of DIC which leads to enhanced thrombosis (75). Warfarin is ineffective in the management of this disorder. Continuous IV heparin or twice-daily subcutaneous heparin may be helpful. Low-molecular-weight heparin may be a reasonable alternative. Ultimately, treatment of the underlying tumor will control the DIC.

7. *Myeloproliferative Disorders and Paroxysmal Nocturnal Hemoglobinuria*

An increased risk for thromboembolic events has been observed in polycythemia vera and essential thrombocytosis. Quantitative and qualitative platelet abnormalities as well as increased blood viscosity secondary to increased red blood cell mass contribute to the pathogenesis of thrombosis in these disorders.

Paroxysmal nocturnal hemoglobinuria (PNH) is characterized by hemolytic anemia, venous thrombosis, and recurrent episodes of abdominal pain, which is presumably secondary to thrombotic events in the intra-abdominal veins and Budd-Chiari syndrome which can occur in 10% to 20% of these patients. Enhanced sensitivity of platelets to the lytic activity of complement exposes the procoagulant surfaces, leading to increased thrombosis (76).

8. *Relationship Between Traditional Risk factors for CAD and Hemostatic Parameters*

Hypercholesterolemia is a major risk factor for atherosclerosis and thrombosis, and is associated with a high incidence of coronary artery disease and stroke. In addition to inducing endothelial dysfunction, high blood cholesterol also alters platelet function (77) and produces a hypercoagulable state, thereby contributing to increased tendency to thrombosis (78).

Vascular homeostasis is maintained by a dynamic equilibrium between prothrombotic and fibrinolytic factors. This balance may be shifted in favor of a prothrombotic state in patients with hyperlipidemia who have high levels of circulating plasma fibrinogen, activated coagulation factor VII (79) and Lp(a) (46), and reduced fibrinolysis related to reduced levels of tissue-type plasminogen activator (t-PA) activity (80) and elevated plasminogen activator inhibitor (PAI-1) activity (80). Impaired antithrombotic activity may also be related to endothelial dysfunction-induced reduced antiplatelet antiaggregatory activity due to decreased nitric oxide and prostacyclin activity and reduced anticoagulant (thrombomodulin) activity in these patients. Reduced antioxidant levels observed in hyperlipidemia can also promote increased platelet aggregability.

Diabetes mellitus, smoking, and hypertension are also characterized by platelet hyperreactivity, hypercoagulable state secondary to increased fibrinogen levels, and impaired fibrinolysis due to augmented PAI-1 activity. Thus, altered platelet function as well as altered coagulation-fibrinolysis associated with the traditional risk factors for CAD may contribute to increased susceptibility to thrombosis in atherosclerosis.

IV. SUMMARY

Although hypercoagulability disorders are not common, they frequently present diagnostic and therapeutic challenge to the cardiologist. The key is to maintain a high index of suspicion. Every patient presenting with a new or recurrent thromboembolic event should be carefully assessed for potential predisposing factors. Most hypercoagulability disorders can be identified through specific hematologic tests, including immunologic and functional assays, which are available in most laboratories. Hematology consultation should be sought if indicated. Most patients with manifest thromboembolic events will require lifelong therapy with antithrombotic agents. Prophylactic therapy should be considered in individuals at high risk for future events.

REFERENCES

1. Davies MJ. Mechanisms of thrombosis in atherosclerosis. In: Colman RW, Hirsh J, Marder VJ, Salzman EW, eds. Hemostasis and Thrombosis: Basic Principles and Clinical Practice. Philadelphia; J. B. Lippincott, 1994;1224–1237.
2. Fuster V, Badimon L, Badimon JJ, Chesebro JH. Coronary artery disease progression and acute coronary syndromes. N Engl J Med 1992; 326:242–250.
3. Lincoff AM, Popma JJ, Ellis SG, Hacker JA, Topol EJ. Abrupt vessel closure complicating coronary angioplasty: clinical, angiographic and therapeutic profile. J Am Coll Cardiol 1992; 19:926–935.
4. Davie EW, Fujikawa K, Kisiel W. The coagulation cascade: initiation, maintenance and regulation. Biochemistry 1991; 30:10363–10370.
5. Walker FJ. The regulation of activated protein C by a new protein: a possible function for bovine protein. J Biol Chem 1980; 68:1370–1373.
6. D'Angelo A, Lockhart MS, D'Angelo SV, et al. Protein S is a cofactor for activated protein C neutralization of an inhibitor of plasminogen activation released from platelets. Blood 1987; 69:231.
7. Rosenberg RD. Actions and interactions of antithrombin and heparin. N Engl J Med 1975; 292:146–151.
8. Thaler E. Antithrombin III deficiency and thromboembolism. Clin Haematol 1981; 10:369–390.
9. Bauer KA, Ashenhurst JB, Chediak J, et al. Antithrombin "Chicago": a functionally abnormal molecule with increased heparin affinity causing familial thrombophilia. Blood 1983; 62:1242–1250.
10. Filip DJ, Eckstein JD, Veltkamp JJ. Hereditary antithrombin III deficiency and thromboembolic disease. Am J. Hematol 1976; 2:343–349.
11. Demers C, Ginsberg JS, Hirsh J, Henderson P, Blajchman MA. Thrombosis in antithrombin-III deficient persons: report of a large kindred and literature review. Ann Intern Med 1992; 116:754–761.
12. Meade TW, Brozovic OR, Chakrabarti R, et al.: An epidemiologic study of hemostatic and other effects of oral contraceptives. Br J Haematol 1976; 34:353–364.
13. Sager S, Thomas DP, Stametakis JD, et al. Oral contraceptives, antithrombin-III activity, and post-operative deep vein thrombosis. Lancet 1976; 1:509–511.
14. Kaufman RH, Veltkamp JJ, Van Thilburg NH, Van Es LA. Acquired antithrombin III deficiency and thrombosis in the nephrotic syndrome. Am J Med 1978; 65:607–613.
15. Vazini ND, Paule P, Toohey J, et al. Acquired deficiency and urinary excretion of antithrombin III in nephrotic syndrome. Arch Intern Med 1984; 144:1802–1803.
16. Lechner K, Niesner H, Thaler E. Coagulation abnormalities in liver disease. Semin Throm Hemostas 1977; 4:40–54.
17. Flinn WR, McDaniel MS, Yao JST, Fahey VA, Green D. Antithrombin III deficiency

as a reflection of dynamic protein metabolism in patients undergoing vascular reconstruction. J Vasc Surg 1984; 1:888–895.
18. Kucuk OF, Kwaan HC, Gunnar W, et al. Thromboembolic complications associated with L-asparaginase therapy. Cancer 1985; 55:702.
19. Rotschild BM. The role of antithrombin III in clinical management of pulmonary embolization. Am J Med 1983; 74:529–531.
20. Gruenberg JC, Smallridge RC, Rosenberg DR. Inherited antithrombin-III deficiency. JAMA 1981; 245:1259–1261.
21. Mannucci PM, Vigano S. Deficiencies of protein C, an inhibitor of blood coagulation. Lancet 1982; 2:463–467.
22. Comp PC, Esmon CT. Familial protein S deficiency is associated with recurrent thrombosis. J Clin Invest 1984; 74:2082–2088.
23. Griffin JH, Evatt B, Zimmerman TS, Kleiss AJ, Wideman C. Deficiency of protein C in congenital thrombotic disease. J Clin Invest 1981; 68:1370–1373.
24. Schwarz HP, Fischer M, Hopmeier P, Batard MA, Griffin JH. Plasma protein S deficiency in familial thrombotic disease. Blood 1984; 64:1297–1300.
25. Gladson CL, Scharrer I, Hach V, Beck KH, Griffin JH. The frequency of type I heterozygous protein S and protein C deficiency in 141 unrelated young patients with venous thrombosis. Thromb Hemostas 1988; 59:18–22.
26. Seligoshn U, Berger A, Abend M, et al. Homozygous protein C deficiency manifested by massive venous thrombosis in the newborn. N Engl J Med 1984; 310:559.
27. Kazimer FJ. Thromboembolism, coumarin necrosis, and protein C. Semin Thromb Hemostas 1984; 10:1099–1121.
28. Svensson F, Dahlback B. Resistance to activated protein C as a basis for venous thrombosis. N Engl J Med 1994; 330:517–522.
29. Coller BS, Owen J, Jesty J, et al. Deficiency of plasma protein S, protein C, or antithrombin III and arterial thrombosis. Arteriosclerosis 1987; 7:456–462.
30. Griffin JH, Evatt B, Wideman C, et al. Anticoagulant protein C pathway defective in majority of thrombophilic patients. Blood 1993; 82:1989.
31. Bertina RM, Koeleman BPC, Koster T, et al. Mutation in blood coagulation factor V associated with resistance to activated protein C. Nature 1994; 369:64.
32. Dahlback B. Inherited thrombophilia: resistance to activated protein C as a pathogenic factor of venous thromboembolism. Blood 1995; 85:607.
33. Ridker PM, Hennekens CH, Lindpaintner K, et al. Mutation in the gene coding for coagulation factor V and the risk of myocardial infarction, stroke, and venous thrombosis in apparently healthy men. N Engl J Med 1995; 332:912.
34. Bauer KA. Pathobiology of the hypercoagulable state: clinical features, laboratory evaluation and management. In: Hoffman R, Benz EJ Jr, Shattil ST, et al., eds. Hematology: Basic Principles and Practice. New York: Churchill Livingstone, 1995; 1781–1795.
35. Vandenbroucke JP, Koster T, Briet E. Increased risk of venous thrombosis in oral-contraceptive users who are carriers of factor V Leiden mutation. Lancet 1944; 344–453.
36. Ridker PM, Miletich JP, Stampfer MJ, Goldhaber SZ, Lindpaintner K, Hennekens CH. Factor V Leiden and risks of recurrent idiopathic venous thromboembolism. Circulation 1996; 92:2800–2802.

37. Aoki N, Moroi M, Sakata Y, Yoshida N, Mutsuda M. Abnormal plasminogen: a hereditary molecular abnormality found in a patient with recurrent thrombosis. J Clin Invest 1978; 61:1186–1195.
38. Mullertz S. Fibrinolysis: an overview. Semin Thromb Hemostas 1984; 10:1–5.
39. Stead NW, Bauer KA, Kinney TR, et al. Venous thrombosis in a family with defective release of vascular plasminogen activator and elevated plasma factor VIII/von Willebrand's factor. Am J Med 1983; 74:33–39.
40. Aznar J, Fernandez Pavon A. Thromboembolic accidents in patients with congenital deficiency of factor XII. Thromb Diath Haemorrh 1974; 31:525–526.
41. Pins MH, Hirsh J. A critical review of the evidence supporting a relationship between impaired fibrinolytic activity and venous thromboembolism. Arch Intern Med 1991; 151:1721.
42. Hamsten A, de Faire U, Walldius G, Dahlen G, Szamosi A, Landou C, Blomback M, Wiman B. Plasminogen activator inhibitor in plasma: risk factor for recurrent myocardial infarction. Lancet 1987; 2:3–9.
43. Stubbs P, Seed M, Moseley D, O'Connor B, Collinson P, Noble M. A prospective study of the role of lipoprotein(a) in the pathogenesis of unstable angina. Eur Heart J 1997; 18(4):603–607.
44. Pearson TA, LaCava J, Weil HF. Epidemiology of thrombotic-hemostatic factors and their association with cardiovascular disease. Am J Clin Nutr 1997; 65(5 suppl): 1674S–1682S.
45. Hajjar KA, Gavish D, Breslow JL, Nachman RL. Lipoprotein (a) moderation of endothelial cell surface fibrinolysis and its potential role in atherosclerosis. Nature 1989; 339:303–305.
46. Miles LA, Fless GM, Levin EG, Scanu AM, Plow EF. A potential basis for the thrombotic risks associated with lipoprotein (a). Nature 1989; 339:301–303.
47. Carrell N, Gabriel DA, Blatt PM, Carr ME, McDonagh J. Hereditary dysfibrinogenemia in a patient with thrombotic disease. Blood 1983; 62:439–447.
48. Sie P, Dupouy D, Pichon J, et al. Constitutional heparin co-factor II deficiency associated with recurrent thrombosis. Lancet 1985; 2:414.
49. Roubey RAS. Autoantibodies to phospholipid-binding plasma proteins: a new view of lupus anticoagulants and other "antiphospholipid" autoantibodies. Blood 1994; 84:2864.
50. Rosove MH, Brewer MC. Antiphospholipid thrombosis: clinical course after the first thrombotic event in 70 patents. Ann Intern Med 1992; 117:303.
51. Khamashta MA, Cuadrado MJ, Mujic F, et al. The management of thrombosis in the antiphospholipid-antibody syndrome. N Engl J Med 1995; 332:993.
52. Harris EN. Antiphospholipid antibodies. Br J Haematol 1990; 74:251.
53. Ginsburg KS, Liang MH, Newcomer L, et al. Anticardiolipin antibodies and the risk for ischemic stroke and venous thrombosis. Ann Intern Med 1992; 117:997–1002.
54. Shortell CK, Ouriel K, Green RM, Condemi JJ, DeWeese JA. Vascular disease in the antiphospholipid syndrome: a comparison with the patient population with atherosclerosis. J Vasc Surg 1992; 15:158–166.
55. Harris EN, Asherson RA, Hughes GRV, Gharavi AE. Antiphospholipid antibodies-autoantibodies with a difference. Annu Rev Med 1988; 39:261–271.
56. Boey ML, Colaco CB, Ghanavi AE, Elkon KB, Lozous S, Hughes GR. Thrombosis in

systemic lupus erythermatosus: striking association with the presence of circulating lupus anticoagulant. Br Med J 1983; 287:1021–1023.
57. Feinstein DI. Lupus anticoagulant, thrombosis, and fetal loss. N Engl J Med 1985; 313:1348–1350.
58. Kaplan SD, Chartash EK, Pizzarello RA, Furie RA. Cardiac manifestations of the antiphospholipid syndrome. Am Heart J 1992; 124:1331–1338.
59. Macik BG, Ortel TL. Clinical and laboratory evaluation of the hypercoagulable states. Clin Chest Med 1995; 16:375–387.
60. Boerger LM, Morris PC, Thumau GR, et al. Oral contraceptives and gender affect protein S status. Blood 1987; 69:692.
61. Godal HC. Report of the International Committee on Thrombosis and Haemostasis: thrombocytopenia and heparin. Thromb Haemostas 1980; 43:222–224.
62. King DJ, Kelton JG. Heparin associated thrombocytopenia. Ann Intern Med 1984; 100:535–540.
63. Laster J, Cikrit D, Walker N, Silver D. The heparin-induced thrombocytopenia syndrome: an update. Surgery 1987: 102:763–770.
64. Greinacher A, Michels I, Mueller-Eckhardt C. Heparin-associated thrombocytopenia: the antibody is not heparin specific. Thromb Haemostas 1992; 67:545–549.
65. Ueland PM, Refsum H, Brattstrom L. Plasma homocysteine and cardiovascular disease. In: Francis RB Jr, ed. Atherosclerotic Cardiovascular Disease, Hemostasis and Endothelial Function. New York: Marcel Dekker, 1993:183–236.
66. Clarke OR, Daly L, Robinson K, et al. Hyperhomocysteinemia: an independent risk factor for vascular disease. N Engl J Med 1991; 324:1149.
67. Engbersen AMT, Franken DG, Boers GHJ, Stevens EMB, Trijbels FJM, Blom HJ. Thermolabile 5,10–methylenetetrahydrofolate reductase as a cause of mild hyperhomocysteinemia. Am J Hum Genet 1995; 56:150.
68. Den Heijer M, Koster T, Blom HJ, et al. Hyperhomocysteinemia as a risk factor for deep-vein thrombosis. New Engl J Med 1996; 334:759–762.
69. Harker LA, Harlan JM, Ross R. Effect of sulfinpyrazone on homocysteine-induced endothelial injury and arteriosclerosis in baboons. Circ Res 1983; 53:731.
70. Starkebaum G, Harlan JM. Endothelial cell injury due to copper-catalyzed hydrogen peroxide generation from homocysteine. J Clin Invest 1986; 77:1370.
71. Lentz SR, Sadler JE. Inhibition of thrombomoulin surface expression and protein C activation by the thrombogenic agent homocysteine. J Clin Invest 1991; 88:1906.
72. Rodgers GM, Conn MT. Homocysteine, an atherogenic stimulus, reduces protein C activation by arterial and venous endothelial cells. Blood 1990; 75:895.
73. Nishinaga M, Ozawa T, Shimada K. Homocysteine, a thrombogenic agent, suppresses anticoagulant heparin sulfate expression in culture porcine aortic endothelial cells. J Clin Invest 1993; 92:1381.
74. Harpel PC, Chang VT, Borth W. Homocysteine and other sulfhydryl compounds enhance the binding of lipoprotein(a) to fibrin: a potential biochemical link between thrombosis, atherogenesis, and sulfhydryl compound metabolism. Proc Natl Acad Sci USA 1992; 89:10193.
75. Sack GH, Levin J, Bell W. Trousseau's syndrome and other manifestations of chronic disseminated coagulopathy in patients with neoplasms: clinical, pathophysiologic, and therapeutic features. Medicine 1977; 56:1–37.

76. Mitus AJ, Barbui T, Shulman LN, et al. Hemostatic complications in young patients with essential thrombocytopenia. Am J Med 1990; 88:371.
77. Schror K. Platelet reactivity and arachidonic acid metabolism in type 11 hyperlipoproteinemia and its modification by cholesterol lowering agents: a review. Eicosanoids 1990; 3:67–73.
78. Lacoste L, Lam JYT, Hung J, Letchacovski G, Solymoss CB, Waters D. Hyperlipidemia and coronary disease. Correction of the increased thrombogenic potential with cholesterol reduction. Circulation 1995; 92:3172–3177.
79. Wada H, Mori Y, Kaneko T, et al. Elevated plasma levels of vascular endothelial cell markers in patients with hypercholesterolemia. Am J Hematol 1993; 44:112–116.
80. Brown SL, Sobel BE, Fujii S. Attenuation of the synthesis of plasminogen activator inhibitor type I by niacin: a potential link between lipid lowering and fibrinolysis. Circulation 1995; 92:767–772.

9

Hematologic Problems in the Cardiac Intensive Care Unit

SVEN DE VOS

Cedars-Sinai Medical Center, Los Angeles, California

I. INTRODUCTION

Only rarely do hematologic problems in the CCU arise due to the cardiovascular disease process itself. Usually, the hematologic problems either are preexistent or are complications of therapeutic interventions (Table 1).

II. HEMATOLOGIC PROBLEMS ASSOCIATED WITH CARDIOVASCULAR DISEASE

Thrombocytopenia has been described in patients with severe congenital cyanotic heart disease (1–3), valvular heart disease (4,5), and disorders characterized by pulmonary hypertension (6). In valvular heart disease the mechanism responsible for platelet consumption is thought to be due to increased platelet–on Willebrand factor interactions at high shear (7).

The cause of mechanical hemolytic anemia with red blood cell fragmentation in the CCU setting usually can be deducted from the clinical circumstances. Traumatic valvular hemolysis, a result from high blood flow through abnormal mitral and aortic valves, can be seen in rheumatic heart disease, infective endocarditis, and aortic stenosis, and with prosthetic valves. Other clinical settings associated with mechanical hemolysis are seen with AV malformations, like AV shunts or hemangioendotheliomas, aortic aneurysm, rupture of sinus of valsalva, and

Table 1 Drugs Commonly Associated with Hematological Dyscrasias (in approx. descending order of incidence)

Aplasia	Agranulocytosis	Thrombocytopenia	Hemolytic anemia
Gold	Antithyroid drugs	Gold	β-Lactams
Phenylbutazone	Phenylbutazone	Heparin	Quinine/quinidine
Chloramphenicol	Sulfonamides	Quinine/quinidine	Thiazides
Penicillamine	Clozapine	Sulfonamides	Sulfonamides
NSAIDs	Phenothiazines	Anticonvulsants	NSAIDs
Sulfonamides	Mianserin	NSAIDs	Rifampicine
Antithyroid drugs	NSAIDs	Diuretics	INH
Sulfonylureas	β-Lactams	Rifampicine	Phenothiazines
Phenothiazines	Captopril	Sulfonylureas	Sulfonylureas
Allopurinol	H_2 antagonists	Cimetidine	Nomifensine

rupture of cordi tendini; with diseases associated with damaged microvasculature, like TTP, vasculitis; and abnormalities of the renal vasculature, like malignant hypertension or glomerulonephritis. The diagnosis relies on the clinical setting and the observation of the red cell morphology. The therapy is primarily directed toward the underlying disease. To optimize compensation of red blood cell production, iron and folic acid replacement are advisable if the patient is deficient. Occasionally it is necessary to replace a prostetic heart valve because of intolerable transfusion requirements.

A. Polycythemia in Congenital Cyanotic Heart Disease

Congenital heart disease with right-to-left shunt can cause secondary polycythemia. Extreme elevations of the hematocrit, up to 86%, have been observed. Above a hematocrit of 55%, the blood viscosity rises logarithmically, leading to rheologic problems. The most common defects producing polycythemia in adults are tetralogy of Fallot and the Eisenmenger syndrome. In neonates this complication is seen in transposition of the great arteries, tricuspid atresia, and persistent truncus arteriosus. Patients present with cyanosis, dizziness, headaches, epistaxes, and an increased incidence of thrombotic complications.

B. Fe^{2+} Deficiency Anemia in Chronic Hemopthysis in Patients with Mitral Stenosis

Hemoptysis in mitral senosis (MS) is due to ruptures of pulmonary-bronchial venous connections secondary to pulmonary venous hypertension. It is seen in patients with elevated left atrial pressures and without marked elevated pulmonary resistance. These patients can present with a microcytic anemia due to chronic blood loss.

C. Malabsorption in Congestive Heart Failure

Congestive heart failure (CHF) can cause impairment of intestinal absorption due to congestion of intestinal veins. In severe cases of right heart failure, even a protein-losing enteropathy can be seen. Malabsorption then can be responsible for anemia due to impaired absorption of iron, vitamin B_{12} and folic acid, and for hemorrhagic problems due to vitamin K malabsorption. Therefore dietary/parenteral supplementation is recommended for patients with severe CHF. Of note, anemia of any cause can demask previously compensated heart disease. Oxygen needs in the presence of anemia can only be met by an increased cardiac output, which might overburden a diseased heart, leading to clinically significant CHF.

D. Post Cardiopulmonary Bypass Surgery

Thrombocytopenia and platelet dysfunction are seen most in patients post cardiopulmonary bypass surgery (8). Still, excessive bleeding is uncommon, occurring in only about 5% of patients. Bleeding, presenting as excessive chest tube blood loss (>100 ml/h), is due to a surgical cause in over 50% of cases, while platelet function abnormalities are responsible for most of the rest (9). The platelet defect is most likely due to effects of platelet activation and fragmentation within the extracorporeal circulation. The severity of the platelet abnormalities is proportional to the bypass time. Following uncomplicated surgery, the platelet function returns to normal within a few hours (8), and the platelet count returns to normal within 3 to 4 days. Patients who have a prolonged bleeding time and excessive bleeding in the postoperative period usually respond well to platelet transfusion (8). The use of desamino-D-arginine-vasopressin (DDAVP) after bypass surgery to diminish blood loss is controversial. Some patients develop acute intravascular hemolysis and neutropenia postsurgery, which are thought to be secondary to lytic complement activation during the blood passage through the oxygenator. Treatment is supportive until the situation corrects itself (10).

III. DRUG-INDUCED HEMATOLOGIC SYNDROMES

Unexpected thrombocytopenia due to drugs through immunological mechanisms can be divided into two different subgroups. One is a syndrome, exemplified by quinine- and quinidin-induced thrombocytopenias, where Fab sites of IgG bind to a drug/platelet-membrane complex; the Fc site is presumably binding to Fc receptors on phagocytes of the reticuloendothelial system, inducing moderate to severe thrombocytopenia. The other subgroup of drug-induced thrombocytopenias is exemplified by heparin-induced thrombocytopenia. Here the Fab sites of

IgG bind to a complex of heparin and platelet factor 4 on the surface of platelets, and the Fc site is bound by Fc receptors on platelets, resulting in platelet activation rather than removal through the reticuloendothelial system with less severe thrombocytopenia.

A. Heparin-Induced Thrombocytopenia (HIT)

Heparin is the most important drug to cause thrombocytopenia, frequently used, with an incidence of HIT of 5% (11), and complicated by potentially life-threatening arterial and venous thromboses (11). HIT is caused by heparin-dependent IgG that activates platelets via their Fc receptors (12,13). The marked difference in clinical complications of HIT is thought to be due to platelet variability to Fc receptor stimulation (14,15) and comorbid clinical factors (16). Low-molecular-weight heparin can cause a similar syndrome with thrombocytopenia and paradoxical thrombosis (17). The thrombocytopenia is usually mild to moderate with mean platelet count nadirs of 50×10^9/L (18), and only rarely the count is as low as 10 to 20×10^9/L. The thrombocytopenia usually begins 5 to 10 days after the initiation of heparin therapy (low-dose or full-dose), with 10% to 30% of thrombocytopenic patients developing thrombotic complications affecting the venous as well as the arterial vasculature (Table 2).

1. Diagnosis

A high level of suspicion is advisable. Every patient receiving heparin should have a prior platelet count. Although thrombocytopenia is usually defined as a platelet count below 150×10^9/L, a sudden drop even with numbers above 150×10^9/L can indicate a platelet-destructive process like HIT. HIT has to be distinguished from another, benign form of heparin-induced thrombocytopenia: About 25% of patients receiving full-dose heparin show a mild and early (after 2 to 14 days of initiation of therapy) drop of their platelet count, thought to be caused by an intrinsic ability of heparin to weakly activate platelets (19). The platelet count usually remains above 100×10^9/L, and heparin therapy can be continued without bleeding risk. HIT is suggested if the platelet count drops below 100×10^9/L from a normal pretreatment level in the absence of another cause of thrombocytopenia (e.g., other drugs, sepsis, DIC). Occasionally thrombosis can precede the throm-

Table 2 Clinical Complications of Heparin-Induced Thrombocytopenia

Arterial thrombosis	Venous thrombosis	Other
stroke	DVT	skin necrosis
acute MI	pulmonary embolism	
limb necrosis	venous limb gangrene	
splanchnic infarcts	cerebral sinus thrombosis	

bocytopenia. The diagnosis has to be made clinically, as laboratory tests to confirm the diagnosis are time-consuming and not always reliable. Most patients with immune thrombocytopenia have elevated platelet-associated IgG (PAIgG), but none of the standard PAIgG assays can reliably distinguish immune from nonimmune thrombocytopenias (20). Recently introduced platelet antibody assays, detecting IgG on individual platelet glycoproteins, may be more useful tests (21–24).

2. *Management/Treatment*

Heparin should be stopped in any patient with HIT. The thrombocytopenia usually resolves within several days after discontinuation of therapy. The choice of further anticoagulation presents a problem, as warfarin has a slow onset of action and can cause complications in some patients with HIT. Low-molecular-weight heparin is not recommended in HIT because of cross-reactivity (25). Heparinoids and ancrod, a defibrinogenating snake venom, have been used successfully in clinical trials of patients with HIT (26,27). It is a dilemma in the United States that there is no FDA-approved treatment available for HIT. The patient with a past history of HIT represents an anticoagulation problem as well, as the risk of recurrence is unclear. In cases of venous and especially arterial thrombosis, the optimal therapy is uncertain. Fibrinolytic therapy or surgical embolectomy should be considered for arterial thrombosis affecting a limb.

3. *Prevention*

HIT cannot be predicted prior to heparinization. But each patient should have a pretreatment count, followed by daily platelet counts while receiving heparin. Any unexplained drop of the platelet count should be investigated. As HIT is quite common and unrelated to the dose of heparin administered, routine heparin–saline flushes of venous catheters may be replaced by saline flushes only.

B. Drug-Induced Immune Thrombocytopenia

A large number of drugs can produce a syndrome that mimics acute ITP (Table 3). Typically, these patients develop severe thrombocytopenia with platelet counts below $20 \times 10^9/L$, together with petechiae and purpura usually within a week, but occasionally within years, of starting drug therapy. These syndromes are much less common than HIT. Almost all patients have elevated PAIgG, but drug-dependent binding of antibodies to platelets can only infrequently be demonstrated (28). Drug-dependent IgG binding is very heterogenous with respect to binding affinity, number of binding sites per platelet, and the range of drug concentration required (29,30).

1. *Diagnosis*

Again, a high index of clinical suspicion is required to make the diagnosis. The sensitivity of in vitro testing for drug-dependent binding to platelets is very low

Table 3 Drugs, Commonly Used in the CCU Setting, That Can Induce Immune Thrombocytopenia Purpura

Positive inotropic drugs	Antihypertensive drugs	Diuretics
amrinone	captopril	furosemide
digoxin	α-methyldopa	HTZ
Antiarrhythmic drugs	H_2 antagonists	spironolactone
amiodarone	cimetidine	Antiepileptic drugs
procainamide	ranitidine	carbamazepine
quinidine	Benzodiazepines	diphenylhydantoin
β Blockers	diazepam	valproic acid
alprenolol		Antibiotics
oxyprenolol		NSAIDs

and sometimes complicated, as metabolites, rather than the parental drug itself, may be responsible for the binding. Therefore the diagnosis is made clinically with laboratory confirmation, if possible.

2. *Management/Treatment*

As many drugs as possible should be discontinued in patients with suspected drug-induced thrombocytopenia. Platelet transfusions should be given to patients with life-threatening bleeding. The lifespan of the transfused platelets is shortened as well, but may also help clearing the circulating drug-dependent antibodies. High-dose intravenous γ-globulin (1 mg/kg given over 6 to 8 h) for 2 consecutive days is generally effective in drug-induced thrombocytopenia (31,32).

3. *Prevention*

As with HIT, drug-induced thrombocytopenia cannot be predicted. A high level of clinical suspicion and regular platelet counts are advisable. Any unexplained drop of the platelet count should be investigated.

C. Drugs Affecting Platelet Function

Many drugs are known to affect platelet function, defined by an abnormality of platelet aggregation or the bleeding time. Whether they contribute to a risk of excessive bleeding is definitively established only for aspirin (33). Among this group of drugs are nonsteroidal antiinflammatory drugs, β-lactam antibiotics, plasma expanders, calcium antagonists, propanolol, nitroglycerine, isosorbide dinitrates, antihistamines, tricyclic antidepressants, and phenothiazines.

Ticlopidine inhibits adenosine diphosophate (ADP)-induced platelet aggregation. The most common side effects are skin rashes, diarrhea, neutropenia, and, rarely, fatal aplastic anemia. Neutropenia occurs in about 1% of treated patients. Regular blood counts are mandatory during treatment with this drug.

More recently, a more complete antiaggregation effect has been accomplished by the use of monoclonal antibodies that bind to the platelet fibrinogen receptor glycoprotein (GP) IIb/IIIa. This receptor becomes activated by platelet stimulation and binds fibrinogen molecules between platelets in the aggregation process. Abciximab, the Fab fragment of an antibody against GP IIb/IIIa, inhibits the final common pathway of platelet aggregation. Side effects include excessive bleeding.

D. Neutropenia

Idiosyncratic drug reactions are a frequent cause of neutropenia, although the exact frequency is not known. Most drug-related neutropenias are due to dose-dependent marrow suppression. Phenothiazines, semisynthetic penicillins, nonsteroidal anti-inflammatory drugs (NSAIDs), aminopyrine derivatives, and antithyroid medications are the most common offenders. Neutropenia may occur at any time but tends to occur relatively early in the course of treatment with drugs to which the patient has previously been exposed. A high level of suspicion and a careful history are critical to identify the offending drug. The differential diagnosis includes acute viral infections, particularly infectious mononucleosis and viral hepatitis, and bacterial sepsis. Recovery usually starts within a few days of stopping the drug, and is preceded by the appearance of monocytes and immature neutrophils in the peripheral blood. Rebound leukocytosis with marrow and peripheral blasts has been reported and can simulate a leukemic state (34,35).

E. Anemia

Drug-induced Coombs-positive hemolytic anemia was commonly seen when penicillin was administered in large doses ($>20 \times 10^6$ U/day) and when α-methyldopa was widely used in the treatment of hypertension. However, the disease is unusual in present day clinical practice (36).

Aplastic anemia is more serious than other hematological dyscrasias because of the high mortality related to the severity of the underlying aplasia (37,38). It is important to discontinue immediately any likely offending agents, as some early-onset drug-induced hypoplasias are completely reversible following drug withdrawal and because many patients may survive marrow hypoplasia if the stem cell damage is incomplete (39,40). Drugs commonly associated with aplastic anemia are gold, phenylbutazone, chloramphenicol, penicillamine, NSAIDs, sulfonamides, antithyroid drugs, sulphonureas, phenothiazines, and allopurinol.

F. Drug-Induced Vitamin K Deficiency

Bacteria in the large intestine produce functional forms of vitamin K. In the absence of dietary vitamin K, small amounts of vitamin K, absorbed from the large intestine, prevent severe vitamin K deficiencies. In patients receiving antibiotics that destroy the intestinal flora, this additional vitamin K source is eliminated. Therefore patients with inadequate vitamin K intake, treated at the same time with antibiotics, can develop vitamin K deficiency with prolonged PT within 1 to 3 weeks.

Drug-induced deficiency of the vitamin K-dependent factors can be seen particularly in patients receiving third-generation cephalosporins that contain the N-methylthiotetrazole side chain (moxalactam, cefamandol, cefotaxime, cefoperazone).

IV. DISSEMINATED INTRAVASCULAR COAGULATION (DIC)

DIC is among the most common disorders of coagulation seen in the intensive care unit. It is an epiphenomenon, almost always caused by a serious illness (Table 4). It is of special interest in the CCU that hematomas can induce DIC. A big, unnoticed retroperitoneal hematoma as a complication of angiography can present with DIC as the leading clinical sign. DIC formerly carried a mortality of up to 67% (41). However, with improvement in treatment, survival now approaches 75% (42). DIC occurs when the hemostatic regulatory systems break down (43). The predominant mediator of DIC is tissue thromboplastin, and almost all forms of DIC lead to activation of both the coagulation and fibrinolytic systems (44,45).

Table 4 Conditions Associated with Disseminated Intravascular Coagulation

1.	Infections		
2.	Obstetrical		
3.	Transfusion reactions —acute hemolysis		
4.	Trauma or burns		
5.	Venoms and toxins		
6.	Hepatic disease		
7.	Vascular disorders		
	—TTP —vasculitis —arteriovenous fistula —malignant hypertension	—angiosarcoma —hereditary telangiectasia —aortic aneurysm —giant hemangioma	—acute myocardial infarction —intracardiac tumor and thrombus
8.	Malignancy		
9.	Prosthetic devices		
	—intra-aortic balloon pump	—leveen shunt	—cardiopulmonary bypass
10.	Shock		
11.	ARDS		
12.	Hematoma		

The degree to which each of these two processes contribute to the coagulopathy varies. Tissue thromboplastin triggers the coagulation cascade with the generation of thrombin and the consequent formation of a fibrin clot. Local vasomotor activity as well as endothelial injury contribute to localizing soluble fibrin. After the soluble fibrin monomers polymerize, the injury to end organs by microvascular thrombi is perpetuated due to inhibition of fibrinolysis. Once activated, plasmin initiates the process of secondary fibrinolysis and also degrades clotting factors (46). Bleeding results from the consumption of coagulation factors and platelets as well as from fibrin degradation products, inhibition of platelets, and impairment of fibrin polymerization. The local endothelial integrity and vasomotor activity influence whether bleeding or thrombosis dominates at a particular site. Still, most patients with acute DIC have little clinical or pathologic evidence for the formation of stable fibrin clots, despite the high level of thrombin activity in their blood (47,48). Evidence of rapid fibrinolysis is the most important predictor of bleeding risk.

A. Diagnosis

DIC can be assumed if there is evidence of accelerated fibrinolysis and also consumption of platelets and clotting factors in a patient with a disorder known to cause DIC. The best screening tests for DIC are measurement of the fibrin degradation products (FDP), prothrombin time (PT), fibrinogen level, and platelet count. If the FDP titer is normal, DIC is unlikely. If screening tests suggest the presence of DIC, useful information can often be obtained by measuring plasma antithrombin III (AT-III), plasminogen, and α_2-antiplasmin (α_2-PI) activity. These provide an index of severity (generally, high-grade DIC is associated with AT-III and plasminogen activities below 60% of normal) and of the balance between coagulation and fibrinolysis, as reflected in the degree of AT III and α_2-PI depletion, respectively. Information about the dynamics of DIC can be obtained by measuring the products of coagulation factor activation. The plasma level of fibrinopeptide A reflects the rate of fibrin formation, it is sensitive for DIC but not very specific. Levels of prothrombin activation peptide (F1·2) are indicators of the rate of thrombin formation and are a very sensitive test for DIC (49). The D-dimer assay measures the subpopulation of FDP derived from cross-linked fibrin. It can be performed on plasma samples and is not susceptible to artifacts caused by incomplete clotting of serum samples, but it is less sensitive than the serum FDP assay (50). The differential diagnosis of DIC includes vitamin K deficiency, thrombocytopenia of sepsis, liver disease, microangiopathy, localized coagulation, lupus anticoagulant, and hemodilution. The presence of liver failure causes the most difficulty in diagnosing DIC because it also results in deficiency of clotting factors and inhibitors, moderate thrombocytopenia, and delayed clearance of FDP, causing mild to moderate elevation of the FDP titer. When liver failure is present, serial testing may be required. If significant DIC is present, the coagulation abnormalities will become progressively more severe.

B. Management/Treatment

Treatment of the underlying cause, removal of the inciting factor, is the key in arresting the vicious cycle of DIC. Therapy aims at minimizing the two major complications—thrombosis and bleeding. Since peripheral vasoconstriction may precipitate or exacerbate tissue necrosis in sepsis, blood pressure should be maintained by aggressive fluid administration rather than α-adrenergic agents, when possible.

1. Replacement of Factors

Clotting factors and inhibitors can be replenished by giving fresh-frozen plasma (FFP). The prothrombin time (PT) is the single best parameter to guide plasma replacement. Cryoprecipitate contains a fivefold to 10-fold higher fibrinogen concentration than FFP.

If significant depletion of clotting factors has occurred, as evidenced by a PT greater than 1.3 to 1.5 times control, plasma replacement may reduce the bleeding risk. When the fibrinogen is <100 mg/dl, 10 U of cryoprecipitate for each 2 or 3 U of plasma should be given. Therapy goal, according to general guidelines, are a PT within 2 to 3 sec of the control and a fibrinogen level >100 mg/dl. AT III concentrates ameliorate experimental DIC, and reports suggest it may be of clinical benefit in humans (51–53). Thrombocytopenia is usually not severe, and most patients do not require platelet transfusions (54,55). Prophylactic platelet transfusion may benefit patients who are severely thrombocytopenic (platelet count below 20×10^9/L), and platelets should be given to bleeding patients if the platelet count is below 50×10^9/L. Platelet and fibrinogen levels should be measured 30 to 60 min posttransfusion and every 6 h thereafter to assess platelet and fibrinogen survival times.

2. Pharmacological Inhibitors

The use of heparin and antifibrinolytic agents in DIC is controversial. These treatments have not been shown conclusively to improve survival in DIC and may exacerbate bleeding (heparin) or thrombosis (antifibrinolytic agents) (56–58). Heparin may be beneficial in any case of DIC associated with thrombosis. In the absence of large vessel thrombosis, a dose of heparin (5 to 10 U/kg/h) may be effective. Higher doses of heparin are of questionable therapeutic value. An exception is the patient with chronic DIC associated with large-vessel thrombosis, in whom heparin should be given in doses sufficient to prolong the activated partial thromboplastin time (PTT) to at least 1.5 times control, as usual in the treatment of deep venous thrombosis. Patients who may benefit from the use of antifibrinolytic drugs, like ε-aminocaproic acid or tranexamic acid, include those in whom there is laboratory evidence of hyperfibrinolysis with depletion of physiologic plasmin inhibitors (α_2-antiplasmin) and who bleed despite replacement therapy (59). Antifibrinolytic agents are usually given in conjunction with heparin to minimize the potential for thrombosis.

V. THROMBOTIC THROMBOCYTOPENIC PURPURA

Thrombotic thrombocytopenic purpura (TTP) is characterized by a triad of consumptive thrombocytopenia, microangiopathic hemolytic anemia, and fluctuating neurological signs. The peak incidence occurs in the fourth decade with a female preponderance of 2:1. The underlying pathophysiologic process is still unclear. Most patients who develop TTP have no known underlying disorder. Autoimmune disorders, infections, drugs, and pregnancy have been associated with TTP. TTP is believed to be triggered by intrusion of one or more platelet-aggregating agents into the circulation. Immunochemical studies of thrombi have revealed an abundance of von Willebrand factor (VWF), with only little fibrinogen/fibrin (60). The VWF multimers are thought to function as multimeric bridges promoting platelet-platelet aggregation. Intravascular platelet aggregation results in organ ischemia and severe thrombocytopenia. Platelet counts are below 20×10^9/L in over 50% of patients. Bleeding into the skin is common. Hemolysis is usually severe, with 90% of patients having hemoglobin values below 10 g/dl. Blood films always show extensive poikilocytosis and erythrocyte fragmentation. Serum LDH is always increased, often to levels five to 10 times normal. Haptoglobin is usually absent. Neurologic abnormalities, which may be transient, occur in 50% to 71% of patients during acute TTP episodes (61,62). Renal dysfunction is present in 50% to 75% of TTP patients during acute episodes (61,62). Symptoms of myocardial ischemia are unusual in the absence of underlying cardiac or coronary artery pathology, unless the acute hemolytic anemia is profound. Angina, CHF with pulmonary edema, or conduction disturbances with cardiac arrhythmias may occur in severely ill patients, however (63).

A. Diagnosis

Diagnosis is based on clinical presentation and a constellation of laboratory and histological features. Microangiopathic changes are seen on peripheral blood smears. The PT, PTT, and fibrinogen levels are usually normal and help distinguishing TTP from DIC. In TTP, there might be a mild elevation in fibrin degradation products; high levels, however, are found in DIC. Large VWF multimers may be present. Biopsy of the gingiva will demonstrate thrombi composed primarily of platelets in contrast to the more fibrin-rich thrombi found in DIC (64).

B. Management/Treatment

In 71% to 91% of patients with TTP, the process can be reversed with intensive plasma manipulation (61,62,65–68). The most effective therapy is plasma exchange at 3 to 4 L/day, started as soon as possible and continued for a minimum of 5 days. In case plasma exchange is not readily available, infusion of FFP at 30 ml/kg/day together with prednisolone 200 mg/day can be used initially. It is recommended that all patients receive pharmacological doses of glucocorticoids until the patient recovers (62). Importantly, platelet transfusions should be avoided, because they may exacerbate production of microthrombi. But if the platelet count is very low and if bleeding is a primary problem, or if intracranial bleeding is demonstrated by CT or MRI, platelet transfusion will be necessary. In a few reports, however, this has been associated with exacerbation of the thrombotic process in the cerebral microcirculation (64,69). If a patient does not respond within the first 5 days of therapy, or deteriorates within the first 2 or 3 days, other therapies should be tried. Splenectomy (65) or immunosuppressive agents like vincristine (70) or azathioprine (64,71) should be considered. The use of antiplatelet agents is controversial; aspirin may exacerbate hemorrhagic complications (72).

VI. PROBLEMS WITH ANTICOAGULATION

A. Heparin Resistance

Patients with inherited antithrombin deficiency usually have 40% to 60% of normal AT III plasma levels, and in most of those patients the PTT responds normally to heparin (73,74). However, in patients with DIC (54), nephrotic syndrome (75), or liver cirrhosis (76) with acquired AT-III levels below 25% of the normal level, even large doses of heparin may not increase the PTT. Patients with massive pulmonary embolism have an increased clearance of heparin and may need large doses of heparin to reach therapeutic PTT levels (77).

B. Heparin Overdose

The anticoagulant effect of heparin disappears within hours after discontinuation of the drug, rarely requiring the use of antagonists. In case of life-threatening hemorrhage, intravenous protamin quickly antagonizes heparin as well as low-molecular-weight heparin. The usual protamin dose is 1 mg/100 U of heparin. An antibody-mediated anaphylactic reaction can occur, as seen in approximately 1% of diabetic patients who had received protamin-containing insulin before (78).

C. Warfarin Resistance

Patients requiring more than 15 to 20 mg/day of warfarin to maintain a therapeutic PT are described as warfarin-resistant. It is important to rule out recent intake of vitamin K as well as the consumption of large amounts of vitamin K-rich vegetables. There are no known antibody responses to warfarin. Patients resistant to the effects of warfarin can still be treated with warfarin, but higher doses are necessary.

D. Warfarin Overdose

In patients with prolongation of PT without signs of bleeding, warfarin can be withheld until the PT reaches the therapeutic level. Patients with life-threatening bleeding must be treated with FFP (2 to 3 U) as a source of vitamin K-dependent coagulation factors. Administration of vitamin K to reverse the effect of warfarin bears several problems. The response to vitamin K is delayed 12 to 24 h due to de novo synthesis of vitamin K-dependent coagulation factors. The PT then tends to normalize, and reanticoagulation with warfarin may become very difficult (warfarin resistance).

ACKNOWLEDGMENT

I am very grateful to Sheila Kar, M.D. for her constructive criticism.

REFERENCES

1. Wedemeyer AL, Edson JR, Krivit W. Coagulation in cyanotic congenital heart disease. Am J Dis Child 1972; 124:656.
2. Goldschmidt B. Platelet functions in children with congenital heart disease. Acta Pediatr Scand 1974; 63:271.
3. Waldmann JD, Czapek EE, Paul MH, et al. Shortened platelet survival in cyanotic heart disease. J Pediatr 1975; 87:77.
4. Jacobsen RJ, Rath CE, Perloff JK. Intravascular hemolysis and thrombocytopenia in left ventricular outflow obstruction. Br Heart J 1973; 35:849.
5. Steele PP, Weily HS, Davies H, Genton E. Platelet survival in patients with rheumatic heart disease. N Engl J Med 1974; 290:537.
6. Edwards BS, Weir EK, Edwards WD, et al. Coexistent pulmonary and portal hypertension: morphologic and clinical features. J Am Coll Cardiol 1987; 10:1233.
7. O'Brien JR. Shear-induced platelet aggregation. Lancet 1990; 335:711.
8. Harker LA, Malpass TW, Branson HE, et al. Mechanism of abnormal bleeding in patients undergoing cardiopulmonary bypass: acquired platelet dysfunction associated with selective alpha-granule release. Blood 1980; 56:824.
9. Khuri SF, Wolfe JA, Josa M, et al. Hematologic changes during and after cardiopulmonary bypass and their relationship to the bleeding time and nonsurgical blood loss. J Thorac Cardiovas Surg 1992; 104:94.
10. Salama A, Hugo F, Heinrich D, et al. Deposition of terminal C5b-9 complement complexes on erythrocytes and leukocytes during cardiopulmonary bypass. N Engl J Med 1988; 318:408.
11. Warkentin TE, Kelton JG. Heparin-induced thrombocytopenia. Prog Hemost Thromb 1991; 10:1.

12. Kelton JG, Sheridan D, Santos A, et al. Heparin-induced thrombocytopenia: laboratory studies. Blood 1988; 72:925.
13. Chong BH, Fawaz I, Chesterman CN, Berndt MC. Heparin-induced thrombocytopenia: mechanism of interaction of the heparin-dependent antibody with platelets. Br J Haematol 1989; 73:235.
14. Warkentin TE, Hayward CPM, Smith CA, et al. Determinants of donor platelet variability when testing for heparin-induced thrombocytopenia. J Lab Clin Med 1992; 120:371.
15. Chong BH, Pilgrim RL, Cooley MA, Chesterman CN. Increased expression of platelet IgG Fc receptors in immune heparin-induced thrombocytopenia. Blood 1993; 81:988.
16. Greinacher A, Michels I, Schäfer M, et al. Heparin-associated thrombocytopenia treated with polysulphated chondroitin sulfate: evidence for immunological cross-reactivity between heparin and polysulphated glycosaminoglycan. Br J Haematol 1992; 81:252.
17. Eichinger S, Kyrle PA, Brenner B, et al. Thrombocytopenia associated with low molecular weight heparin. Lancet 1991; 337:1425. Letter.
18. Warkentin TE, Kelton JG. Interaction of heparin with platelets, including heparin-induced thrombocytopenia. In: Bounameaux (ed): Low-Molecular-Weight Heparins in Prophylaxis and Therapy of Thromboembolic Diseases. New York: Marcel Dekker, 1994.
19. Rothrock JF, Hart RG. Antithrombotic therapy in cerebrovascular disease. Ann Intern Med 1991; 115:885.
20. Kelton JG, Murphy WG, Lucarelli A, et al. A prospective comparison of four techniques for measuring platelet-associated IgG. Br J Haematol 1989; 71:97.
21. Kiefel V, Santoso S, Weisheit M, Mueller-Eckhardt C. Monoclonal antibody-specific immobilization of platelet antigens (MAIPA): a new tool for the identification of platelet-reactive antibodies. Blood 1987; 70:1722.
22. Kiefel V. The MAIPA assay and its application in immunohaematology. Tranf Med 1992; 2:181.
23. Wood VL Jr, Oh EH, Mason D, McMillan OR. Autoantibodies against the platelet glycoprotein IIb/IIIa complex in patients with chronic ITP. Blood 1984; 63:368.
24. Woods VL Jr. Kurata Y, Montgomery RR, et al. Autoantibodies against platelet glycoprotein Ib, in patients with chronic immune thrombocytopenic purpura. Blood 1984; 64:156.
25. Warkentin TE, Kelton JG. Heparin-induced thrombocytopenia. Annu Rev Med 1989; 40:31.
26. Demers C, Ginsberg JS, Brill-Edwards P, et al. Rapid anticoagulation using ancrod for heparin-induced thrombocytopenia. Blood 1991; 78:2198.
27. Magnani HN. Heparin-induced thrombocytopenia (HIT): an overview of 230 patients treated with Orgaran (Org 10172). Thromb Haemost 1993; 70:554.
28. Kelton JG, Meltzer D, Moore J, et al. Drug-induced thrombocytopenia is associated with increased binding of IgG to platelets both in vivo and in vitro. Blood 1981; 58:524.
29. Christie DJ, Weber RW, Mullen PC, et al. Structural features of the quinidine and quinine molecules necessary for binding of drug-induced antibodies to human platelets. J Lab Clin Med 1984; 104:730.

30. Christie DJ, Diaz-Arauzo H, Cook JM. Antibody-mediated platelet destruction by quinine, quinidine and their metabolites. J Lab Clin Med 1988; 112:92.
31. Redell MA, Moore BR, Fass L. Use of i.v. immune globulin for presumed quinidine-induced thrombocytopenia, letter. Clin Pharm 1989; 8:89.
32. Raj JB, Brereton WF, Nullet FR. Intravenous immune globulin for the treatment of presumed quinidine-induced thrombocytopenia. DICP 1989; 24:693.
33. Steering Committee of the Physician's Health Study Research Group. Final report of the aspirin component of the ongoing physician's health study. N Engl J Med 1989; 321:129.
34. Rudvic OR, Jelic S. Haematologic aspects of drug-induced agranulocytosis. Scand J Haematol 1972; 9:18.
35. Levine P, Weintraub L. Pseudo-leukemia following recovery from dapsone-induced agranulocytosis. Ann Intern Med 1968; 68:1060.
36. Danielson DA, Douglas SW III, Herzog P, et al. Drug-induced blood disorders. JAMA 1984; 252:3257.
37. Williams DM. Pancytopenia, aplastic anemia and pure red cell aplasia. In: Lee GR, Bithell TC, Foerster J, et al., eds. Wintrobe's Clinical Haematology. Philadelphia; Lea and Febinger, 1993: 911–943.
38. Camitta BM, Storb R, Thomas ED. Aplastic aneamia. Pathogenesis, diagnosis, treatment and prognosis. N Engl J Med 1982; 306:645.
39. Kay AGL. Myelotoxicity of gold. BMJ 1976; 1:1266.
40. Patten WN, Murray JA, Blake DR, et al. How should we monitor gold therapy? Lancet 1988; 1:581.
41. Baker WF Jr. Clinical aspects of disseminated intravascular coagulation: a clinician's point of view. Semin Thromb Hemost 1989; 15:1.
42. Feinstein DI. Treatment of disseminated intravascular coagulation. Semin Thromb Hemost 1988: 14:351.
43. Müller-Berghaus G. Pathophysiologic and biochemical events in disseminated intravascular coagulation: dysregulation of procoagulant and anticoagulant pathways. Semin Thromb Hemost 1989; 15:58.
44. Merskey C, Johnson AJ, Kleiner G, Wohl H. The defibrination syndrome: clinical features and laboratory diagnosis. Br J Haematol 1967; 13:528.
45. Harker L, Slichter S. Platelet and fibrinagen consumption in man. N Engl J Med 1972; 287:999.
46. Bick RL. Disseminated intravascular coagulation and related syndromes: a clinical review. Semin Thromb Hemost 1988; 14:299.
47. McKay D, Müller-Berghaus G. Therapeutic implications of disseminated intravascular coagulation. Am J Cardiol 1967; 20:392.
48. Mant M, King E. Severe, acute disseminated intravascular coagulation. A reappraisal of its pathophysiology, clinical significance and therapy based on 47 patients. Am J Med 1979; 67:557.
49. Bauer K, Rosenberg R. Thrombin generation in acute promyelocytic leukemia. Blood 1984; 64:791.
50. Carr JM, McKinney M, McDonagh J. Diagnosis of disseminated intravascular coagulation. Role of D dimer. Am J Clin Pathol 1989; 91:280.
51. Fourrier F, Lestavel P, Chopin C, et al. Meningococcemia and purpura fulminans in

adults: acute deficiencies of proteins C and S and early treatment with antithrombin III concentrates. Intens Care Med 1990 16:121.

52. Schipper H, Jenkins C, Kahle L, Ten Cate J. Antithrombin III transfusion in disseminated intravascular coagulation. Lancet 1978; 1:854.
53. Delshammar M, Lasson A, Nilsson I-M, et al. Abnormal proteolysis (DIC)—successful treatment with antithrombin III concentrate and a concentrate containing fXIII and native von Willebrand factor. J Intern Med 1989; 225:21.
54. Spero J, Lewis J, Hasiba U. Disseminated intravascular coagulation. Findings in 346 patients. Thromb Haemost 1980; 43:28.
55. Rosner F, Ritz N. The defibrination syndrome. Arch Intern Med 1966; 117:17.
56. Marciniak E, Wilson H, Marlar R. Neonatal purpura fulminans: a genetic disorder related to the absence of protein C in the blood. Blood 1985; 65:15.
57. Feinstein D. Diagnosis and management of disseminated intravascular coagulation: the role of heparin therapy. Blood 1982; 60:284.
58. Charytan C, Purtillo D. Glomerular capillary thrombosis and acute renal failure after epsilon-amino caproic acid therapy. N Engl J Med 1969; 280:1102.
59. Williams E. Plasma α-2 antiplasmin activity: role in the evaluation and management of fibrinolytic states and other bleeding disorders. Arch Intern Med 1989; 149:1769.
60. Asada Y, Sumiyoshi A, Hayashi T, et al. Immunohistochemistry of the vascular lesion in thrombotic thrombocytic purpura, with special reference to factor VIII related antigen. Thromb Res 1985; 38:469.
61. Rock GA, Sumak KH, Buskard NA, et al. Comparison of plasma exchange with plasma infusion in the treatment of thrombotic thrombocytic purpura. N Engl J Med 1991; 325:393.
62. Bell WR, Braine HG, Ness PM, Kickler TS. Improved survival in thrombotic thrombocytopenic purpura-hemolytic-uremic syndrome—clinical experience in 108 patients. N Engl J Med 1991; 325:398.
63. Ridolfi RL, Hutchins GM, Bell WR. The heart and conductive system in thrombotic thrombocytopenic purpura. Ann Intern Med 1979; 91:357.
64. Byrnes JJ, Moake JL. Thrombotic thrombocytopenia purpura and hemolytic syndrome: evolving concepts of pathogenesis and therapy. Clin Hematol 1986; 15:413.
65. Thompson CE, Damon LE, Ries CA, Linker CA. Thrombotic microangiopathies in the 1980's: clinical features, response to treatment, and the impact of the human immunodeficiency virus epidemic. Blood 1992; 80:1890.
66. Bukowsky RM, Hewlett JS, Reimer RR, et al. Therapy of thrombotic thrombocytic purpura: an overview. Semin Thromb Hemost 1981; 7:1.
67. Shepard KV, Bukowski RM. The treatment of thrombotic thrombocytopenic purpura with exchange transfusions, plasma infusions, and plasma exchange. Semin Hematol 1987; 24:178.
68. Byrnes JJ. Plasma infusion in the treatment of thrombotic thrombocytopenic purpura. Semin Thromb Hemost 1981; 7:9.
69. Gordon LI, Kwaan HC, Rossi EC. Deleterious effects of platelet transfusions and recovery thrombocytosis in patients with thrombotic microangiopathy. Semin Hematol 1987; 24:194.
70. Gutterman LA, Stevenson TD. Treatment of thrombotic thrombocytopenic purpura with vincristine. JAMA 1982; 247:1433.

71. Moake JL, Rudy CK, Troll HJ, et al. Therapy of chronic relapsing thrombotic thrombocytopenic purpura with predisone and azathioprine. Am J Hematol 1985; 20:73.
72. Rosove MH, Ho WG, Goldfinger D. Ineffectiveness of aspirin and dipyridamole in the treatment of thrombotic thrombocytopenic purpura. Ann Intern Med 1982; 96:73.
73. Leclerc JR, Geerts W, Panju A, et al. Management of antithrombin III deficiency during pregnancy without administration of anti-thrombin III. Thromb Res 1986; 41:567.
74. Nielsen LE, Bell WR, Borkon AM, Neill CA. Extensive thrombus formation with heparin resistance during extracorporeal circulation. A new presentation of familial antithrombin II deficiency. Arch Intern Med 1987; 147:149.
75. Kauffman RH, Veltkamp JJ, van Tilburg NH, van Es LA. Acquired antithrombin III deficiency and thrombosis in the nephrotic syndrome. Am J Med 1978; 65:607.
76. Knot E, ten-Cate JW, Drijhout HR, et al. Antithrombin III metabolism in patients with liver disease. J Clin Pathol 1984; 37:523.
77. Hirsh J, van Aken WG, Gallus AS, et al. Heparin kinetics in venous thrombosis and pulmonary embolism Circulation 1976; 53:691.
78. Weiss ME, Nyhan D, Peng ZK, et al. Association of protamin IgE and IgG antibodies with life-threatening reactions to intravenous protamine. N Engl J Med 1989; 320:886.

10

The Cardiologist and Coagulation Cascade

SAMUEL A. BERKMAN

University of California, Los Angeles, School of Medicine, Los Angeles, California

I. INTRODUCTION

The coagulation cascade is of major relevance to the field of cardiology. Not only do disturbances in the cascade cause thrombotic disorders requiring cardiologist intervention, but these very interventions may result in perturbations in the cascade. It will be the purpose of this article to take a detailed look at the clotting cascade with particular relevance as to how disturbances involving clotting factors influence clinical situations encountered by the cardiologist. These perturbations will be caused either by a disease process or by cardiologist interventions to treat thrombotic disease.

The cascade or waterfall hypothesis was promulgated in 1964 by MacFarland et al. (1,2) (Fig. 1). The purpose was to demonstrate a schematized relationship between component coagulation factors. In this way, deficiencies could be correlated with clinical disease entities.

Both intrinsic and extrinsic activation systems were identified and felt to function independently. The extrinsic pathway was initiated by a factor VII–tissue factor complex and measured by the prothrombin time. Activation of the intrinsic pathway was initiated by plasma binding to a negatively charged surface causing activation of factor XII, high-molecular-weight kininogen, and prekallikrein. This system was measured by the partial thromboplastin time.

Both mechanisms were viewed as independent means of activating clotting

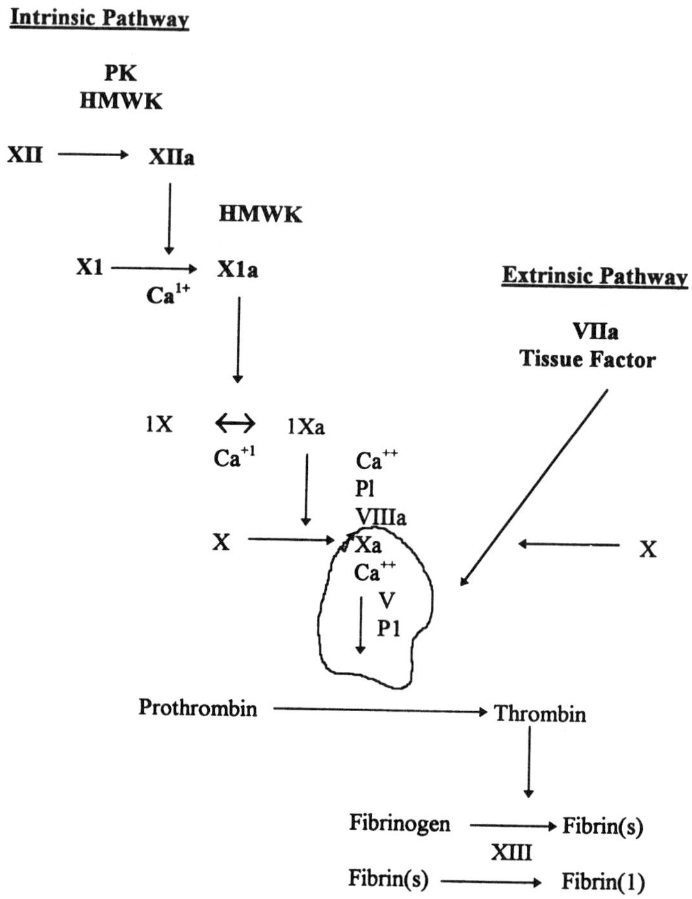

Figure 1 The classical coagulation cascade or waterfall hypothesis was promulgated in 1964 by MacFarlane, Davey, and Ratnoff. While extremely useful and quite accurate today, there are some questions left unanswered by this schema (see text).

factor Xa from its inactive precursor. The second major step in coagulation is the activation of thrombin from its precursor prothrombin with the assistance of the prothrombin activator complex (Fig. 1). This complex consists of clotting factor Va, factor Xa, platelet phospholipid, and calcium. The third major step involves the activation of fibrin from fibrinogen by thrombin.

This 1960s model of the cascade, while a laudable beginning and in many ways still accurate, does not address certain basic questions in hematology. For example, the cascade does not explain why people with hemophilia bleed. If the extrinsic system is an equally efficient activation system as the intrinsic one for factor Xa activation, why do hemophiliacs bleed? Since their factor VII and tissue factor levels are adequate, they should be able to compensate for their lack of factor VIII by using the extrinsic system to activate factor Xa.

However, we know that hemophiliacs do bleed seriously despite their normal extrinsic systems. The 1964 model of the cascade does not explain why. The explanation given at the time was that the intrinsic system was more important in activation. This point of view is no longer held. Furthermore, people with factor XII deficiency do not have a bleeding diathesis. On the contrary, a deficiency of this factor has been linked with thrombotic predisposition probably on the basis of factor XII's crucial involvement in the fibrinolytic pathway (3). Deficient levels of factor XII have led to deficient thrombolysis of clot. Myocardial infarction and pulmonary embolism have been associated with this deficiency (4,5).

By contrast, people with factor XI deficiency do bleed under surgical or traumatic situations. If the only way to activate factor XI were through factor XII, as the cascade indicates, then people with factor XII deficiency should have an accompanying XI deficiency and be susceptible to hemorrhage. We know, however, this is not the case. Therefore there must be an alternative pathway to the activation of factor XI. The MacFarland model does not explain what that may be.

The 1960 model does not include the systems of naturally occurring anticoagulants which play an important role in the balance of hemostasis and thrombosis. These include the antithrombin III system, the protein C and S system, the tissue factor pathway inhibitor system, and the fibrinolytic system characterized by the interaction between tissue plasminogen activator (tPA) and plasminogen activator inhibitor (PAI). The current model of the cascade including these four anticoagulant systems is presented in Figure 2.

II. PLATELETS

One cannot ignore platelets in addressing the clotting cascade since platelets interact with coagulation proteins in several locations. The activated platelet surface is an essential catalytic surface for several coagulation reactions that generate thrombin. There is an important interaction as well between the platelet and fibrinogen via the IIb-IIIa receptor, and with von Willebrand's factor (VWF) by the same receptor (6).

The fluid shear stress of blood flow in atherosclerotic or spasmodic arteries may influence platelet activation by leading to spontaneous platelet aggregation (7). Spontaneous platelet activation has been strongly correlated with arterial thrombotic disorders. It has been observed to increase the risk of mortality in myocardial infarction by fivefold and the recurrence rate by more than a factor of 3 (8).

In addition, platelet phospholipid is an important component of the prothrombin activator complex otherwise known as prothrombinase (Fig. 1). Furthermore,

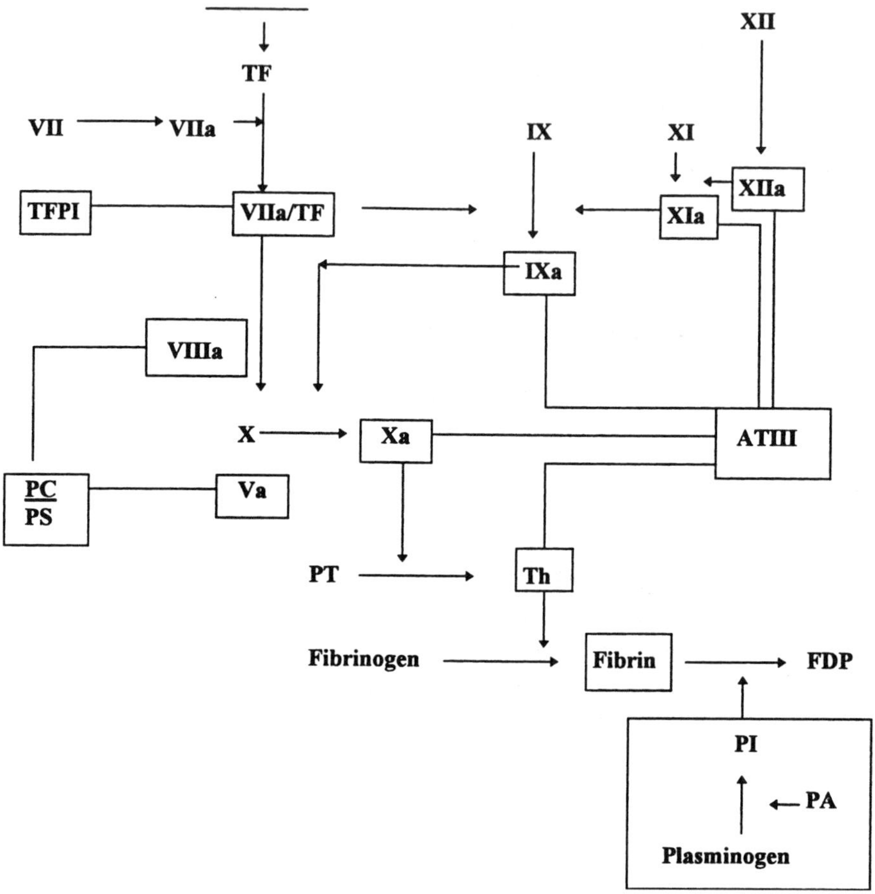

Figure 2 The revised coagulation cascade shows the interrelationship between the extrinsic and intrinsic systems as well as the sites of action of the major antithrombotic pathways. From Ref. 73.

thrombin exerts an extremely potent aggregating effect on platelets. Therefore any process either pathological or interventional which affects platelets may affect thrombotic risk.

β Thromboglobulin, a release product of platelet granules, has been shown to portend an increased risk of carotid atherosclerosis (9,10). Shear stress-induced platelet aggregation depends upon the binding to VWF to platelet GPIIb/IIIa receptor (11). On the other hand, platelet aggregation under low shear conditions is mediated by a fibrinogen-GPIIb/IIIa interaction (12). Elevated levels of fibrinogen and VWF have been associated with increased risk of atherosclerosis (13,14).

Interventions at inhibiting the platelet have been helpful in preventing and treating cardiac disease. Patients undergoing coronary bypass (15), those with unstable angina (16), chronic stable angina (17), myocardial infarction (18), atrial fibrillation (19), and those who have experienced transient ischemic attacks (20) have demonstrated benefit from aspirin to some degree. Even healthy males over the age of 50 without hypertension have profited from small doses of aspirin (21). The interruption of synthesis of thromboxane by inhibition of prostaglandin G/H synthetase appears to be the main mechanism by which aspirin exerts its antiplatelet effects (22). This inhibition results in the loss of the enzyme's cyclo-oxygenase catalytic activity and ability to generate thromboxane (23).

However, there have been reports of non-cyclo-oxygenase-related inhibition (24) and even platelet independent antithrombotic actions of aspirin (25). While doses vary in different studies and no optimal dosage is widely acknowledged, 160 mg/day of a rapidly absorbable preparation would appear adequate to achieve rapid effective antithrombotic activity in most circumstances and 80 to 16 mg/day for maintenance (26). The minimal effective daily dose is approximately 40 mg/day (27). Interestingly, even on 30 mg/day, a 2.5% incidence of hemorrhage has been observed which included gastrointestinal as well as hemorrhagic stroke (28). Therefore this is not an innocuous drug even at small doses.

While the inhibition of thrombaxane is useful in inhibiting platelet aggregation, more potent inhibitors of platelet action are in use today. Ticlopidine is an antiplatelet agent that inhibits both the primary and secondary waves of adenosine diphosphate (ADP)-induced platelet aggregation (29). It has demonstrated itself to be superior to aspirin as well as placebo in the prevention of thrombotic strokes in patients who have experienced transient ischemic attacks, amaurosis fugax, and reversible ischemic neurological defects (30,31). In addition, it may be effective in a reducing stroke recurrence in patients who have experienced a completed thrombotic stroke (32).

Maximal platelet inhibition occurs after 8 to 10 days of treatment. The bleeding time becomes maximally prolonged at 5 days after initiation of therapy and returns to normal a week to 10 days after treatment is stopped (33). Bleeding time prolongations are generally greater than those achievable with aspirin (34). Because over 50% of treated patients will experience at least one untoward reaction to ticlopidine and because its average cost is significantly greater than that of aspirin, it is often used in patients who have not benefited from or cannot tolerate aspirin (35).

A typical candidate for ticlopidine would be an individual with a history of transient ischemic attacks and a history of gastrointestinal intolerance to aspirin. Diarrhea is the most common complication reported with ticlopidine, and neutropenia the most serious (36). Disturbingly, there has been a question of number of cases of thrombotic thrombocytopenic purpura have been reported with this medication (37).

Careful monitoring of the blood count is necessary during the first 3 months of therapy to monitor against the development of neutropenia. Ticlopidine has been also shown to be beneficial in unstable angina (38). However, because of its delayed onset of action, it may not be prudent to rely on it as the sole agent for this indication. Ticlopidine has also been used successfully in conjunction with aspirin alone and with aspirin and low-molecular-weight heparin in stent angioplasty situations (39,40).

Abciximab, or c7E3Fab, is a monoclonal antibody Fab fragment that inhibits platelet aggregation by blocking the glycoprotein IIb/IIIa receptor on the platelet surface. One can achieve an 80% inhibition of aggregation with this drug, which cannot be achieved with any of the other antiplatelet drugs (41). With this degree of inhibition, ADP release can be totally inhibited. It is administered both with aspirin and with heparin. It has been shown to be a useful adjunct to angioplasty for the prevention of acute ischemic complications in patients at high risk for closure of the treated vessel (42). The criteria of high risk are well known to cardiologists (43).

Severe bleeding, defined as a drop in hemoglobin of greater than 5 g/dl or central nervous system hemorrhage, has been a problem with this drug. Fourteen percent of patients in the EPIC trial who received the drug both by bolus and continuous infusion experienced severe bleeding. It did not increase the rate of intracerebral bleeding or fatal bleeding; however, there were increases in hematemesis and retroperitoneal hemorrhage.

Most bleeding was found at interventional sites. Such patients may require platelet and packed red blood cell infusions. Platelet transfusion improves the bleeding time and partially restores aggregation, but plasma does not. This is despite the fact that 7E3Fab bound to circulating platelets redistributes to newly transfused uncoated platelets very rapidly after transfusion (44). The management of bleeding should involve local measures including the direct pressure and frequent palpation for hematoma formation (45,46). If bleeding from the catheter site cannot be controlled or if other serious bleeding is occurring, the infusion should be stopped. Consideration should also be given to decreasing or even stopping the dose of heparin. Newer studies using lower doses of heparin which are weight-adjusted are expected to be associated with less hemorrhage.

Patients at very high risk of bleeding from Abciximab include patients over 80 years old, patients under 77 kg, and patients with a recent history of bleeding, surgery, or thrombolytic therapy or coumadin unless the INR is under 1.3. The drug should be used with extreme caution or not at all in such patients.

The cardiologist's main involvement with the platelet will be through the use of a treatment to inhibit platelet activity. However, on occasion clinical situations arise involving the platelet which warrant the cardiologist's attention.

Certain drugs used to control arrhythmias such as quinidine or pronestyl may elicit the formation of an antibody that destroys platelets immediately and can cause profound thrombocytopenia. This emergency situation with its attendant risk of intracerebral hemorrhage requires the use of high-dose steroids. In fact, more than 100 drugs have been reported to cause immune-mediated thrombocytopenia (47).

By far the main medication used by the cardiologist resulting in thrombocytopenia is heparin. There are two types of heparin-induced thrombocytopenia. The first and most common type is a self-limited suppression of the platelet count with the second (and more rare) type being a progressive delayed drop in the platelet count due to aggregation induced by heparin and an antibody directed against heparin and platelet factor 4 (48,49).

The risk of heparin-induced thrombocytopenia is between 1% and 5%; that of the rare type II is about 0.6% (50,51). Type 2 heparin-induced thrombocytopenia is unique in its predisposition to life-threatening thrombotic complications. Patients with this condition tend to produce procoagulant microparticles which are not seen in other immune conditions such as quinidine-induced thrombocytopenia (52). There is a 25% risk of loss of life and a substantial risk of loss of limb as well (53).

This complication, which rarely occurs before day 6 in first-time recipients of the medication, has been reported with minidose heparin, full-dose heparin, heparin-coated catheters, and even flushing doses of heparin (54,55). In fact, many hospitals have eliminated the use of heparin from flushing catheters due to this problem. There seems to be a particular propensity for this problem to occur after cardiac surgery, cardiac interventions, or even any surgical situation as opposed to medical indication for heparin therapy (56,57).

Heparin-induced thrombocytopenia has been defined as a platelet count of under 100,000 in a patient on heparin. This definition does not take into account the magnitude of the drop from baseline, and has been criticized that it should include a 30% drop from baseline (58). A serotonin release assay is confirmatory but not always instantly available (59). Newly developed solid-phase assays that use complexes of heparin and platelet factor 4 are more sensitive than serotonin release methods (60).

This syndrome is characterized by ischemic interruption of blood flow to the extremities as well as the cerebral or coronary arteries. It is actually more common for thrombosis to occur in the veins than the arteries. A common scenario is massive thrombosis in the leg veins with pulses attainable but gangrene development nevertheless. It is therefore most important to monitor platelet counts every other day on patients taking heparin in the hospital and to stop the drug if a 33% drop in the baseline platelet count is noted. Twenty percent of patients who develop significant thrombocytopenia on heparin will develop the white clot syndrome (61). Early commencement of coumadin allows one to discontinue heparin before day 6, avoiding the high-risk period. This strategy is particularly relevant in pulmonary embolism and deep venous thrombosis patients where prolonged use of heparin has been customary (62).

The patient with the white clot syndrome frequently presents with three daunting simultaneous problems. The first entails the obstructed artery or vein caused by the white clot syndrome. Secondly, the issue arises as to which form of anticoagulation should be used in lieu of heparin. Thirdly, if the platelet count is severely decreased, the patient may be at risk for bleeding. Fortunately bleeding does not seem to be a major risk in this situation despite significant thrombocytopenia.

Surgery is frequently necessary to handle the first problem if it is arterial. Thrombolytic therapy is the most likely course if one is dealing with major venous thrombosis. Frequently the infusion will need to be infused through two ports due to the large length of clot involved. Unfortunately at this time there are no FDA-approved drugs in the United States appropriate for use in the white clot syndrome. As a consequence, many doctors utilize antiplatelet agents that have some utility but probably have an ancillary role.

Ancrod, a potent defibrinating agent, has been shown to be useful in this regard in the past and was widely used in Canada but has fallen into disfavor because of concerns of lack of efficacy (63). ORG 10172, otherwise known as Organon, is a heparinoid available for compassionate use in the United States with no cross-reactivity against heparin. It consists of heparin sulfate, chondroitin sulfate, and dermatan sulfate (64). Direct antithrombin inhibitors such as hirudin, Hirulog, or Argantroban may be the optimal agents for this condition.

While low-molecular-weight heparin is less likely to provoke the white clot syndrome and less likely to elicit the formation of antibody than unfractionated heparin, its use is not recommended once this complication has occurred due to its high cross-reactivity with heparin (65,66). As mentioned, early commencement of coumadin will allow discontinuation of heparin, preventing many cases of the white clot syndrome. However, should one encounter the white clot syndrome, the immediate administration of warfarin is contraindicated since the large initial drops of protein C engendered by coumadin are likely to aggravate clotting.

Other causes of thrombocytopenia that may present themselves to the cardiologist include the thrombocytopenia of sepsis seen in patients with major infections (67). A patient with acute or subacute bacterial endocarditis could well have this problem based on an antibody synthesized against the platelet which bears some relationship to an antigen on the infecting bacterium. Some of these patients may develop disseminated intravascular coagulation, which would warrant calling a hematologist for management assistance.

Disseminated intravascular coagulation (DIC) is not a condition the cardiologist will be called on to treat but which may occur in a patient under his or her care. Elderly patients who develop a serious infection may develop this complication and manifest diffuse oozing. The widespread hemorrhage characteristic of this condition results from four different disturbances in the coagulation cascade. Most important is the inhibitory action of fibrin degradation products on the fibrinogen to fibrin reaction in the same way it is caused by fibrinolytic therapy. In addition quantitative thrombocytopenia, qualitative platelet defect, and consumption of coagulation factors result in prolongations of the partial thromboplastin time and prothrombin time (68).

The underlying disturbance with the coagulation cascade in disseminated intravascular coagulation stems from the excessive activation of thrombin by the underlying disease process. This excessive thrombin reactivity leads to a reciprocal hyperactivity of the thrombolytic system, causing the formation of fibrin degradation products. The treatment of the condition therefore always entails successful treatment of the underlying cause of the excessive generation of thrombin (69). A particular dilemma arises in cardiology in the elderly patient maintained on coumadin for a prosthetic valve or atrial fibrillation who develops disseminated intravascular coagulation secondary to severe infection.

While possibly initially attributable to the warfarin, diffuse oozing is uncommon with this medication. Thrombocytopenia and a prolonged partial thromboplastin time will also be noted, both of which are distinctly uncharacteristic of coumadin therapy. Elderly patients with ischemic bowel disease, diverticulitis, or sepsis are particularly predisposed to this complication.

The issue often arises as to how to handle the patient's warfarin which is being prescribed for prevention of thrombosis. It should be emphasized that disseminated intravascular coagulation is a clotting disorder as well as a hemorrhagic one. While each case must be taken on its own merits, the optimal plan is usually to persist with low-dose coumadin to protect against thromboembolism. In addition, treatment of the underlying cause of disseminated intravascular coagulation should be undertaken. Platelets and fresh-frozen plasma may also be necessary depending on the degree of bleeding, but the warfarin should be maintained if possible in a dosage to ensure an INR of at least 2.

Another important cause of thrombocytopenia with possible cardiac implications is the disorder of thrombotic thrombocytopenic purpura. This rare illness is in some cases related to gastrointestinal *E. coli* 0157: H7 infections (70). It is characterized by a pentad consisting of thrombocytopenia, microangiopathic hemolytic anemia, fever, renal failure, and CNS signs (71). Frequently these signs are fleeting and may consist of hemiparesis or seizures. The microangiopathy rarely presents as myocardial infarction but is more likely to produce arrhythmias due to involvement of the microvasculature supplying the conduction system (72). Congestive heart failure secondary to the arrhythmias is not unusual. It is most important to identify TTP as the cause of the arrhythmia since the treatment is plasma exchange, which would be different from any other cause of arrhythmias.

III. ISSUES REGARDING THE CASCADE

As mentioned earlier, it was not clear from the 1964 cascade why people with hemophilia bleed if two independent pathways exist to activate factor X. If a person has a major deficiency in clotting factors indigenous to the intrinsic pathway, an intact extrinsic pathway should be able to effectively compensate.

A. Tissue Factor, Tissue Factor Pathway Inhibitor, and Factor VII

We now know about tissue factor and tissue factor pathway inhibitor. While tissue factor's existence was known at the time of the 1964 cascade, tissue factor pathway inhibitor hadn't yet been well defined. Factor VII is activated by tissue factor. Tissue factor–factor VII complex serves to activate factor X to Xa. However, what is now known is that in addition to this activity, tissue factor VIIa also activates the intrinsic pathway by directly activating factor IXa (73). A four-component complex then forms among tissue factor, factor 7, factor X, and tissue factor pathway inhibitor. This complex limits further clotting initiated through the extrinsic pathway (74). (See Figure 2.)

Factor IX in conjunction with factor VIII also initiates factor X activation, and it is mainly through this pathway that clotting is maintained. The intrinsic pathway is between 10 and 50 times more efficient in activating factor X than is the extrinsic tissue factor–factor VII pathway (74).

Therefore the reason hemophiliacs bleed is because without sufficient factor VIII or IX levels, coagulation cannot proceed by the intrinsic pathway. Since coagulation along the extrinsic pathway is by and large limited by tissue pathway factor inhibitor, an intact intrinsic pathway is necessary for hemostasis. Consequently, the mild or moderate hemophiliac will experience severe hemorrhages in surgery, and trauma and spontaneous hemorrhages are noted frequently in severe hemophilia.

It should also be noted that the back activation of factor XI by thrombin is most important in replenishing the supply of factor IX to activate factor X (75). This back-activation is also the explanation why people with factor XII deficiency do not necessarily also have a factor XI deficiency.

Activated factor VII has been shown to be a very strong and somewhat underemphasized risk factor for myocardial infarction. Studies at the Northwick Park Institute have indicated the incidence of myocardial infarction and death were three and eight times higher, respectively, for levels of VII coagulant activity of over 119% of control as compared with those with levels under 98% (76). Factor VII levels have been shown to correlate with fibrinogen levels and to be sensitive to varying the amount of fat in the diet (77). Most patients with elevated factor VII levels have elevated triglycerides and may well also have decreased levels of tissue plasminogen activator (78). These components may all be parts of Reaven's syndrome of low-HDL cholesterol, elevated triglycerides, and obesity with insulin resistance (79). This hypothesis is supported by the relation in some studies of activated factor VII levels to postprandial lipidemia (80). It may therefore be that insulin resistance has more and broader implications involving more factors than has been previously realized.

The use of warfarin in a dosage of 3 mg/day has reduced factor VII levels by 26% and moved levels into a much safer zone from pretreatment ones (81). Factor VII may exercise its atherothrombotic predisposition by interacting with the monocyte tissue factor in which atherosclerotic plaque is so rich (82). Individuals with high activated factor VII levels and hypercholesterolemia, diabetes, or other predisposing factors to coronary plaquing should be viewed at high risk for ischemic events. Retinoic acid and other oxidizing agents have been shown to diminish monocyte tissue factor production and tissue factor–factor VIIa-dependent arterial thromboses formation (83,84).

In practice, more attention has been focused on the causes of the plaquing by addressing risk factors such as hypercholesterolemia through diet, exercise, and medication. However, the issue of activated factor VII has been relegated to secondary status in viewing the severity of risk factors.

Consequently, any patient with significant risk factors for plaquing should also have an activated factor VII level performed. Should that level be found to be elevated, consideration should be given to maintaining such patients on 3 mg coumadin along with antioxidants. Such a low dose of warfarin allows for the coadministration of aspirin (81). Warfarin has generally been employed to prevent venous disease and has not been thought of as an arterial protective agent. However, its effect on factor VII may be very helpful in preventing a life-threatening atherothrombotic event stemming from the ominous combination of significant plaque rich in tissue factor and high activated factor VII levels.

It has also been demonstrated that one of the actions of heparin is to increase the activity of tissue factor pathway inhibitor (85). Interestingly, when heparin binds to tissue pathway factor inhibitor, factor Xa is inhibited even when it is attached to prothrombin activator complex. Heparin, on the other hand, only neutralizes factor Xa unbound in plasma (86). It is possible that the tissue factor mechanism is as efficient in binding activated factor Xa as the antithrombin III-related mechanism. This observation may explain why people with antithrombin III deficiency are sensitive to relatively normal doses of heparin. It is not clear how much of heparin's anticoagulant activity is exercised through tissue factor pathway inhibitor; however, it seems apparent that it is not minimal.

B. Factors X and Xa

Factor Xa is a pivotal coagulation protein that exerts its action at the junction of the intrinsic and extrinsic pathways. Both pathways have as their purpose the formation of activated factor X(Xa) from factor X precursor. While the intrinsic pathway is 10 times more efficient in this activation process than the extrinsic, the initial activation of factor X is more commonly via the extrinsic pathway. Activated factor X is a component of the prothrombin activator complex along with clotting factor V, calcium, and platelet phospholipid. A sensitive means of measuring factor Xa activity is by a measurement of prothrombin fragment I+II (87) (Fig. 3). Another is through the enzyme inhibitor complex thrombin–antithrombin III (TAT). These are both measures of factor Xa activity or thrombin generation (88).

Fragment I+II is increased in situations of increased factor Xa activity such as hypercoaguable states. Patients with antithrombin III deficiency, protein C deficiency, protein S deficiency, or resistance to activated protein C frequently have elevated levels of prothrombin fragment I+II (89). One of the effective uses of this test is to determine if a patient with a history of thrombotic events remains at risk for further thrombotic events. The finding of an elevated level of fragment I+II would suggest that a chronic, ongoing hypercoaguable state remains. This information could assist the practitioner in deciding whether indefinite prophylactic anticoagulation is warranted.

Proteins C and S are naturally occurring anticoagulants to be discussed in detail later. It has been established that protein S is a cofactor for protein C in the inhibition of activated coagulation factors V and VIII (90). It has now been established that in addition Protein S has independent actions involving direct inhibition of factor X (91). In a series of 36 patients under the age of 40 with cerebrovascular accidents, five were found to have protein S deficiency (92). This finding would be difficult to attribute to lack of protein S's supporting of protein C-induced inhibition of factors 5 and 8.

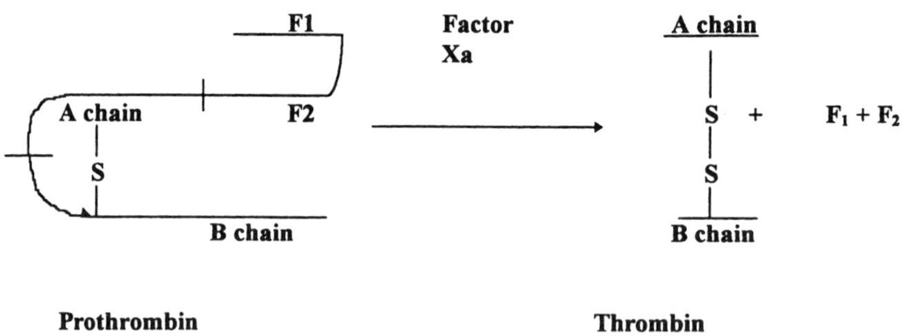

Figure 3 Peptide F1 + F2 is generated along with thrombin as a consequence of factor Xa's conversion of prothrombin to thrombin. It consequently serves as a marker of thrombin generation and hypercoagulability and is increased in thrombotic disorders such as protein C and protein S deficiency, as well as resistance to activated protein C.

Protein C protects against venous disease rather than arterial because it is activated by thrombin binding to thrombomodulin. There is much more contact between capillary endothelial thrombomodulin and blood thrombin than in the venous circulation. Consequently any quantitative or qualitative abnormality in thrombomodulin, protein C, or protein S reflects itself in the venous system, where the thrombomodulin generation of protein C is less efficient to begin with (93).

Consequently, disorders such as protein C deficiency, hereditary resistance to activated protein C, or thrombomodulin disturbances cause venous clots. Likewise, any deficiency in protein S should also mainly be associated with venous clots since the heretofore described action of protein S is to assist protein C. The association of protein S deficiency with arterial thrombosis confirms a significant protein C-independent action of protein S. Therefore young adults with cerebrovascular accidents should be monitored for protein S deficiency as well.

To summarize, the salient features of coagulation factor Xa are these:

1. It sits at the convergence of both pathways and belongs to the common pathway.
2. It is more effectively activated by the intrinsic pathway.
3. Its activity is measured by the PT and APTT but more specifically by levels of prothrombin fragment I+II.
4. It is a major site of inactivation by the major anticoagulants including coumadin, heparin, and low-molecular-weight heparin, to be discussed later.
5. It is effectively inhibited by tissue factor pathway inhibitor.

It has also been widely postulated that a major site of action of antiphospholipid antibodies is the phospholipid component of prothrombin activator complex of which factor Xa is a member (94). It has also been suggested that this antibody exerts its thrombogenic potential by binding to complexes of phospholipid and protein C or S (95). Patients with antiphospholipid syndrome, 50% of whom have systemic lupus, may present to the cardiologist with deep venous thrombosis, pulmonary embolism, or cerebrovascular accident as well as cardiac abnormalities. Those cardiac abnormalities associated with antiphospholipid antibodies include valvular lesions, ventricular dysfunction, mass lesions, and myocardial infarction (96,97). In certain instances intracardiac mass lesions have disappeared with anticoagulant therapy (98). While patients with the antiphospholipid syndrome frequently have an abnormality in the PTT and a normal PT, both pathways are abnormal. This can be illustrated by performing the prothrombin time with dilute thromboplastin which will reveal prolongation of the prothrombin time (99). Patients with seemingly normal partial thromboplastin times can have their defects demonstrated by the Russell viper venom test, which will illustrate a prolongation of the partial thromboplastin time (100).

C. Thrombin and Fibrinogen (factors II and I)

Thrombin and fibrinogen—factors II and I, respectively—are crucial coagulation factors to the cardiologist. Much of the anticoagulant and thrombolytic armamentarium is directed at disrupting the activity of these two coagulation proteins. Thrombin is a protein that is well named as it has numerous procoagulant actions. These include (Table 1):

1. Cleaving of fibrinogen into fibrinopeptides A and B.
2. Promoting aggregation of platelets.
3. Activation of cytokines.
4. Changing of the endothelium from nonmitotic to mitotic.
5. Activation of factor XI.
6. Activation of clotting factors V and VIII.
7. Increases synthesis of plasminogen activator inhibitor type 2.
8. Activation of factor XIII (101,102).

As mentioned, it also has a major anticoagulant action by binding to endothelium thrombomodulin and activating protein C. Activated protein C then inactivates clotting factors V and VIII.

Thrombin is a major site of action of heparin, which binds to its active site with the assistance of antithrombin III. One of the limitations of antithrombin III-mediated thrombin inhibition is that clot-bound thrombin is not inactivated by heparin (103). Direct thrombin inhibitors have been produced which bind to either the active site of thrombin or the processing, or anion binding, site. These inhibitors are able to inactivate thrombin even when bound to fibrin (104) (Fig. 4). The direct thrombin inhibitors include hirudin, hirugen, hirulog, D-phenylalanyl-

Table 1 Major Procoagulant Actions of Thrombin[a]

1. Catalyzes fibrinogen to fibrin
2. Activates factors V and VIII
3. Activates platelet aggregation
4. Activates cytokines; mediates vascular inflammation
5. Activates factor XI
6. Activates factor XIII
7. Changes phenotype from antithrombotic to thrombotic
8. Induces adhesion molecules on endothelial cell surface
9. Mitogenic for smooth muscle cells and fibroblasts

[a]Thrombin has numerous procoagulant actions which cause it to be a target of numerous therapeutic anticoagulant drugs such as heparin, low-molecular-weight heparin, the heparinoids, and the direct thrombin inhibitors.

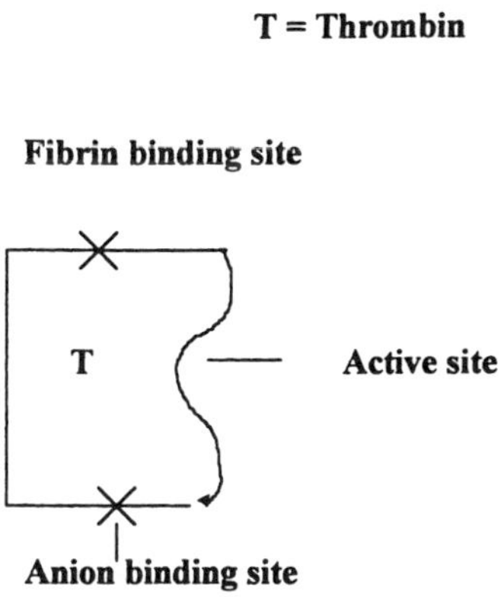

Figure 4 Thrombin possesses a catalytic or active site, a substrate recognition or anion binding site, and a site for fibrin binding. Heparin and antithrombin III will normally bind to the active site but cannot bind to clot-bound thrombin. By contrast, direct thrombin inhibitors can bind to clot-bound thrombin. Hirudin and Hirulog bind to both the active site and substrate recognition site. Argantroban binds to the active site alone.

L-propyl-L arginyl chlorommethyl ketone (PPACK), and argantroban. While hirudin and hirulog bind to both of the above receptors, argantroban and PPACK bind only to the active site (105). Hirudin has been compared to heparin in angioplasty patients with fewer early cardiac events but no apparent benefit in long-term follow-up (106). It has also reduced thromboembolic complication in a study of 1119 hip surgery patients to 8.54% from 19.6% in heparin-prophylaxed patients (107).

As mentioned previously, an important potential role of the direct thrombin inhibitors is in heparin-induced thrombocytopenia. At this time there is no FDA-approved medication for this condition in the United States. As mentioned, Canadians may choose between Organon (a heparinoid) and Ancrod (a defibrinating agent), and tend to prefer the former. Currently an international protocol is under way using argantroban for heparin-induced thrombocytopenia.

D. Fibrinogen and Fibrin

Thrombin converts fibrinogen to fibrin via cleaving fibrinopeptides A and B from fibrinogen. Fibrin monomers then coalesce to form fibrin polymers which are stabilized in their cross-linkages by factor XIII. The possibility of the dissolution of fibrin and the importance of the fibrin clot in the pathogenesis of arterial thrombosis has rendered fibrinolytic therapy a mainstay in cardiovascular practice (108). Fibrinolytic therapy has revolutionized the initial treatment of myocardial infarction (109). However, when thrombolytic therapy is used to dissolve life-threatening coronary thrombi, secondary hyperactivity of the hemostatic mechanism can be elicited (110).

It has been postulated that the dissolution of fibrin allows more clot-bound thrombin to become activated and create the numerous procoagulant actions of thrombin already mentioned (104). Plasmin has been shown to directly activate coagulation factors (111). Plasminogen activator inhibitor 1 synthesized by endothelial cells and platelets has been induced by cytokines during fibrinolysis (112). Because of this seemingly paradoxical hypercoaguability, heparin is a necessary adjuvant to the use of thrombolytic therapy, particularly with tissue plasminogen activator (113). Due to thrombin's potent procoagulant effect on platelets, aspirin is used routinely as an adjunct with thrombolytic therapy and heparin (114).

Fibrinogen has been strongly implicated as a risk factor for coronary artery disease and for stroke (115). In one study fibrinogen was viewed as a greater risk factor for the development of stroke than high blood pressure, although both were considered important (116). Fibrinogen is the major determinant of plasma viscosity and induces reversible red cell aggregation. It strongly affects hemostasis, rheology, platelet, endothelial, and smooth muscle cell function (117). Fibrinogen has also been related to plasma insulin levels and seems to be elevated by cigarette smoking and by season of the year (118,119). Hyperfibrinogenemia has been determined to be an independent risk factor for further cardiovascular disease in survivors of strokes.

There appears to be a correlation between fibrinogen and factor VII levels; however, unlike factor VII, fibrinogen does not appear to be influenced by a low-fat diet (120). However, like factor VII, fibrinogen has been linked to high triglyceride levels (121). Ticlopidine, β blockers, and fibrates have been reported to lower fibrinogen levels along with regular exercise (122). It has been shown to be a greater risk factor in younger than older men as well as in blacks versus Caucasians. It has been also related to job stress (123).

E. Naturally Occurring Anticoagulants

The four anticoagulant systems are relevant in their interaction with clotting factors in the coagulation cascade. These include antithrombin III, protein C/protein S, tissue factor pathway inhibitor, and tissue plasminogen activator. Deficiencies in many of these systems have resulted in predisposition to hypercoagulability.

Antithrombin III neutralizes several coagulation factors of the intrinsic coagulation pathway; however, its most important actions are against coagulation factors Xa and IIa (124). Both heparin and low-molecular-weight heparin exert their activity through antithrombin III. Unfractionated heparin neutralizes factors IIa and Xa comparably, while low-molecular-weight heparin inactivates clotting factor Xa to a greater degree than factor IIa (125). They are both efficacious in the prevention of deep venous thrombosis in medical and surgical settings. While unfractionated heparin has been widely used in coronary syndromes, low-molecular-weight heparin has been shown to have utility in these areas as well (126).

LMW heparin does not require monitoring. This is because of its superior bioavailability and longer half-life (127). These advantages, which make its levels much more predictable than unfractionated heparin, stem from its lack of binding to plasma proteins, endothelial cells, and leukocytes which regularly bind to unfractionated heparin (128).

With respect to the treatment of deep venous thrombosis, subcutaneous low-molecular-weight heparin has demonstrated equivalent efficacy to unfractionated heparin delivered by continuous infusion (129). In addition, it has been used to treat deep venous thrombosis at home equally effectively as hospitalizing patients for the treatment of deep venous thrombosis (130). Consequently, large amounts of money may be saved by avoiding hospitalizations through the use of this medication in this condition; however, the cost-effectiveness has not yet been rigorously established (131). The medication has not yet received FDA clearance for use in this indication in the United States, and at this time one preparation has been approved for the prophylaxis of deep venous thrombosis in hip and knee surgery, and another for general surgery.

Deficiency states of antithrombin III are seen in between 1 in 2000 and 1 in 5000 people in the general population (132). Such individuals are heterozygote and thrombose in about 65% of cases before the age of 30 (133). Arterial thrombosis is most unusual but has been reported (134). Young individuals with idiopathic deep venous disease and pulmonary emboli should be viewed as candidates for this disease. Heparin is useful in treating this problem despite low levels of antithrombin III, possibly because it also works through enhancing the activity of tissue factor pathway inhibitor. Approximately 5% of a population of patients with thrombophilia will have antithrombin III deficiency. AT-III-deficient patients usually have AT-III levels that are 40% to 60% of normal adult values (135).

IV. PROTEIN C AND PROTEIN S

The protein C pathway has received major attention in the last few years. The main mechanism of action of activated protein C is to inactivate activated clotting factors V and VIII with the assistance of protein S (136). It is such a powerful anticoagulant that a 50:50 mixture of protein C and normal plasma will prolong the partial thromboplastin time to two times control values in normal patients (137). Protein C is activated by thrombin, which binds to a capillary endothelial protein known as thrombomodulin (138) (Fig. 5). This binding generates activated protein C which then drifts downstream into the veins and cleaves activated

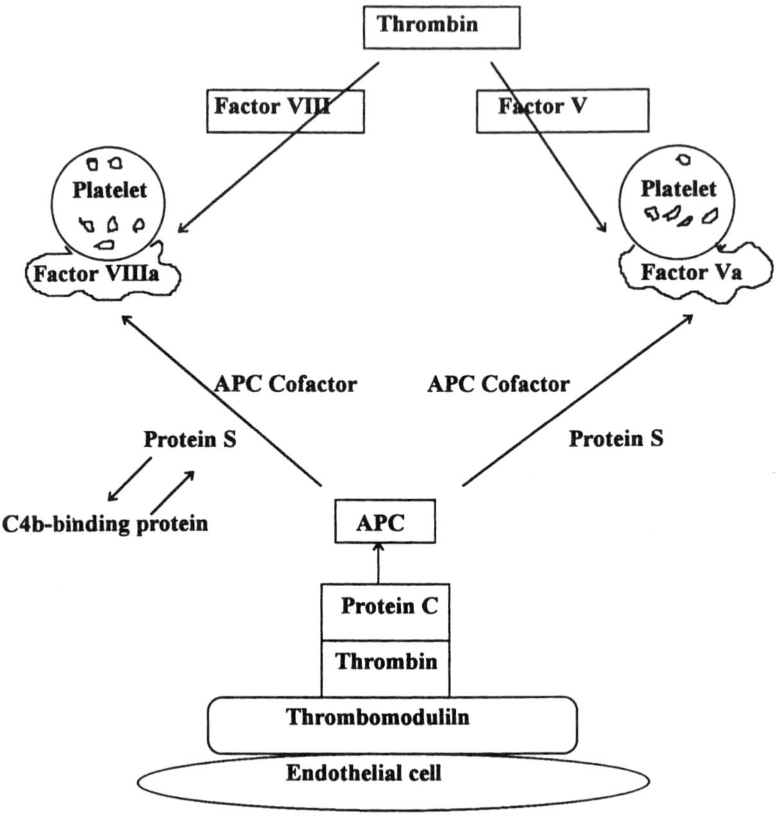

Figure 5 Thrombin's main anticoagulant action involves binding to the endothelial cell receptor thrombomodulin. This binding activates protein C which, with protein S and inactive factor V or APC cofactor II, inactivates platelet-bound activated factors 5 and 8. Taken from Ref. 138.

platelet-bound clotting factors V and VIII. It requires two cofactors, unbound protein S and inactive factor V, to produce this action (139).

The incidence of protein C deficiency is approximately 1 in 300 in the population. However, the vast majority of these patients are asymptomatic (140). Protein C is a vitamin K-dependent protein like coagulation factors 2, 7, 9, and 10 with a short half-life of approximately 7 h. It can therefore drop precipitously on initiation of warfarin (141). Thrombotic complications such as skin or breast necrosis have been reported in people with protein C deficiency receiving large initial doses of warfarin (142).

Deficiency of protein S, protein C, and antithrombin III might make up approximately 15% of a cohort of patients with thrombophilia (143). In the past 2 years a condition has been uncovered with a much higher incidence of deep venous thrombosis, known as resistance to activated protein C (144). This condition occurs in as many as 7% of a general population and 45% of individuals, with thrombophilia. It is due to a mutation in the factor V molecule. The defect appears to be at least 10 times as common in thrombophilic patients as any of the other known inherited deficiencies in anticoagulant proteins (145)

While the mutation does not affect the procoagulant role for factor V, it does affect its anticoagulant affect. While homozygotically affected individuals have a 10-fold higher risk of clotting than heterozygotes, only about 60% of affected homozygotes clot (146). This observation implies that while this condition is much more prevalent than protein C or protein S deficiency states, it is a less severe deficiency. Homozygotically affected individuals with such deficiencies invariably demonstrate pupura fulminans at birth (147). This disorder tends to complicate the use of the birth control pill in women as well as pregnancy (148). While primarily venous disease has been described with this disorder, rare cases of arterial disorders have been described (149,150).

With respect to protein S, the salient features have been mentioned and will be summarized. It is a vitamin K-dependent cofactor for the action of protein C. In addition, it possesses an independent anticoagulant action antagonizing factor X. Deficiency states are associated with a thrombotic predisposition which, like protein C deficiency, comprises about 5% of cases of familial thrombophilia. The treatment of thrombotic disease in deficiencies of proteins C or S or resistance to activated protein C consists of heparin followed by warfarin to an INR of 2 or 3 indefinitely. Asymptomatic affected individuals with any of these states do not necessarily require treatment but should receive prophylaxis in high-risk settings such as surgery.

V. FIBRINOLYTIC SYSTEM

Hypercoagulable states due to defects of the fibrinolytic system have not been as well characterized as those due to defects in protein C, protein S, or the antithrombins. There have been reports showing various abnormalities in the fibrinolytic pathway being associated with thrombosis. These include hypoplasminogenemia, dysplasminogenemia, decreased release of tissue plasminogen activator, and increased concentrations of plasminogen activator inhibition (151–154). Patients studied 3 years after a myocardial infarction have been fond to have higher PA-I levels than a control population and lower tPA levels. Interestingly, they also tend to show higher triglyceride levels. Whether these changes had antedated these patients' infarction or represented a complication is unclear. Levels of tissue plasminogen activator have been shown to rise steadily with increased moderate alcohol consumption, implying one reason for the French paradox (155).

Therefore, the coagulation cascade and its ramifications provide many challenges for the cardiologist. Excesses in some of the factors result, such as fibrinogen and factor VII result in atherosclerosis. Deficiencies in naturally occurring anticoagulants result in venous disease. The use of fibrinolytic therapy produces a hypercoagulable state due to increased generation of clot bound thrombin. The platelet and its interaction with the cascade are relevant as well, particularly with respect to antiplatelet therapy. Other cardiac risk factors not mentioned in this article such as a homocysteine and lipoprotein (a) interact with the cascade to produce much of their atherothrombotic disturbance which cardiologists are called upon to prevent and treat.

REFERENCES

1. Macfarlane RG. An enzyme cascade in the blood clotting mechanism and its function as a biochemical amplifier. Nature 1964; 202:498.
2. Davie, EW, Ratnoff OD. Waterfall sequence for intrinsic blood clotting: Science 1964; 145:1310.
3. Mandle RJ, Kaplan AP. Hageman factor dependent fibrinolysis. Generation of fibrinolytic activity by the interaction of human activated factor XI and plasminogen. Blood 1979; 54:850.
4. Glueck HI, Roehill W. Myocardial infarction in a patient with a Hageman (factor XII) defect. Ann Intern Med 1966; 64(2):390–395.
5. Ratnoff, OD, Busse RJ Jr, Sheon RP. The demise of John Hageman. N Engl J Med 1968; 279:760.
6. Report of a meeting of physicians and scientists, University of Texas Health Science Center at Houston and Texas Heart Institute, Houston. Lancet 1994; 344:991–995.
7. Brown CH, Leverett LB, Lewis CW, Alfrey CP, Hellums JD. Morphological, biochemical and functional changes in human platelets subjected to shear stress. J Lab Clin Med 1975; 86:462–471.
8. Trip MD, Cats VM, van Capelle FJ, Vreeken J. Platelet hyperactivity and prognosis in survivors of myocardial infarction. N Engl J Med 1990; 323:1549–1554.
9. Atherosclerosis Risk in Community (ARIC) Study: Design and objectives. ARIC investigators. Am J Epidemiol 1989; 129:687–702.
10. Cortes J, Stinson V, Salomaa V, et al. Platelet activation and early carotid atherosclerosis: the ARIC study. Thromb Haemost 1993; 69:1155. Abstract.
11. Moake JL, Turner NA, Stahhopoulos NA, Nolasco LH, Hellums JD. Involvement of large plasma Von Willebrand factor (vWF) multimers and unusually large vWF forms derived from endothelial cells in shear stress induced platelet aggregation. J Clin Invest 1986; 78:1456–1461.
12. De Marco L, Girolami A, Zimmerman TS, Ruggeri ZM. Von Willebrand factor interaction with the glycoprotein IIb/IIIa complex. Its role in platelet function as

demonstrated in patients with congenital afibrinogenemia. J Clin Invest 1986; 77: 1272–1277.

13. Resch KL, Ernst E, Matrai A, Paulsen H. Fibrinogen and viscosity as risk factors for subsequent cardiovascular events in stroke survivors, Ann Intern Med 1992; 117:371–375.
14. Jansson JH, Nilsson TK, Johnson O. Von Willebrand factor in plasma: a novel risk factor for recurrent myocardial infarction and death. Br Heart J 1991; 66: 351–355.
15. Chesebro JH, Clements IP, Fuster V, et al. A platelet inhibitor drug trial in coronary artery bypass operations: benefit of perioperative dipyridamole and aspirin therapy on early postoperative graft patency. N Engl J Med 1982; 307:73–78.
16. Lewis HD Jr, Davis JW, Archibald DG, et al. Protective effects of aspirin against myocardial infarction and death in men with unstable angina: results of a Veterans Administration cooperative study. N Engl J Med 1983; 309:396–403.
17. Ridker PM, Manson JET, Gaziano JM, Buring JET, Hennekens CH. Low dose aspirin therapy for chronic stable angina. A randomized, placebo controlled clinical trial. Ann Intern Med 1991; 114:835–839.
18. Aspirin after myocardial infarction. Lancet 1980; 1:1172–1173.
19. Stroke Prevention in Atrial Fibrillation Investigators. Warfarin versus aspirin for prevention of thromboembolism in atrial fibrillation: stroke prevention in atrial fibrillation I study. Lance 1994; 343:687–691.
20. Dutch TIA Trial Study Group. A comparison of two doses of aspirin (30 mg vs. 283 mg a day) in patients after a transient ischemic attack or minor ischemic stroke. N Engl J Med 1991; 325(18):1261–1266.
21. Steering Committee of the Physician's Health Study Research Group. Final report on the aspirin component of the ongoing physicians' health study. N Engl J Med 1989; 321:129–135.
22. Smith WL. Prostanoid biosynthesis and mechanism of action. Am J Physiol 1992; 263:F181–F191.
23. Patrano C. Aspirin as an antiplatelet Drug. N Engl J Med 1994; 330(18):1287–1294.
24. Gaspari F, Vigano G, Orisio S, Bonati M, Livio M, Remuzzi G. Aspirin prolongs the bleeding time in uremia by a mechanism distinct from platelet cyclooxygenase inhibition. J Clin Invest 1987; 79:1788–1797.
25. Lekstrom JA, Bell WR. Aspirin in the prevention of thrombosis. Medicine 1991; 70: 161–178.
26. Kearon C, Hirsh J. Optimal does for starting and maintaining low dose aspirin. Arch Intern Med 1993; 153:700–702.
27. Burch JW, Stanford N, Majerus PW. Inhibition of platelet prostaglandin synthetase by oral aspirin. J Clin Invest 1978; 61:5181–5184.
28. Mills JA. Aspirin the ageless remedy? N Engl J Med 1991; 325(18):1303–1304.
29. Hardisty RM, Powling MJ, Nokes TJC. The action of ticlopidine on human platelets: studies on aggregation, secretion calcium mobilization and membrane glycoproteins. Thromb Haemost 1990; 64:150–155.
30. Gent M, Blakeley JA, Easton JD, CATS Group. The Canadian American Ticlopidine Study (CATS) in thromboembolic stroke. Lancet 1989; 1:1214–1220.

31. Hass WK, Easton JD, Adams HP, et al. A randomized trial comparing ticlopidine hydrochloride with aspirin for the prevention of stroke in high risk patients. N Engl J Med 1989; 321:501–507.
32. Murray JC, Kelly MA, Gorelick PB. Ticlopidine: a new antiplatelet agent for the secondary prevention of stroke. Clin Neuropharmacol 1994; 17:23–31.
33. McTavish D, Faulds D, Goa KL. Ticlopidine. An updated review of its pharmacology and therapeutic uses in platelet dependent disorders. Drugs 1990; 40(2): 238–259.
34. David JL, Monfort F, Sheri F, et al. Compared effects of three dose levels of ticlopidine on platelet function in normal subjects. Thromb Res 1979; 14:35–49.
35. Handin RI, Editorial. N Engl J Med 1996; 334(17): 1126–1128.
36. TIMAD Study Group. Ticlopidine treatment reduces the progression of non proliferative diabetic retinopathy. Arch Ophthalmol 1990; 108:1577–1583.
37. Coller BS. Education session. Platelets Newer Antiplatelet Agents. 1995 American Society of Hematology annual meeting. Dec 2–15. Seattle, Washington.
38. Balsano F, Rizzon P, Violi F, et al. Antiplatelet treatment with ticlopidine in unstable angina: a controlled multicenter clinical trial. Circulation 1990; 82:17–26.
39. Monca MC, Bourdonnec C, Valeix B, et al. Coronary stenting without coumadin. Phase II. Eur Heart J 1994; 15:536. Abstract 2939.
40. Schoemig A, Neumann F-J, Kastrati A, et al. A randomized comparison of antiplatelet and anticoagulant therapy after the placement of coronary artery stents. N Engl J Med 1996; 334(17):1084–1089.
41. Ellis SG, Navetta FI, Tcheng JT, et al. Safety and antiplatelet effect of murine monoclonal antibody 7E3Fab directed against platelet glycoprotein IIb/IIIa in patients undergoing coronary angioplasty: an initial experience. Coron Artery Dis 1993; 4:167–175.
42. EPIC Investigators. Use of a monoclonal antibody directed against the platelet glycoprotein IIb/IIa receptor in high risk coronary angioplasty. N Engl J Med 1994; 330(14):956–961.
43. Ellis SG, Bates ER, Schaible T, Weisman HF, Pitt B, Topo EJ. Prospects for the use of antagonists to the glycoprotein IIb/IIIa receptor to prevent post angioplasty restenosis and thrombosis. J Am Coll Cardiol 1991; 17(suppl B):89B–95B.
44. Christopoulous C, Mackie R, Lahiri A, Machin S. Flow cytometric observations on the in vivo use of Fab fragments of chimaeric monoclonal antibody to platelet glycoprotein IIb-IIIa. Blood Coagul Fibrinol 1993; 4:729.
45. Abciximab, package insert.
46. Brezina K, Murphy M, Stonner T. Care of the patient receiving RheoPro following angioplasty. J Invas Cardiol 1994; 6(suppl A):38A.
47. Hackett T, Kelton JG, Powers P. Drug induced platelet destruction. Semin Thromb Hemost 1982; 8:116.
48. Miller MM. Heparin induced thrombocytopenia. Cleve Clin J Med 1989; 56(5): 483–490.
49. Amiral J, Bridey F, Dreyfus M, et al. Platelet factor 4 complexed to heparin is the target for antibodies generated in heparin induced thrombocytopenia. Thromb Haemost 1992; 68:95–96.

50. Warkentin TE, Kelton JG. Heparin induced thrombocytopenia. Prog Hemost Thromb 1991; 10:1–34.
51. Makhoul RS, McCann RL, Austin EH, Greenberg CS, Lowe JE. Management of patients with heparin associated thrombocytopenia and thrombosis requiring cardiac surgery. Ann Thorac Surg 1987; 43:617–661.
52. Warkentin TE, Hayward CPM, Boshkov LK, et al. Sera from patients with heparin induced thrombocytopenia generate platelet derived microparticles with rocoagulant activity: an explanation for the thrombotic complications of heparin induced thrombocytopenia. Blood 1994; 84(11):3691–3699.
53. Aburahma AF, Boland JP, Witsberger T. Diagnostic and therapeutic strategies of white clot syndrome. Am J Surg 1991; 162(2):175–179.
54. Laster JL, Nichols K, Silver D. Thrombocytopenia associated with heparin coated catheters, in patients with heparin associated antiplatelet antibodies. Arch Intern Med 1989; 149:2285–2290.
55. Makhoul RG, Greenberg CS, McCann RL. Heparin associated thrombocytopenia and thrombosis: a serious clinical problem and potential solution. J Vasc Surg 1986; 4(6):521–528.
56. Boshkov LK, Warkentin TE, Hayward CPM, Andrew M, Kelton JG. Heparin induced thrombocytopenia and thrombosis: clinical and laboratory studies. Br J Hematol 1993; 84:332–338.
57. Warkentin TI. Heparin induced thrombocytopenia, Western Regional Meeting of Argantroban Investigators, Newport Beach, Calif., June 1, 1996.
58. Singer RL, Mannion JD, Bauer TL, Armenti FR, Edie RN. Complications from heparin induced thrombocytopenia in patients undergoing cardiopulmonary bypass. Chest 1992; 102(2):73S.
59. Sheridan D, Carter C, Kelton JG. A diagnostic test for heparin induced thrombocytopenia. Blood 1986; 67:27–30.
60. Amiral J, Bridey F, Wolf M, et al. Antibodies to macromolecular platelet factor 4 complexes in heparin induced thrombocytopenia. A study of 44 cases. Thromb Haemost 1995; 73:21–28.
61. Warkentin TE, Kelton JG. Heparin and platelets. Hematol Oncol Clin North Am 1990; 4(1): 243–264.
62. King DJ, Kelton JG. Heparin associated thrombocytopenia. Ann Intern Med 1984; 100:535–540.
63. Zulys V, Teasdale SJ, Michel ER, et al. Ancrod as an alternative to heparin anticoagulation for cardiopulmonary bypass. Anesthesiology 1989; 71:870–877.
64. Cong BH, Ismail F, Cade J, Gallus AS, Gordon S, Chesterman CN. Heparin induced thrombocytopenia: studies with a new low molecular weight heparinoid. Org 10172. Blood 1989; 73:1592–1596.
65. Warkentin THE, Levine MN, Hirsh J, et al. Heparin induced thrombocytopenia in patients treated with low molecular weight heparin or unfractionated heparin. N Engl J Med 1995; 332:1330–1335.
66. Leroy J, Leclerc MH, Delahousse B, et al. Treatment of heparin associated thrombocytopenia and thrombosis with low molecular weight heparin (CY 216). Semin Thromb Hemost 1985; 11:326–329.

67. Neame PB, Kelton JG, Walker IR, et al. Thrombocytopenia in sepsis. The role of disseminated intravascular coagulation. Blood 1980; 56:88.
68. Deykin D. The clinical challenge of disseminated intravascular coagulation. N Engl J Med 1970; 283(12):636–644.
69. Marder VJ, Feinstein DI, Francis CW, Colman RW. Consumptive thrombohemorrhagic disorders. In: Colman RW, Hirsh J, Marder VJ, Salzman E, eds. Hemostasis and Thrombosis. Philadelphia: Lippincott, 1982:844–856.
70. Sue C, Brandt LJ. *Escherica coli* 015:H7 infection in humans. Ann Intern Med 1995; 1233:698–714.
71. Bell W. Thrombotic thrombocytopenic purpura. JAMA 1991; 265(1):91–94.
72. Ridolfi RL, Hutchins GM, Bell WR. The heart and conduction system in thrombotic thrombocytopenic purpura. A clinicopathologic study of 17 autopsied patients. Ann Intern Med 1979; 91:357–363.
73. Schaefer AI. Hypercoagulable states: molecular genetics to clinical practice. Lancet 1994; 344:1739–1742.
74. Broze GJ. A revised coagulation cascade. American Society of Hematology Annual Meeting, St. Louis, Missouri, Dec. 1993.
75. Naito K, Fujikawa K. Activation of human blood coagulation factor XI independent of factor XII. Factor XI is activated by thrombin and factor Xia in the presence of negatively charged surfaces. J B Biol Chem 1991; 266:7353–7358.
76. Meade TW, Mellows S, Brozovic M, et al. Haemostatic function and ischemic heart disease: principal results of the Northwick Park Heart Study. Lancet 1986; 2:533.
77. Vaisanen S, Rankinen T, Penttila I, Rauramaa R. Factor VII coagulant activity in relation to serum lipoproteins and dietary fat in middle aged men. Thromb Hemost 1995; 73(3):435–438.
78. Simpson HCR, Meade TW, Stirling Y, Mann JI, Chakrabarti R, Woolf L. Hypertriglyceridemia and hypercoaguability. Lancet 1983; 1:786–789.
79. Reaven GM. Role of insulin resistance in human disease. Diabetes 188; 37:1595–1607.
80. Silveira A, Karpe F, Biobaeck, Steiner G, Walldius G, Hamsten A. Activation of coagulation factor VII during alimentary lipemia. Atheroscler Thromb 1994; 14: 60–69.
81. Raskob GE, Durica SS, Morrissey JH, Own WL, Comp PC. Effect of treatment with low dose warfarin-aspirin on activated factor VII. Blood 1995; 85(11):3034–3039.
82. Wilcox JN, Smith KM, Schwartz SM, Gordon D. Localization of tissue factor in normal vessel wall and in the arteriosclerotic plaque. Proc Natl Acad Sci USA 1989; 86:2839.
83. Barstad RM, Hamers JAG, Stephens RW, Sakariassen KS. Retinoic acid reduces induction of monocyte tissue factor and tissue factor VIIa dependent arterial thrombus formation. Blood 1995; 86(1): 212–218.
84. Brisseau GF, Dackiw APB, Cheung PYC, Christie N, Rotstein OD. Posttranscriptional regulation of macrophage tissue factor expression by antioxidant. Blood 1995; 86:1025–1035.
85. Sandset PM, Abildgaard U, Larsen ML. Heparin induces release of extrinsic pathway inhibitor (EPI). Thromb Res 1988; 50:803.

86. Mast AE, Broze GJ Jr. Physiological concentrations of tissue factor pathway inhibitor do not inhibit prothrombinase. Blood 1996; 87(5):1845–1850.
87. Aronson DL, Stevan L, Ball AP, Franza BR Jr, Finlayson JS. Generation of the combined prothrombin activation peptide ($F_{1p}l_2$) during the clotting of blood and plasma. J Clin Invest 1977; 60:1410–1418.
88. Baglin TP, Luddington R, Jennings I, Richards EM. Thrombin generation and myocardial infarction during infusion of tissue plasminogen activator. Lancet 1993; 341:504–505.
89. Bauer KA. New markers for in vivo coagulation. Curr Opin Hematol 1994; 1: 341–346.
90. Walter FJ. Regulation of activated protein C by a new protein S. J Biol Chem 1980; 255:5521.
91. Heeb MJ, Rosing J, Bakker HM, Fernandez JA, Tans G, Griffin JH. Protein S binds to and inhibits Xa. Proc Natl Acad Sci USA 1994; 91:2728.
92. Barinagarrementeria F, Cantu-Brito C, De La Pena A, Izaguirre R. Prethrombotic states in young people with idiopathic stroke. Stroke 1994; 25(2):287–290.
93. Clouse LH, Comp PC. The regulation of hemostasis. The protein C system. N Engl J Med 1986; 314(20):1298–1303.
94. Galli M, Beguin S, Lindhout T, Hemker CH. Inhibition of phospholipid and platelet dependent prothrombinase activity in the plasma of patients with lupus anticoagulants. Br J Haematol 1989; 72:549.
95. Oosting JD, Derksen RHWM, Bobbink IWG, Hackeng TM, Bouma BN, de Groot PG. Antiphospholipid antibodies directed against a combination of phospholipids with prothrombin, protein C, protein S. An explanation for their pathogenic mechanism? Blood 1993; 81:2618–2625.
96. Leung WH, Wong KL, Lau CP, Wong CK, Liu HW. Association between antiphospholipid antibodies and cardiac abnormalities in patients with systemic lupus erythematous. Am J Med 1990; 89:411–419.
97. Kattwinkel N, Villanueva AG, Labib SB, et al. Myocardial infarction caused by cardiac microvasculopathy in a patient with the primary antiphospholipid syndrome. Ann Intern Med 1992; 116:974–976.
98. O'Neill D, Magaldi J, Dobkins D, Greco T. Dissolution of intracardiac mass lesions in the primary antiphospholipid antibody syndrome. Arch Intern Med 1995; 155: 325–327.
99. Exner T. Comparison of two simple test for the lupus anticoagulant. Am J Clin Pathol 1985; 83:215.
100. Thiagarajan P, Pengo V, Shapiro S. The use of the dilute Russell viper venom time for the diagnosis of lupus anticoagulants. Blood 1986; 68(4):869–874.
101. Leung L. Education session. American Society of Hematology National Meeting. St. Louis, Missouri, Dec. 1993.
102. Ritchie H, Jamieson A, Booth N. Thrombin modulates synthesis of plasminogen activator inhibitor type 2 by human peripheral blood monocytes. Blood 1995; 86(9): 3432–3435.
103. Hogg PJ, Jackson CM. Fibrin monomer protects thrombin from inactivation by heparin-antithrombin III. Implications for heparin efficacy. Proc Natl Acad Sci USA 1989; 86:3619–3623.

104. Weitz JI, Hudoba M, Massel D, Maraganore J, Hirsh J. Clot bound thrombin is protected from inhibition by heparin-antithrombin III but is susceptible to inactivation by antithrombin III independent inhibitors. J Clin Invest 1990; 86: 385–389.
105. Weitz J. Activation of blood coagulation by plaque rupture. Mechanisms and prevention. Am J Cardiol 1995; 75:18B–32B.
106. Serruys P, Herrmann J-PR, Simon R, et al. A comparison of hirudin with heparin in the prevention of restenosis after coronary angioplasty. N Engl J Med 1995; 333(12): 757–763.
107. Eriksson BI, Ekman S, Kalebo P, Zachrisson B, Bach D, Close P. Prevention of deep vein thrombosis after total hip replacement: direct thrombin inhibition with recombinant hirudin. CGP 39393. Lancet 1996; 347:635–638.
108. DeWood MA. Prevalence of total coronary occlusion during the early hours of transmural myocardial infarction. N Engl J Med 1980; 303:897.
109. Gruppo Italiano per lo Studio Streptochinasi nell' infarto Miocardico (GISSI). Effectiveness of intravenous thrombolytic treatment ion acute myocardial infarction. Lancet 1986; 1:397–402.
110. Merlini PA, Ardissino D, Bauer KA, et al. Activation of the hemostatic mechanism during thrombolysis in patients with unstable angina pectoris. Blood 1995; 86(9): 3327–3332.
111. Lee CD, Mann KG. Activation/inactivation of human factor V by plasmin. Blood 1989; 73:185.
112. Handt S, Jerome WG, Tietze L, Hantgan RR. Plasminogen activator secretion by endothelial cells increases fibrinolytic resistance of an in vitro clot. Evidence for a key role of endothelial cells in thrombotic resistance. Blood 1996; 87:4204–4213.
113. deBono D, Simmons M, Tijssen J, et al. Early intravenous heparin improves coronary patency in thrombolysis with tissue plasminogen activator. Br Heart J 1992; 67:122–128.
114. ISIS-2 Collaborative Group. Randomized trial of intravenous streptokinase, aspirin, both or neither among 17187 cases of suspected acute myocardial infarction. Lancet 1988; ii:349–60.
115. Kannel WB, Wolf PA, Castelli WP, D'Agostino RB. Fibrinogen and risk of cardiovascular disease. JAMA 1984; 258(9):1183–1186.
116. Wilhelmsen L, Svardsdudd K, Bengsten KK, et al. Fibrinogen as a risk factor for stroke and myocardial infarction. N Engl J Med 1984; 311(8):501–505.
117. Ernst E, Reich KL. F fibrinogen as a cardiovascular risk factor: a meta analysis and revue of the literature. Ann Intern Med 1993; 118:956–963.
118. Kannel WB, D'Agostino RB, Belanger AJ. Fibrinogen cigarette smoking and risk of cardiovascular disease insights from the Framingham study. Am Heart J 1987; 113: 1006–1110.
119. Woodhouse PR, Khaw KT, Plummer M, Foley A, Meade TW. Seasonal variations of plasma fibrinogen and factor VII activity in the elderly; winter infections and death from cardiovascular disease. Lancet 1994; 343:435–439.
120. Miller GJ, Martin JC, Webster J, et al. Association between dietary fat and plasma factor VII coagulant activity. A predictor of cardiovascular mortality. Atherosclerosis 1986; 60:269–277.

121. Simpson HRC, Meade TW, Stirling Y, Mann JI, Chakrabarti R, Woolf L. Hypertriglyceridemia and hypercoaguability. Lancet 1983; 1:786–789.
122. Koenig W, Resch KL, Ernst E. Fibrinogen and cardiovascular risk. Primary Cardiol 1994; 20(4):39–44.
123. Markowe HLJ, Marmot MG, Shipley MJ, et al. Fibrinogen: a possible link between social class and coronary heart disease. Br Med J 1985; 291:1312–1314.
124. Blajchman MA, Austin RC, Fernandez-Rachubinski F, Sheffield WP. Molecular basis of inherited human antithrombin deficiency. Blood 1992; 80(9):2159–2171.
125. Hirsh J, Levine MN. Low molecular weight heparin. Blood 1992; 79(1):1–17.
126. Gurfinkel EP, Manos EJ, Mejail RI, et al. Low molecular weight heparin versus regular heparin or aspirin in the treatment of unstable angina and silent ischemia. JACC 1995; 26(2):313–318.
127. Buckley MM, Sorkin EM. Enoxaparin. A review of its pharmacology and clinical applications in the prevention of thromboembolic disorders in patients undergoing hip replacement. Drugs 1992; 44(3):465–497.
128. Triplett DA. Low molecular weight heparin. Is smaller better? Arch Intern Med 1993; 153:1525–1526.
129. Lensing AWA, Prins MH, Davidson BL, Hirsh J. Treatment of deep venous thrombosis with low molecular weight heparin. Arch Intern Med 1995; 155:601–607.
130. Levine M, Gent M, Hirsh J, et al. A comparison of low molecular weight heparin administered primarily at home with unfractionated heparin administered in the hospital for proximal deep vein thrombosis. N Engl J Med 1996; 334:677–681.
131. Schafer AI. Low molecular weight heparin, an opportunity for home treatment of venous thrombosis. N Engl J Med 1996; 334:724–725.
132. Prochownik EV. Molecular genetics of inherited antithrombin III deficiencies. Am J Med 1989; 87(suppl 3B):15S–18S.
133. Hirsh J, Piovella F, Pini M. Congenital antithrombin III deficiency. Am J Med 1989; 87(3B):34S–38S.
134. Menache D, Grossman BJ, Jackson CM. Antithrombin III: physiology, deficiency and replacement therapy. Transfusion 1991; 32(6):580–588.
135. Mitchell L, Piovella F, Ofosu F, Andrew M. Alpha 2 macroglobulin may provide protection from thromboembolic events in antithrombin III deficient children. Blood 1991; 78(9):2299–2304.
136. Stenflo J. Structure and function of protein C. Semin Thromb Hemost 1984; 10: 109–121.
137. Griffin JH, Evatt B, Widerman C, Fernandez JA. Anticoagulant protein C pathway defective in majority of thrombophilic patients. Blood 1993; 82(7):1989–993.
138. Bauer KA. Hypercoagulability–a new cofactor in the protein C anticoagulant pathway. N Engl J Med 1994; 330(8):566–577.
139. Dahlback B, Hildebrand B. Inherited resistance to activated protein C is corrected by anticoagulant cofactor activity found to be a property of factor V. Proc Natl Acad Sci USA 1994; 91:1396–1400.
140. Militech J, Sherman L, Broze G. Absence of thrombosis in subjects with heterozygotic protein C deficiency. N Engl J Med 1987; 317:991.
141. Rick M. Protein C and protein S. Vitamin K dependent inhibitors of blood coagulation. JAMA 1990; 263(5):701–703.

142. Broekmans AW, Bertina RM, Loelinger RA, Hofmann V, Klingemann HG. Protein C and the development of skin necrosis during anticoagulant therapy. Thromb Haemost 1985; 49:251.
143. Bauer KA. Pathobiology of the hypercoaguable state; clinical features, laboratory evaluation and management. In: Hoffman R, Benze EJ Jr, Shattil SJ, Furie B, Cohen HJ, eds. Hematology: Basic Principles and Clinical Practice. New York: Churchill Livingstone, 1991:1415–1430.
144. Dahlback B, Carlsson M, Svensson PJ. Familial thrombophilia due to a previously unrecognized mechanism characterized by poor anticoagulant response to activated protein C. Prediction of a cofactor to activated protein C. Proc Natl Acad Sci USA 1993; 90:1004–1008.
145. Svensson PJ, Dahlback B. Resistance to activated protein C as a basis for venous thrombosis. N Engl J Med 1994; 330(8): 517–521.
146. Dahlback B. Inherited thrombophilia: resistance to activated protein C as a pathogenic factor of venous thromboembolism. Blood 1995; 85(3):607–614.
147. Seligsohn U, Berger A, Abend A, et al. Homozygous protein C deficiency manifested by massive thrombosis in the newborn. N Engl J Med 1984; 310:559.
148. Hellgren M, Svensson PJ, Dahlback B. Resistance to activated protein C as a basis for venous thromboembolism associated with pregnancy and oral contraceptives. Am J Obstet Gynecol 1995; 173(1):210–213.
149. Ridker PM, Hennekens CH, Lindpaintner K, Stampfer MJ, Eisenberg PR, Militech JP. Mutation in the gene coding for coagulation factor V and the risk of myocardial infarction, stroke and venous thrombosis in apparently healthy men. N Engl J Med 1995; 392:912–917.
150. Holm J, Zoller B, Svensson PJ, Berntorp E, Erhardt L, Dahlback B. Myocardial infarction in two young women associated with homozygous resistance to activated protein C. Lancet 1994; 344:952.
151. Lottenberg R, Dolly FR, Kitchens CS. Recurring thromboembolic disease and pulmonary hypertension associated with severe hypoplasminogenemia. Am J Hematol 1985; 19:181–193.
152. Aoki N, Moroi M, Sakata Y, Yoshida N, Matsuda M. Abnormal plasminogen. A hereditary molecular abnormality found in a patient with recurrent thrombosis. J Clin Invest 1978; 61:1186–1195.
153. Nilsson IM, Ljungner H, Tengborn L. Two different mechanisms in patients with venous thrombosis and defective fibrinolysis: low concentrations of plasminogen activator or increased concentration of plasminogen activator inhibitor. BMJ 1985; 1453–1456.
154. Hamster A, Wiman B, deFaire U, Blomback B. Increased plasma levels of a rapid inhibitor of tissue plasminogen activator in young survivors of myocardial infarction. N Engl J Med 1985; 313:1557–1563.
155. Ridker PM, Vaughan DE, Stampfer MJ, Glynn RJ, Hennekens CH. Association of moderate alcohol consumption and plasma concentration of endogenous tissue type plasminogen activator. JAMA 1994; 272(12):929–933.

11

Gastrointestinal Hemorrhage and Mesenteric Ischemia in Cardiac Patients

ANDERSON ROWE

University of California, Los Angeles, School of Medicine, and Cedars-Sinai Medical Center, Los Angeles, California

JONATHAN D. KAUNITZ

University of California, Los Angeles, School of Medicine, Los Angeles, California

I. INTRODUCTION

Of all the problems experienced by cardiac patients, gastrointestinal complications constitute a relatively small subset. Despite their relative rarity, the syndromes of acute and chronic mesenteric ischemia, upper gastrointestinal hemorrhage in critically ill patients, and bleeding from angiodysplasia comprise well-defined syndromes that can be treated effectively if promptly diagnosed. The purpose of this chapter is to describe the most common gastrointestinal problems encountered in patients with cardiac disease in order to increase the likelihood that a prompt diagnosis can be made and that effective therapies can be instituted.

II. MESENTERIC ISCHEMIA SYNDROMES

The celiac axis, superior mesenteric artery, and inferior mesenteric artery provide almost all of the blood flow to the digestive tract. In some areas such as the duodenum and rectum, there is abundant collateral circulation, and hence ischemic injury in these areas is unusual. In other areas, such as the splenic flexure and sigmoid, fewer collaterals exist, producing watershed areas that are more susceptible to ischemic damage. Due to the presence of these extensive collaterals, the diagnosis of chronic ischemia requires angiographic documentation of narrowing of at least two of the three of the major abdominal vessels. Chronic ischemia most commonly occurs in patients with significant atherosclerotic disease. Acute ischemia can result from embolic occlusion of a major artery or branch vessel, vasculitis, mesenteric vasoconstriction, or low flow states, especially with associated thrombotic narrowing (1). Acute ischemia due to emboli, thrombosis, low flow states, and mesenteric vasoconstriction is the primary form of damage associated with cardiovascular disease. In these settings, two factors operate to produce intestinal damage: hypoxia during the ischemic period, and reperfusion injury when flow is reestablished. Thus, the injury after 3 h of ischemia and 1 h of reperfusion is more severe than after 4 h of ischemia. Nevertheless, as the ischemic period lengthens, damage due to oxygen deprivation outweighs that due to reperfusion (2). Thus, complete occlusion associated with emboli will produce transmural necrosis whereas low flow states associated with, for example, congestive heart failure (CHF), may produce only mucosal damage if cardiac function can be improved (2).

A. Chronic Ischemia

Intestinal ischemia can be classified as acute or chronic and of venous or arterial origin. In chronic forms of intestinal ischemia, viability is not compromised but blood flow is inadequate to sustain metabolic function. Atherosclerotic narrowing of at least two of the major arterial trunks and gradually evolving mesenteric venous thrombosis are the common etiologies of chronic intestinal ischemia. Narrowing of the major mesenteric vessels is almost always due to a plaque at the aortic ostium or in the 1 to 2 cm of the artery distal to the aortic takeoff. The most consistent clinical feature is abdominal discomfort or pain that most commonly occurs 10 to 30 min after eating, gradually increases in severity, reaches a plateau, then abates over 1 to 3 h. The pain is typically a periumbilical or epigastric, can be dull or cramping, and can occur in a bandlike fashion. Initially the pain only follows large meals, but it may progress to occurring after small meals. The pain of chronic mesenteric ischemia almost invariably occurs within 3 min of eating (3). The patient often eats progressively smaller meals and may avoid food completely to avoid the pain. A hallmark of this syndrome is weight loss due to fear of eating, which should be distinguished from weight loss due to other causes such as anorexia or early satiety. Diagnosis is based on a typical clinical history, angiographic demonstration of >50% narrowing of two of the three mesenteric vessels, and exclusion of other forms of disease. Although chronic mesenteric ischemia has not been considered to require urgent therapy, there is a risk of eventual complete occlusion of one or more of the mesenteric vessels, producing the syndrome of acute mesenteric ischemia. Surgical revascularization is performed on patients with typical symptoms, weight loss, and angiography. It is generally successful in reversing the ischemic signs and symptoms, and may reduce the probability of a future occurrence of acute mesenteric ischemia.

B. Acute Ischemia

Acute mesenteric ischemia is much more common than chronic ischemia and is generally associated with arterial, rather than venous, pathology. Arterial forms of acute mesenteric ischemia include mesenteric arterial embolus, nonocclusive mesenteric ischemic, mesenteric thrombosis, and focal segmental ischemia. The venous forms include acute mesenteric venous thrombosis and focal segmental ischemia caused by strangulation. Acute mesenteric ischemia is more common in patients aged 50 or older with a history of congestive heart failure, recent myocardial infarction (MI), or a severe episode of hypotension (4). The exact incidence of acute mesenteric ischemia is unknown, but is estimated at 0.1% of admissions to tertiary referral centers (5). In most series reported, embolic occlusion of the superior mesenteric artery and nonocclusive mesenteric ischemia were responsible for 70% to 80% of cases of acute ischemia. Again, these are also the most common forms of mesenteric ischemia seen in cardiac patients.

Superior mesenteric artery emboli account for 40% to 50% of cases of acute mesenteric ischemia (6). Emboli arise most commonly from the left atrium, ventricle, or aorta. Associated conditions include: atrial fibrillation; a history of a large, transmural anterior wall MI; ventricular aneurysm; and bacterial endocarditis. Angiography and percutaneous transluminal coronary angioplasty (PTCA) have been associated with dislodging aortic thrombi, producing superior mesenteric artery (SMA) emboli (7). Paradoxical emboli to the mesenteric vessels are associated with atrial and ventricular septal defects. Other rare causes include intra-aortic balloon pumps and thrombolytic therapy (8). Emboli have been associated with streptokinase and recombinant tissue plasminogen activator (9). The mechanism is thought to be degradation of the platelet fibrin thrombus covering the intimal plaque, exposing ulcerated surfaces, which allows cholesterol embolization to occur. Many patients with embolic occlusion of the SMA have had previous peripheral arterial emboli, and roughly 20% have synchronous emboli to other arteries. The emboli typically lodge at points of normal arterial narrowing usually just distal to a major branch point. Ten percent to 15% of SMA emboli lodge in distal branches.

Nonocclusive mesenteric ischemia accounts for 20% to 30% of acute mesenteric ischemia and often results from splanchnic vasoconstriction consequent to a cardiovascular event. Precipitating events include: acute MI, CHF, valvular heart lesions, cardiac arrhythmias, shock, and major cardiac surgery (10). The common thread of these conditions is a low flow state. The patients at risk for nonocclusive mesenteric ischemia include those with preexisting occlusive arterial disease, low ejection fraction, preexisting CHF, and age >70 years. Though a rare complication of each entity listed, the mortality rate remains high due to delays in diagnosis and the debilitated state of the patients. The mortality rate for all forms of acute intestinal ischemia is 70% to 80% (5).

Despite extensive evaluation, the pathophysiologic basis for nonocclusive mesenteric ischemia has not been elucidated, although several theories predominate. Mesenteric vasoconstriction remains at the forefront of current theories. In the face of cardiogenic shock, many organs become hypoxic and gangrenous due to low flow states. With hypovolemic shock, severe mesenteric vasoconstriction shunts blood into the central venous system. Data from animal models suggest that activation of adrenergic or angiotensin receptors produce this profound vasoconstriction (11). Although mesenteric ischemia occurs in the face of low cardiac output with associated mesenteric vasoconstriction, intestinal ischemia will frequently continue despite optimization of cardiac function (10). Several investigators have shown that persistent vasoconstriction occurs in the smaller branches of the SMA in experimental models of low cardiac output. The precise mechanism is unclear, but it has been shown to be reversible by intra-arterial papaverine.

The second predominant theory addressing tissue injury in nonocclusive mesenteric ischemia involves ischemia/reperfusion injury (10). The initial injury results from hypoxia (oxygen uptake $<50\%$ of normal), which is equivalent to a flow rate of 20 ml/min/100 g tissue. Intestinal oxygen uptake in the canine mesenteric circulation becomes flow-dependent at a rate of 30 ml/min/100 g tissue. Intestinal mucosal injury occurs after blood flow decreases to the point that oxygen extraction (the percent of oxygen extracted from hemoglobin) can no longer increase. Oxygen extraction then becomes flow-dependent. Hypoxic tissue initially attempts to maintain its integrity through anaerobic metabolism. As a consequence, xanthine dehydrogenase is converted to xanthine oxidase. Hypoxanthine is not metabolized to uric acid due to low intracellular pO_2. During reperfusion, with the influx of oxygenated blood, the large load of intracellular hypoxanthine is converted to uric acid by xanthine oxidase, not xanthine dehydrogenase, in a reaction that generates toxic oxygen free radicals (10). Several studies have shown that this damage can be prevented by pretreatment with free radical scavengers (12). It is theorized that nonocclusive mesenteric ischemia is initiated by mesenteric vasoconstriction associated with a low flow state. After resuscitation, reperfusion produces oxygen free radicals and further tissue damage. During total vascular occlusion, ischemic injury with transmural necrosis occurs. This injury is not reversible, is not worsened by reperfusion, and is not preventable using free-radical scavengers (10). Although there are data supporting the role of free-radical scavengers in the prevention of damage due to mesenteric ischemia, these experimental studies are not supported by clinical data.

The most common symptom in acute mesenteric ischemia is abdominal pain, which occurs in 75% to 98% of patients. The severity, location, and nature of the pain are variable. In patients with acute embolic occlusion, the pain is typically out of proportion to the physical findings early in the course. Sudden severe abdominal pain accompanied by a rapid forceful bowel movement suggests acute arterial occlusion. In contrast, up to 25% of patients with nonocclusive mesenteric ischemia will not have pain. Bloody stools are found in up to 75% of patients, especially in colonic ischemia, which usually presents with sudden crampy left lower abdominal pain, a strong urge to defecate, and passage of bright red or maroon-colored stool. With any cause of intestine ischemia, development of peritoneal signs such as guarding and rebound indicates transmural infarction.

Laboratory findings in acute mesenteric ischemia are nonspecific. Roughly 75% of patients develop leukocytosis, and about 50% have metabolic acidosis; the latter usually indicates intestinal infarction, as opposed to ischemia (13). Elevations of lactate dehydrogenase (LDH) and creatine kinase (CK-MM) have also been reported in mesenteric ischemia (14). With transmural infarction, fever, hypovolemic shock, and peritoneal signs develop. Radiographs of the abdomen are usually unhelpful. Occasionally, x-ray films will demonstrate "thumbprinting" thickening of the intestinal wall, intramural air, portal venous air, or free intraperitoneal air. Unfortunately these findings often occur late in the disease course, after the transmural infarction.

As indicated above, laboratory evaluation and abdominal x-rays do not provide specific evidence of mesenteric ischemia. Angiography is considered the "gold standard" and should generally be performed soon after the clinical presentation. Prompt resuscitation of the patient is necessary prior to the diagnostic angiography since mesenteric vasoconstriction is a normal physiologic response to hypertension or hypovolemia of any cause. If abdominal symptoms persist despite fluid resuscitation, broad-spectrum antibiotics, and nasogastric decompression, mesenteric angiography should be pursued. In nonocclusive ischemia, the classic angiographic appearance is spasm of the mesenteric arteries, accompanied by the angiographic visualization of fewer than normal distal branching vessels. Vessel arcades next to the intestinal wall are frequently not visualized (15). In patients with acute occlusion due to embolus, angiography will demonstrate a typical "cutoff" of flow at the site of occlusion (16).

Mesenteric angiography serves both a diagnostic and a therapeutic purpose. In nonocclusive mesenteric ischemia in patients without signs of peritonitis or overt intestinal infarction, intra-arterial infusion of papaverine can be instituted in an attempt to reverse vasoconstriction. In patients with acute embolization, papaverine therapy should be started immediately after documentation of the embolus. Patients with minor emboli to SMA branches or to the SMA distal to the ileocolic artery and no peritoneal signs can be managed with papaverine alone (6).

Relief of mesenteric vasoconstriction is essential in treatment of emboli, thrombosis, and low flow states. Papaverine (1 mg/ml) is infused through the angiographic catheter which is left in place after angiography, at a rate of 30 to 60 ml/h (17). Though papaverine is mostly metabolized by the first pass through the liver, blood pressure, heart rate, and rhythm must be monitored continually. Papaverine infusions have been maintained for up to 5 days without complications. Some patients with liver disease may develop hypotension while receiving standard doses, but the most common cause of hypotension during infusion is catheter displacement. Patients who develop hypotension should have the papaverine infusion replaced by saline and a plain radiograph of the abdomen performed. If catheter displacement has occurred, the catheter should be repositioned and the infusion of the papaverine restarted. Duration of the infusion should be based on clinical response. The infusion should initially be maintained for 24 h, then replaced by saline and an angiogram performed within 30 min. The papaverine is restarted and angiograms are repeated daily until there is no radiographic evidence of vasoconstriction and the patient's symptoms have resolved (17).

Patients with major emboli—i.e., emboli above the ileocolic artery—and those with peritoneal signs should undergo exploratory laparotomy. Even when the decision to operate has been made on clinical grounds, an angiogram should be performed. Infusion of papaverine through the angiographic catheter can be used to relieve vasospasm both preoperatively and postoperatively (17). Laparotomy is performed to restore arterial blood flow or to resect necrotic intestine. In cases of borderline viability, embolectomy, thrombectomy, or arterial bypass is attempted. Intestine initially appearing infarcted may show surprising recovery after restoration of blood flow. Segments of intestine are resected if they are nonviable or of questionably viability after revascularization. If extensive portions of intestine are of questionable viability, only the necrotic areas are resected, and a second-look laparotomy is performed within 12 to 24 h. In these cases, papaverine infusion should be maintained and cardiovascular function optimized. If no second-look operation is planned, papaverine infusion is continued for 12 to 24 h. Arteriography is then performed to exclude persistent vasopasm before the catheter is removed. If a second-look procedure is performed, the papaverine infusion is continued through the second operation and until no vasospasm is present on a subsequent angiogram (17). Thrombolytic agents, infused through selectively placed catheters, have been used to successfully treat SMA embolus, although this approach is still considered experimental. Moreover, thrombolytic agents may require up to 36 h to lyse a clot, during which time there can be continued ischemic damage (18).

Mortality rates of 70% to 80% for acute mesenteric ischemia were reported through the 1980s (5). Several studies over the past 10 years have suggested a lower mortality rate with an aggressive approach similar to that outlined above. Diagnosis by early angiography prior to development of an acute surgical abdomen is essential.

C. Colonic Ischemia

Colonic ischemia differs from acute mesenteric ischemia in that a precipitating factor is often not identified and abnormalities on angiography seldom correlate with clinical disease. In the resting state, colonic blood flow is lower than any other intestinal segment. Colonic blood flow decreases during digestion in contrast to the small intestine, which experiences increased blood flow during digestion. This combination of normally low blood flow with further decreases during periods of activity may predispose the colon to ischemic injury. Colonic ischemia is one of the more common disorders of the large intestine in elderly patients. Greater than 90% of cases occur in patients older than 60 years, and no sex predilection exists (19). The exact incidence of this disorder is difficult to quantitate, since many cases are undiagnosed antemortem. Most colonic ischemia is not associated with either an occlusion of a major vessel or a period of low cardiac output such as hemorrhage, shock, MI, or arrhythmia. The most commonly involved sites include the splenic flexure, descending colon, and sigmoid. Systemic low flow states commonly affect the right colon, and local nonocclusive ischemic injury typically involves the watershed areas of the splenic flexure and rectosigmoid, and occlusion of the inferior mesenteric artery affects the sigmoid colon.

If colonic ischemia is suspected and the patient has no signs of peritonitis, early colonoscopy or barium enema with flexible sigmoidoscopy should be performed. The intestine should be unprepared and the study performed within 48 h of the onset of symptoms (20). Air insufflation during the course of barium enema or colonoscopy can decrease colonic blood flow and increase the risk of perforation. If possible, CO_2 should be used for insufflation as it is more rapidly absorbed from the intestine and has vasodilatory properties (21). Angiography is rarely indicated, as it seldom reveals significant lesions in colonic ischemia.

Symptoms of colonic ischemia usually subside within 24 to 48 h, and healing is seen within 2 weeks. Two-thirds of patients with reversible disease have intramural and submucosal hemorrhage, and one-third have transient colitis (19). These findings can be visualized endoscopically and, if segmental in location, are most consistent with ischemic colitis. Irreversible damage occurs in up to 50% of patients and is characterized by segmental colitis, strictures, or gangrene. These complications can remain silent for weeks or months after the initial event and can present as protein-losing colopathy with persistent diarrhea or intestinal obstruction.

Management of colonic ischemia is dependent on the severity of the disease. In mild to moderate cases, patients are followed expectantly with intravenous fluids, nothing by mouth, and broad-spectrum antibiotics to treat infection due to fecal flora. Serial abdominal x-rays and endoscopic procedures are used to follow the patients. As noted above, the initial endoscopy should be performed within 48 h of onset of symptoms. Repeat examinations are based on the clinical status of the patient. Most patients with mild to moderate symptoms will resolve within 1 to 2 weeks without further therapy. In patients with severe disease (i.e., signs of infarction and perforation), exploratory laparotomy should be performed.

III. GASTROINTESTINAL HEMORRHAGE

A. Bleeding from the Upper GI Tract in Critically Ill Patients

1. Post-MI and Postbypass

The incidence of GI bleeding after MI has been the subject of a limited number of studies. One study retrospectively reviewed all patients admitted to a tertiary referral center for myocardial infarction over a 6-year period and found a 1.2% incidence of overt gastrointestinal bleeding and a 0.2% prevalence of occult bleeding within 3 weeks of the MI. Of the 86 patients in this study, 36 underwent endoscopy, which revealed 11 duodenal ulcers, four gastric ulcers, and four instances of hemorrhagic gastritis (22). Gastrointestinal complications of cardiopulmonary bypass procedures are rare, with a reported incidence of 0.6% to 2.6%; however, the mortality rate is reported to be as high as 50% (23). Papers from the 1980s and early 1990s report bleeding as the most common GI complication, accounting for up to 45% of gastrointestinal complications of cardiopulmonary bypass surgery (4). Several authors have suggested the use of the prophylactic use of H_2 blockers after cardiopulmonary bypass procedures, and retrospective reviews have shown a lower incidence of bleeding and a lower mortality rate.

2. Stress Ulceration

Stress ulceration with significant gastrointestinal bleeding has been classically associated with burns and central nervous system (CNS) trauma with coma. In cases of respiratory failure with prolonged mechanical ventilation, coagulopathy, shock, or prolonged hypotension from any cause, renal failure, hepatic decompensation, severe trauma, or multiorgan failure are also correlated with stress-induced bleeding. Stress ulceration develops as a function of the severity of the underlying illness. Ulceration with bleeding predicts a high mortality. Stress-related ulceration is most likely due to disruption of mucosal defense and repair mechanisms since acid secretion is usually normal, with the exception of CNS lesions, which are associated with cholinergically mediated acid hypersecretion. Compared with bleeding from non-stress-related peptic ulcer, stress ulcer bleeding is associated with a higher rebleeding rate, transfusion requirement, length of hospitalization in an ICU, and mortality. Many of these factors reflect the severity of the underlying illness in stress ulcer bleeding patients, including the presence of associated coagulopathies, but it also indicates that stress ulcers per se have more features that are associated with severe and recurrent bleeding than do normal peptic ulcers. Due to this high morbidity and mortality, much attention has been focused on prophylactic therapy of stress ulceration. A meta-analysis of 16 trials showed that the rate of overt GI bleeding in an ICU setting was reduced from 16.1% in the placebo group to 5.3% in the group treated with prophylactic H_2 receptor antagonists (24). Sucralfate and antacids have also been found to be effective in prophylaxis against stress ulceration. Sucralfate has a theoretical advantage over H_2 receptor antagonists and antacids in that it does not lead to gastric alkalization, which may increase the risk for nosocomial pneumonia, although few data have supported this contention. Prophylactic therapy is not recommended for uncomplicated MI, which is considered to be low risk for stress ulceration.

Initial management of patients with gastrointestinal bleeding should focus on stabilization and, if possible, localization of the bleeding source to the upper or lower tract. Two large-bore intravenous catheters (18 gauge or larger) should be inserted. Fluid resuscitation would begin immediately with crystalloid such as normal saline. If the patient has a history of CHF or if the ejection fraction is <40% postinfarction, a Swan-Ganz catheter should be placed. Intravenous H_2 receptor antagonists are traditionally instituted with an acute gastrointestinal hemorrhage; however, no study has documented a decrease in mortality, rebleed rate, or transfusion requirement when H_2 receptor antagonists are used in this fashion. Initial laboratory evaluation includes a complete blood count (CBC), prothrombin time (PT), partial thromboplastin time (PTT), type and cross of at least four units, and an electrolyte panel. In initial evaluation, the hemoglobin and hematocrit can be falsely elevated due to lack of vascular volume equilibration. The most important determinants of the volume of blood loss are the vital signs. A sustained tachycardia >120 beats/min denotes a 20% blood loss, orthostatic hypotension (systolic <100 mm Hg), a 30% blood loss, and shock at 50% blood loss. A large-volume bleed is also indicated if the patient is having hematemesis and hematochezia concurrently. In these situations, the patient should be transfused without waiting for the results of the CBC. For smaller-volume hemorrhage, the patient should be transfused to maintain a hematocrit >30 and hemoglobin >10. If a coagulopathy exists, it should be corrected with fresh-frozen plasma to a PT <15 sec or International Normalized Ratio (INR) of <1.4. If the patient is receiving heparin therapy, it should be discontinued immediately and reversed with protamine if possible. Thrombocytopenia should be corrected to a platelet count >50,000. Antiplatelet agents should also be discontinued. No data exist on the use of platelet transfusions to correct the effects of antiplatelet agents in acute GI bleeding; this practice is thus not recommended. After initial stabilization of the patient, a nasogastric tube should be placed and the gastric contents aspirated to aid in localizing the source and to assess whether the patient is actively bleeding. Aspiration of material resembling coffee grounds or bright red blood localized the source of the bleeding to the upper gastrointestinal tract (or in rare instances, the upper airway). When the aspirate is negative for blood but appears bilious, an upper gastrointestinal source of hemorrhage is excluded with a sensitivity of 90%. If the aspirate is negative for both blood and bile, the sensitivity falls to 60%. The aspirate is also useful in assessing whether the patient is actively bleeding. If the aspirate cannot be cleared of bright red blood with 2 L of lavage fluid, the patient is considered to be actively bleeding and should undergo endoscopy immediately after stabilization.

Few data exist on the safety and efficacy of endoscopy for GI bleeding post-MI. Previously, the safety was extrapolated from data obtained in patients who underwent surgery in the post-MI period. These studies demonstrated that surgery within 6 weeks of MI is associated with increased mortality and should be performed only when absolutely necessary (25). In 1993, two retrospective studies were published on the safety and efficacy of esophagogastroduodenoscopy (EGD) and colonoscopy post-MI. Thirty-six patients underwent EGD, nine flexible sigmoidoscopies, and nine colonoscopy. Two patients developed complications from EGD, two from flexible sigmoidoscopy, and one with colonoscopy. All complications occurred in the most unstable patients in each group. The authors concluded that significantly ill patients are at increased risk from endoscopy, and that post-MI patients are particularly susceptible to cardiopulmonary complications. In relatively stable patients with significant bleeding post-MI, however, endoscopy is not contraindicated (26,27).

B. Intestinal Angiodysplasia and Heart Disease

An association of gastrointestinal bleeding from angiodysplasia and aortic stenosis, first noted in 1958, has subsequently become known as Heyde's syndrome. Several case reports have described cessation of bleeding after aortic valve replacement with a porcine-derived aortic valve (28,29). Imperiale in 1988 called into question this association, citing flaws in methodology and statistical analysis in supporting articles (30). A possible explanation of the association was put forth by Warkentin et al. in 1992 (31). The authors noted that aortic stenosis can be complicated by acquired von Willebrand's disease type IIA, which corrects after valve replacement. Since angiodysplasia and aortic stenosis are common in elderly patients, the acquired von Willebrand's promoted bleeding in preexisting gastrointestinal angiodysplasia. Regardless of the possible association, a history of gastrointestinal bleeding necessitates use of a porcine valve in valve replacement surgery so that chronic anticoagulant therapy is obviated.

IV. SUMMARY

The three most common gastrointestinal complications encountered in cardiac patients are chronic and acute mesenteric ischemia, upper gastrointestinal bleeding due to stress ulceration, and bleeding from angiodysplasia in patients with aortic stenosis. Awareness of the existence of these syndromes and of the appropriate diagnostic and therapeutic options available will help ensure that these complications are optimally recognized and treated.

REFERENCES

1. Horton JW, White DJ. Cardiac contractile injury after intestinal ischemia-reperfusion. Am J Physiol 1991; 261:H1164–H1170.
2. Albes JM, Schistek R, Baier R, Unger F. Intestinal ischemia associated with cardiopulmonary bypass surgery: a life threatening complication. J Cardiovasc Surg 1991; 32:527–533.
3. Poole JW, Sammartano RJ, Boley SJ. Hemodynamic basis of the pain of chronic mesenteric ischemia. Am J Surg 1987; 153:171–178.
4. Christenson JT, Schmuzinger M, Maurice J, Simonet F. Gastrointestinal complications after coronary artery bypass graft. J Thorac Cardiovasc Surg 1994; 108: 899–906.
5. Guttormson NI, Brubeck MP. Mortality from ischemic colitis. Dis Col Rect 1983; 26:449–461.
6. Boley SJ, Feinstein FR, Sammartano R, Brant LJ, Sprayregen S. New concepts in the management of superior mesenteric artery emboli. Surg Genycol Obstet 1981; 153:561.
7. Oweida SW, Roubin GS, Smith RB, Salam AA. Post catheterization vascular complications associated with percutaneous transluminal coronary angioplasty. J Vasc Surg 1990; 12:310–315.
8. Belli AM, Cumberland DC, Knox AM, Procter AE, Welsh CL. The complication rate of percutaneous peripheral balloon angioplasty. Clin Radiol 1990; 41:380–383.
9. Turnbull RG, Hayashi AH, McLean DR. Multiple spontaneous intestinal perforations from atheroemboli after thrombolytic therapy: a case report. Can J Surg 1994; 37: 325–328.
10. Wilcox MG, Howard TJ, Plaskon LA, Unthank JL, Madura JA. Current theories of pathogenesis and treatment if nonocclusive mesenteric ischemia. Dig Dis Sci 1995; 40:709–716.
11. Cohn CE, Floyd CF, Dresden CF, Bornside CE. Strangulation obstruction in germ free rats. Ann Surg 1962; 156:692–701.
12. Horton JW, White DJ. Free radical scavengers prevent intestinal ischemia-reperfusion-mediated cardiac dysfunction. J Surg Res 1993; 55:282–289.
13. Kurlan B, Brant LJ, Delany HM. Diagnostic tests for intestinal angina. Surg Clin North Am 1992; 72:85–92.
14. Cavaliere F, Martinelli I, Guarneri S, Morelli M, Possati GF. Creatine kinase isoenzyme pattern in colonic infarction. J Cardiovasc Surg 1993; 34:263–265.
15. Siegelman SS, Sprayregen S, Boley SJ. Angiographic diagnosis of mesenteric arterial vasoconstriction. Radiology 1974; 122:533–542.
16. Boley SJ, Sprayregen S, Siegelman SS, Veith FJ. Initial results from aggressive roentgenological and surgical approach to acute mesenteric ischemia. Surgery 1977; 82:848–856.
17. Clark RA, Gallant TE. Acute mesenteric ischemia: angiographic spectrum. Am J Radiol 1984; 142:555–563.
18. Vujic I, Stanley J, Gobien RP. Treatment of acute embolus of the superior mesenteric artery by topical infusion of streptokinase. Cardiovasc Intervent Radiol 1984; 7:94–98.

19. Brant LJ, Boley SJ, Goldberg L, Mitsudo S, Berman A. Colitis in the elderly. Am J Gastro 1981; 76:239–249.
20. Scowcroft SW, Sanowski RA, Kozarek RA. Colonoscopy in ischemic colitis. Gastrointest Endosc 1981; 27:157–163.
21. Brant SJ, Boley SJ, Sammartano RJ. Carbon dioxide and room air insufflation of the colon. Gastrointest Endosc 1986; 32:324–329.
22. Cappell MS. A study of the syndrome of simultaneous upper gastrointestinal bleeding and myocardial infarction in 36 patients. Am J Gastroenterol 1995; 90:1444–1449.
23. Huddy SP, Joyce WP, Pepper JP. Gastrointestinal complications in 4473 patients who underwent cardiopulmonary bypass surgery. Br J Surg 1991; 78:293–296.
24. Cook DJ, Witt LG, Cook RJ, Guyatt GH. Stress ulcer prophylaxis in the critically ill: a meta-analysis. Am J Med 1991; 91:519–527.
25. Rourk RM, Caldwell HS, Barritt AS, McCallum RW. Endoscopy for gastrointestinal bleeding after myocardial infarction. Va Med Q 1994; 121:246–248.
26. Cappell MS. Safety and clinical efficacy of flexible sigmoidoscopy and colonoscopy for gastrointestinal bleeding after myocardial infarction. Dig Dis Sci 1994; 39: 473–480.
27. Cappell MS. The safety and clinical utility of esophagogastroduodenoscopy for acute gastrointestinal bleeding after myocardial infarction. Am J Gastroenterol 1993; 88: 344–350.
28. Oneglia C, Sabatini T, Rusconi C, et al. Prevalence of aortic valve stenosis in patients affected by gastrointestinal angiodysplasia. Eur J Med 1993; 2:75–78.
29. Natowitz L, Defraigne JO, Limet R. Association of aortic stenosis and gastrointestinal bleeding (Hedye's syndrome). Report of two cases. Acta Chirurg Belg 1993; 93:31–33.
30. Imperiale TF, Ransohoff DF. Aortic stenosis, idiopathic gastrointestinal bleeding, and angiodysplasia: is there an association? A methodologic critique of the literature. Gastroenterology 1988; 95:1670–1676.
31. Warkentin TE, Moore JC, Morgan DG. Aortic stenosis and bleeding gastrointestinal angiodysplasia: is acquired von Willebrand's disease the link? Lancet 1992; 340:35–37.

12

Drug Interactions in the Cardiac Intensive Care Unit

CHARLES F. LACY and SYLVIA MARTIN

Cedars-Sinai Medical Center, Los Angeles, California

I. INTRODUCTION

The number of drugs available for the treatment of critically ill patients in the cardiac intensive care unit (CCU) is growing in an exponential fashion. The desire of the pharmaceutical manufacturer and prescribing clinician is to provide the most progressive therapies which offer therapeutic benefits to patients while reducing the potential for adverse drug-induced reactions. However, the sheer number of drugs prescribed to patients in the critical care setting increases the likelihood that a toxic reaction may occur. For this reason, increasing emphasis has been placed on the clinical significance of potential interactions between concurrently administered medications. These drug-drug interactions may endanger a patient or enhance the therapeutic benefits of a drug regimen.

In the intensive care setting there are many opportunities for these interactions to occur. Some drug interactions in the CCU setting are difficult to predict and can result in serious consequences. Fortunately, such interactions are relatively rare, and many of the more serious reactions are frequently avoidable simply by changing one drug in the combination to an equally effective, noninteractive alternative. An awareness of significant drug interactions in the cardiac patient can minimize the risk and maximize the benefit of drug therapy.

II. TYPES OF INTERACTIONS

When two or more drugs are taken concurrently and an effect is observed that cannot be explained by either drug's single mechanism of action, a drug interaction is said to have occurred. The usual result of this interaction is an increase or a decrease in the effects of one of the drugs involved, which may or may not be desirable. Drugs interact with each other through a variety of mechanisms, most of which can be classified as pharmacokinetic or pharmacodynamic.

Pharmacokinetic interactions involve the absorption, distribution, metabolism, or excretion of drugs. Drug absorption may be affected by a number of factors including drug dissolution properties, rate of gastric motility and emptying, gastric pH, available surface area, and gastrointestinal blood flow. Drug distribution throughout the body is affected primarily by protein binding. Interactions may involve competition for binding sites, which may result in an increase in unbound or "active" drug. These displacement interactions are usually of little clinical importance, except when the displaced drug is normally highly protein-bound, is slowly eliminated, or has a narrow therapeutic index. Metabolism of drugs occurs primarily via the enzyme system known as the mixed-function oxidase system or cytochrome P450 system. This system may be induced or inhibited by a variety of drugs, which has significant implications in terms of interactions. As metabolism is accelerated, the therapeutic efficacy of a drug may decrease. Similarly, as metabolism is decreased, the toxic effects of a drug may be magnified. Lastly, renal elimination may be affected by concurrently administered medications, resulting in clinically relevant changes. Interactive mechanisms involve changing the glomerular filtration rate, degree of tubular secretion, or urinary acidity. Fortunately, only a handful of these interactions result in clinically relevant changes, some of which are desirable.

Pharmacodynamic interactions involve potentiation, synergy, and antagonism. Potentiation occurs when the action of a drug is increased by the concomitant administration of an additional agent. The two agents given separately do not produce the same degree of pharmacological effect. On the other hand, synergy is defined as an enhanced pharmacological effect which is greater than what would be expected from a mere additive effect. Synergistic interactions are often employed when single-drug therapies offer inadequate therapeutic results. Antagonism occurs when two drugs with opposing pharmacological effects are given together. This may be beneficial in the case of poisonings treated with antidotes, or detrimental in cases where the desired effect is antagonized.

III. DRUG CLASSES USED IN THE CCU

A. Antiarrhythmics

The potential for antiarrhythmic drugs to induce or exacerbate arrhythmias has been appreciated for many years. Most antiarrhythmic drugs produce changes in conduction and, under the right conditions, might produce arrhythmias rather than abolish them. The aggravation of arrhythmias through a proarrhythmic effect has been reported with most every antiarrhythmic agent. This situation is complicated by the possibility that drug interactions can worsen the proarrhythmic effects of these agents when the antiarrhythmic drug level rises as a result of a pharmacokinetic alteration.

1. Lidocaine

Lidocaine has a narrow antiarrhythmic spectrum. It is almost exclusively intended for the treatment of ventricular arrhythmias. Lidocaine is especially useful against arrhythmias caused by acute myocardial infarction, open heart surgery, and digoxin toxicity.

Lidocaine has few cardiovascular toxicities, although it can adversely affect hemodynamics. The hemodynamic effects of lidocaine are most commonly observed in the elderly population or in patients with congestive heart failure (CHF) and are usually manifested as depression of myocardial contractility, reduced automaticity, and depressed AV conduction.

The noncardiovascular reactions observed with lidocaine are attributable to its action on the CNS and include slurred speech, drowsiness, paresthesias, muscle twitching, convulsions, respiratory depression, and coma.

a. Lidocaine and β Blockers. The results of many controlled studies demonstrate that lidocaine clearance can be significantly reduced by the concurrent use of β blockers. The reduction of lidocaine clearance may be due to a reduction in hepatic blood flow by the β blocker, thereby producing reduced liver extraction of the active compound. This effect can also be attributed to a reduction in cardiac output and β-blocker-induced inhibition of hepatic microsomal enzymes. Whatever the primary mechanism, the result is that as lidocaine's clearance is reduced, its serum level rises and the potential for lidocaine toxicity increases. Lidocaine toxicity has been reported to occur when it is combined with propranolol therapy. In a study by Ochs, propranolol reduced the clearance of lidocaine by 40% and the mean steady-state lidocaine levels rose from 3.02 μg/ml to 3.9 μg/ml, for an average increase of 30% (1).

At least two other beta-blockers have been shown to affect lidocaine clearance. Metoprolol and nadolol have increased lidocaine levels by 20% to 30%. Concomitant lidocaine and metoprolol therapy has been shown to reduce lidocaine clearance by 31% by one pretreatment dose of metoprolol 200 mg. However, this effect was less than the 47% decrease induced by propranolol (2).

In other studies, propranolol, metoprolol, and nadolol have been reported to reduce lidocaine clearance by 15% to 45%. This difference is of clinical significance and therefore, the dose of lidocaine requires adjustment when it is coadministered with a beta-blocker. Additionally, the negative inotropic effects of the beta-blockers may be enhanced by lidocaine, possibly precipitating heart failure in the susceptible patient (3).

b. Lidocaine and H_2 Antagonists. Lidocaine clearance may be reduced by the concomitant administration of cimetidine and may be associated with symptoms of toxicity. The interaction between cimetidine and lidocaine has been demonstrated by several well-designed studies (4,5). However, the quantifiable effects cimetidine has on lidocaine clearance have varied. Cimetidine reportedly can decrease lidocaine clearance by 25% to 30%, decrease its volume of distribution, decrease its protein binding, increase its peak levels, and prolong its half-life; lidocaine levels have increased by as much as 75%. An increased incidence of drug-induced neurotoxicity has been reported as a result of these increases. Ranitidine, another H_2 antagonist, does not appear to alter lidocaine's metabolism significantly and therefore can be utilized instead of cimetidine when the need arises.

c. Other Antiarrhythmics and Lidocaine. The concomitant administration of lidocaine with other antiarrhythmics can be synergistic, additive, or antagonistic. Most often when the effects are additive, an adverse cardiac event occurs. For example, when administered concurrently with lidocaine, amiodarone can have potent suppressive effects that are additive on the sinus node. This interaction has been shown to result in bradycardia (6,7).

When disopyramide and lidocaine are used together, not only can their actions increase the possibility of a proarrhythmic effect, but they may also have additive cardiodepressant properties manifesting as an exacerbation or precipitation of heart failure (8).

In patients with liver dysfunction or reduced liver extraction abilities due to reduced hepatic blood flow, such as patients receiving cimetidine (9), propranolol (2), or halothane anesthesia (10), the elimination of lidocaine is reduced such that lidocaine toxicity is significantly more likely. This may be manifested as sinoatrial arrest, especially in the presence of quinidine therapy (11) (Table 1).

B. Procainamide

Procainamide is a class I antiarrhythmic with properties similar to quinidine. Originally approved in 1950, procainamide has become a widely used agent in the control of ventricular arrhythmias.

The cardiovascular effects of procainamide are very similar to those of the other class 1a antiarrhythmics (e.g., quinidine). While procainamide can induce a negative inotropic effect with hypotension similar to the other class 1a antiarrhythmics, the proarrhythmic risk of procainamide appears to be less than that of quinidine or disopyramide (12). These effects occur most frequently with high-dose intravenous administration; however, hypotension has been reported to occur after oral dosing as well (13).

Severe procainamide intoxication has resulted in profound hypotension, life-threatening arrhythmias, and in some cases an inability to electrically pace the

Table 1 Drug Interactions with Lidocaine

Interacting drugs	Interactive mechanism(s)	Potential consequence
Amiodarone	Additive sinus node suppression	Sinus bradycardia
β blockers	β Blockers decrease liver blood flow, decreasing lidocaine clearance	Lidocaine toxicity
Cimetidine and other H_2 antagonists	Decreased hepatic metabolism of lidocaine, which can increase lidocaine levels	Lidocaine toxicity
Disopyramide	Additive cardiodepressant effects	Arrhythmias, exacerbated heart failure in predisposed patients
Gentamicin and other aminoglycoside antibiotics	Additive neuromuscular blocking properties	Neuromuscular blockade, possible respiratory depression
Halothane	Halothane decreases liver blood flow, decreasing lidocaine clearance	Lidocaine toxicity
Phenytoin	Additive cardiac depressant effects and decreased metabolism of lidocaine	Lidocaine toxicity
Succinylcholine	Succinylcholine effects may be increased; increased neuromuscular blockade	Respiratory depression

Source: Refs. 1–11.

heart due to high pacing thresholds with failure to capture (14). When drugs known to increase the serum concentrations of procainamide are given concurrently, this risk is amplified.

A major metabolite of procainamide is N-acetylprocainamide (NAPA), which also possesses antiarrhythmic properties. However, more importantly, it is believed that many of the toxicities ascribed to procainamide are actually due to this metabolite. The NAPA metabolite is highly dependent on the kidney for its elimination, and patients with impaired renal function can therefore experience a marked increase in their serum NAPA levels. Additionally, drugs shown to interact with NAPA can also increase the drug metabolite levels and, thus, the potential for toxicity.

1. Procainamide Drug Interactions

The addition of amiodarone to procainamide therapy has resulted in as much as 57% greater serum concentrations of procainamide and its active metabolite NAPA, resulting in clinical toxicity (15). This effect is thought to occur as a result of amiodarone's ability to inhibit the hepatic metabolism and renal elimination of procainamide, thereby reducing its total clearance (16).

Concurrent administration of procainamide with other antiarrhythmic agents has also resulted in additive effects. Concomitant lidocaine and procainamide therapy has been reported to result in possible additive CNS toxicity; their pharmacologic effects on the heart may be additive as well (17–19).

Procainamide appears to potentiate or prolong the effects of both the depolarizing and the nondepolarizing neuromuscular blocking agents. Although the clinical significance of this interaction remains uncertain, patients receiving procainamide following surgery should be monitored closely for prolonged neuromuscular blockade (20).

Trimethoprim and procainamide both undergo renal tubular secretion. As a result, each drug can interfere with the renal clearance of the other. In a report by Kosoglou et al. (21), it was demonstrated that the concurrent use of procainamide and trimethoprim resulted in significant increases in the average serum concentrations for both procainamide (62%) and NAPA (52%). The renal clearance of procainamide and NAPA decreased by 47% and 13%, respectively. It appears that trimethoprim increases the concentration of procainamide and NAPA in the blood by decreasing the renal clearance (22). Although it is not necessary to avoid concomitant use of these two drugs, lower doses of procainamide may be necessary during trimethoprim administration. Procainamide and NAPA serum concentrations should be monitored closely, as the dose may require readjustment following trimethoprim discontinuation.

The histamine H_2 receptor antagonists, such as cimetidine and ranitidine, can inhibit the renal tubular secretion of procainamide (23). Concomitant cimetidine and procainamide administration has been reported to reduce procainamide elimination, possibly by reduction in renal blood flow induced by cimetidine or competition for active tubular secretion (24–26). The clearance of procainamide does not appear to be inhibited by famotidine. (Table 2).

C. Quinidine

Quinidine is a natural alkaloid prepared from the bark of the cinchona tree. It is considered by many to be the prototypical antiarrhythmic agent. Quinidine is a class 1A antiarrhythmic agent used for the management of atrial fibrillation, atrial flutter, atrial tachycardia, premature atrial contractions, paroxysmal supraventricular tachycardia, and ventricular tachycardia. Significant interactions and their mechanisms are listed in Table 3.

Table 2 Drug Interactions with Procainamide

Interacting drugs	Interactive mechanism(s)	Potential consequence
Amiodarone	Decreased clearance of procainamide and NAPA; additive electrophysiologic effects	Procainamide-associated toxicities
Captopril	Additive immune effects	Increased risk of neutropenia and possibly glomerulopathy
Cimetidine	Decreased renal clearance of procainamide and possibly NAPA	Enhanced procainamide effects and increased potential for toxicity
Quinidine	Competitive inhibition of procainamide elimination via organic base pathway	Increase procainamide levels; increased QT interval
Rantidine	Same as cimetidine only reduced potential; decreased renal clearance of procainamide and its metabolites	Enhanced procainamide effects; increased toxicity potential
Trimethoprim	Trimethoprim decreases the renal clearance of procainamide and NAPA	Increased procainamide levels; increased QT interval

Source: Refs. 12–26, 140, 141.

D. Amiodarone

Drug interactions associated with amiodarone may be pharmacodynamic or pharmacokinetic in nature. The pharmacodynamic interactions associated with amiodarone occur primarily with other antiarrhythmics and are a consequence of additive or synergistic electrophysiologic effects. Manifestations are primarily in the form of QT prolongation. Because of the long half-life of amiodarone, drug interactions may be significantly delayed. Noteworthy interactions are listed in Table 4.

E. Disopyramide

The greatest incidence of Torsades de Pointe seen with the use of disopyramide occurs when disopyramide is combined with other QT interval-prolonging drugs such as those listed in Table 5.

Table 3 Drug Interactions with Quinidine

Interacting drugs	Interactive mechanism(s)	Potential consequence
Acetazolamide and alkalinizing agents (142)	Acetazolamide, sodium bicarbonate, and other urinary alkalinizers can increase the urinary reabsorption of quinidine, increasing its levels	Increased quinidine toxicities such as hypotension, dysrhythmias, or aggravated heart failure
Amiodarone (143,144)	Amiodarone decreases the renal elimination of quinidine, increasing quinidine levels	Increased quinidine toxicities such as hypotension, dysrhythmias, or aggravated heart failure
Pentobarbital or phenobarbital (145)	Increased clearance of quinidine and decreasing its drug levels	Loss of arrhythmia control
Phenytoin (145)	Increased clearance of quinidine and decreasing its drug levels	Loss of arrhythmia control
Propranolol and other β blockers (146)	Additive cardiovascular effects; Increased β blockade; increased quinidine effects	Bradycardia; hypotension; increased QT and PR intervals
Bretylium (170)	Reduced quinidine membrane effects and bretylium antagonism	Reduced antiarrhythmic efficacy, causing breakthrough arrhythmias
Disopyramide (147)	Additive QT prolongation	Torsade de pointes
Procainamide (170)	Competitive inhibition of procainamide elimination via organic base pathway	Increase procainamide levels; increased QT interval
Propafenone (148)	Quinidine increases propafenone levels by inhibiting its hepatic metabolism	Increased propafenone levels
Verapamil and other calcium channel blockers (149,150)	Verapamil with quinidine can cause hypotension; nifedipine reduces quinidine levels	Hypotension with verapamil; loss of arrhythmia control with nifedipine
Imipramine and other tricyclic antidepressants (151)	Tricyclic antidepressants share the QT-prolonging properties of the antiarrhythmics	QT interval prolongation, possibly causing dysrhythmias
Phenothiazines (170)	Certain phenothiazine drugs share the QT, prolonging properties of the antiarrhythmics	QT interval prolongation, possibly causing dysrhythmias

Table 3 Continued

Interacting drugs	Interactive mechanism(s)	Potential consequence
Digoxin (152)	Quinidine can significantly increase the serum concentrations of digitalis glycosides	Digitalis toxicity
Cimetidine and other H_2 antagonists (153)	Cimetidine and possibly rantidine can decrease the metabolism of quinidine, increasing its levels in the blood	Increased quinidine toxicities such as hypotension, dysrhythmias, or aggravated heart failure
Ketoconazole (154)	Ketoconazole can decrease the metabolism of quinidine, increasing its levels in the blood	Increased quinidine toxicities such as hypotension, dysrhythmias, or aggravated heart failure
Warfarin (170)	Quinidine may produce additive hypoprothombinemic effects with warfarin	Increased PT and INR
Rifampin (152)	Increased clearance of quinidine, decreasing its drug levels	Loss of arrhythmia control

IV. ANGIOTENSIN-CONVERTING ENZYME INHIBITORS

The angiotensin converting enzyme (ACE) inhibitors are used widely in the treatment of hypertension and CHF, but there is little information available on the potential interactions that may occur when an ACE inhibitor is administered concurrently with other cardiovascular or noncardiovascular agents. In general, these agents have few drug interactions (27). To avoid excessive first-dose hypotension and the risk of renal impairment in patients with CHF, it is conventional to give a small test dose of the ACE inhibitor, particularly to patients already diuresed.

In patients taking thiazide diuretics (such as hydrochlorothiazide) or loop diuretics (such as furosemide), the possibility of becoming sodium-depleted or volume-depleted is real (28). When ACE inhibitors are added to a regimen containing a thiazide diuretic or a loop diuretic, an excessive drop in blood pressure with symptomatic hypotension can ensue. Patients with hyponatremia or hypovolemia may become hypotensive or may develop reversible renal insufficiency when given ACE inhibitors and diuretics concomitantly. The therapeutic

Table 4 Amiodarone Drug Interactions

Interacting drugs	Interactive mechanism(s)	Potential consequence
Calcium channel blockers (155)	Additive electrophysiological effects	Bradycardia; sinus arrest; AV block
Digoxin (156)	Decreased digoxin clearance	Increased effects and toxicity of digoxin
Disopyramide (157)	Additive QT prolongation	Torsade de pointes
Flecainide (148)	Unknown; possibly decreased metabolism or renal clearance of flecainide or changes in flecainide absorption/distribution	Increased flecainide levels and potential toxicity
Iodinated contrast media (158)	Unknown	Fatal respiratory distress syndrome
Metoprolol and other β blockers (159)	Decreased hepatic metabolism of metoprolol or a decrease in its first-pass metabolism	Increased metoprolol effects and toxic potential
Phenothiazines (160)	Additive QT prolongation	Torsade de pointes
Phenytoin (161)	Decreased metabolism of phenytoin	Phenytoin toxicity
Procainamide (162)	Unknown pharmacokinetic interactions	Increased procainamide and NAPA levels, increasing potential for toxicity
Quinidine (162)	Additive proarrhythmic effects	Potential fatal arrhythmias, including torsade de pointes, due to greatly increased quinidine serum levels
Sotalol (163)	Additive QT prolongation	Torsade de pointes
Tricyclic antidepressants (162)	Additive QT prolongation	Torsade de pointes
Warfarin (164)	Inhibition of warfarin metabolism	Hypoprothrombinemia due to increase of warfarin effects

benefits of the ACE inhibitors may also be enhanced when combined with a diuretic, but dosage must be adjusted accordingly.

The ACE inhibitors decrease aldosterone secretion and therefore can cause a small increase in serum potassium levels. When these agents are given to patients receiving drugs that may also increase serum potassium concentrations, including potassium-sparing diuretics (such as triamterene, amiloride, or spironolactone), significant hyperkalemia can occur (29). The risk of hyperkalemia is greatest in patients who are predisposed to potassium accumulation by virtue of impaired

Table 5 Disopyramide Drug Interactionse

Interacting drugs	Interactive mechanism(s)	Potential consequence
Amiodarone (165)	Additive pharmacodynamic effects by prolonging impulse conduction through the myocardium	Excessive QT prolongation; torsade de pointes
Phenobarbital (166)	The barbiturates stimulate liver enzymes which thereby increase the metabolism of disopyramide	Loss of antiarrhythmic activity
Phenytoin (167)	Increased metabolism and accumulation of metabolites	Loss of antiarrhythmic activity; increased anticholinergic effects
Propranolol and other β blockers (168)	Additive negative inotropic effects on the heart	Reduced cardiac output
Erythromycin (169)	Erythromycin inhibits disopyramide clearance, increasing disopyramide levels	Cardiac toxicities of disopyramide such as arrhythmias

renal function (30), high amounts of potassium in the diet, concurrent use of potassium supplements (31), or severe diabetes (32).

Captopril and possibly other ACE inhibitors can enhance the activity of oral antidiabetic agents. The ACE inhibitors appear to increase insulin-mediated glucose uptake in skeletal muscle. Hypoglycemia has occurred when captopril was added to either glyburide or metformin therapy (33). Therefore, caution should be observed when captopril is added to an antidiabetic regimen containing one or both of these drugs.

In patients receiving nonsteroidal antiinflammatory drugs (NSAIDs), the antihypertensive effects of the ACE inhibitor may be reduced. NSAIDs inhibit the synthesis of vasodilatory prostaglandins, which is thought to be one of the primary mechanisms for ACE inhibitor antihypertensive effects (34). Because of these opposing actions, when an NSAID such as indomethacin is coadministered with an ACE inhibitor, the blood pressure-lowering capacity of the ACE inhibitor may be attenuated (35). Additionally, the NSAIDs tend to decrease renal blood flow and, when added to a regimen containing an ACE inhibitor, can further decrease the glomerular filtration rate, thereby increasing the risk of hyperkalemia (36).

Concomitant use of ACE inhibitors and cyclosporine may decrease renal function. Two reported cases involved renal transplant patients receiving enalapril concurrently with cyclosporine and furosemide (37). Upon discontinuation of the ACE inhibitor, renal function improved. Because enalapril was associated with acute renal impairment in only two patients receiving cyclosporine, additional evidence will be needed to establish a causal relationship. Until further evidence is available, it is probably advisable to cautiously monitor patients receiving cyclosporine and ACE inhibitors concurrently.

Serum digoxin concentrations can increase by as much as 30% in patients with CHF who are receiving digoxin and captopril concurrently (38). However, enalpril has not been shown to share this effect (39). Additionally, catopril-induced hyperkalemia can offset the increased digoxin concentrations, and captopril and digoxin have been administered to patients with CHF without any apparent ill effects (40). It is unlikely that the dose of digoxin will need adjustment in most patients; however, it would seem prudent to monitor these patients for evidence of increased serum digoxin levels, especially in patients demonstrating a reduction of renal function while receiving ACE inhibitors.

Table 6 ACE Inhibitor Drug Interactions

Interacting drugs	Interactive mechanism(s)	Potential consequence
Hydrochlorothiazide	High renin levels in excessively diuresed patients	Hypotension and increased risk of renal dysfunction
Furosemide	High renin levels in excessively diuresed patients	Hypotension and increased risk of renal dysfunction
Triamterene, amiloride, or spironolactone	Additive potassium retention especially in patients with renal dysfunction or those receiving potassium supplements	Hyperkalemia
Indomethacin or other NSAIDs	Inhibition of prostaglandin synthesis	Renal impairment; Reduced antihypertensive effects
Cyclosporine	Additive reductions in glomerular filtration rates	Renal impairment
Lithium	Lithium induced sodium depletion causing increased tubular reabsorption of lithium	Lithium toxicity
Digoxin	Captopril decreases the renal clearance of digoxin	Increased digoxin levels and possibility of digoxin toxicity

Source: Refs. 27–41.

Several case reports suggest that the ACE inhibitors may increase the risk of serious lithium toxicity. Lithium and sodium ions are competitively reabsorbed in the proximal tubule of the nephron. Because ACE inhibitors cause a loss of sodium and fluid volume, less sodium is available and more lithium is retained (41) (Table 6).

V. CALCIUM CHANNEL BLOCKERS

The calcium channel blockers have gained a prominent role in the treatment of many cardiovascular disorders. This class of drugs has also been explored in the management of noncardiovascular disorders such as migraine headache, preterm labor, and gastrointestinal diseases.

The calcium channel blockers, including nifedipine, nicardipine, verapamil, and diltiazem, inhibit the influx of extracellular calcium through myocardial and vascular channels. While verapamil and diltiazem exert a balanced effect on the calcium channels in the SA node, AV node, and the vasculature, nifedipine and other dihydropyridine calcium channel blockers act predominantly on the vasculature, making these agents more potent peripheral vasodilators. The decrease in intracellular calcium inhibits the contractile processes of smooth muscle, causing dilation of the coronary and systemic arteries. This results in increased oxygen delivery to the myocardium, decreased total peripheral resistance, decreased systemic blood pressure, and decreased afterload.

Over the years, investigators have documented that several markers of metabolic clearance can be affected by the calcium channel blockers (42). Specifically, the clearance of antipyrine is reduced by 20% to 30% when given with diltiazem (43) or verapamil, but not with nifedipine (44). These data support the idea that certain calcium channel blockers have the potential to inhibit the clearance of drug metabolized by the liver, such as antipyrine.

A. Calcium Channel Blockers and Digoxin

The combined use of digoxin and verapamil has proven beneficial in controlling the ventricular rate and exercise tolerance in patients with chronic atrial flutter or atrial fibrillation (45). However, adverse reactions including fatal cardiovascular sequelae have been attributed to a verapamil-digoxin interaction (49). Initiation of verapamil therapy has caused, in the majority of cases, a >60% rise in plasma digoxin concentrations among patients previously stabilized on digoxin (46). Verapamil and digoxin interact both pharmacokinetically and pharmacodynamically. Verapamil reduces the renal and nonrenal clearance of digoxin, and both drugs slow conduction through the AV node, thereby providing the beneficial effects already stated. More recently, investigations have indicated either that verapamil has no effect on the renal clearance of digoxin or that any inhibitory effect is transient, lasting less than 6 weeks (47). However, dosages should still be adjusted according to the clinical response, since digoxin serum concentrations may not accurately reflect response in the presence of verapamil.

Digoxin levels may be increased by as much as 45% with concomitant administration of nifedipine. This is thought to occur as a result of nifedipine decreasing both the renal and nonrenal clearance of digoxin. Despite some reports showing no effects on digoxin, plasma levels of digoxin should be monitored carefully when nifedipine is administered (48).

Conflicting reports have been published regarding the potential drug interactions between digoxin and diltiazem. Some studies have found that diltiazem increases steady-state serum digoxin concentrations by nearly 60% (49). It is believed that diltiazem decreases the renal and nonrenal clearance of digoxin, causing an increase in serum digoxin levels. All patients receiving both agents should be monitored for signs of digoxin toxicity, and digoxin dosage reductions should be made if necessary.

Overall, it appears that the newer dihydropyridine calcium channel blockers are less likely to cause significant interactions with the cardiac glycosides. To date, this reaction has not been reported with nicardipine.

B. Calcium Channel Blockers and Antihypertensives

The calcium channel blockers, while being effective blood pressure-lowering agents as monotherapy, can have additive effects when combined with other antihypertensive agents. This may be desirable, but dosages should be adjusted carefully. For example, when verapamil is combined with agents like clonidine, the combination can lead to excessive bradycardia, cardiac conduction abnormalities, heart block, and CHF. However, the concomitant use of nifedipine with a β-adrenergic blocker can reduce angina and improve exercise tolerance. Generally speaking, the concomitant use of the calcium channel blocking agents and other antihypertensive agents can produce additive effects on hypotension as well as increase the possibility of orthostatic hypotension. More severe sequelae are relatively rare if the dosages of the combined agents are reduced appropriately (180).

Diltiazem has been shown to inhibit the metabolism of some β blockers to a greater degree than other calcium channel blockers, particularly the dihydropyridines. As a result, additive effects on AV conduction (bradycardia) and blood pressure (hypotension) can occur.

Although concomitant therapy with calcium channel blockers and β blockers is generally well tolerated and can even be beneficial by inhibiting calcium channel blocker-induced reflex tachycardia, the combined use of β blockers can induce excessive bradycardia and hypotension. This combination can cause additive negative inotropic effects; angina has been reportedly worsened when β blocking agents are withdrawn abruptly and calcium channel blocker therapy is initiated

(50). Therefore, it is recommended that a gradual downward titration of the β-blocking agent dose be instituted during the initiation of calcium channel blocker therapy to minimize or eliminate this interaction.

It is important to note that calcium channel blocking agents and β blockers are frequently used together without adverse reactions. However, patients should be monitored carefully for excessive bradycardia, cardiac conduction abnormalities, or hypotension when these drugs are given concomitantly. In general, these reactions are more likely to occur with verapamil or diltiazem than with nifedipine or nicardipine.

C. H_2 Antagonists and Calcium Channel Blockers

Cimetidine and, to a lesser degree, ranitidine have been shown to decrease the clearance and increase the oral bioavailability of most of the calcium channel blockers. However, clinically significant changes in hemodynamic response are most apparent only with nifedipine or diltiazem (153).

These drugs can affect the disposition of the calcium channel blocking drugs due to their inhibitory effects on liver cytochrome P450 and thereby increase the calcium channel blocker's serum concentrations. Therefore, lower doses of the calcium channel blocker may be required during concomitant therapy with H_2 antagonists.

The interaction between H_2 antagonists and verapamil is more controversial, with some reports indicating enhanced oral bioavailability (171) and increased elimination half-life of verapamil (172), while others indicate no kinetic interactions at all (173). Nonetheless, it would still be prudent to monitor those patients receiving this combination for the toxic effects of verapamil, especially early in therapy or after any dosage changes.

D. Calcium Channel Blockers and Cyclosporine

Concurrent administration of diltiazem, verapamil, and nicardipine has been reported to significantly increase the blood concentrations of cyclosporine, probably as a result of inhibition of cyclosporine metabolism by the calcium channel blocker (128).

Cyclosporine levels were raised by 17% to 400% as early as 3 days after diltiazem therapy with a daily dose of 90 to 720 mg (175). A 33% to 50% dose reduction of cyclosporine may be necessary in diltiazem-treated patients to maintain proper cyclosporine blood levels. Increases in cyclosporine blood levels in both cardiac patients and renal transplant patients have been observed after the addition of verapamil for the treatment of hypertension or an arrhythmia. In one report, increases in cyclosporine levels did not occur until the dosage of verapamil was increased from 240 mg/day to 360 mg/day, suggesting that this interaction may possibly be dose-dependent (176). A rise in cyclosporine levels can be seen within 1 week of beginning verapamil therapy, and levels usually return to their pretreatment values 1 week after discontinuation of verapamil.

Introduction of nicardipine into cyclosporine therapy has increased the cyclosporin levels by 350% within 30 days of staring the calcium channel blocker. The cyclosporine levels usually returned to prenicardipine values within 1 to 7 days following discontinuation (122).

The clinical significance of these interactions is not yet fully understood. Renal toxicities, as a result of pharmacokinetic interactions with cyclosporine and diltiazem, nicardipine, or verapamil, have been reported. However, the administration of diltiazem or verapamil concurrently with cyclosporine has been shown to have a protective effect against cyclosporine-induced nephrotoxicity, has improved early graft function, and has reduced early rejection episodes in renal transplant recipients (174).

As a result, cyclosporine levels and indicators of renal function should be closely monitored with the introduction of a calcium channel blocker to cyclosporine therapy to ensure optimal therapeutic outcomes. Upon cessation of any of the calcium channel blockers, the dose of cyclosporine may require upward titration if the levels fall below the desired therapeutic range.

E. Rifamycins and Calcium Channel Blockers

Rifampin and rifabutin are the only rifamycin antimicrobials available in the United States. Although the grand majority of case reports of drug interactions between a rifamycin and the calcium channel blockers have been with rifampin, rifabutin has been shown to be a potent inducer of liver enzymes like rifampin, and therefore has the potential to alter the activity of susceptible drugs when administered concurrently.

Rifampin significantly reduces the oral bioavailability of verapamil and certain other calcium channel blockers, presumably by increasing the first-pass metabolism of these agents. Rifampin also enhances the hepatic metabolism of these agents by stimulating the cytochrome 450 enzyme system. The concomitant use of rifampin and certain calcium channel blockers has resulted in a lowering of the serum drug concentrations of the calcium antagonist and attenuation of the patient's cardiovascular stability, including worsening hypertension and angina and loss of expected electrocardiographic findings (51).

The mean plasma drug concentrations, maximum drug concentrations, and bioavailability of orally administered verapamil, but not intravenous verapamil, were lowered by more than 90% in subjects who had been receiving rifampin as part of a treatment regimen for tuberculosis (52). Discontinuation of the rifampin resulted in about a fourfold increase in the serum verapamil levels. Additionally, failure of verapamil 480 mg given every 6 h to control paroxysmal supraventricular tachycardia in a patient receiving rifampin therapy for pulmonary tuberculosis further justifies the concern over prescribing this combination of agents in patients without very closely monitoring the patient's clinical response and drug levels, where available (53).

Exacerbation of variant angina in a patient has also been reported during concurrent administration of nifedipine and rifampin (54). The drug levels of nifedipine were decreased by an average of 50% in the presence of rifampin therapy. In a report by Tada et al., a 75-year-old hypertensive woman whose hypertension had been well controlled with nifedipine was started on rifampin therapy after developing tuberculosis (55). After initiation of the rifampin therapy, the patient's nifedipine peak plasma concentrations and average drug concentrations decreased to about 40% of their previous levels. The control of her hypertension was significantly affected, and although the patient was switched to another calcium channel blocker, nicardipine, her blood pressure remained elevated.

When rifampin is initiated for patients receiving calcium channel blockers, clinicians should be aware that the patient's therapeutic response may be markedly compromised and that dosage increases of the calcium channel blocker or replacement of rifampin may be necessary to achieve the desired therapeutic outcome.

Other enzyme inducers, such as phenytoin and phenobarbital, also have this effect on verapamil serum concentrations, and similar effects have been observed when rifampin, phenobarbital, or phenytoin was added to diltiazem therapy (56).

F. Neuromuscular Blocking Agents and Calcium Channel Blockers

Prolonged neuromuscular blockade has been observed when the nondepolarizing neuromuscular blocking agents vecuronium, pancuronium, or tubocurarine were administered to patients who had been maintained on verapamil therapy. Reversal of the blockade was promptly achieved only by edrophonium but not with neostigmine. A negative inotropic effect of nifedipine has also been reported in patients treated with pancuronium and fentanyl.

G. Miscellaneous Drug Metabolism and Calcium Channel Blockers

Verapamil can inhibit the hepatic metabolism of carbamazepine, midazolam, doxorubicin, valproic acid, and theophylline (178). The interaction between verapamil and midazolam has only been reported with the oral formulation of midazolam. If administered to patients receiving carbamazepine, verapamil can cause carbamazepine toxicity within 36 to 96 h in some patients (177). Verapamil appears to decrease the clearance of carbamazepine, and carbamazepine doses should therefore be reduced if verapamil is added. The moderate alterations in theophylline metabolism by verapamil do not cause a clinically significant consequence.

The addition of diltiazem to a patient stabilized on lithium therapy will increase

Table 7 Calcium Channel Blocker Drug Interactions

Interacting drugs	Interactive mechanism(s)	Potential consequence
Carbamazepine	Decrease in carbamazepine clearance	Neurotoxicity
Phenytoin	Increased serum phenytoin levels	Neurotoxicity
Lithium		Lithium toxicity
Midazolam	Decreased clearance of midazolam	Significantly prolonged excessive sedation
Metoprolol	Decreased clearance of metoprolol	Enhanced efficacy; possible decreased heart rate
Propranolol	Decreaased clearance of both drugs	Bradycardia, heart block, and worsening CHF
Digoxin	Decreased clearance of digoxin	Increased digoxin levels; bradycardia; syncope; possible increase in PR interval

Source: Refs. 42–56.

the potential for lithium-induced neurotoxicity or psychosis (178). However, the interaction between verapamil and lithium is less predictable. Verapamil administration has been associated with both decreased lithium concentrations and lithium toxicity (179). Verapamil may substantially lower serum lithium concentrations when administered to patients stabilized on lithium therapy. This effect may be offset somewhat by the fact that calcium channel blocking agents share some neuropharmacological actions with lithium. Some preliminary data suggest that verapamil is effective in controlling an acute manic episode either as monotherapy or in combination with lithium. Concurrent therapy, however, may lead to neurotoxicity, even without a measurable increase in lithium serum concentrations (179). Because verapamil has been associated with both decreased lithium concentrations and with lithium toxicity, verapamil should be avoided in patients receiving lithium until further data are available (Table 7).

VI. β BLOCKERS

Propranolol is the prototype of the β-adrenergic receptor antagonists. Like other β blockers, propranolol competes with adrenergic neurotransmitters for binding at sympathetic receptor sites in the heart, lungs, vasculature, and many other tissue sites. The pharmacodynamic consequences of β blockade include a decrease in both resting and exercise heart rate and cardiac output, and a decrease in both systolic and diastolic blood pressure. The fall in cardiac output induced by beta blockade is often countered by a moderate reflex increase in the peripheral vascular resistance.

A. β Blockers and Other Antihypertensive Agents

As described in our discussion regarding calcium channel blocker interactions, orthostatic hypotension may be more likely if β blockers are coadministered with a dihydropyridine calcium channel blocker such as nifedipine (50).

In general, β blockers can be administered safely with most antihypertensives although it may be wise to avoid their use with agents that cause catecholamine depletion such as guanethidine, reserpine, or other rauwolfia alkaloids. β Blockade can interfere with reflex tachycardia and can worsen orthostatic hypotension (181).

If a β blocker is to be substituted for clonidine in an antihypertensive regimen, clonidine should be gradually tapered and the β blocker gradually increased over several days to avoid the possibility of rebound hypertension. The administration of β blockers during the withdrawal of clonidine can precipitate severe increases in blood pressure as a result of unopposed α stimulation. It is possible to administer clonidine and β blockers concurrently without sequelae, although the hypotensive effects can be additive (181).

B. β Blockers and Antiarrhythmics

While additive effects are possible if a β blocker is administered with any other antiarrhythmic agent, particular attention should be given to using β blockers in combination with the cardiac glycosides (see the following section on the cardiac glycosides). Additionally, the use of β blockers with the other antiarrhythmics may significantly suppress AV nodal conduction and can lead to AV block.

Amiodarone appears to significantly decrease the clearance of those β blockers significantly eliminated by hepatic clearance (e.g., metoprolol, propranolol) and severe cardiovascular reactions have been reported when propranolol was administered to patients receiving amiodarone. Propafenone has been shown to increase the plasma concentrations and prolong the elimination half-life of propranolol (182).

Additive negative inotropic effects are possible if β blockers are used with disopyramide, quinidine, verapamil, or diltiazem. Quinidine may also inhibit the clearance of propranolol (183).

Propranolol and flecainide each appear to inhibit the clearance of each other, and both drugs possess negative inotropic effects (57). Therefore, when propranolol and flecainide are used in combination, patients should be monitored for increased effects of both drugs and negative inotropic effects on the heart.

C. β Blockers and Adrenergic Agonists

The concurrent use of β-blocking agents with adrenergic agonists or sympathomimetics can result in antagonism of the desired therapeutic effect of either agent or may lead to excessive α-adrenergic pharmacodynamic effects. The concomitant use of epinephrine and β blockers can lead to excessive α tone, which may cause a hypertensive response. Epinephrine stimulates both α and β receptors; however, the overall hemodynamic effects mainly reflect its β activity. Patients on propranolol may exhibit marked hypertension followed by bradycardia when epinephrine is administered. It is thought that the severity of the response is due to β-2 receptor blockade, which accompanies nonselective β blocker use (e.g., propranolol). Trials comparing the effects of epinephrine on metoprolol (a selective β blocker) versus propranolol have substantiated this mechanism (58).

VII. NITRATES

The nitrate drugs have been used to relieve anginal pain for over 100 years. The first organic nitrate, nitroglycerin, was synthesized in 1846, and its use was clearly established shortly thereafter. However, the duration of action of nitroglycerin is short and is best suited for the acute relief of anginal attacks when administered sublingually. Its short duration of action gave way to the development of longer-acting preparations such as the isosorbide salts.

The nitrates relax vascular smooth muscle, producing vasodilation in peripheral veins, peripheral arteries, and the coronary arteries. The venodilation decreases blood return to the heart, which reduces ventricular filling pressures. Myocardial work and oxygen demand are decreased, relieving anginal pain. Patients with severe congestive heart failure particularly benefit from intravenously administered nitroglycerin.

The hypotension induced by the nitrates may be additive with other agents that can cause hypotension such as other vasodilators including diuretics, certain antidepressants, phenothiazine neuroleptics, some opiate analgesics, the benzodiazepine hypnotics, and some antiarrhythmics such as quinidine or procainamide. Patients should be monitored more closely for hypotension if nitroglycerin is used concurrently with any of these drugs.

The ergot alkaloids, such as ergotamine or dihydroergotamine, can precipitate angina and thus oppose the vasodilatory actions of nitroglycerin. Additionally, nitroglycerin can increase the bioavailability of dihydroergotamine by decreasing its first-pass hepatic metabolism (184). This drug combination should be avoided whenever possible, but, if it is absolutely necessary, patients requiring the combination should be closely monitored for increased ergot alkaloid effects and ergotism, and dosages should be adjusted accordingly.

Some reports suggest that intravenous nitroglycerin can decrease the anticoagulant effects of heparin; however, other reports have not been able to document any interaction. Until the potential for this interaction is evaluated fully, clinicians should be alert to the possible reduction in heparin's effectiveness when intravenous nitroglycerin is coadministered (185).

Administration of epinephrine, phenylephrine, or other sympathomimetics can result in antagonism of the antianginal effects of nitroglycerin. In addition, nitroglycerin may block the adrenergic effects of epinephrine, possibly precipitating tachycardia and severe hypotension.

Limited data suggest that patients receiving aspirin in high doses can exhibit an exaggerated response to sublingual nitroglycerin. Although hypotension and tachycardia were more significant during concomitant therapy, no special precautions appear necessary.

VIII. NITROPRUSSIDE

Nitroprusside is an intravenous hypotensive agent effective in the acute management of hypertensive crisis and in the management of congestive heart failure. It is an extremely potent vasodilator with a rapid onset and a short titratable duration of action.

Nitroprusside is metabolized to cyanide and thiocyanate, which, although they do not contribute to the drug's antihypertensive action, have the potential to cause severe toxic reactions (186). In addition to the toxic potential of its metabolites, nitroprusside's primary mode of action can result in severe hypotension, especially when not monitored closely or when given to patients who are receiving potentially interactive drugs (187). Additive hypotensive effects may occur when nitroprusside is used concomitantly with other antihypertensive agents, negative inotropic agents, general anesthetics, or ganglionic blocking agents (186).

Pressor agents that may directly stimulate myocardial tissue, such as epinephrine, may cause an increase in blood pressure during nitroprusside infusions. Sympathomimetics such as dopamine, dobutamine, norepinephrine, epinephrine, metaraminol, phenylephrine, phenylpropanolamine, or cocaine may antagonize the hypotensive effects of nitroprusside when administered concomitantly. Therefore, patients should be monitored closely to confirm that the desired antihypertensive effect is achieved. Conversely, the concomitant use of certain pressors (e.g., dobutamine) with nitroprusside can have therapeutically beneficial effects. This combination has been shown to result in a reduced pulmonary wedge pressure and an enhanced cardiac output (188). Additionally, the combined use of dobutamine with nitroprusside has been shown to be significantly more effective at increasing the cardiac index and stroke volume index and decreasing the systemic vascular resistance than when either drug is used alone (188).

IX. DIURETICS

The diuretics can be divided into thiazide diuretics like hydrochlorothiazide; the loop or high-ceiling diuretics like ethacrynic acid, furosemide, bumetanide, and torsemide; the potassium-sparing diuretics like amiloride, spironolactone, and triamterene; and the carbonic anhydrase inhibitors like acetazolamide.

All diuretics affect electrolyte transport at the nephron epithelium. The thiazides inhibit sodium reabsorption at the distal loop of Henle, metolazone acts in the proximal tubule in addition to the distal tubule, the loop diuretics operate in the ascending loop of Henle, and the carbonic anhydrase inhibitors work as their name suggests, by interfering with the actions of the carbonic anhydrase enzyme in the renal cortex to enhance the clearance of sodium and bicarbonate (121).

In patients receiving concurrent digoxin and diuretics, diuretic-induced electrolyte disturbances such as hypokalemia and/or hypomagnesemia can predispose the patient to digitalis toxicity, possibly resulting in fatal arrhythmias. Therefore, electrolyte imbalances should be corrected prior to initiating with a cardiac glycoside. In the absence of any electrolyte imbalances, diuretics and digoxin can be used together safely (111).

The concomitant use of metolazone and a loop diuretic can cause severe electrolyte loss. Metolazone, a long-acting thiazide diuretic, should be used only in combination with a loop diuretic in patients who are refractory to the loop diuretic alone (189). Close monitoring of serum electrolytes and cardiac function is highly advisable in these patients. In patients with reduced glomerular filtration (creatine clearances <30 mL/min), the combination of a loop diuretic with a thiazide diuretic has a greater potential to result in profound fluid and electrolyte loss. Loop diuretics should therefore be used with much caution in combination with a thiazide diuretic, especially in the presence of renal impairment (189). Conversely, the potassium-sparing diuretics such as triamterene, amiloride, or spironolactone can counteract the hypokalemia induced by a loop diuretic. These agents have been effectively used in place of potassium supplements in patients receiving loop diuretics. Furthermore, the potassium-sparing diuretics may also counteract the magnesium wasting that occurs as a result of loop diuretic therapy (189).

Additive hypotension is possible if a loop diuretic is used in combination with any other antihypertensive agent including calcium channel blockers, β blockers, nitrates, and direct-acting vasodilators. Hyponatremia or hypovolemia predisposes patients to acute hypotensive episodes following initiation of an ACE inhibitor like captopril (31). While the ACE inhibitors and diuretics are routinely administered together, especially for the treatment of heart failure, doses should be conservative when first initiated to avoid this possible interaction.

Lithium clearance may be decreased in patients receiving diuretics; however, clinical data supporting this possibility are scarce. Nonetheless, careful monitoring of lithium serum drug levels is recommended when these drugs are used concurrently (191).

The NSAIDs, as exemplified by indomethacin, have been shown to reduce the diuretic and antihypertensive effects of diuretics. The NSAIDs inhibit prostaglandin synthesis, which can lead to fluid retention and an increased peripheral vascular resistance. The risk of renal failure can be increased in patients receiving an NSAID and a diuretic concurrently. This interaction appears to occur as a result of a decrease in renal blood flow caused by inhibition of renal prostaglandin synthesis (190).

Despite the widespread belief that furosemide enhances the ototoxic effects of the aminoglycoside antibiotics (e.g., gentamicin), there is little evidence to support this. The risk of ototoxicity during combined therapy with an aminoglycoside and a loop diuretic is most likely to occur with ethacrynic acid. Furosemide alone, however, can be ototoxic, particularly when given in high doses over too short of an administration period. Since ototoxicity is very difficult to assess, when it does happen, it is probably best to reduce its potential by avoiding high-risk combinations when possible.

Concomitant administration of furosemide to patients receiving neuromuscular blocking agents has been reported to cause prolonged neuromuscular blockade. However, the data are conflicting. Low doses of furosemide have been reported to enhance the neuromuscular blockade of tubocurarine and succinylcholine, while high doses (1 to 4 mg/kg) of furosemide have been reported to antagonize neuromuscular blockade (59).

The use of other nephrotoxic agents with loop diuretics should be avoided or minimized since there is the possibility of additive nephrotoxicity, especially in the presence of preexisting renal impairment. Agents to avoid administering with a loop diuretic include amphotericin B, cyclosporine, the aminoglycoside antibiotics, acyclovir, and cisplatin (Table 8).

X. NEUROMUSCULAR BLOCKING AGENTS

Once confined to the operating room, neuromuscular blockers have become ever present as adjunctive therapy in the intensive care setting to facilitate endotracheal intubation and to optimize mechanical ventilation. There are two subgroups of neuromuscular blockers: the depolarizing and the nondepolarizing agents. Succinylcholine is the only depolarizing agent currently marketed and because of its extremely rapid onset and short duration of action (1 min and 8 min, respectively), it is used primarily in rapid endotracheal intubation. Long-term paralysis is maintained with nondepolarizing agents such as pancuronium, vecuronium, atracurium, and rocuronium, which exhibit a slower onset and longer duration of action than succinlycholine.

Delayed recovery from paralysis, a well-recognized adverse effect of neuro-

Table 8 Diuretic Drug Interactions

Interacting drugs	Interactive mechanism(s)	Potential consequence
Acyclovir	Additive nephrotoxicity	Renal dysfunction
Aminoglycoside antibiotics	Additive nephrotoxicity and ototoxicity	Renal dysfunction; hearing loss
Amphotericin B	Additive nephrotoxicity	Renal dysfunction
Calcium channel blockers	Additive hypotensive effects; hyponatremia; hypovolemia	Hypotension
Cisplatin	Additive nephrotoxicity	Renal dysfunction
Cyclosporine	Additive nephrotoxicity	Renal dysfunction
Digoxin	Diuretic-induced electrolyte disturbance	Digitalis toxicity
Indomethacin and other NSAIDs	Prostaglandin inhibition reduces renal blood flow	Reduced antihypertensive effects
Lithium	Competitive inhibition of lithium clearance	Lithium toxicity
Neuromuscular blockers	Unknown	Prolonged neuromuscular blockade

muscular blockade, can be exacerbated by the coadministration of a number of agents with a neuromuscular blocker. Conversely, some agents may make patients more resistant to neuromuscular blockade. Because of the prevalence of non-depolarizing agents in therapeutic paralysis, the interactions covered here will emphasize the agents most commonly seen in the intensive care unit—namely, atracurium, cisatracurium, doxacurium, vecuronium, pancuronium, and rocuronium.

A. Neuromuscular Blocking Agents and Antibiotics

High-dose antibiotic therapy has been associated with prolonged neuromuscular blockade (60). In combination with neuromuscular blocking agents, lower doses of antibiotics can precipitate a similar prolonged paralysis (61). Certain antibiotics can potentiate the effects of neuromuscular blockers by inhibiting presynaptic acetycholine release and by stabilizing the postjunctional membrane (62). The classes of agents most frequently associated with this interaction are the aminoglycosides (gentamicin, tobramycin), the polymyxins, vancomycin, and the lincosamides (clindamycin) (63–65). The penicillins and cephalosporins have not been shown to affect the neuromuscular junction. When antibiotic-associated neuromuscular blockade occurs, calcium is intermittently successful in reversing the paralysis, but its use is not recommended because of its unpredictable and unsustained effects (66).

B. Neuromuscular Blocking Agents and Electrolytes/Acid/Base

It is important to remember that serum concentrations of electrolytes often do not reflect the intracellular concentrations of the electrolytes and that multiple electrolyte disturbances can coexist. This makes the prediction of neuromuscular blocking effects in the presence of altered electrolytes or acid/base status a definite challenge.

Sodium and potassium are the primary electrolytes involved in depolarization and repolarization of ion channels, and their concentrations thus have the greatest potential to affect the degree of neuromuscular blockade produced. Hyponatremia and hypokalemia impose a similar effect on nondepolarizing blocking agents by hyperpolarizing cell membranes and thereby increasing their sensitivity to pharmacological blockade. Conversely, the lowered resting membrane potential found in the setting of hyperkalemia causes the reverse effect and may require that higher doses of a blocking agent be administered. It is important to recognize that drugs affecting electrolyte balance (e.g., furosemide) may indirectly interact as well.

The efficacy of neuromuscular blocking agents can be decreased by the administration of calcium, which enhances release of acetylcholine (ACh) from the nerve ending. Similarly, blockade of calcium channels may potentiate the effects of pharmacological paralysis by antagonizing the release of acetylcholine (67).

Magnesium potentiates the effects of neuromuscular blocking agents by inhibiting presynaptic ACh release and stabilizing the postjunctional membrane. To minimize this effect, it is recommended that infusions of magnesium sulfate be discontinued 30 min before the administration of paralytic agents.

Acid/base dysregulation may also have profound effects on neuromuscular blockade. Because of the association between acid/base balance and intracellular electrolyte concentrations, it is sometimes difficult to predict the clinical effect of alkalosis or acidosis. As the hydrogen ion concentration decreases extracellularly and the serum becomes alkalotic, protein binding of neuromuscular blocking agents is maximized, making them less available for activity at the neuromuscular junction. Therefore, in cases of alkalosis, higher doses of neuromuscular blocking agents may be required. Conversely, in acidosis the activity of the agent is potentiated as the degree of protein binding decreases. It is critical to acknowledge the concurrent electrolyte disturbances that may have opposing effects. For example, alkalosis is often associated with hypokalemia; these two states have opposite effects on the efficacy of the neuromuscular blocking agents. It is therefore important to accurately monitor the degree of paralysis with a peripheral nerve stimulator in individual patients (Table 9).

Table 9 Agents That Antagonize Neuromuscular Blocking Agents (NMBA)

Agent	Mechanism
Alkalosis	Increased protein binding of NMBA, therefore decreasing concentration of "active" agent.
β Blockers	Unclear; may also potentiate effects of NMBA's.
Carbamazepine	Unclear; possible altered metabolism of NMBA's.
Corticosteroids	Unclear mechanism.
Hypercalcemia	Increased release of acetylcholine from nerve ending.
Hyperkalemia	Decreased resting membrane potential and subsequent decreased sensitivity to pharmacological blockade.
Loop diuretics	Unclear; possibly enzyme inhibition.
Phenytoin	Unclear; perhaps altered metabolism.
Theophylline	Accumulation of cAMP potentiating the release of certain neurotransmitters.

Source: Refs. 60–68.

C. Neuromuscular Blocking Agents and Anticonvulsants

Because of the multiple effects of phenytoin, including postjunctional and prejunctional blocking, decreased synthesis of acetylcholine, and stabilization of the neuronal membrane, an additive effect may be seen when phenytoin is coadministered with nondepolarizing agents. Although this reaction is not likely to be clinically significant when phenytoin is used appropriately, it may be of greater importance in cases of phenytoin toxicity (68). Other reports have demonstrated an antagonism of the effects of neuromuscular blockade in the presence of anticonvulsants such as carbamazepine and phenytoin.

D. Neuromuscular Blocking Agents and Antiarrhythmics

Procainamide, quinidine, and propranolol have demonstrated an increased neuromuscular blocking effect when administered with nondepolarizing agents. Although not necessarily related to serum drug levels of these agents, a greater than therapeutic level may augment this interaction.

E. Neuromuscular Blocking Agents and Theophylline

Theophylline, a potent agent used for the treatment of hyperreactive airway disorders, such as asthma, and bronchorestrictive disorders, such as chronic bronchitis, has been shown to exert its clinical effects by mediating the actions of a circulating enzyme called cyclic AMP (cAMP). cAMP has been shown to potenti-

Table 10 Agents That Potentiate NMBAs

Agent	Mechanism
Acidosis	Decreased protein binding of NMBA, leading to increased "active" drug concentrations
Antibiotics	Inhibition of presynaptic acetylcholine release and membrane stabilization
β blockers	Unclear; may antagonize NMBAs
Calcium blockers	Decrease acetylcholine release due to blockade of calcium channel
Hypocalcemia	Hyperpolarize cell membranes, increasing sensitivity to pharmacological blockade
Hypokalemia	Hyperpolarize cell membranes, increasing sensitivity to pharmacological blockade
Lithium	Unclear mechanism
Magnesium	Inhibition of presynaptic acetylcholine release and stabilization of postjunctional membrane
Loop diuretics	Unclear; possibly hypokalemia
Nitroglycerine	Unclear mechanism
Phenytoin	Decreased ACh synthesis; stabilization of membrane; post-prejunctional effects
Procainamide	Possibly altered metabolism
Quinidine/quinine	Possible synergistic effects

Source: Refs. 60–68.

ate the release of certain neurotransmitters. Consequently, due to the accumulation of intracellular cAMP during theophylline therapy, pharmacological paralysis may be more difficult to induce in asthmatic patients receiving theophylline therapy.

These interactions can be applied to all nondepolarizing neuromuscular blocking agents, as no one particular agent appears to interact more or less than any other. Proper monitoring of the patient's paralytic state is essential to minimize these interactions (Table 10).

XI. CARDIAC GLYCOSIDES

Awareness of significant drug interactions is critical in cases where a narrow therapeutic window exists and calls for careful monitoring and clinical evaluation. Cardiac glycoside toxicity or underdigitalization is commonly a consequence of any one of a number of drug interactions identified to date. Inadequate digitalization in cases of heart failure or arrhythmia is as worrisome as toxicity, making an understanding of relevant interactions a priority.

A. Digitalis Pharmacokinetics

The oral absorption of digoxin is most complete with the elixir or encapsulated gel formulation. Digoxin tablets are approximately 70% absorbed (69). Digoxin is roughly 25% protein-bound and undergoes extensive distribution in body tissues. In patients with normal renal function, the half-life approaches 1.5 days, resulting in a period of 4 to 7 days to reach steady serum concentrations. Renal filtration and secretion are the primary means of elimination while extensive metabolism to inactive metabolites occurs in only 10% to 15% of patients. This metabolism is the result of bacterial activity in the colon by *Eubacterium lentum*.

The cardiac glycoside digitoxin is more completely absorbed and has greater lipophilicity. It differs from digoxin in that it is highly albumin-bound and demonstrates a much longer half-life—7 days. Additionally, hepatic metabolism plays a greater role in its elimination.

These properties are essential components of the therapeutic efficacy of the cardiac glycosides and are susceptible to alteration due to drug interactions. The reactions most relevant to those seen in the cardiac intensive care unit include interactions with antiarrhythmics, antihypertensive agents, antibiotics, and a number of drugs used for symptom control.

B. Digoxin and Amiodarone

A proactive 50% reduction in the dose of digoxin is recommended in patients initiating amiodarone therapy to avoid toxicity. Increases in serum digoxin levels during amiodarone loading may result in gastrointestinal (e.g., vomiting), central nervous system (e.g., visual disturbances), and cardiac (e.g., sinus bradycardia/arrest) effects. Hypokalemia due to concurrent diuretic use in cardiac patients may exacerbate the digoxin toxicity precipitated by the addition of amiodarone. With a half-life of 20 to 60 days, amiodarone may interact with digoxin for a significant period of time following discontinuation. The mechanism of the interaction involves a reduction in both renal and nonrenal clearance of digoxin and a displacement from tissue-binding sites by amiodarone (70).

C. Digoxin and Quinidine

As in the case of amiodarone, a 50% reduction in digoxin dose is recommended at the initiation of concurrent digoxin/quinidine therapy. Serum digoxin concentrations begin to increase during the first 24 h of therapy. Multiple mechanisms contribute to this increase: decreased volume of distribution, decreased renal and nonrenal clearance, and increased bioavailability. The clinical manifestation of this interaction includes symptoms of digoxin toxicity and a reduced beneficial effect on sinus rhythm (71).

D. Digoxin and Antacids

Orally administered digoxin is susceptible to interaction with antacids (e.g., aluminum and magnesium hydroxide, and magnesium trisilicate), kaolin-pectin, and sucralfate. Kaolin-pectin and sucralfate have known adsorptive properties. Altered absorption via an unclear mechanism, separate from binding or altered gut transit time, is the primary mechanism for the interaction with antacids. This interaction can be minimized by the use of antacid tablets rather than liquid or the use of digoxin capsules. In the absence of these options, separation of administration times of the antacid or adsorptive agent and digoxin by 2 h or more is recommended (72). Additionally, serum digoxin levels should be evaluated periodically.

E. Digoxin and Antibiotics

Concurrent treatment with amphotericin B and digoxin may lead to digoxin toxicity in the presence of therapeutic serum levels. Manifested as arrhythmias, this interaction is due to the hypokalemia often associated with amphotericin B rather than a direct effect on digoxin levels.

Treatment with erythromycin or tetracycline may result in a significant increase in serum digoxin concentrations in a small subpopulation of patients. These patients, termed "nonexcretors," are colonized with *Eubacterium lentum*, which is responsible for extensive metabolism of digoxin. These patients often require higher maintenance doses of digoxin (73). As the colonic flora is altered by antibiotic therapy, namely, erythromycin and tetracycline, the serum digoxin concentrations rise, often necessitating a dose reduction. It is not known whether other antibiotics cause a similar interaction (74).

Neomycin and rifampin both reduce serum digoxin concentrations, albeit via differing mechanisms. The mechanism of the neomycin interaction is unclear, but is not eliminated by temporally spacing the medications (75). Rifampin, a known hepatic enzyme inducer, enhances the hepatic metabolism of digoxin and digitoxin, resulting in lower, perhaps subtherapeutic serum drug concentrations (76).

F. Digoxin and Calcium Channel Blockers

The interaction between digoxin and verapamil is well established. Due to a reduction in renal and nonrenal clearance by verapamil, serum digoxin concentrations gradually increase and may result in toxicity-related conduction disturbances. The principal route of nonrenal elimination is biliary clearance, which is inhibited by verapamil. Thus, in patients with hepatic dysfunction, the verapamil/digoxin interaction is magnified (77). Serum digoxin concentrations should be frequently monitored in patients on combination therapy.

Although some studies suggest a slight increase in serum digoxin levels in healthy subjects taking nifedipine and digoxin concurrently, the interaction appears to be clinically insignificant. Nifedipine does not appear to interact significantly with digoxin in cardiac patients (78).

Diltiazem does not appear to cause a clinically significant increase in serum digoxin concentrations. However, patients with renal or hepatic insufficiency, who are more prone to toxic digoxin levels, should be monitored closely.

G. Digoxin and Diuretics

Spironolactone, a potassium sparing diuretic, interacts with the radioimmunoassay procedure used to quantify serum digoxin concentrations, causing spuriously elevated serum levels (79). An inconsistent interference, more commonly seen in patients with hepatic dysfunction, has been demonstrated in vivo and in vitro and appears to be related to spironolactone itself as well as its metabolites (80). Serum digoxin concentrations require careful evaluation in these patients. Amiloride and triamterene do not significantly impact serum digoxin concentrations.

Diuretics such as furosemide and hydrochlorothiazide cause potassium and magnesium wasting. These electrolyte imbalances predispose cardiac patients to arrhythmias in the setting of normal digoxin levels. Potassium and magnesium supplementation and sodium restriction are recommended to minimize the risk of digoxin toxicity (81).

H. Digoxin and CNS Agents

The benzodiazepines appear to alter digoxin elimination. Both alprazolam and diazepam, given concurrently with digoxin, have demonstrated an increase in serum digoxin concentrations (82). Although the mechanism is unclear, elderly patients appear more susceptible to toxicity.

Due to hepatic enzyme induction, phenytoin and phenobarbital significantly increase the metabolism of digoxin. An increase in dose and careful monitoring of serum concentrations to avoid underdigitalization is recommended.

I. Digoxin and Propafenone

A 25% reduction in digoxin dose is recommended in patients receiving concurrent propafenone. A decrease in volume of distribution together with a decrease in nonrenal clearance contributes to the increase in serum digoxin concentrations. Clinical signs of toxicity such as prolonged QRS intervals were demonstrated (83).

J. Digoxin and Cyclosporine

Cyclosporine has been shown to increase serum digoxin concentrations in cardiac transplant patients. Plasma clearance and volume of distribution were decreased, resulting in symptoms of digoxin toxicity such as vomiting and arrhythmias. Digoxin levels should be closely monitored following transplantation, and doses should be decreased upon initiation of cyclosporine (83,84).

K. Digoxin and Metoclopramide

Metoclopramide, a gastric motility agent, may cause a decrease in serum digoxin concentrations. The bioavailability of digoxin tablets is dependent on disintegration and dissolution of the tablet as well as the absorption in the upper gastrointestinal tract. With decreased intestinal transit time, inadequate absorption occurs, leading to subtherapeutic serum levels. This interaction can be avoided by administering digoxin in capsule form (85).

L. Digoxin and NSAIDs

Indomethacin has demonstrated a significant effect on serum digoxin levels, which have been shown to increase up to 40% during concomitant therapy. Decreased renal function secondary to indomethacin is not a likely explanation, as studies show a constant serum creatinine during therapy (86). Although the mechanism of the interaction is unclear, reduction in digoxin dose would be prudent.

Conflicting results make establishing a true interaction with ibuprofen difficult. It is possible that digoxin levels may increase as a result of renal dysfunction secondary to NSAID therapy. Additionally, heart failure patients are more susceptible to decreased glomerular filtration rates, which may be exacerbated by NSAID therapy. Nevertheless, careful monitoring of clinical status and serum levels is recommended.

Although first-line therapy for a number of disease states, cardiac glycosides possess a very narrow therapeutic window. Interactions are well established and warrant diligent monitoring of clinical status and serum levels (Tables 11, 12).

XII. THROMBOLYTIC AGENTS

The dissolution of thrombi and emboli is the primary goal of thrombolytic therapy. The fibrin clots are dissolved via the action of plasmin, generated from the precursor, plasminogen. Together with aspirin, thrombolytic therapy has played an integral part in improving morbidity and mortality following acute myocardial infarction (87). Both the beneficial and adverse effects of thrombolytic therapy can be altered by interactions with other medications. The consequences of this range from inadequate thrombolysis to excessive bleeding.

There are four thrombolytics commercially available: alteplase, streptokinase, anistreplase, and urokinase. Because of the dependence of alteplase on hepatic blood flow (HBF) for clearance, it is most susceptible to interaction with agents

Table 11 Interactions Leading to Digoxin Toxicity

Drug	Mechanism
Amiodarone	Decreased renal and nonrenal clearance; displacement of digoxin from tissues
Quinidine	Decreased renal and nonrenal clearance; increased bioavailability; decreased volume of distribution
Antacids (magnesium and aluminum hydroxide) kaolin-pectin, sucralfate	Altered absorption; adsorption
Amphotericin B	Hypokalemia
Erythromycin/tetracycline	Altered colonic flora and bacterial metabolism
Verapamil	Decreased renal and non-renal clearance
Diuretics (furosemide/ hydrochlorothiazide)	Hypokalemia and hypomagnesemia
Benzodiazepines	Unclear
Propafenone	Decreased volume of distribution and nonrenal clearance
Cyclosporine	Decreaased clearance and volume of distribution
Indomethacin	Unclear

Source: Refs. 69–86.

altering HBF. The clearance of the remaining thrombolytics is not closely related to HBF. Anticoagulants, platelet inhibitors, and other agents often used concurrently with thrombolytics have been shown to have a potentiating yet beneficial effect on outcome, and will therefore not be discussed as interactions.

A. Alteplase and Hepatic Blood Flow

It has been demonstrated that the clearance of recombinant tissue-type plasminogen activator (tPA) is highly dependent on HBF. Therefore, any concurrent medication that alters HBF will alter the effects of tPA (88). As clearance of tPA decreases, plasma concentrations increase, and vice versa. Drug interactions with

Table 12 Interaction Leading to Underdigitalization

Drug	Mechanism
Phenytoin	Hepatic enzyme induction
Phenobarbital	Hepatic enzyme induction
Metoclopramide	Increased gastric motility

Source: Ref. 75.

tPA are more common during the short-term administration and tend to diminish with long-term treatment (89). It is also important to assess the effect of the disease state on HBF; in cases of forward heart failure due to ischemia, HBF may be significantly decreased and the properties of alteplase altered.

B. Alteplase and Nitroglycerin

An unclear interaction has been shown between alteplase and nitroglycerin. Nitroglycerin, a common component of the treatment of myocardial ischemia, is a potent vasodilator. Presumably, this effect increases HBF and increases the rate of degradation of tPA. Consequently, a reduction in reperfusion rate and increase in reocclusion rate have been demonstrated in patients receiving combination therapy (90). Conversely, it has been demonstrated that nitroglycerin causes only a transient increase in HBF followed by a more sustained decrease (91). The effect of nitroglycerin on the efficacy of tPA remains unclear.

C. Alteplase and Calcium Channel Blockers/β Blockers

Calcium channel blockers have been shown to increase HBF (92). Acute administration is associated with a more pronounced effect than chronic administration, as in the long-term treatment of angina or hypertension. Acutely administered β blockers cause a decrease in HBF (93). An increase in plasma concentrations of alteplase would be expected. Definitive clinical outcomes have not been demonstrated.

XIII. ANTIBIOTICS

The predominant infectious processes found in the critical care setting include pneumonia, urinary tract infections, catheter sepsis, and wound infections. Less common infections involve the abdomen, sinuses, and meninges (94). Successful treatment is contingent upon appropriate empiric therapy and, when diagnostic tests permit, subsequent tailoring of the regimen to the most effective antibiotics. Multiple interactions, ranging from decreased antibiotic efficacy to toxic serum concentrations of an object drug, are possible when antibiotics are a component of the therapeutic regimen. Awareness of potential interactions and careful monitoring of potentially toxic combinations is critical in maximizing the benefits of antibiotic therapy. Several classes and their interactions with other medications commonly seen in the CCU will be discussed in this section.

A. Quinolone Antibiotics

Ciprofloxacin, ofloxacin, enoxacin, norfloxacin, and lomefloxacin are members of the quinolone family. Because of the ideal pharmacological properties of the quinolones, including bactericidal action, broad spectrum, and optimal kinetics, they are a common choice in the treatment of infection in the hospitalized patient. The interactions covered in this section will apply to all quinolones unless stated otherwise.

1. Quinolones and Antacids/Sucralfate

Although all quinolones interact with antacids to some degree, the strongest interaction occurs with norfloxacin followed by ciprofloxacin and enoxacin (95). The cations present in antacids, namely calcium, magnesium, and aluminum, form a complex with the quinolones, which significantly decreases the oral bioavailability. This results in suboptimal serum and urinary concentrations (96). Because the interaction is precipitated by the formation of complexes rather than an increase in pH, ranitidine and other H_2 antagonists do not affect quinolone absorption. Aluminum and magnesium products appear to have the greatest binding potential and therefore affect absorption the most. To maximize quinolone absorption in the presence of antacids, it is recommended that the quinolone be given at least 2 h before or 6 h after the antacid. If possible, concomitant administration of these products should be avoided.

It is also important to remember that certain medication may be formulated with a "built-in" buffer which may interact. Didanosine tablets contain magnesium-aluminum hydroxide and have been shown to decrease ciprofloxacin absorption (97). Dietary sources of cations, such as milk and yogurt, should also be considered as concurrent ingestion has been shown to reduce absorption of ciprofloxacin (98).

Sucralfate contains a significant amount of aluminum which, upon dissolution, complexes with the quinolone. Ciprofloxacin serum concentrations have been shown to drop dramatically in the presence of sucralfate (99). If concurrent administration is unavoidable, the quinolone should be given several hours prior to the sucralfate.

2. Quinolones and Theophylline

Quinolones are potent inhibitors of the cytochrome P450 enzyme system and are therefore capable of causing serious toxicity when given concurrently with agents metabolized predominantly via this pathway. Theophylline toxicity, manifesting as seizures, has been reported in patients receiving ciprofloxacin or norfloxacin and theophylline (100). Enoxacin and ciprofloxacin have the greatest effect on theophylline clearance, although norfloxacin is also capable of precipitating toxicity in sensitive patients (101,102). Because of the negligible effect of ofloxacin and lomefloxacin on theophylline clearance, these agents can be used if quinolones must be given. Regardless of the quinolone chosen, careful monitoring of theophylline levels and clinical signs of toxicity is prudent.

3. *Quinolones and Warfarin*

Conflicting reports exist with respect to this interaction. Some studies indicate an unpredictable and questionably significant interaction between quinolones and warfarin. Other case reports describe significant bleeding events from concurrent administration (103). The complications appeared more common in elderly patients and were seen anytime between 2 and 16 days after initiation of quinolone therapy. A proposed mechanism involves inhibited metabolism of the less active R-stereoisomer of warfarin, an effect also seen with cimetidine, a well-recognized interaction (104). Although this study was restricted to healthy patients and did not demonstrate an increased risk of bleeding, caution must be exercised when applying these results to the elderly or any patient with organ dysfunction. Further studies are required to fully elucidate the interaction between the quinolones and warfarin and to identify patients at risk for bleeding complications. Until then, monitoring of prothrombin time and the INR is recommended (Tables 13, 14).

B. Macrolide Antibiotics

The macrolide antibiotics include erythromycin, troleandomycin, azithromycin, and clarithromycin. The majority of interactions involve the inhibition of hepatic enzymes required to metabolize the object drug. This results in a variety of clinical consequences ranging from insignificant to toxic. The mechanism of hepatic enzyme inhibition is complex, such that interactions are sometimes not seen for several days following the addition of the interacting drug (105).

Some variation among the degree of enzyme inhibition exists among the different macrolides. Azithromycin appears to have the least, if any, effect

Table 13 Interactions Decreasing Efficacy of Quinolones

Interacting drug	Mechanism
Antacids (calcium, magnesium, and aluminum containing)	Reduced absorption due to complexation with cations
Didanosine	Buffers in tablet formulation bind quinolones
Iron	Similar to antacid interaction; reduced absorption due to complexation
Sucralfate	Reduced absorption due to complexation with aluminum

Source: Ref. 95.

Table 14 Quinolone Interactions Leading to Toxicity of Object Drug

Object drug	Mechanism	Consequence
Cyclosporine	Unclear association	May increase cyclosporine levels and increase risk of nephrotoxicity; conflicting data
Theophylline	Inhibition of cytochrome P450; enoxacin > ciprofloxacin > norfloxacin > lomefloxacin	Increased theophylline levels, leading to seizures
Warfarin	Inhibition of metabolism of R-isomer of warfarin	Hypoprothrombinemic response; more studies needed

Source: Ref. 95

on hepatic drug metabolism. It does not appear to interact with any of the other agents known to interact with clarithromycin and erythromycin, such as theophylline, terfenadine, and carbamazepine. Clarithromycin, erythromycin, and troleandomycin are known to affect the metabolism of many of the same drugs and are therefore viewed as equipotent enzyme inhibitors with respect to drug interactions.

1. Macrolides and Antihistamines

A well-documented and life-threatening interaction exists between erythromycin and the nonsedating antihistamines, terfenadine and astemizole. Because of the extensive first-pass metabolism of both terfenadine and astemizole, they are particularly sensitive to any inhibition of hepatic enzymes. Erythromycin- and clarithromycin-induced enzyme inhibition results in increased serum concentrations of astemizole and terfenadine. This has been associated with the development of torsade de pointe (106). Although loratadine is similarly affected by erythromycin, it is not cardiotoxic at higher serum concentrations.

2. Macrolides and Theophylline

The macrolides have a significant impact on the metabolism of theophylline, which can quickly lead to toxic plasma levels. Erythromycin reduces the clearance of theophylline by 20% to 40% (107). A similar reduction in clearance has been identified with clarithromycin (108). It is important to remember that due to the complexity of the inhibition mechanism, it may take 5 to 7 days for the effect on serum theophylline concentrations to be realized (109).

3. Macrolides and Carbamazepine

Macrolide administration is known to inhibit the metabolism of carbamazepine, leading to increased serum concentrations and potential toxicity. In cases where a macrolide is indicated in a patient stabilized on carbamazepine, the recommended agent is azithromycin, as it does not appear to interfere with hepatic drug metabolism.

4. *Macrolides and Digoxin*

A small (10%) subsection of patients experience a unique interaction when erythromycin is administered with digoxin, which can lead to toxic serum levels of digoxin (110). *Eubacterium lentum* is an organism present in the colon of these patients which extensively metabolizes digoxin. It is believed that antibiotic therapy may alter the colonic flora such that bacterial metabolism of digoxin is decreased and serum levels rise. It is unknown whether other antibiotics cause a similar reaction.

5. *Macrolides and Warfarin*

Warfarin is extensively metabolized by the hepatic enzyme system, which predisposes it to interactions with any agent that affects this system. Since macrolides inhibit these enzymes, a hypoprothrombinemic effect can be precipitated with concomitant therapy. The interaction appears to be more commonly seen in the elderly and in patients with predisposing factors such as liver disease or enhanced bleeding tendency. Careful monitoring of signs of bleeding, prothrombin time, and INR is recommended (Table 15).

Table 15 Significant Interactions with Macrolide Antibiotics

Interacting drug	Mechanism	Effect
Astemizole/terfenadine	Decreased first-pass metabolism; increased serum levels of astemizole/terfenadine	Cardiac arrhythmias (i.e., torsade de pointe)
Carbamazepine	Inhibition of hepatic metabolism	Potential carbamazepine toxicity
Digoxin	Altered colonic flora, leading to decreased metabolism of digoxin	Potential digoxin toxicity in small subpopulation of patients
Theophylline	Inhibition of theophylline metabolism	Potential theophylline toxicity
Warfarin	Inhibition of warfarin metabolism	Enhanced hypoprothrombinemic response; potential bleeding complications

Source: Refs. 108,109.

C. The Penicillins

Penicillin and its derivatives are involved in very few interactions (106). Those that are significant usually involve an effect of the renal tubular secretion of the penicillins. For example, concomitant administration of probenicid and penicillin results in decreased elimination of penicillin. This interaction is often used to prolong the effect of penicillin in the treatment of sexually transmitted diseases such as gonorrhea. Conversely, this interaction may lead to toxicity if large doses of penicillins are administered. Competition for renal tubular secretion occurs in instances where methotrexate, even in small doses, is given with penicillin. A reduction in methotrexate is recommended as toxicity has been reported (112).

Nafcillin and dicloxacillin have been reported to decrease the anticoagulant effect of warfarin. Whether this interaction is seen with other penicillin derivatives is unknown. It is recommended that patients be monitored for decreased hypoprothrombinemic response during antibiotic therapy. If an increase in warfarin is required, doses should be reduced upon completion of antibiotic therapy to avoid excessive anticoagulation (113).

D. The Tetracyclines

Tetracyclines are sensitive to chelation by divalent and trivalent cations in the gastrointestinal tract. Antacids, as well as sucralfate, can significantly decrease the efficacy of tetracycline therapy due to decreased absorption (114). To maximize tetracycline therapy, antacids or any other cation-containing agent (e.g., milk, yogurt) should be given at least 2 h after the tetracycline.

Hepatic enzyme inducers and inhibitors have little effect on tetracycline therapy. However, doxycycline, a tetracycline derivative, is sensitive to enzyme inducers such as carbamazepine, phenobarbital, phenytoin, and rifampin. Concurrent administration has been shown to decrease plasma concentrations significantly (115–117). Clinical sequelae as a consequence of lower serum levels are unclear; however, it is recommended that another antibacterial agent be used if possible.

E. The Cephalosporins

The four generations of cephalosporins are a mainstay of therapy in the intensive care setting. Like the penicillins, they are involved in few significant interactions. The absorption of the orally administered cephalosporins is sensitive to the effects of antacids and H_2 receptor antagonists. The oral cephalosporins cefpodoxime and cefuroxime have demonstrated a pH-dependent absorption and should not be administered with antacids or H_2 blockers (118–120).

A potential interaction exists between anticoagulants and the N-methylthiotetrazole (NMTT) side-chain-containing cephalosporins. Cefamandole, cefoperazone, cefotetan, cefmetazole, and moxalactam contain this side chain and have been associated with hypoprothrombinemia and bleeding. This may be exacerbated in the presence of anticoagulants. These NMTT side-chain-containing agents also produce a disulfiram reaction (i.e., flushing, tachycardia, nausea) in the presence of alcohol. This should be monitored in patients receiving drugs diluted in an alcohol base (e.g., nitroglycerin IV) (121).

F. Trimethoprim/Sulfamethoxazole (TMP/SMX)

Both components of this combination product are responsible for interacting with other medications. Interactions with TMP/SMX are a result of both renal and hepatic mechanisms (122).

Renally, TMP/SMX interacts with procainamide and methotrexate. Concentrations of procainamide and its metabolite NAPA increase significantly due to competition with trimethoprim for tubular secretion. This interaction is significant enough to cause procainamide toxicity, and it is recommended that levels and clinical parameters be monitored in patients treated with TMP/SMX. As always, a reevaluation of procinamide dosage should be carried out following completion of antibiotic therapy (123).

Methotrexate appears to compete with TMP/SMX for renal tubular secretion, which has resulted in toxicity in some patients (124). It is unclear which component of TMP/SMX is responsible for the interaction, and it is recommended that concurrent therapy be avoided. In cases where concurrent therapy is the only option, careful attention should be given to signs of methotrexate toxicity.

Due to inhibition of hepatic metabolism by TMP/SMX, phenytoin toxicity and excessive anticoagulation are potential consequences of concomitant therapy. Phenytoin serum levels and signs of toxicity should be monitored and doses should be adjusted to compensate for the increase in plasma levels when TMP/SMX is added (125). The combination of warfarin and TMP/SMX should be avoided because of the well-documented risk of hypoprothrombinemia and bleeding (126) (Table 16).

G. Metronidazole

Metronidazole is an inhibitor of hepatic drug metabolism due to the imidazole ring found in its structure. The most significant interaction with metronidazole involves warfarin, the result of which is a significantly hypoprothrombinemic state (127). Patients stabilized on warfarin, in whom metronidazole therapy is initiated, should be carefully monitored with respect to prothrombin time, INR, and signs of bleeding for a period of up to 2 weeks. Changes in anticoagulation may occur between 3 and 14 days of adding metronidazole. Single-dose metronidazole is less likely to result in significant changes in bleeding tendencies (128).

Table 16 Interactions with Trimethoprim/Sulfamethoxazole

Interacting drug	Mechanism	Consequence
Phenytoin	Inhibition of phenytoin metabolism	Potential phenytoin toxicity; incidence not established
Procainamide	Decreased clearance of procainamide and NAPA	Potential procainamide toxicity; incidence not established
Sulfonylurea hypoglycemics	Inhibition of metabolism	Hypoglycemia
Warfarin	Inhibition of warfarin metabolism	Bleeding complications

Source: Ref. 111.

XIV. ANTICOAGULATION

Anticoagulants have revolutionized the medical management of deep vein thrombosis, pulmonary embolism, atrial fibrillation, and prosthetic heart valves, but therapy is often long-term if not lifelong, and this predisposes a patient to many potential drug interactions. Heparin, aspirin, and warfarin exert their therapeutic benefits by interfering with different steps of the clotting cascade. Each agent, with its unique mechanism, has the potential to interact with a variety of drugs.

The most significant interactions in patients requiring anticoagulant therapy occur in those prescribed oral anticoagulants. Warfarin exerts its pharmacological activity by interfering with the vitamin K-dependent coagulation factors (factors II, VII, IX, X). Agents affecting metabolism or binding of warfarin as well as those affecting vitamin K synthesis contribute to interactions. Warfarin therapy must be tightly controlled to minimize the potential of hemorrhage or inadequate anticoagulation. In all cases, clinical parameters as well as laboratory parameters (PT, INR, hematocrit) should be closely monitored.

Significant interactions involving heparin and aspirin are limited to potentiated anticoagulant effects when given in combination with oral anticoagulants or thrombolytics. Often this interaction is beneficial in optimizing the anticoagulant and thrombolytic effects of these agents. However, in all cases, careful monitoring is critical to minimize the potential for hemorrhage.

A. Warfarin and Amiodarone

Amiodarone, an antiarrythmic agent indicated for treatment of recurrent ventricular fibrillation or tachycardia, causes a significant interaction with warfarin. Because warfarin is hepatically metabolized, it is sensitive to any agent that inhibits this metabolism. Amiodarone decreases the metabolism of warfarin, causing a hypoprothrombinemic effect which may lead to a significant risk of bleeding. It is recommended either that the two agents not be coadministered or that the dose of warfarin be decreased by one-half (129). Monitoring for prolonged PT and elevated INR should continue for a period of weeks following discontinuation of amiodarone due to the prolonged effects on the metabolism of warfarin (130).

B. Warfarin and Antibiotics

Several antibiotics cause significant interactions with warfarin. Some cephalosporins, the quinolones, erythromycin, metronidazole, antifungals, and TMP/SMZ can lead to clinically significant bleeding events if given concurrently with warfarin.

The cephalosporins having the NMTT side chain have the potential to increase bleeding, especially in the presence of anticoagulants. Cefamandole, cefoperazone, cefotetan, cefmetazole, and moxalactam have been associated with hypoprothrombinemia and bleeding. In addition, the second- and third-generation cephalosporins interfere with the hepatic interconversion of vitamin K (131). A reduction in warfarin dose or a change in antibiotic choice may be warranted in patients being considered for concomitant therapy.

Conflicting reports exist concerning the significance of the interaction between warfarin and the quinolones. Bleeding complications have been reported primarily in the elderly. The mechanism involves the inhibition of metabolism of the R-stereoisomer of warfarin (104). Until more definitive studies concerning the interaction and its clinical consequences are available, elderly patients and those with organ dysfunction should be closely monitored.

The macrolide antibiotics, specifically erythromycin and clarithromycin, as well as metronidazole and the azole antifungal agents inhibit the hepatic P450 enzyme system. Consequently, warfarin metabolism is decreased, leading to a hypoprothrombinemic effect. Careful monitoring and dose reduction, when appropriate, are recommended in cases where patients are initiating or terminating concurrent therapy with these agents.

Cotrimoxazole (TMP/SMZ) appears to affect warfarin through inhibition of hepatic metabolism and altered protein binding. Several cases of hypoprothrombinemia have been reported. For this reason, concurrent therapy is not recommended. If no alternative antibiotic therapy is available, clinical and laboratory parameters should be carefully monitored (132).

C. Warfarin and Cimetidine or Omeprazole

Cimetidine causes varying degrees of hypoprothrombinemia in anticoagulated patients. Upon addition of cimetidine, the prothrombin time increases gradually over a period of 1 to 2 weeks; baseline prothrombin times return within approximately 1 week following discontinuation of cimetidine (133). The primary mechanism, as with most agents interacting with warfarin, is inhibition of hepatic metabolism. The metabolism of the less active R-isomer of warfarin is preferentially inhibited. It is suggested that patients requiring H_2 receptor antagonist therapy be treated with ranitidine or similar agent, rather than cimetidine (134).

Omeprazole appears to have some inhibitory effect on the metabolism of warfarin in vitro (135). A slight hypoprothrombinemic effect was seen in healthy subjects treated with 20 mg omeprazole daily (136). It is unclear how significant the interaction is in the clinical setting or in patients with comorbid disease states. Until the interaction has been fully elucidated, patients on concurrent therapy should be closely monitored.

D. Warfarin and Enzyme Inducers

Drugs that enhance the activity of the hepatic enzyme system will consequently produce a decrease in the therapeutic hypoprothrombinemia caused by warfarin. Well-known enzyme inducers include carbamazepine, phenobarbital, and rifampin. Concurrent therapy may antagonize the effects of warfarin, leading to inadequate anticoagulation (137). Increased doses may be required, and frequent monitoring is recommended as the metabolic effects of these agents may change over a prolonged time.

Phenytoin, with some enzyme-inducing properties, may inhibit the hypoprothrombinemic response in patients on chronic phenytoin therapy. However,

Table 17 Interactions Potentiating the Effects of Warfarin

Drug	Mechanism
Amiodarone	Decreased hepatic metabolism leading to increased PT/INR; prolonged effects following discontinuation of amiodarone
Antibiotics Antifungals Cephalosporins Erythromycin Metronidazole Quinolones TMP/SMX	Various mechanisms; antifungals inhibit hepatic metabolism; cephalosporins have NMTT side chain and also inhibit hepatic vitamin K synthesis; macrolides inhibit cyt P450; TMP/SMX and quinolones inhibit metabolism of R-isomer
Aspirin	Platelet inhibition leads to increased potential for bleeding
Carbamazepine Phenobarbital Rifampin	Enzyme induction leads to increased hepatic metabolism and decreased anticoagulant effects
Phenytoin	May decrease protein binding, leading to increased anticoagulant effects; may also increase metabolism, leading to decreased anticoagulation

Source: Ref. 137.

upon initiation of phenytoin therapy in a patient on stable warfarin therapy, the hypoprothrombinemic response may be transiently enhanced. One week to 2 weeks later, an inhibited hypoprothrombinemic response may prevail (138). Mechanisms include altered protein binding leading to displacement of warfarin, and subsequent enhanced anticoagulation, followed by hepatic enzyme induction leading to decreased anticoagulant effects (139). The interaction between phenytoin and warfarin remains unclear, warranting careful monitoring of both drugs during concurrent therapy (Table 17).

REFERENCES

1. Ochs HR, Carstens G, Greenblatt DJ. Reduction in lidocaine clearance during continuous infusion and by coadministration of propranolol. N Engl J Med 1980; 303:373–377.
2. Conrad KA, Byers JM III, Finley PR, Burnham L. Lidocaine elimination: effects of metoprolol and of propranolol. Clin Pharmacol Ther 1983; 33:133.
3. Schneck DW, Luderer JR, Davis D. Effects of nadolol and propranolol on plasma lidocaine clearance. Clin Pharmacol Ther 1984; 36:584–587.
4. Jackson JE, Bentley Jackson JE, Bentley JB, Glass SJ. Effects of histamine-2 receptor blockade on lidocaine kinetics. Clin Pharmacol Ther 1985; 37:544–548.
5. Feely J, Wilkinson GR, McAllister CB. Increased toxicity and reduced clearance of lidocaine by cimetidine. Ann Intern Med 1982; 96:592–594.
6. Siegmund J, Wilson J, Imhoff T. Amiodarone interaction with lidocaine. J Cardiovasc Pharmacol 1993; 21:513–515.
7. Keidar S, Grenadier E, Palant A. Sinoatrial arrest due to lidocaine injection in sick sinus syndrome during amiodarone administration. Am Heart J 1982; 104:1384–1385.
8. Kappenbeger L, Schwartz PJ. Comparative evaluation of antiarrhythmic therapy. Drugs 1985; 29:86.
9. Feely J, Wilkinson GR, McAllister CB. Increased toxicity and reduced clearance of lidocaine by cimetidine. Ann Intern Med 1982; 96:592–594.
10. Boyce JR, Cervenno FW, Wright FJ. Effects of halothane on the pharmacokinetics of lidocaine in digitalis-toxic dogs. Can Anaesth Soc J. 1978; 25:323–328.
11. Jeresaty RM, Kahn AH, Landry AB Jr. Sinoatrial arrest due to lidocaine in a patient receiving quinidine. Chest 1972; 61:683–685.
12. Au PK, Bhandaru Ak, Bream R. Proarrhythmic effects of antiarrhythmic drugs during programmed ventricular stimulation in patients without ventricular tachycardia. J Am Coll Cardiol 1987; 9:389–397.
13. Kosowsky BD, Taylor J, Lown B. Long-term use of procainamide following acute myocardial infarction. Circulation 1973; 47:1204–1210.
14. Gay RJ, Brown DF. Pacemaker failure due to procainamide toxicity. Am J Cardiol 1974; 34:728–732.
15. Saal AK, Werner JA, Greene HL. Effect of amiodarone on serum quinidine and procainamide levels. Am J Cardiol 1984; 53:1264–1267.

16. Windle J, Prystowsky EN, Miles WM. Pharmacokinetic and electrophysiologic interactions of amiodarone and procainamide. Clin Pharmacol Ther 1987; 41: 603–610.
17. Ilyas M, Owens D, Kvasnicka G. Delirium induced by a combination of anti-arrhythmic drugs. Lancet 1969; 2:1368–1369.
18. Koch-Weser J. Antiarrhythmic prophylaxis with procainamide in acute myocardial infarction. N Engl J Med 1971; 285:1024–1025.
19. Gianelly RE, von der Groeben JO, Spivack AP. Effect of lidocaine on ventricular arrhythmias in patients with coronary heart disease. N Engl J Med 1967; 277:1215–1219.
20. Viby-Mogensen J. Interaction of other drugs with muscle relaxants. Semin Anesth 1985; 4:52–64.
21. Kosoglou T, Rocci ML Jr, Vlasses PH. Trimethoprim alters the disposition of procainamide and N-acetylprocainamide. Clin Pharmacol Ther 1988; 44:467–477.
22. Vlasses PH, Kosoglou T, Chase SL. Trimethoprim inhibition of the renal clearance of procainamide and N-acetylprocainamide. Arch Intern Med 1989; 149:1350–1353.
23. Somogyi A, Bochner F. Dose and concentration dependent effect of ranitidine on procainamide disposition and renal clearance in man. Br J Clin Pharmacol 1984; 18: 175–181.
24. Somogyi A, Heinzow B. Cimetidine reduces procainamide elimination. N Engl J Med 1982; 307:1080.
25. Higbee MD, Wood JS, Mead RA. Procainamide-cimetidine interaction: a potential toxic interaction in the elderly. J Am Geriatr Soc 1984; 32:162–164.
26. Baciewicz AM, Baciewicz FA Jr. Effect of cimetidine and ranitidine on cardiovascular drugs. Am Heart J 1989; 118:144–154.
27. Mignat C, Unger T. ACE inhibitors. Drug interactions of clinical significance. Drug Safety 1995; 12(5):334–347.
28. De Lepeleire I, Van Hecken A, Verbesselt R. Interaction between furosemide and the converting enzyme inhibitor benazepril in healthy volunteers. Eur J Clin Pharmacol 1988; 34:465–468.
29. Speirs CJ, Dollery CT, Inman WH, Rawson NS, Wilton LV. Postmarketing surveillance of enalapril. II. Investigation of the potential role of enalapril in deaths with renal failure. BMJ 1988; 297:830–832.
30. Textor SC, Bravo EL, Fouad FM, Tarazi RC. Hyperkalemia in azotemic patients during angiotensin-converting enzyme inhibition and aldosterone reduction with captopril. Am J Med 1982; 73:719–725.
31. Burnakis TG, Mioduch HJ. Combined therapy with captopril and potassium supplementation. A potential for hyperkalemia. Arch Intern Med 1984; 144:2371–2372.
32. Goldfarb S, Cox M, Singer I, Goldberg M. Acute hyperkalemia induced by hyperglycemia: hormonal mechanisms. Ann Intern Med 1976; 84:426–432.
33. Rett K, Wicklmayr M, Dietze GJ. Hypoglycemia in hypertensive diabetic patients treated with sulfonylureas, biguanides and captopril. N Engl J Med 1988; 319:1609.
34. Moore TJ, Crantz FR, Hollenberg NK, et al. Contribution of prostaglandins to the antihypertensive action of captopril in essential hypertension. Hypertension 1981; 3:168–173.

35. Fujita T, Yamashita N, Yamashita K. Effect of indomethacin on antihypertensive action of captopril in hypertensive patients. Clin Exp Hypertens 1981; 3:939–952.
36. Nichols MG. Angiotensin converting enzyme inhibitors and renal function in heart failure. ACE Rep 1988; 56:1–5.
37. Murray BM, Venuto RC, Kohli OR. Enalapril-associated acute renal failure in renal transplants: possible role of cyclosporine. Am J Kidney Dis 1990; 16:66–69.
38. Cleland JG, Dargie HJ, Pettigrew A, Gillen G, Robertson JI. The effects of captopril on serum digoxin and urinary urea and digoxin clearances in patients with congestive heart failure. Am Heart J 1986; 112:130–135.
39. Douste-Blazy P, Blanc M, Montastruc JL, Conte D, Cotonat J, Galinier F. Is there any interaction between digoxin and enalapril? Br J Clin Pharmacol 1986; 22: 752–753.
40. Magelli C, Bassein L, Ribani MA, Liberatore S, Ambrosioni E. Lack of effect of captopril on serum digoxin in congestive heart failure. Eur J Clin Pharmacol 1989; 26:99–100.
41. Baldwin CH, Safferman AZ. A case of lisinopril-induced lithium toxicity. DICP 1990; 24:946–947.
42. Rosenthal T, Ezra D. Calcium antagonists. Drug interactions of clinical significance. Drug Safety 1995; 13(3):157–187.
43. Klockowski PM, Lener ME, Sirgo MA, Rocci ML Jr. Comparative evaluation of the effects of isradipine and diltiazem on antipyrine and indocyanine green clearances in elderly volunteers. Clin Pharm Ther 1990; 48:375–380.
44. Bauer LA, Stenwall M, Horn JR, Davis R, Opheim K, Greene L. Changes in antipyrine and indocyanine green kinetics during nifedipine, verapamil, and diltiazem therapy. Clin Pharm Ther 1986; 40:239–242.
45. Klein HO, Pauzner H, Di Segni E, David D, Kaplinsky E. The beneficial effects of verapamil in chronic atrial fibrillation. Arch Intern Med 1979; 139:747–749.
46. Klein HO, Lang R, Weiss E, Di Segni E, Libhaber C, Guerrero J. The influence of verapamil on serum digoxin concentration. Circulation 1982; 65:998–1003.
47. Rodin, SM, Johnson BF, et al. Comparative effects of verapamil and isradipine on steady state digoxin kinetics. Clin Pharm Ther 1988; 43:668–672.
48. Belz GG. Digoxin plasma concentrations and nifedipine. Lancet 1981; 1:844.
49. Mannani B, Malini PL. Cardiac glycosides: drug interactions of clinical significance. Drug Safety 1995; 12(2):97–109.
50. Dargie HJ, Lynch PG, Krikler DM. Nifedipine and propranolol: a beneficial drug interaction. Am J Med 1981; 71:676–682.
51. Rahn KH, Mooy J, Bohm R, v.d. Vet A. Reduction of bioavailability of verapamil by rifampin. N Engl J Med 1985; 312:920–921.
52. Barbarash RA, Bauman JL, Fischer JH, Kondos GT, Batenhorst RL. Near-total reduction in verapamil bioavailability by rifampin. Electrocardiographic correlates. Chest 1988; 94:954–959.
53. Barbarash RA. Verapamil-rifampin interaction. Drug Intell Clin Pharm 1985; 19:559–560.
54. Tsuchihashi K, Fukami K, Kishimoto H, Sumiyoshi T, Haze K, Saito M. A case of variant angina exacerbated by administration of rifampin. Heart Vessels 1987; 3:214–217.

55. Tada Y, Tsuda Y, Otsuka T. Case report: nifedipine-rifampin interaction attenuates the effect on blood pressure in a patient with essential hypertension. Am J Med Sci 1992; 303:25–27.
56. Drda KD. Effects of debrisoquine hydroxylation phenotype and enzyme induction with rifampin on diltiazem pharmacokinetics and pharmacodynamics. Pharmacotherapy 1991; 11:278–281.
57. Holtman JL, Kvam DC, Berry DA, Mottonen L, Borrell G, Harrison LI. The pharmacodynamic and pharmacokinetic interaction of flecainide acetate with propranolol: effects on cardiac function and drug clearance. Eur J Clin Pharmacol 1987; 33:97–99.
58. Houben H, Thien T, van't Laar A. Effect of low-dose epinephrine infusion on hemodynamics after selective and nonselective beta-blockade in hypertension. Clin Pharm Ther 1982; 31:685–690.
59. Scappaticci KA, Ham JA, John YJ. Effects of furosemide on the neuromuscular junction. Anesthesiology 1982; 57:381–388.
60. Osama AA, Bevan DR. Clindamycin induced neuromuscular blockade. Can J Anaesth 1995; 42(7):614–617.
61. Jedeikin R, Dolgunski E, Kaplan R, Hoffman S. Prolongation of neuromuscular blocking effect of vecuronium by antibiotics. Aneasthesia 1987; 42:858–860.
62. Sokoll MD, Gergis AD. Antibiotics and neuromuscular function. Anesthesiology 1982; 61:313–316.
63. Richardson FJ, Agoston S. Neuromuscular blocking agents and skeletal muscle relaxants. In: Dukes MNG, ed. Meyler's Side Effects of Drugs. New York: Elsevier, 1984.
64. Huang KC, Heise A, Shrader AK, Tsueda K. Vancomycin enhances the neuromuscular blockade of vecuronium. Anesth Analg 1990; 71:194–196.
65. Dupuis JY, Martin R, Tetrault JP. Atracurium and vecuronium interactions with gentamicin and tobramycin. Can J Anaesth 1989; 36(4):407–411.
66. Isenstein DA, Venner DS, Duggan J. Neuromuscular blockade in the intensive care unit. Chest 1992; 102:1258–1266.
67. Dickens MD. Pharmacology of neuromuscular blockade: interactions and implications for concurrent drug therapies. Crit Care Nurs Q 1995; 18(2):1–12.
68. Gray H, Slater RM, Pollard BJ. The effect of acutely administered phenytoin on vecuronium-induced neuromuscular blockade. Anaesth 1989; 44:379–381.
69. Magnani B, Malini PL. Cardiac glycosides: drug interactions of clinical significance. Drug Safety 1995; 12(2):97–109.
70. Nademanee K, Kannan R, Hendrickson J, Ookhtens M, Kay I, Singh BN. Amiodarone-digoxin interaction: clinical significance, time course of development, potential pharmacokinetic mechanisms and therapeutic implications. J Am Coll Cardiol 1984; 4(1):111–116.
71. Aronson JK. Cardiac glycosides and drugs used in dysrhythmias. In: Dukes MNG, ed. Meyler's Side Effects of Drugs. New York; Elsevier, 1984.
72. Brown DD, Juhl RP. Decrease bioavailability of digoxin due to antacids and kaolinpectin. N Engl J Med 1976; 295:1034–1037.
73. Rodin SM, Johnson BF. Pharmacokinetic interactions with digoxin. Clin Pharm 1988; 15:227–244.

74. Maxwell DL, Gilmour-White SK. Digoxin toxicity due to interactions of digoxin with erythromycin. BMJ 1989; 298:572.
75. Hooymans PM, Merkus FW. Current status of cardiac glycoside interactions. Clin Pharm 1985; 4:404–413.
76. Gault H, Longerich L, Dawe M, et al. Digoxin-rifampin interaction. Clin Pharmacol Ther 1984; 35:750–754.
77. Rosenthal T, Ezra D. Calcium antagonists: drug interactions of clinical significance. Drug Safety 1995; 13(3):157–187.
78. Garty M, Shamir E, Ilfeld D, et al. Non-interaction of digoxin and nifedipine in cardiac patients. J Clin Pharmacol 1986; 26:304–305.
79. Silber B, Sheiner LB, Powers JL, et al. Spironolactone associated digoxin radioimmunoassay interference. Clin Chem 1979; 25:48–50.
80. Dipiro JT, Cote JR, Dipiro CR, et al. Spironolactone interference with digoxin radioimmunoassay in cirrhotic patients. Am J Hosp Pharm 1980; 37:1518–1521.
81. Drug Interactions; Facts and Comparisons. Facts & Comparisons, Inc. St. Louis, Missouri. Updated monthly.
82. Tollefson G, Lesar T, Grothe D, Garvey M. Alprazolam-related digoxin toxicity. Am J Psychiatry 1984; 141:1612–1614.
83. Nolan P, Marcus F, Erstad B, et al. Effects of coadministration of propafenone on the pharmacokinetics of digoxin in healthy volunteer subjects. J Clin Pharmacol 1989; 29:46–52.
84. Dorian P, Strauss M, Cardella C, et al. Digoxin-cyclosporine interaction: severe digitalis toxicity after cyclosporine treatment. Clin Invest Med 1988; 11:108–112.
85. Manninen V, Apajalahti A, Melin J, Karesoja M. Altered absorption of digoxin in patients given propantheline and metoclopramide. Lancet 1973; 1:398–400.
86. Jorgensen HS, Christensen HR, Kampmann JP. Interaction between digoxin and indomethacin or ibuprofen. Br J Clin Pharmacol 1991; 31:108–110.
87. ISIS-2 (Second International Study of Infarct Survival) Collaborative Group. Randomised trial of intravenous streptokinase, oral aspirin, both or neither among 17,187 cases of suspected acute myocardial infarction. Lancet 1988; 2:356–360.
88. de Boer A, van Griensven JM. Drug interactions with thrombolytic agents. Clin Pharm 1995; 28(4):315–326.
89. Meredith PA, Pasanini F, Elliott HL. Verapamil pharmacokinetics and apparent hepatic and renal blood flow. Br J Clin Pharm 1985; 20:235–237.
90. Nicoloni FA, Ferrini D, Ottani F, Galvani M. Concurrent nitroglycerin therapy impairs tissue-type plasminogen activator-induced thrombolysis in patients with acute myocardial infarction. Am J Cardiol 1994; 74:662–666.
91. Svensson CK, Cumella JC, Tronolone M, Middleton E, Lalka D. Effects of hydralazine, nitroglycerin, and food on estimated hepatic blood flow. Clin Pharmacol Ther 1985; 37:464–468.
92. Bauer LA, Stenwall M, Horn JR. Changes in antipyrine and indocyanine green kinetics during nifedipine, verapamil, and diltiazem therapy. Clin Pharmacol Ther 1986; 40:239–242.
93. Parker G, Ene MD, Daneshmend TK. Do beta-blockers differ in their effects on hepatic microsomal enzymes and liver blood flow? J Clin Pharmacol 1984; 24:493–499.
94. Marino PL. The ICU Book. Malvern, PA: Lea & Febiger, 1991.

95. Borcherding SM, Stevens OR, Nicholas RA, et al. Quinolones: a practical review of clinical uses, dosing considerations and drug interactions. J Family Pract 1996; 42(1):69–78.
96. Nex DE, Watson WA, Lener ME, et al. Effects of aluminum and magnesium antacids and ranitidine on the absorption of spirofloxacin. Clin Pharmacol Ther 1989; 46: 700–705.
97. Sahai J, Gallicano K, Oliveras L, et al. Cations in the didanosine tablet reduce ciprofloxacin bioavailability. Clin Pharm Ther 1993; 53:292–297.
98. Neuvonen PJ, Kivisto KT, Lehto P. Interference of dairy products with the absorption of ciprofloxacin. Clin Pharmacol Ther 1991; 51:498–502.
99. Garrelts JC, Godley PJ, Peterie JD, et al. Sucralfate significantly reduces ciprofloxacin concentrations in the serum. Antimicrob Agents Chemother 1990; 34:931–933.
100. Grasela TH, Dreis MW. An evaluation of the quinolone-theophylline interaction using the Food and Drug Administration spontaneous reporting system. Arch Intern Med 1992; 152:617–621.
101. Ho G, Tierney MG, Dales RE. Evaluation of the effect of norfloxacin on the pharmacokinetics of theophylline. Clin Pharmacol Ther 1988; 44:35.
102. Wijnands WJA, Vree TB, Van Herwaarden CLA. The influence of quinolone derivatives on theophylline clearance. Br J Clin Pharmacol 1986; 22:677–683.
103. Jolson HM, Tanner LA, Green L, Grasela TH. Adverse reaction reporting of interaction between warfarin and fluoroquinolones. Arch Intern Med 1991; 151:1003–1004.
104. Toon S, Hopkins KJ, Garstang FM, et al. Enoxacin-warfarin interaction: pharmacokinetic and stereochemical aspects. Clin Pharmacol Ther 1987; 42:33–41.
105. Horn JR, Hansten PD. Drug interactions with antibacterial agents. J Family Pract 1995; 41(1):81–90.
106. Honig P, Wortham D, Zamani K, et al. Effect of clarithromycin, erythromycin and azithromycin on the pharmacokinetics of terfenadine. Clin Pharmacol Ther 1993; 53:161.
107. May DS, Jarboe CH, Ellenburg DT, et al. The effects of erythromycin on theophylline elimination in normal males. J Clin Pharmacol 1982; 22:125–130.
108. Periti P, Mazzei T, Mini E, Novelli A. Pharmacokinetic drug interactions of macrolides. Clin Pharm 1992; 23:106–131.
109. Ludden TM. Pharmacokinetic interactions of the macrolide antibiotics. Clin Pharm 1985; 10:63–79.
110. Lindenbaum J, Rund DG, Butler VP, et al. Inactivation of digoxin by the gut flora: reversal by antibiotic therapy. N Engl J Med 1981; 305:789–794.
111. Brater DC, Morelli HF. Digoxin toxicity in patients with normokalemic potassium depletion. Clin Pharm Ther 1977; 22:21.
112. Mayall B, Poggi G, Parkin JD. Neutropenia due to low-dose methotrexate therapy for psoriasis and rheumatoid arthritis may be fatal. Med J Austr 1991; 155:480–484.
113. Davis RI, Berman W Jr, Wernly JA, Kelly HW. Warfarin-nafcillin interaction. J Pediatr 1991; 118:300–303.
114. Neuvonen PJ. Interactions with the absorption of tetracycline. Drugs 1976; 11: 45–54.

115. Pentilla O, Newvonen PJ, Aho K, Lehtovarra R. Interaction between doxycycline and some antiepileptic drugs. BMJ 1974; 2:470–472.
116. Neuvonen PJ, Penttila F. Interaction between doxycycline and barbiturates. BMJ 1974; 1:535–536.
117. Neuvonen PJ, Penttila O, Lehtovaara R, Aho K. Effect of antiepileptic drugs on the elimination of various tetracycline derivatives. Eur J Clin Pharmacol 1975; 9: 147–154.
118. Saathoff N, Lode H, Neider K, et al. Pharmacokinetics of cefpodoxime proxetil and interactions with an antacid and an H_2 receptor antagonist. Antimicrob Agents Chemother 1992; 36:796–800.
119. Schentag JJ. Cefmetazole sodium: pharmacology, pharmacokinetics and clinical trials. Pharmacotherapy 1991; 11:2–19.
120. Sommers DE, Van Wyk M, Moncrieff J, et al. Influence of food and reduced gastric acidity on the availability of bacampicillin and cefuroxime axetil. Br J Clin Pharmacol 1984; 18:535–539.
121. Costanzo LS. Mechanism of action of thiazide diuretics. Semin Nephrol 1988; 8: 234–241.
122. Bourbigot B, et al. Nicardipine increases cyclosporine blood levels. Lancet 1986; 1:1447.
123. Kosoglou T, Rocci ML, Vlasses PH. Trimethoprim alters disposition of procainamide and NAPA. Clin Pharmacol Ther 1988; 44:467–477.
124. Thomas MH, Gutterman LA. Methotrexate toxicity in a patient receiving TMP/SMX. J Rheumatol 1989; 40:440–441.
125. Hansen JM, Kampmann JP, Siersback-Nielsen K, et al. The effects of different sulfonamides on phenytoin metabolism in man. Acta Scand 1979; 624:106–110.
126. O'Reilly RA. Stereoselective interactions of TMP/SMX with the separated enantiomorphs of racemic warfarin in man. N Engl J Med 1980; 302:33–35.
127. O'Reilly RA. The stereoselective interaction of warfarin and metronidazole in man. N Engl J Med 1976; 295:354–357.
128. Baciewicz AM, Baciewicz FA. Cyclosporine pharmacokinetic drug interactions. Am J Surg 1989; 157:264–271.
129. O'Reilly RA, Trager WF, Rettie AE, et al. Interaction of amiodarone with racemic warfarin and its separated enantiomorphs in humans. Clin Pharmacol Ther 1987; 42: 290–294.
130. Kerin NZ. The incidence, magnitude and time course of the amiodarone-warfarin interaction. Arch Intern Med 1988; 148:1779.
131. Bechtold H, Andrassy K, Jahnchen E, et al. Evidence for impaired hepatic vitamin K metabolism in patients treated with NMTT cephalosporins. Thrombos Hemostas 1984; 51:358–361.
132. Greenlaw CW. Drug interaction between co-trimoxazole and warfarin. Am J Hosp Pharm 1979; 36:1155.
133. Serlin MJ. Cimetidine: interactions with oral anticoagulants in man. Lancet 1979; 2:317.
134. Serlin MJ. Lack of effect of ranitidine on warfarin action. Br J Clin Pharmacol 1981; 12:791.

135. Jensen JC. Inhibition of human liver cytochrome P450 by omeprazole. Br J Clin Pharmacol 1986; 21:328.
136. Sutfin T. Stereoselective interaction of omeprazole with warfarin in healthy men. Ther Drug Monit 1989; 11:176.
137. Hirsch J, Fuster V. Guide to anticoagulant therapy Part 2: oral anticoagulants. Circulation 1994; 89(3):1469–1480.
138. Nappi JM. Warfarin and phenytoin interaction. Ann Intern Med 1979; 90:852.
139. Solomon GE. Coagulation defects caused by diphenylhydantoin. Neurology 1972; 22:1165.
140. Hill GS. Drug-associated glomerulopathies. Toxicol Pathol 1986; 14:37–44.
141. Katsutani N, Shionoya H. Drug-specific immune responses induced by immunization with drugs in guinea pigs and mice. J Toxicol Sci 1992; 17:169–183.
142. Gerhardt RE, Knouss RF, Thyrum PT. Quinidine excretion in aciduria and alkaluria. Ann Intern Med 1969; 71:927–933.
143. Rotmensch HH, Belhassen B. Amiodarone in the management of cardiac arrhythmias: current concepts. Med Clin North Am 1988; 72:321–358.
144. Tartini OR, Kappenberger L, Steinbrunn W. Dangerous interaction between amiodarone and quinidine. Lancet 1982; 1:1327–1329.
145. Rodgers GC, Balckman MS. Quinidine interactions with anticonvulsants. Drug Intell Clin Pharm 1983; 17:819–820.
146. Sinn AF, ed. Evaluations of Drug Interactions. New York; Macmillan Publishing Co., 1989.
147. Baker BJ, Gammill J, Massengill J. Concurrent use of quinidine and disopyramide: evaluation of serum concentrations and electrocardiographic effects. Am Heart J 1983; 105:12–15.
148. Funck-Brentano C, Kroemer HK, Pavlou H. Genetically-determined interaction between propafenone and low dose quinidine: role of active metabolites in modulating net drug effect. Br J Clin Pharmacol 1989; 27:435–444.
149. Oates NS, Feher MD, Perry HE. Influence of quinidine on nifedipine plasma pharmacokinetics. Br J Clin Pharmacol 1988; 25:675.
150. Bailey DG, Freeman DJ, Melendez LJ. Quinidine interaction with nifedipine and felodipine: pharmacokinetic and pharmacodynamic evaluation. Clin Pharmacol Ther 1993; 53:354–359.
151. Steiner E. Dumont E, Spina E. Inhibition of desipramine 2-hydroxylation by quinidine and quinine. Clin Pharmacol Ther 1988; 43:577–581.
152. Bussey HI, Merritt GJ, Hill EG. The influence of rifampin on quinidine and digoxin. Arch Intern Med 1984; 144:1021–1023.
153. Baciewicz AM, Baciewicz FA Jr. Effect of cimetidine and ranitidine on cardiovascular drugs. Am Heart J 1989; 118:144–154.
154. McNulty RM, Lazor JA, Sketch M. Transient increase in plasma quinidine concentrations during ketoconazole-quinidine therapy. Clin Pharm 1989; 8:222–225.
155. Lee TH, Friedman PL, Goldman L, Stone PH. Sinus arrest and hypotension with combined amiodarone-diltiazem therapy. Am Heart J 1985; 109:163–164.
156. Nademanee K, Kannan R, Hendrickson J, et al. Amiodarone-digoxin interaction: clinical significance, time course of development, potential pharmacokinetic mechanism and therapeutic implications. J Am Coll Cardiol 1984; 4:111.

157. Marcus FI. Drug interactions with amiodarone. Am Heart J 1983; 106:924–930.
158. Malden ES, Tartar VM, Gutierrez FR. Acute fatality following pulmonary angiography in a patient on an amiodarone regimen. Angiology 1993; 44:152–155.
159. Leor J, Levartowsky D, Sharon C, Farfel Z. Amiodarone and beta adrenergic blockers: an interaction with metoprolol but not atenolol. Am Heart J 1988; 116:206–207.
160. Niemann JT, Bessen HA, Rothstein RJ, Laks MM. Electrocardiographic criteria for tricyclic antidepressant cardiotoxicity. Am Heart J 1986; 57:1154–1159.
161. Shackleford EJ, Watson FT. Amiodarone-phenytoin interaction. Drug Intell Clin Pharm 1987; 21:921.
162. Saal AK, Werner JA, Greene HL. Effect of amiodarone on serum quinidine and procainamide levels. Am J Cardiol 1984; 53:1264–1267.
163. Warren R, Vohra J, Hunt D. Serious interactions of sotalol with amiodarone and flecainide. Med J Aust 1990; 152:277.
164. Kerin NZ, Blevins RD, Goldman L. The incidence, magnitude, and time course of the amiodarone-warfarin interaction. Arch Intern Med 1988; 148:1779–1781.
165. James MA. Combined therapy with disopyramide and amiodarone: a report of 11 cases. Int J Cardiol 1986; 13:248.
166. Kapil RP. Disopyramide pharmacokinetics and metabolism: effect of inducers. Br J Clin Pharmacol 1987; 24:781.
167. Kessler JM. Disopyramide and phenytoin interaction. Clin Pharm 1982; 1:263.
168. Cathcart-Rake WF. The pharmacodynamics of concurrent disopyramide and propranolol. Clin Pharmacol Ther 1979; 25:217.
169. Ragosta M. Potentially fatal interaction between erythromycin and disopyramide. Am J Med 1989; 86:465.
170. DeAzedo IM, Wanatabe Y, et al. Electrophysiologic antagonism on quinidine and bretylium tosylate. Am J Cardiol 1974; 33:633–638.
171. Smith MS, Benyanes MC, et al. Influence of cimetidine on verapamil kinetics and dynamics. Clin Pharmacol Ther 1984; 36:551–554.
172. Loi CM, Rollins DE, et al. Effect of cimetidine on verapamil disposition. Clin Pharmacol Ther 1985; 37:654–657.
173. Abernathy DR, Schwartz JB, Todd EL. Lack of interaction between verapamil and cimetidine. Clin Pharmacol Ther 1985; 38:342–349.
174. Citterio F, Serino F, et al. Verapamil improves gandimmune immunosuppression, reducing acute rejection episodes. Transplant Proc 1996; 28:2174–2176.
175. Bleck JS, Thiesemann C, Kliem V, et al. Diltiazem increases blood concentrations of cyclized cyclosporine metabolites resulting in different cyclosporine metabolite patterns in stable male and female allograft recipients. Br J Clin Pharm 1996; 41: 551–556.
176. Campara C, Regazzi MB, et al. Clinically significant drug interactions with cyclosporin. An update. Clin Pharmacokin 1996; 30:141–179.
177. Beattie B, Biller J, Mehlhaus B, et al. Verapamil-induced carbamazepine neurotoxicity: a report of two cases. Eur Neurol 1988; 28:104–105.
178. McInnes GT. Clinical pharmacology of verapamil. Br J Clin Practice, Supp 1988; 60:3–8.
179. Dubovsky SL, Franks RD, Allen S. Verapamil: a new antimanic drug with potential interactions with lithium. J Clin Psych 1987; 48:371–372.

180. Vercruysse I, Massart DL, et al. Increase in plasma propranolol caused by nicardipine is dependent on the delivery rate of propranolol. Eur J Clin Pharmacol 1995: 49(1–2):121–125.
181. Kyle MC. In: Freis, ed. Serial measurements of systolic time intervals: effects of propranolol alone and combined with other agents in hypertensive patients. Hypertension 1980; 2(1):111–117.
182. Hinderling PH, Tendolkar A, Dee CM, et al. Single-dose interactin study of diprafenone HCL in healthy volunteers. J Clin Pharm 1995; 35:721–729.
183. Loon NR, Wilcox CS, Folger W. Orthostatic hypotension due to quinidine and propranolol. Am J Med 1986; 81:1101–1104.
184. Bobik A et al. Low oral bioavailability of dihydroergotamine and first-pass extraction in patients with orthostatic hypotension. Clin Pharmacol Ther 1981; 30:673.
185. Pye M, Oldroyd KG, Conkie JA, et al. A clinical and in vitro study on the possible interaction of intravenous nitrates with heparin anticoagulation. Clin Cardiol 1994; 17:658–661.
186. Shah PK. Ventricular unloading in the management of heart disease: role of vasodilators. Am Heart J 1977; 93:256–260, 403–406.
187. Cohen IM et al. Danger in nitroprusside therapy. Ann Intern Med 1976; 85:205.
188. Coddens J, Delooft , Vandenbrouke G. Effects of dobutamine and/or nitroprusside on the pulmonary circulation in patients with pulmonary hypertension secondary to end-stage heart failure. J Cardiothor Vasc Anesth 1993; 7:321–325.
189. Epstein M, Lepp BA, et al. Potentiation of furosemide by metolazone in refractory edema. Curr Ther Res 1977; 21:656.
190. Wilkins MR, Woods KL, Kendall MJ. The effects of selective and non-selective inhibition of cyclo-oxygenase on frusemide-stimulated natriuresis. Int J Clin Pharmacol Ther Toxicol 1986; 24:55–57.
191. Singer I, Rotenberg P. Mechanisms of lithium action. N Engl J Med 1973; 289:254.

13

Pulmonary Embolus and Pulmonary Infarction in Cardiac Patients

BOJAN CERCEK

Cedars-Sinai Medical Center and University of California, Los Angeles, School of Medicine, Los Angeles, California

I. EPIDEMIOLOGY OF PULMONARY EMBOLISM

Pulmonary embolism (PE) is strongly associated with deep venous thrombosis (DVT). More than two-thirds of the patients with clinically symptomatic PE are found to have asymptomatic DVT, and PE is detected in about half of the patients with documented DVT. Each year DVT occurs in approximately 2 million Americans, and approximately 600,000 Americans develop PE that is fatal in 60,000 of them (1). In a most recent population-based study of DVT and PE by Anderson et al. from the Worcester County, the most prominent risk factors for development of DVT and PE were cancer and heart disease, notably congestive heart failure and myocardial infarction. Approximately one-third of the patients hospitalized in 1985 and 1986 with a DVT and PE also had congestive heart failure (CHF). The only other risk factor with such high prevalence of PE was cancer (2). Several decades ago, when patients with myocardial infarction were subjected to prolonged bed rest, significant pulmonary embolism was found at autopsy in more than 20% of patients with AMI. With anticoagulation it was reduced to 5% (3). The incidence of DVT and PE in patients with myocardial infarction is currently estimated to be approximately 1% to 8%. (4,5).

II. PATHOGENESIS AND NATURAL COURSE OF DVT AND PE

Venous thrombi are composed predominantly of fibrin, red cells, and a component of platelets. They usually form in the regions with stagnant blood flow or large venous sinuses, or in the valve cusp pockets in the deep veins of the calf. Another factor that promotes thrombus formation is the damaged vessel wall. The damage can be either direct, mechanical damage or activation of the endothelial cells by cytokines, primarily interleukin-1 (IL-1) and tumor necrosis factor-α (TNF-α) released locally or systemically as the result of tissue injury or inflammation (6). The third factor that promotes thrombus formation is hypercoagulability, best divided as primary and secondary (7). Primary are the deficiencies of antithrombin-III (AT-III), proteins C and S, and presence of lupus anticoagulant and anticardiolipin antibodies. The secondary hypercoagulable states are the consequences of systemic diseases such as cancer and nephrotic syndrome, or they develop during pregnancy or with therapy with oral contraceptives. In hospitalized cardiac patients, the immobility with blood stasis is the predominant factor.

The natural course of undetected DVT is mostly asymptomatic, especially those that develop in the calf veins. If untreated, proximal extension occurs in approximately 20% to 30% and may produce symptoms due to obstruction of the venous flow and inflammation of the vein walls and local tissues, and in 40% to 50% the extension is associated with embolization to the pulmonary circulation. Spontaneous, complete lysis occurs in less than 10% of cases, while incomplete lysis results in many patients in postthrombotic syndrome. If treated, the prognosis of DVT is good with clinical significant recurrent events during 3 months in only 5%. Still approximately one-third of the patients will have a recurrence of a thrombosis within the 8-year follow-up (6).

III. PATHOPHYSIOLOGY OF PE AND PULMONARY INFARCTION

Dislodged venous thrombi float through the venous system to the pulmonary arterial circulation. Very large thrombi may lodge in the bifurcation of pulmonary artery, forming a saddle embolus. More commonly, one of the major pulmonary vessels is occluded. Besides purely mechanical obstruction to the flow caused by the thrombus, the locally lodged thrombi in the pulmonary circulation release substances that cause vasoconstriction and possibly bronchospasms, thromboxane A2, serotonin, and platelet-derived growth factor, among others. In patients with no previous cardiopulmonary disease, the occlusion of approximately 25% of the pulmonary vascular causes significant increase in right ventricular afterload and right ventricular chamber dilatation. In a echocardiographic study Jardin et. al. (8) have shown that during massive pulmonary embolism, low cardiac output and shock are primarily due to the decrease in preload of the left ventricle by the obstruction of the pulmonary bed. In addition, the decreased compliance of the left ventricle due to ventricular interdependence and leftward septal displacement also contributed to the decreased left ventricular end-diastolic dimensions (8). In patients with preexistent cardiopulmonary compromise, smaller thrombi occluding only pulmonary segment can have a similar hemodynamic effect. Especially at risk are patients with preexistent pulmonary hypertension secondary to chronic obstructive lung disease or failing left ventricle.

IV. CLINICAL PRESENTATION

PE mimics a variety of cardiopulmonary diseases, and it is often only the clinical suspicion of PE that leads the diagnostic testing (9). In several autopsy studies the nonspecific clinical presentation is reflected in between 30% and 62% overdiagnosis or as high as 82% underdiagnosis of PE, respectively. In patients with CHF, PE was not suspected in 40% of patients prior to the patients' death (10). Because of this nonspecific clinical presentation, whenever there is a clinical suspicion, further objective testing for PE is necessary to establish the diagnosis and to initiate appropriate treatment.

In both the Urokinase, Streptokinase Pulmonary Embolism Trial (UPET) (11) and the Prospective Investigation of Pulmonary Embolism Diagnosis (PIOPED) study (12), the most sensitive symptom and sign were dyspnea or tachypnea, over 80%. The chest pain that was described in over 70% of patients was largely pleuritic. Dyspnea, tachypnea, and chest pain had a combined sensitivity of 97%. Other common symptoms/signs—cough, hemoptysis, diaphoresis, apprehension, accentuated P2 secondary to pulmonary hypertension, tachycardia, fever, and cyanosis are present in less than half of the patients.

About 15% patients present with syncope. Syncopal episodes are often vagally mediated (13). The occasional patient will present with brochospastic wheezing or paradoxical embolism. The differential diagnosis of PE consists therefore of CHF, myocardial infarction (MI), unstable angina, pneumonia, asthma, chronic obstructive pulmonary disease (COPD), rib fracture, pneumothorax, and even musculoskeletal pain. An entity of PE is pulmonary infarction. It evolves 3 to 7 days after the onset of embolism provided small distal peripheral pulmonary arteries are occluded that in conjunction with bronchoconstriction lead to decreased collateral blood flow from the bronchial arteries. The decreased nutritional perfusion of the lung tissue leads to necrosis and pulmonary infarction. The patient can present with hemoptysis or intense pleuritic chest pain.

The clinical presentation is more evident in patients with massive PE. The consequences of sudden pulmonary hypertension usually mean pulmonary pressure of no more than 40 mm Hg, are severe—sudden dyspnea, signs of acute cor pulmonale, and shock, possibly cardiac arrest. The differential diagnosis of massive PE includes cardiogenic shock, superior vena cava syndrome, tamponade, and constrictive pericarditis or right ventricular infarction (9).

V. CHEST X-RAY

The important sign of a large PE is an enlargement of the hilar arteries. The enlargement is observed predominantly on the right side because the main pulmonary artery often obscures the pulmonary artery in the left hilum. The abrupt tapering of the vessel, the "knuckle sign," is rarely noted. More common but less specific signs are diminished volume of a pulmonary lobe, elevation of the hemodiaphragm, or hyperlucency on a plain film. In pulmonary infarction the parenchymal consolidation is observed. The classical wedged-shape density in the peripheral region with apex expanding toward the hilum, the Hampton hump, is rarely seen. Parenchymal consolidation can occasionally lead to air bronchogram.

Overall, the chest radiography is an insensitive and nonspecific screen test for PE. It does play a major diagnostic utility in conjunction with ventilation-perfusion scan and to exclude other diseases that may mimic PE—i.e., pneumonia, heart failure, or pneumothorax (14).

VI. ELECTROCARDIOGRAPHY

With massive PE the ECG can display signs of an acute cor pulmonale with S1, Q3, T3, new right bundle branch block, or new right axis deviation. The electrocardiogram is nevertheless poorly sensitive; only 15% to 20% of patients will display ECG changes except for nonspecific sinus tachycardia or T-wave changes (15).

VII. ECHOCARDIOGRAPHY

Several findings on the echocardiogram are suggestive of PE: right ventricular (RV) dilatation and hypokinesia, abnormal septal position in diastole and paradoxical septal systolic motion, pulmonary artery (PA) dilatation, unusual degree of tricuspid and pulmonary regurgitation, and increased pulmonary artery systolic and diastolic pressures (16). The RV dilatation and hypokinesia are due to increased RV afterload. Mean RV diameter with significant PE has been reported at 2.8 ± 1.5 cm, in three of four patients' mean RV diameter with PE has been reported at > 2.7 cm. The dimension are best measured in apical four-chamber view. In absence of previous cardiac disease, LV dimensions and pressure are reduced secondary to decreased LV preload. Bulging of the septum in diastole into the cavity of the left ventricle is present even during cardiac arrest after PE; this is different to normal nonbeating heart, where the septum usually occupies the central position. In systole the septum often moves paradoxically. The E-F slope of the mitral valve is often reduced. Increase in the right atrial (RA) pressure can be assessed from the decreased respiratory variations in the dimensions of the vena cava. Normally the diameter of the vena cava decreases during expiration to $< 40\%$ of the maximal diameter during inspiration. Absence of the decrease in collapse to $< 40\%$ correlates very well with RA pressure > 8 mm Hg. This finding is significant as RA pressure correlates with the extent of the pulmonary bed obstruction better than the RV pressure. The use of Bernoulli equations permits quantification of RV/PA peak systolic blood pressure with excellent correlation with invasive measurements. These measurements have largely replaced non-specific signs of pulmonary hypertension recorded on M-mode echo. More than 90% of patients with PE will have detectable tricuspid insufficiency. In acute PE, mean pulmonary pressure is seldom > 40 mm Hg because of the inability of the RV to generate higher pressures acutely. In 52 of 60 patients with significant PE, the maximum velocity of tricuspid regurgitant jet was > 2.6 m/sec. Many patients also develop pulmonary insufficiency, which allows calculation of the PA diastolic pressure by the same principle. The detection of the peak velocity of the pulmonary regurgitant jet is technically more difficult than the one of tricuspid regurgitant jet and may lead to significant underestimation of the PA diastolic pressure. The transthoracic echo allows occasionally the detection of thrombi trapped in or traveling through RA or RV (17). These thrombi have high potential for embolization to the lungs, and the finding mandates aggressive treatment. Transesophageal echo has much better resolution than transthoracic, and can permit detection of not only RA/RV thrombi but also thrombi in the central pulmonary artery (18). The test requires sedation and may be of risk in the hypoxic, hemodynamically unstable patient.

The sensitivity of the echo for detection of significant PE is unknown. In a study from the Netherlands, 90% of patients with major PE had at least one sign of increased RV pressure or volume load (19). The sensitivity is low in patients with PE with only marginal hemodynamic consequences. The echocardiographic study is ideal, though, for following the effects of therapy: it is noninvasive and can be repeated as needed. The use of transesophageal echo should be reserved for patients with a high degree of diagnostic uncertainty when pulmonary angiography is contraindicated or unavailable.

VIII. ANALYSIS OF ARTERIAL BLOOD GASES

Although arterial hypoxia is an expected consequence of PE, 10% to 26% of patients with documented PE had normal PaO_2 while breathing room air (20). The sensitivity of the arterial blood gas analysis was over 90% in presence of either hypoxemia ($paO_2 < 80$ mm Hg) or hypocapnia ($PaCO_2 < 36$ mm Hg). The sensitivity of increased $P(A\text{-}a)O_2$ was $> 90\%$ and increased to $> 95\%$ when combined with hypocapnia. The study did not assess the specifity of the measurements, likely to be very low.

IX. BLOOD TESTS

A very sensitive but unspecific test is the determination of the fibrin degradation products, D-dimers in the blood. Degradation of the fibrin at any site, hematomas, catheter insertion sites, DVT, etc. is the potential source of the D-dimers. In one study, D-dimers were present in 89% of patients who had PE and at the same time in 56% of those who did not (21).

X. VENTILATION PERFUSION LUNG SCANS

Ventilation-perfusion lung scan remains the cornerstone of the diagnosis of PE (22). Since many pulmonary diseases like pneumonia, neoplasms, and COPD cause a decrease in blood flow to an affected lung zone, a ventilation scan performed in conjunction with perfusion scan increases the specificity of the scintigraphy. In regions where the chest radiograph is normal, abnormalities in the perfusion that are matched by zones of abnormal ventilation are less likely to represent PE than in those that are not.

For the perfusion imaging, injected radiolabeled macroaggregated human albumin particles are trapped in approximately 500,000 pulmonary arterioles. Since the total capacity of the lungs is over 600 million arterioles, the effects are physiologically insignificant. The occlusion is only temporary as the material degrades. The dose of radioactivity injected is low, approximately 4 mCi distributed among 500,000 particles. The ventilation studies are performed with radioactive xenon or crypton gas or radioactive aerosol. Ideally, the ventilation study would be performed after the perfusion study because it would be performed only in patients with indeterminate abnormalities on the perfusion scan.

The normal ventilation-perfusion scan has a homogeneous pattern of matched ventilation and perfusion. In patients with pulmonary embolism the perfusion is typically more compromised than ventilation. Vascular occlusion of any etiology, emboli of nonthrombotic material, air, amniotic fluid, fat, thrombosis in situ, and pulmonary vasculitis will also cause a more pronounced decrease in perfusion than ventilation and can mimic PE. Pulmonary consolidation, bronchial obstructive disease, and pulmonary infarction usually equally impair ventilation and perfusion and cause a matched ventilation-perfusion defect. Emphysema and restrictive lung disease can affect the perfusion more than ventilation, yet the pattern of generalized abnormalities helps to exclude pulmonary embolism (23).

The hallmark of PE is a wedge-shaped perfusion defect based on the pleura in areas with normal ventilation and clear chest radiography. Criteria used in the past

Table 1 Criteria Used in the Interpretation of Ventilation/Perfusion Scans for PE

High probability	Intermediate probability	Low probability
> 2 Large V/Q mismatches (2 large V/Q are borderline high prob) or 1 Large V/Q and ⩾ 2 mod V/Q mismatches or ⩾ 4 Mod V/Q mismatches Mod: 25–75% Seg Large: >75% Seg V/Q mismatch = Nl V and Nl x-ray or Q > V or x-ray in region of Q defect	⩾ 1 Q << x-ray defect or ⩾ 2 V/Q matches with NIx-ray and some areas of normal perfusion in lung or Perfusion defects due to pleural effusion, cardiomegaly, enlarged aorta, hilum, mediastinum, and elevated diaphragmor ⩾ 1 Small Q with Nl x-ray	1 Large ± 1 mod V/Q mismatch or 1 to 3 Mod V/Q mismatches or 1 Matched V/Q with Nl x-ray (2 large V/Q mismatches are borderline, intermediate, to high prob)

Adapted with permission from Ref. 22.

to diagnose a perfusion scan as high, intermediate, or low probability yielded similar results as current criteria developed on the basis of revised PIOPED study (24). The criteria are given in Table 1.

Among the general population of 1493 patients with suspected PE evaluated in the PIOPED study (12), a random sample of 933 patients was prospectively evaluated. Of all patients, with or without definitive angiogram, high probability scan occurred in 13% of patients, intermediate probability scan in 39%, low probability scan in 34%, and near normal/normal ventilation perfusion scan in 14%. Of 755 who had pulmonary angiography, 33% had demonstrated PE. Almost all patients with PE had scans of high, intermediate, or low probability—sensitivity of 98%. As many patients without PE also had one of the three categories of abnormal scan, the specificity of an abnormal scan was only 10%. Of 116 patients with high-probability scan and definitive angiogram, 88% had pulmonary embolism, sensitivity of 97%. Because only a minority of patients with PE had high probability scans, the sensitivity of the high probability scan was only 41%. Of 332 patients with intermediate probability scans and definitive angiogram, 33% had PE, and so had 12% of patients with low probability scans.

In patients with associated cardiopulmonary disease the likelihood of uninformative ventilation/perfusion scan increased. The intermediate probability scan was present in 60% patients with chronic obstructive pulmonary disease, in 43% patients with history of any prior cardiac or pulmonary disease, and in only 32% of patients without prior cardiac or pulmonary disease. In patients with normal chest radiograph, 18% had intermediate probability scan. The value of ventilation/ perfusion scan was similar among elderly as was in younger patients. The interobserver variability was excellent for high probability, very low probability, and normal scans—over 90%. It was only 75% and 70% for the intermediate and low probability scans, respectively.

In the PIOPED study, the clinical assessment for prior probability of PE before the scan was compared with the status as determined by pulmonary angiography. A clinical assessment of high likelihood, 80% to 100%, of PE was made in only 10% of patients and was correct in 61 of 90—68%. A clinical assessment of low likelihood, 0% to 19%, was made in 26% of patients and was correct in 91%—207 of 228 patients. The clinical assessment was therefore more often correct in excluding than in identifying PE. In a majority of the patients, 64%, 569 of 887 patients, clinical assessment was of intermediate likelihood, 20% to 79%, which was noncommittal and did not help in management (12).

Combination of clinical assessment and the findings of ventilation/perfusion scan strengthen the diagnostic value of the noninvasive assessment. In PIOPED, among patients with clinical assessment of high probability and high probability lung scan, the diagnosis of PE was confirmed angiographically in 96%. Similarly, if both clinical assessment and the ventilation/perfusion scan were of low probability, diagnosis of PE was excluded in over 90% of the patients. The concordant diagnostic combinations were uncommon, occurring in only about 28% of the patients with suspected PE. The degree of certainty was much lower when either clinical assessment or ventilation/perfusion scan was of intermediate or low probability. If the clinical assessment was of high probability of PE and the scan was only of intermediate probability, only 66% of such patients had PE by angiography. Conversely, if the scan was rated as being of high probability and the clinical science probability was of only intermediate probability, then 88% of such patients had PE. If both assessments were of intermediate probability, only 28% of such patients had PE. Overall, the lower the probability of the scan for the likelihood of PE, the lesser was the value of clinical probability. PIOPED investigators pointed out that the prior clinical assessment in this study was done by the physicians experienced and interested in PE. The clinical assessment is likely less accurate in daily clinical practice.

In a separate study Quinn and Butler (25) showed that if all patients with the intermediate probability scan were treated, there would be a 97% chance of survival and about 86% chance of survival without major complications. If none of such patients were treated, survival would be 90%. Angiography would increase the survival to 97% and the complications-free survival to 94%. The authors conclude that the optimal strategy in patients with suspected PE and intermediate lung scan is pulmonary angiography (25).

XI. PULMONARY ANGIOGRAPHY

The generally agreed indication for pulmonary angiography in patients with suspected PE is an intermediate probability scan. The technique is considered the gold standard for diagnosis of acute PE. The criteria for identification of pulmonary embolus are either the identification of the trailing edge of an embolus obstructing a pulmonary vessel or the outline of an filling defect within the vessel surrounded by contrast material. The study should be performed within day or 2 after the initial symptoms. If delayed more, the partial or complete lysis may prevent the definitive identification of the thrombus in the pulmonary artery, and the study cannot confirm or exclude PE. The most common angiographic technique currently used in the United States is the selective angiography with a rapidly changed cut film or fluoroscopic spot films (26).

The safety of the procedure is still of concern to many clinicians in spite of the fact that in the PIOPED study fatal complications occurred in only five patients, 0.5%. All patients who died were seriously ill with underlying disease; one was moribund. Nonfatal major complications were reported in 1% of patients, and minor in 5%. The interobserver variability is very good, and in the PIOPED study the agreement was 98% with lobar PE, 96% with segmental, and only 66% with subsegmental embolism. The relatively low interobserver agreement in vessels graded as subsegmental indicates a need for subsegmental injections in this situation (12).

Several techniques have been used, including the superselective injection, wedged technique, flow-guided balloon studies, and balloon occlusion angiography. All these techniques decrease the dilution of the contrast by unopacified blood. Another technique that is used in efforts to improve the resolution is the subtraction angiogram. The technique requires patient cooperation to avoid movement artifacts, and some studies report an unacceptably high 25% of technically inadequate studies (26).

XII. DIAGNOSIS OF DVT

DVT is intimately associated with PE. Although not tested in a prospective manner, many physicians include presence or absence of DVT in their decision-making process in patients with suspected PE (27). Most of the thrombi detected in patients with a first episode of DVT have extended proximally, and these patients are at high risk for PE. Approximately 50% of the patients with proven DVT have scintigraphic evidence of silent PE. The isolated calf thrombosis is less often associated with PE, yet approximately 25% will extend proximally and become a threat for PE (6).

The gold standard for the diagnosis of DVT is still the contrast venography.

The test is very sensitive; out of 106 patients with a negative study, only two returned within 5 days with fully developed DVT, and none developed PE. The disadvantage of the method is that inadequate venograms occur in 20% patients. In addition, it is an invasive study with the use of contrast media.

Of the noninvasive tests venous ultrasonography or compression sonography is mostly used. The test allows visualization of the deep venous system of the legs. The single criterion of noncompressibility of the vein on pressure with the probe is the most accurate for detection of DVT, sensitivity, and specificity of 97%.

The Doppler ultrasonography utilizes the detection of the venous flow with the Doppler signal. The venous flow is typically low-pitched, changes with respiration, and can be augmented by squeezing the leg. With obstruction, the venous flow is constant and loses the relationship to respiration. These signs are sensitive for DVT in 65% to 100% range and specific in 72% to 100%. The comparison between the compression ultrasonography and Doppler sonography showed superiority of the real-time compression ultrasonography over the Doppler sonography. The addition of a color Doppler to conventional ultrasound equipment allows direct visualization of the flow. The combination of the two has not, however, been shown to be superior to standard compression ultrasonography alone.

Another noninvasive test used is impedance pletysmography. It is based on the principle that changes in blood volume lead to changes in the electrical resistance. A cuff inflated to 30 mm Hg is placed around the calf to occlude the venous flow. The changes in impedance during inflation and after release are recorded.

Indirect methods for detection of DVT depend either on incorporation of the radiolabeled fibrin into the accumulating thrombus or detection of products of fibrin degradation (D-dimers) (21).

XIII. DIAGNOSTIC STRATEGY

The Council on Thrombosis of the American Heart Association has developed the guidelines for the management of DVT and PE (28). As diagnostic approach to DVT they recommend the use of venous ultrasound in conjunction with clinical assessment. Note that in patients with high clinical probability of DVT, 24% of patients with negative venous ultrasound will still have venous thrombi detected on venography or serial testing.

The recommendations for diagnostic approach in patients with suspected PE are shown in Figure 1. In patients in whom initial evaluation, history and physical examination, electrocardiogram and chest radiography, possibly cardiac 2-D echo-Doppler study suggest alternative diagnosis, the further workups should be directed toward this diagnosis, and perfusion scan is not needed. Without alternative diagnosis, patients with clinically low, intermediate, or high probability for PE should have the lung scan performed. Normal or near-normal scan excludes PE. Abnormal scan of high probability concordant with clinical probability is

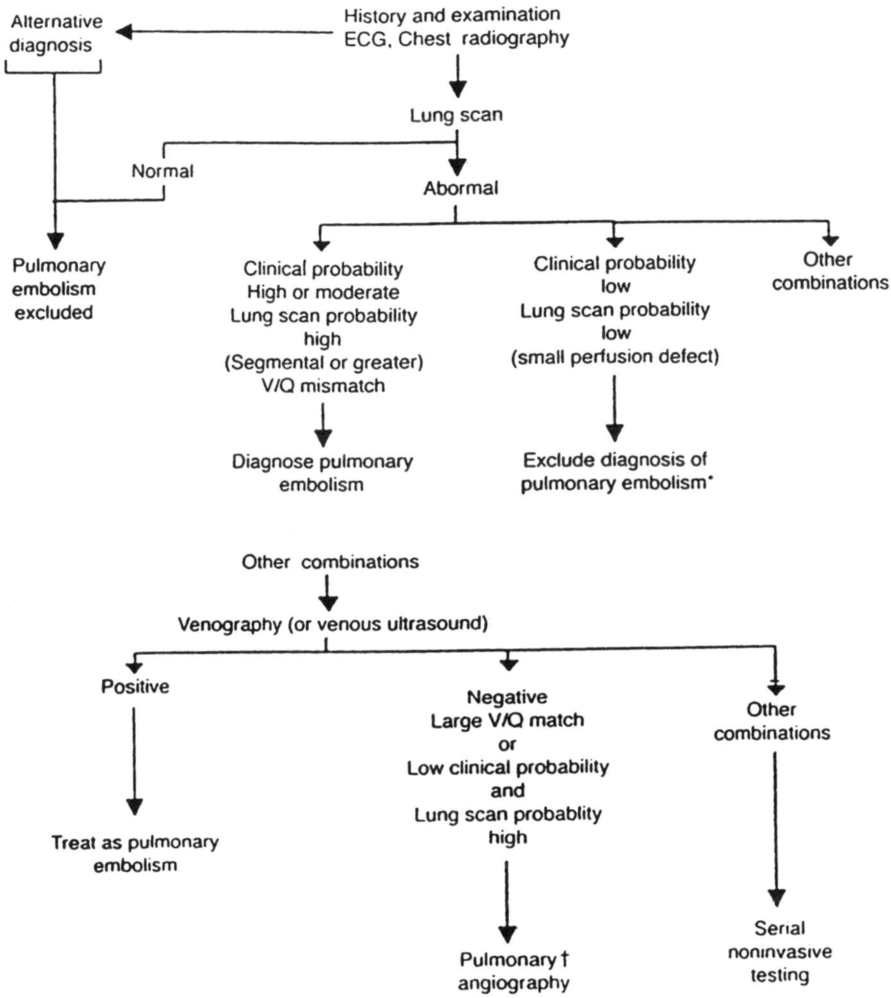

Figure 1 Recommendation for diagnostic approach in patients with suspected PE (From Ref. 28.)

diagnostic of PE. If the patient has a low clinical and lung scan probability for PE, most physicians will continue the workup with venous ultrasound to exclude DVT before excluding the diagnosis of PE. All other patients with suspected PE should have a venous ultrasound.

In the presence of DVT, the patient should be treated for PE. Pulmonary angiogram is reserved for patients with negative venous ultrasound who have intermediate or low probability lung scan irrespective of clinical probability for PE. Presence of high probability lung scan in patients with low clinical probability is also an indication for pulmonary angiography. Combinations of negative venous ultrasound and low clinical probability and intermediate lung scan or intermediate clinical probability and low probability scan are best managed by serial noninvasive testing.

XIV. TREATMENT

The objective of treatment of PE is to prevent local extension of the thrombus and recurrent thrombus embolization and to accelerate the spontaneous lysis of the thrombus. Spontaneous thrombolysis is the net effect between endogenous thrombolysis induced by locally released plasminogen activators and new fibrin deposition on the surface of the partially lysed thrombus. Anticoagulants indirectly promote lysis by prevention of new fibrin formation. Although there are no good randomized trials between anticoagulants and placebo, there is no doubt about the role of anticoagulants in DVT and PE. Studies done before introduction of anticoagulation reported mortality of approximately 20% in patients with PE (29). In comparison, the mortality in heparin arm of UPET trial (11) was only 9%.

Heparin is still the most widely used anticoagulant in early stages of PE (30). It acts immediately by catalyzing the inhibition of activated coagulation factor Xa and thrombin, by antithrombin factor III (AT-III). High doses are needed to inhibit the high local concentrations of thrombin, generated by the thrombus. Heparin should be initiated with an intravenous bolus of 5000 U followed by the intravenous infusion of about 1400 U/h. Weight-adjusted dose could also be used. This regimen consists of an intravenous bolus of 80 U/kg followed by an infusion of 18 U/h. The adequacy of anticoagulation/antithrombotic effect of heparin should be tested about 6 h after the bolus. The most commonly used test is activated partial thromboplastin time (aPTT). The therapeutic range is 1.5 to 3.0 times mean laboratory normal range or heparin level 0.2 to 0.4 U/ml measured by thrombin/protamine titration or 0.3 to 0.7 U/ml antifactor Xa. Twenty-four hours after the heparin bolus, the oral anticoagulation with warfarin should be started. Warfarin inhibits the synthesis of γ-carboxylated vitamin K-dependent coagulation factors (II, V, VII). Factor VII has a half-life of only 6 h, similar to the half-life of natural anticoagulant protein C. As the factor II has a half-life of 60 h, during the first 2 days the anticoagulant effect of warfarin reflects primarily the effects on factor VII. There is a possibility of transient hypercoagulable state with reduced levels of protein C and preserved activities of factor II during the first 24 h. The concept that antithrombotic effect of warfarin reflects its effect on factor II is the rationale for at least 4 days of overlap between heparin and coumadin therapy. Therefore the heparin infusion should be given for at least 5 days. Warfarin should be started with 10 mg/day. The effect of warfarin is routinely followed by prothrombin time

(PT). PT should be performed daily and adjusted warfarin dose to maintain INR between 2 and 3. Once therapeutic the PT should be checked three times during the first week, twice for the next 2 weeks, and then every other week. Therapy with warfarin should be continued for at least 6 weeks to 3 months if the patient has a reversible risk factor for DVT. The duration should be extended to 3 to 6 months in patients with idiopathic venous thrombosis or PE.

Subcutaneous heparin can be used safely and with efficacy after initial adequate starting dose of intravenous heparin of 5000 U heparin. The dose of subcutaneous heparin should be above 15,000 units to assure adequate bioavailability. The usual dose is 17,500 U/twice daily subcutaneously. The aPTT is performed 6 h after the morning injection and adjusted to maintain the midinterval aPTT at 1.5 to 3.0 times the control value. The subcutaneous administration of heparin is less advisable in patients in shock or in heart failure because of the poor and unreliable resorption.

Low-molecular-weight heparins (LMWH) prepared by the depolymerization of standard heparin have molecular weights of 4000 to 5000, in contrast to 12,000 to 16,000 of standard heparin (31). The bioavailability of subcutaneous LMWH is approximately 90% of the intravenous dose. In randomized trials, weight-adjusted subcutaneous LMWH (1 mg/kg/12 h) compared favorably to standard therapy with heparin for treatment and prophylaxis of DVT. Currently the drug is approved in the United States only for DVT prophylaxis after knee surgery in dose of 30 mg every 12 h (32).

Thrombin within the thrombus is poorly accessible to inhibition with heparin-AT-III because of the size of the complex. New antithrombins hirudin and hirulog that directly inhibit thrombin easily gain access to thrombin bound in the thrombus. These drugs are still experimental, tested primarily for the use in patients with coronary artery disease. Before treatment with anticoagulants, hemoglobin and platelet count should be obtained. Platelet count should be followed daily until heparin is stopped because of the possibility of heparin-induced thrombocytopenia. There are two forms—an early, benign reversible nonimmune thrombocytopenia, and a late, IgG-mediated immune thrombocytopenia. The mechanism of the early form is weak activation of platelets by heparin. The immune-mediated form is complicated by strong IgG-mediated plated activation and thrombotic complications, primarily DVT, less commonly intra-arterial thrombosis. Its incidence is approximately 1% at 7 days and 3% at 14 days in patients receiving infusion of heparin (3).

XV. THROMBOLYTIC THERAPY FOR PE

Although thrombolytic therapy with plasminogen activators seems very reasonable in patients with PE, the initial randomized study of urokinase and heparin, UPET, failed to show any difference in total mortality—7% and 9%, respectively

(11). The rate of recurrence was also similar. The urokinase accelerated the resolution rate of thrombi at 24 h but was associated with higher rate of bleeding—45%, compared to 27% with heparin. Similar outcomes were reported from a randomized trial of streptokinase and heparin (33). TPA, given 100 mg over 2 h or 0.6 mg/kg bolus over 2 min also did not improve survival compared to standard dose of heparin (34–36). Again, the perfusion was improved early after administration, within 24 h. At 7 days the perfusion was similar in the two groups of patients (37). Randomized trials also failed to show any benefit of one thrombolytic agent over the other (38–40).

The trials did not have the power to assess the effect of thrombolytic therapy on mortality. With presumptive rate of mortality of PE at 9%, more than 1000 patients would be needed to show the difference in mortality. In patients with PE presenting in shock, the mortality is over 30%, yet fewer than 10% of patients with PE present in shock (41). Furthermore, according to the Thrombolysis in Pulmonary Embolism (TIPE) survey (42), only about half of patients presenting with PE would be eligible for thrombolytic therapy. Therefore very large studies are needed to address the issue of total mortality in patients with PE, similar to the recent megatrials in patients with myocardial infarction. In the recent AHA guidelines, thrombolytic therapy is recommended for massive PE and for patients with major PE and syncope, hypotension, severe hypoxemia, or heart failure. Thrombolytic therapy should also be considered for patients with submassive embolism and underlying heart or pulmonary disease (28).

Of the thrombolytic agents that were approved for use in patients with PE, streptokinase is recommended to be started with 250,000 U over 30 min, followed by 100,000 U/h over 24 h. For urokinase, the standard dose is 4400 IU/kg over 10 min followed by the same dose per kilogram per hour for the next 12 to 24 h. The experience with single bolus dose of urokinase is still limited. TPA has been approved in a dose of 100 mg over 2 h. Bolus dose of TPA appears very appealing because of its ease of use.

In general, thrombolytic therapy has not gained very wide acceptance for the treatment for PE mainly because there is no clear-cut advantage over treatment with heparin.

XVI. CAVAL INTERRUPTION

Anticoagulation is a standard treatment for acute DVT and PE with adjunct thrombolytic therapy for massive PE or hemodynamic instability. The caval interruption either surgical or by intercaval devices is used only exceptionally (43).

The indications for the venous interruptions that are largely agreed on are contraindications to anticoagulation, anticoagulation-induced bleeding, PE in spite of adequate anticoagulation, and after pulmonary embolectomy. More controversial are the indications for prophylactic use in high-risk patients with extensive and progressive DVT, in patients with minimal cardiopulmonary reserve or severe pulmonary hypertension, cor pulmonale, severe heart failure, or following surgical pulmonary embolectomy.

The transvenous devices are currently used in the vast majority of the patients considered for caval interruption. The initial experience was with the Mobin/Uddin umbrella filter. Although most of the patients were anticoagulated, the PE recurrent rate was high; about 12% and the thrombotic occlusion of the inferior vena cava occurred in up to 45%. The rate of proximal migration of the filter was 0.4%. The Greenfield filter is currently used most. The device is commonly placed percutaneously through the right femoral vein. Clinically evident recurrent PE rate occurs on average in 2% to 3%, and occlusion rate in only 5%. Other devices that are occasionally used are Bird Nest Filter, Simon Nitinol Filter, or interruption of the vena cava flow with Hunter's balloon. The surgical ligation of the inferior vena cava with an external clip placed via laparatomy has been considered for septic embolizations only because with intracaval devices small thrombi can pass the obstruction and cause septic emboli to the lungs. The second possibility is the potential for paradoxical embolization through patent foramen ovale or atrium septum defect when small thrombi could cause devastating neurological defects.

XVII. SURGICAL THROMBECTOMY

Surgical removal of PE is of limited benefit. The mortality is extremely high, and most institutions do not have the resources or personnel for this type of surgery. This is in contrast to elective pulmonary endarterectomy in patients with embolic pulmonary hypertension. This operation has been available for years, especially from the group in San Diego, which has the largest experience with the procedure (44).

XVIII. CATHETER EMBOLECTOMY

The use of the catheter pulmonary embolectomy is performed either with the disruption of the embolus by catheter during selective angiography or by retrieval of the embolus with a balloon-tip catheter from more distal segments of pulmonary arteries. There are many reports of a successful hemodynamic recovery of the patients after this procedure (45). Nevertheless, the procedure is experimental and reserved for centers with a special interest in the procedure.

REFERENCES

1. Alpert JS, Dalen JE. Epidemiology and natural history of venous thromboembolism. Prog Cardiovasc Dis 1994; 36(6):417–422.
2. Anderson FA, Jr, Wheeler HB, Goldberg RJ, et al. A population-based perspective of

the hospital incidence and case-fatality rates of deep vein thrombosis and pulmonary embolism. Arch Intern Med 1991; 151:933–938.

3. Cairns JA, Hirsh J, Lewis HD, Resnekov L, Theroux P. Antithrombotic agents in coronary artery disease. Chest 1992; 102:456S–481S.
4. Dalen JE. Pulmonary embolism and systemic in patients with acute myocardial infarction. In: Francis GS, Alpert JS eds. Coronary Care. 2nd ed. Little, Brown, Company, Boston: 1995:361–365.
5. Grines CL. Non-thrombolytic pharmacologic therapy for acute myocardial infarction. In: Anderson JL, ed. Modern Management of AMI in the Community Hospital. New York: Marcel Dekker, 1991:119–135.
6. Carter CJ. The natural history and epidemiology of venous thrombosis. Prog Cardiovasc Dis 1994; 36(6):423–438.
7. Nachman RL, Silverstein R. Hypercoagulable states. Ann Intern Med. 1993; 119: 819–827.
8. Jardin F, Dubourg O, Gueret P, Delorme G, Bourdarias JP. Quantitative two-dimensional echocardiography in massive pulmonary embolism: emphasis on ventricular interdependence and leftward septal displacement. Am J Coll Cardiol 1987; 10(6):1201–1206.
9. Stein PD, Saltzman HA, Weg JG. Clinical characteristics of patients with acute pulmonary embolism. Am J Cardiol 1991; 68:1723–1724.
10. Rubinstein I, Murray D, Hoffstein V. Fatal pulmonary emboli in hospitalized patients. Arch Intern Med 1988; 148:1425–1426.
11. Urokinase Pulmonary Embolism Trial Study Group. Urokinase Pulmonary Embolism Trial. JAMA 1970; 214:2163–2172.
12. PIOPED Investigators. Value of the ventilation/perfusion scan in acute pulmonary embolism. JAMA 1990; 263:2753–2759.
13. Simpson RJ, Podolak RP, Mangano CA, et al. Vagal syncope during recurrent pulmonary embolism. JAMA 1983; 249:390–394.
14. Markisz JA. Radiologic and nuclear medicine diagnosis. In: Goldhaber SZ ed. Pulmonary Embolism and Deep Vein Thrombosis. Philadelphia: W.B. Saunders Company, 1985:41–44.
15. Stein PD, Dalen JE, McIntyre KM, et al. The electrocardiogram in acute pulmonary embolism. Prog Cardiovasc Dis 1975; 17:247–254.
16. Come PC. Echocardiographic evaluation of pulmonary embolism and its response to therapeutic interventions. Chest 1992; 101:151S–171S.
17. Farfel Z, Shechter M, Vered Z, Rath S, Goor D, Gafni J. Review of echocardiographically diagnosed right heart entrapment of pulmonary emboli-in-transit with emphasis on management. Am Heart J 1986; 113:171–178.
18. Chan RKM, Johns JA, Calafiore P. Clinical implications of the morphological features of central pulmonary artery thromboemboli shown by transoesophageal echocardiography. Br Heart J 1994; 72:58–62.
19. Cheriex EC, Sreeram N, Eussen YFJM, Pieters FAA, Wellens HJJ. Cross sectional Doppler echocardiography as the initial technique for the diagnosis of acute pulmonary embolism. Br Heart J 1994; 72:52–57.
20. Cvitanic O, Marino PL. Improved use of arterial blood gas analysis in suspected pulmonary embolism. Chest 1989; 95:48–51.

21. Koopman MMW, van Beek EJR, ten Cate JW. Diagnosis of deep vein thrombosis. Prog Cardiovasc Dis 1994; 37:1–12.
22. Stein PD, Gottschalk A. Critical review of ventilation/perfusion lung scans in acute pulmonary embolism. Prog Cardiovasc Dis 1994; 37(1):13–24.
23. Goldhaber SZ. Strategies for diagnosis. In: Goldhaber SZ, ed. Pulmonary Embolism and Deep Vein Thrombosis. Philadelphia: W.B. Saunders Company, 1985: 79.
24. Stein PD, Hull RD, Saltzman HA, Pineo G. Strategy for diagnosis of patients with suspected acute pulmonary embolism. Chest 1993; 103:1553–1559.
25. Quinn RJ, Butler SP. A decision analysis approach to the treatment of patients with suspected pulmonary emboli and an intermediate probability lung scan. Nucl Med 1991; 2050–2055.
26. Greenspan RH. Pulmonary angiography and the diagnosis of pulmonary embolism. Prog Cardiovasc Dis 1994; 37:93–106.
27. Henschke CI, Mateescu I, Yankelevitz DF. Changing practice patterns in the workup of pulmonary embolism. Chest 1995; 107:940–945.
28. Hirsh J, Hoak J. Management of deep vein thrombosis and pulmonary embolism. Circulation 1996; 93:2212–2245.
29. Pineo GF, Hull RD. Classical anticoagulant therapy for venous thromboembolism. Prog Cardiovasc Dis 1994; 37:59–70.
30. Levine M, Gent M, Hirsh J, et al. A comparison of low molecular weight heparin administered primarily at home with unfractioned heparin administered in the hospital for deep vein thrombosis. N Engl J Med 1996; 334:677–681.
31. Leclerc JR, Geerts WH, Desjardin L, et al. Prevention of venous thromboembolism after knee arthroplasty. A randomized, double-blind trial comparing enoxaparin with warfarin. Ann Intern Med 1996; 124:619–626.
32. Tibbut DA, Davies JA, Anderson JA, et al. Comparison by controlled clinical trial of streptokinase and heparin in the treatment of major pulmonary embolism. Br Med J 1974; 1:343–347.
33. Goldhaber SZ. Tissue plasminogen activator in acute pulmonary embolism. Chest 1989; 95:282S–289S.
34. Levine M, Hirsh J, Weitz J, et al. A randomized trial of a single bolus dosage regimen of recombinant tissue plasminogen activator in patients with acute pulmonary embolism. Chest 1990; 98:1473–1479.
35. PIOPED Investigators. Tissue plasminogen activator for the treatment of acute pulmonary embolism. Chest 1990; 97:528–533.
36. Goldhaber SZ, Haire WD, Feldstein ML, et al. Alteplase versus heparin in acute pulmonary embolism: a randomized trial assessing right ventricular function and perfusion. Lancet 1993; 341:507–511.
37. Urokinase Pulmonary Embolism Group. Urokinase-streptokinase embolism trial. JAMA 1974; 229:1606–1613.
38. Goldhaber SZ, Kessler CM, Heitt JA, et al. Randomized controlled trial of recombinant tissue-type plasminogen activator versus urokinase in the treatment of acute pulmonary embolism. Lancet 1988; 2:293–298.
39. Goldhaber SZ, Kessler CM, Heitt JA, et al. Recombinant tissue-type plasminogen activator versus a novel dosing regimen of urokinase in acute pulmonary embolism: a randomized controlled multicenter trial. J Am Coll Cardiol 1992; 20:24–30.

40. Carson JL, Kelley MA, Duff A, et al. The clinical course of pulmonary embolism. N Engl J Med 1992; 326:1240–1245.
41. Terrin M, Goldhaber SZ, Thompson B, TIPE Investigators. Selection of patients with acute pulmonary embolism for thrombolytic therapy. Chest 1989; 95:279S–281S.
42. Bergqvist D. The role of vena caval interruption in patients with venous thromboembolism. Prog Cardiovasc Dis 1994; 37(1):25–37.
43. Viner SM, Bagg BR, Auger WR, Ford GT. The management of pulmonary hypertension secondary to chronic thromboembolic disease. Prog Cardiovasc Dis 1994; 37: 79–92.
44. Timsit JF, Reynaud P, Meyer G, Sors H. Pulmonary embolectomy by catheter device in massive pulmonary embolism. Chest 1991: 100:655–658.

14

Acute Renal Failure in the CCU

KHAJA R. AHMED, MINHTRI NGUYEN, and JEREMY SCHWIEGER

University of California, Los Angeles, School of Medicine, Los Angeles, California

JULIEN BOHÉ

Centre Hospitalier Lyon-Sud, Lyon, France

I. INTRODUCTION

Acute renal failure frequently complicates the course of patients with severe underlying cardiovascular disease. Although the differential diagnosis can be divided as usual into prerenal, renal, and postrenal categories and include most common causes of renal insufficiency such as various causes of renal hemodynamic insults (i.e., volume depletion secondary to overdiuresis), drug toxicity, and obstructive uropathy in an older medicated group of patients, certain diagnoses are more specific to this patient population. The presence of congestive heart failure (CHF) is the most common cardiac disease affecting renal function. CHF may be defined in a broad sense as an inability of the heart to maintain adequate tissue perfusion under various physiological conditions. The impairment of tissue perfusion may occur as a result of a decrease in cardiac output or an increase in the capacity of the vascular tree (high output failure). The causes of congestive heart failure may be acute as in myocardial infarction (MI), rupture of chordae-tendinae, pulmonary embolism, and cardiac arrhythmias or chronic as in some cardiomyopathies and when secondary to hypertensive and valvular heart disease. Regardless of the etiology, impaired perfusion of the kidneys results in renal insufficiency that is described as prerenal azotemia. Early in CHF several neural, endocrine, and structural compensatory mechanisms are activated that tend to ameliorate congestive heart failure and preserve glomerular filtration rate

(GFR). However, a further decline in myocardial function or an additional renal insult may overwhelm these compensatory phenomena and frank prerenal azotemia develops. Other common causes of renal failure in this setting are cardiac catheterization which may lead to radio contrast-induced acute tubular necrosis (1,2) or atheroembolic renal disease. Major vascular surgery (i.e., involving the aorta) may cause renal ischemia from suprarenal aortic clamping and intravascular blood loss. Coronary artery bypass surgery may result in decreased renal perfusion from preoperative volume depletion, intraoperative blood loss, and hypotension during anesthesia and prolonged bypass (3,4). Unfortunately, cardiac patients are often predisposed to postoperative ischemic renal failure because of preexisting renal insufficiency, volume depletion, and age. When sufficiently severe, hemodynamic renal insults in the surgical or nonsurgical cardiac case can lead to acute tubular necrosis (ATN), a not immediately reversible form of ischemic renal injury: patchy tubular obstruction from sloughed tubular cell debris of mainly proximal and thick ascending limb of Henle origin, and back leak of glomerular filtrate across a now damaged tubule leads to a marked reduction in GFR. Recovery of GFR may take days to a few weeks, and the absence of adequate renal function markedly complicates the clinical management of the cardiac patient in the coronary care unit.

The cellular mechanisms by which ischemic injury occurs are complex and will not be described here. The reader is referred to several excellent reviews on the subject (5,6). Rather, in this chapter we will concentrate on reviewing the physiological determinants of renal blood flow and GFR under normal conditions, then the complex systemic as well as renal compensatory mechanisms that come into play to maintain cardiac output and GFR in the setting of CHF. Table 1 describing the diagnostic features of prerenal azotemia vs ATN follows. The last section is devoted to the management of renal failure in cardiac patients. It includes a brief analysis of some of the more common forms of drug therapy as well as the crucial role of renal replacement therapies including hemodialysis, peritoneal dialysis, and, finally, continuous methods of ultrafiltration (i.e., fluid removal) and dialysis in patients with severe underlying cardiac disease.

II. BACKGROUND

A. Regulation of Plasma Volume

1. *Role of the Kidney*

Sodium and its attendant anion chloride constitute the major extracellular osmoles, hence the extracellular fluid (ECF) volume and the plasma volume are proportional to the amount of sodium chloride present in the body. The kidney plays a central role in sodium homeostasis and therefore in regulation of the plasma volume. A fall in effective arterial volume, in CHF, or a decrease in plasma volume in volume depletion is sensed by pressure receptors in the vasculature as well as receptors in the kidney leading to activation of the renin-aldosterone-

Table 1 Differential Diagnosis of Acute Renal Failure in CHF

	Prerenal failure	ATN	Cortical necrosis	
Pathophysiology	Renal adaptation to hypoperfusion No structural kidney damage	Patchy, tubular cell necrosis	Severe cortical necrosis Loss of kidney function	
Reversibility	Complete and rapid with reperfusion	Usually complete after reperfusion, but delayed (few days to few weeks) until tubular cell regeneration	Irreversible	
GFR (ml/min)	> 20	> 20		
Urine output (ml/day)	low	< 400 (oliguric) > 400 (nonoliguric)		
Urine osmolality (mOsm/kg H_2O)	> 500	Isosthenuria		Considerable overlap between groups
U/P urea	> 8	< 3		Predominantly of value in oliguric patients
U/P creatinine	> 40	< 20		
U_{Na} (mEq/L)	< 20	> 40		Highly influenced by diuretics
Renal failure index (RFI) (%): $U_{Na}/(U/P)_{Creat}$	< 1	> 1		Little overlap when oliguric patients are compared
Fractional excretion of filtered Na: (FE_{Na}) (%): $(U/P)_{Na}/(U/P)_{Creat}$	< 1	> 1		Little overlap when oliguric patients are compared
Urinary sediments	normal	Granular casts Tubular epithelial cells Tubule cell casts		

angiotensin (RAA) system, the sympathetic nervous system, and increased production of antidiuretic hormone or ADH. These pressor stimuli not only increase cardiac output and peripheral vascular resistance, but also inhibit sodium excretion by the kidneys, thus tending to restore the plasma volume. The vasoconstrictive effects of increased AII, epinephrine, endothelin, and ADH are counteracted by the increased production of vasodilatory mediators including prostaglandins, nitric oxide, and atrial natriuretic peptide or ANP. These agents have a vasodilatory and natriuretic effect and play a particularly important role in preserving renal blood flow. Conversely, an elevated renal interstitial hydrostatic pressure as a result of increased renal perfusion pressure promotes natriuresis (7,8). A similar phenomenon can be seen as a result of increased hepatic interstitial hydrostatic pressure (9), although the precise mechanisms remain unclear. A number of excellent reviews have been published on these subjects.

2. *Arterial and Venous Baroreceptors*

Receptors on the arterial as well as the venous side sense the filling of the vascular tree and convey neural impulses to the central nervous system (CNS). Subsequent efferent stimuli to the kidneys alter renal blood flow, GFR, and tubular reabsorption so as to conserve or excrete sodium in the case of circulatory underfilling or overfilling, respectively.

Low-pressure venous receptors (10,11) are present in the atria and the large veins of the heart and sense what has been referred to as the "central blood volume." Overfilling of the venous circulation results in receptors stretching and increased afferent stimuli to the CNS that in turn exerts a negative feedback on the efferent vasoconstrictive sympathetic impulses, leading to a decrease in renal vascular tone, an increase in renal blood flow, GFR, and natriuresis. The physiological role of these receptors can be demonstrated by several experimental maneuvers (i.e., head-out water immersion (12), supine position, negative pressure breathing, and weightlessness) which increase the central blood volume and initiate a brisk natriuresis. Conversely, maneuvers that decrease central blood volume (i.e., erect posture, application of leg tourniquets, and positive pressure) lead to sodium retention.

High-pressure stretch receptors in the major arteries such as the aortic arch and carotids sense the fullness of the arterial system as reflected by the "effective arterial volume," a term introduced by Peter (13) to describe the relationship of the arterial blood volume to the vascular capacity. A fall in effective arterial volume leads to afferent stimuli to the CNS that result in increased sympathetic outflow, increased renin and ADH production, and inhibition of natriuresis.

In CHF, the high-pressure arterial receptors play a dominant role despite chronic distension of the atria and veins and in part because of the gradual desensitization of the low-pressure receptors. The venous circulation distension should lead to natriuresis as described above. However, impulses arising from the arterial receptors which sense a fall in effective arterial volume override the venous stimuli, leading to further volume retention (14,15). This was elegantly demonstrated by Epstein et al. (16) in patients who developed traumatic arteriovenous fistulae. Despite a decrease in venous filling, temporary closure of the fistulae led to a brisk natriuresis following the increase in arterial filling. When the fistulae were allowed to reopen, sodium retention recurred, although the venous circulation reexpansion should have led to natriuresis. Furthermore, surgical or pharmacological denervation of efferent pathways from the arterial receptors inhibit the natriuretic response to volume expansion, also demonstrating the role of the arterial receptors in volume regulation (17,18).

B. Renal Hemodynamics

Three key steps are involved in maintaining renal solute and water homeostatic functions: renal blood flow must be sufficient to adequately perfuse the glomeruli; a glomerular filtrate must be produced through ultrafiltration of renal plasma across the glomerular capillaries; and modulation of tubular reabsorption of solutes and water must reflect underlying hemodynamic conditions. We will briefly review these concepts to provide an understanding of the impact of altered cardiac function on renal function.

1. *Regulation of Renal Blood Flow*

The kidney receives 20% of the total cardiac output, approximately 1250 ml/min. Renal blood flow (RBF) is determined by the cardiac output and the ratio of the systemic and intrarenal vascular resistance. Renal vascular resistance occurs at mainly two sites in the glomerulus—the afferent artery (R_A), and the efferent artery (R_E). The sum of these resistances ($R_A + R_E$) determines the total blood flow to the individual nephron (Q_A) and therefore the single nephron glomerular filtration rate (SNGFR). The difference in these two resistances ($R_E - R_A$) determines the intraglomerular capillary hydrostatic pressure (P_{GC}), also an important determinant of the SNGFR. Under normal circumstances, two-thirds of the resistance occurs at the afferent arteriole. Several local, hormonal, and neurogenic factors can affect the vascular smooth muscle tone and hence the resistances offered by the efferent and afferent artery (see Table 2).

2. *Regulation of GFR*

The glomerulus produces a relatively protein-free plasma. The main determinants of GFR include the difference between the hydrostatic and oncotic pressures that exist across the glomerular capillaries. The SNGFR is derived from the following formula proposed by Brenner (19,20) (Fig. 1):

$$SNGFR = K_f[(P_{GC} - P_T) - (\overline{\Pi}_{GC} - \Pi_T)]$$

Table 2 Hormonal Factors Affecting Renal Vasculature and Sodium Excretion in Heart Failure

Vasoconstrictors and/or antinatriuretic	Vasodilators and/or natriuretics
Renin, angiotensin II	Atrial natriuretic peptide
Norepinephrine	Prostaglandin E_2, I_2
Vasopressin	Kinins
Endothelin	Endothelial-derived relaxing factor (NO)
Thromboxane A_2	Dopamine

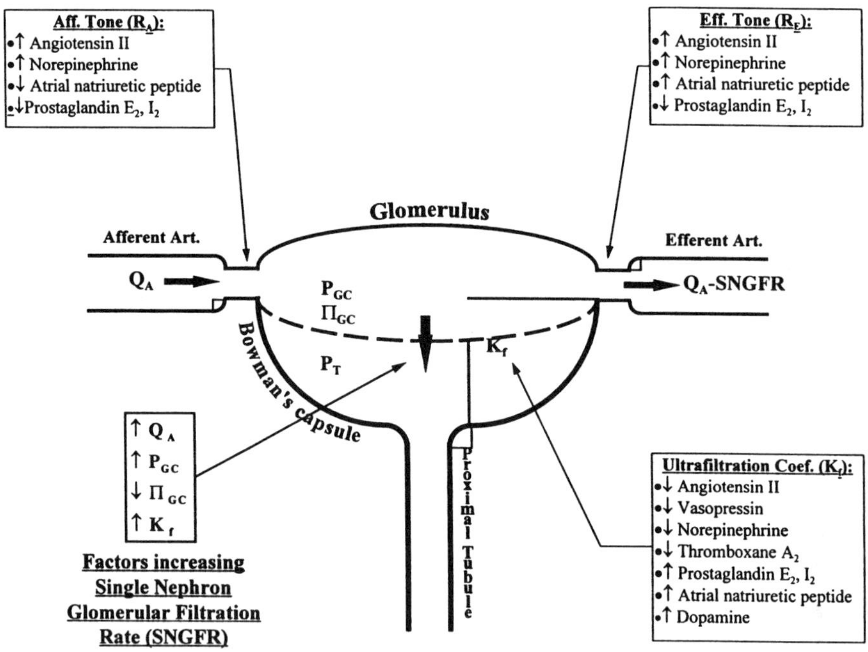

Figure 1 Glomerular hemodynamics. (Figures 1–4: various factors affecting afferent and efferent arterial tone, ultrafiltration coefficient and SNGFR. K_f, ultrafiltration coefficient; P_{GC}, glomerular capillary hydrostatic pressure; P_T, Bowman's space hydrostatic pressure; Π_{GC}, glomerular oncotic pressure; Q_A, glomerular blood flow; R_A, afferent arteriolar resistance; R_E, efferent arteriolar resistance; SNGFR, single nephron glomerular filtration rate.)

where SNGFR is the SNGFR, K_f the ultrafiltration coefficient, P_{GC} the glomerular capillary hydrostatic pressure, P_T the Bowman's space hydrostatic pressure, $\overline{\Pi}_{GC}$ the mean glomerular oncotic pressure, and Π_T the Bowman's space oncotic pressure. P_{GC} and Π_T are forces favoring filtration; P_T and $\overline{\Pi}_{GC}$ are forces opposing filtration. P_{GC} is thus the main driving force for ultrafiltration and is derived from the systemic arterial pressure. It results from the difference between efferent arteriolar resistance and afferent arteriolar resistance ($R_E - R_A$). The vascular tone of these vessels, and hence the R_A and R_E, are regulated by AII, PG, catecholamines, kinins, nor epinephrine, and several other factors. Since Bowman's space hydrostatic pressure (P_T) is relatively constant in experimental models, the net transglomerular hydrostatic gradient (DP) tends to remain within a narrow range under normal physiologic conditions (33 to 35 mm Hg).

Since under these same conditions only trivial amounts of protein are filtered, the Bowman's space oncotic pressure or $\Pi_T \approx O$. However, Π_{GC} increases along the length of the glomerular capillary as plasma is extracted through ultrafiltration and the intracapillary protein concentration increases. Thus when Π_{GC} equals DP, filtration ceases. The ultrafiltration coefficient (K_f) reflects the intrinsic permeability of the glomerular capillary and is proportional to the water and small solute permeability of the capillary wall and the capillary surface area available for filtration.

In summary, SNGFR varies directly with Q_A, Δ_P, and K_f and inversely with Π_{GC}.

3. *Regulation of Tubular Absorption*

The oncotic and hydrostatic pressures with the peritubular vessels that perfuse the renal tubules exert a powerful influence on tubular reabsorption of water and solutes through Starlings forces (21,22). Because the peritubular vessels arise distally from the efferent arteriole, alterations in the hydrostatic and oncotic pressures in the efferent arteriole are reflected downstream in the peritubular vessels. As blood flows from the afferent to the efferent arteriole, extraction of plasma water in the glomerulus leads to a gradual increase in the protein concentration of the capillary. Similarly, vasoactive components that result in an increase or a decrease in glomerular hydrostatic pressure can have a significant impact on tubular sodium and water reabsorption (23,24). In particular, increased angiotensin II levels selectively exert a powerful vasoconstrictive effect on the efferent arteriole resulting in a fall in RBF but preservation of GFR, thus creating an increase in the glomerular filtration fraction (FF = GFR/RBF), an increase in efferent arteriolar protein concentration, and a fall in efferent hydrostatic pressure. These changes in efferent and therefore the peritubular vessels favor tubular reabsorption of fluid and solutes in the proximal tubule. The opposite sequence of events occurs in the case of volume expansion.

Renal blood flow through the vasa recta, which are also branches of the efferent arterioles, affects the medullary concentration gradient. The higher this gradient, the greater the reabsorption of sodium and water in the medulla. Decreased medullary blood flow, resulting from norepinephrine (NE) and AII-induced vasoconstriction tends to preserve the medullary osmotic gradient and enhance sodium and fluid reabsorption. Prostaglandins, on the other hand, increase medullary blood flow leading to washout of the medullary concentration gradient and a decrease in tubular reabsorption.

III. RENAL ADAPTATION TO CARDIAC FAILURE

Several counterregulatory mechanisms are called into play in CHF. These include the sympathetic nervous system, the renin-angiotensin-aldosterone (RAA) system, atrial natriuretic peptide, and urodilatin, prostaglandins, and endothelin. We will briefly review their roles in maintaining renal perfusion and function in the setting of cardiac disease.

A. Sympathetic System

The kidney is richly innervated by the sympathetic system. In CHF, as cardiac output falls, the sympathetic system is activated (25–27), possibly by depression in the baroreflex and perhaps cardioreflex control of sympathetic nerve activity (28,29). The pressor and inotropic effects of NE serve to maintain effective arterial volume. In the kidney NE facilitates sodium retention by: 1. the reduction of RBF and GFR by directly causing afferent and efferent arteriolar vasoconstriction and by stimulating the release of renin; 2. the enhanced proximal tubular reabsorption of solutes and water, an effect that is magnified by the potentiating actions of AII (30); 3. the increased sodium reabsorption in the loop of Henle by decreasing medullary blood flow and preserving the medullary concentration gradient. NE also stimulates ADH production and thus water retention (31) (Fig. 2).

Although the increased adrenergic stimulation has an initial beneficial hemodynamic effect in early CHF, the resultant increase in afterload and the pro-arrythmogenic effect of NE over the long term impact negatively on the cardiovascular system as a whole. NE levels correlate directly with the severity of CHF and are also predictive of worse outcome (8,32–34). Some studies have shown that the judicious use of β-blockers in CHF can have a beneficial effect on these patients (35,36).

B. Renin Angiotensin System

The RAA system is also activated early in CHF and renin production by the kidney increases in response to three main stimuli: baroreceptor stimulation; sympathetic nerve stimulation; and a fall in chloride concentration in the macula

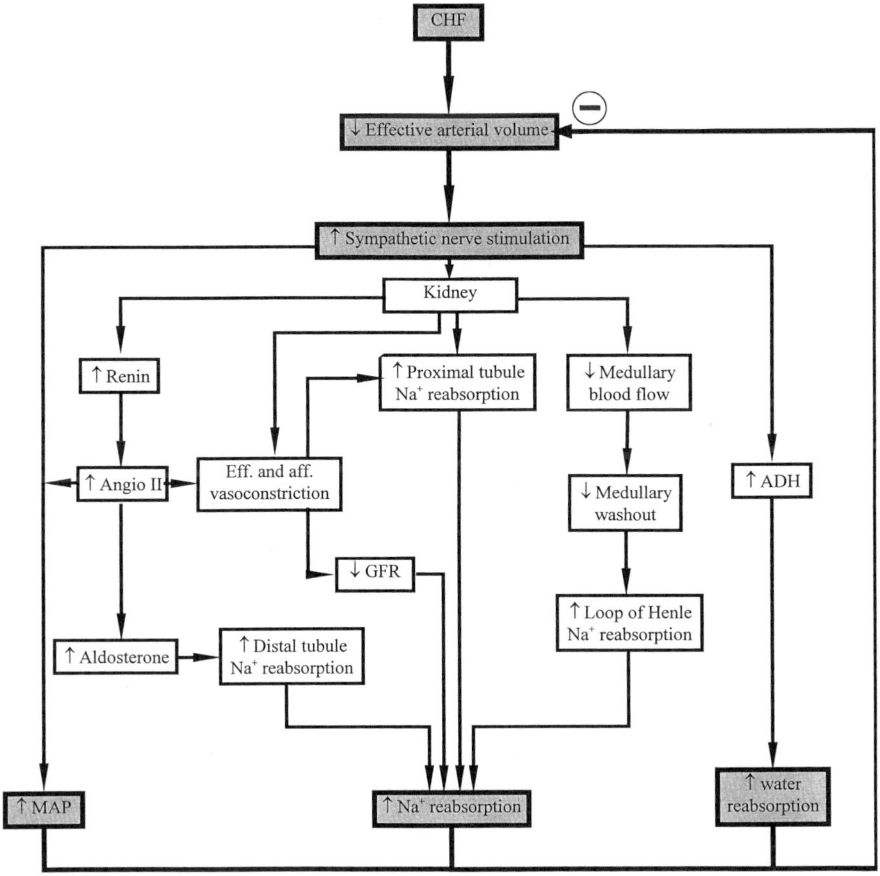

Figure 2 Activation of sympathetic nervous system in CHF.

densa. Renin converts angiotensin substrate produced in the liver to angiotensin I that is then converted by angiotensin-converting enzyme (ACE), produced by endothelial cells, to AII. AII is a pleiotropic hormone, best known as a powerful vasoconstrictor. This constrictor effect of AII also occurs at three sites in the glomerulus: at the efferent and afferent arterioles, and at the mesangial cells. As discussed above, the preferential effect on the efferent vs. the afferent arteriole serves to maintain GFR despite a fall in glomerular blood flow (37) and Kf due to mesangial cell contraction. However, high AII levels result in increased afferent arteriolar responsiveness to its effects (38) which further reduces glomerular blood flow. AII also directly stimulates sodium reabsorption in the proximal tubule (39) by enhancing the activity of the Na^+/H^+ exchanger and the Na/K-ATPase (39,40); indirectly by the resulting efferent arteriolar vasoconstriction (41); and by augmenting norepinephrine release (42). Its other effects include modulation of the tubuloglomerular feedback mechanism (43), a powerful dipsogen effect, and stimulation of renal prostaglandin production. The latter effect serves to counterbalance some of AII's vasoconstrictive and sodium- and water-retaining effects (Fig. 3).

Activation of the RAA system in CHF thus has complex effects. AII has been shown to be a proliferative and angiogenic agent. Although it serves to maintain

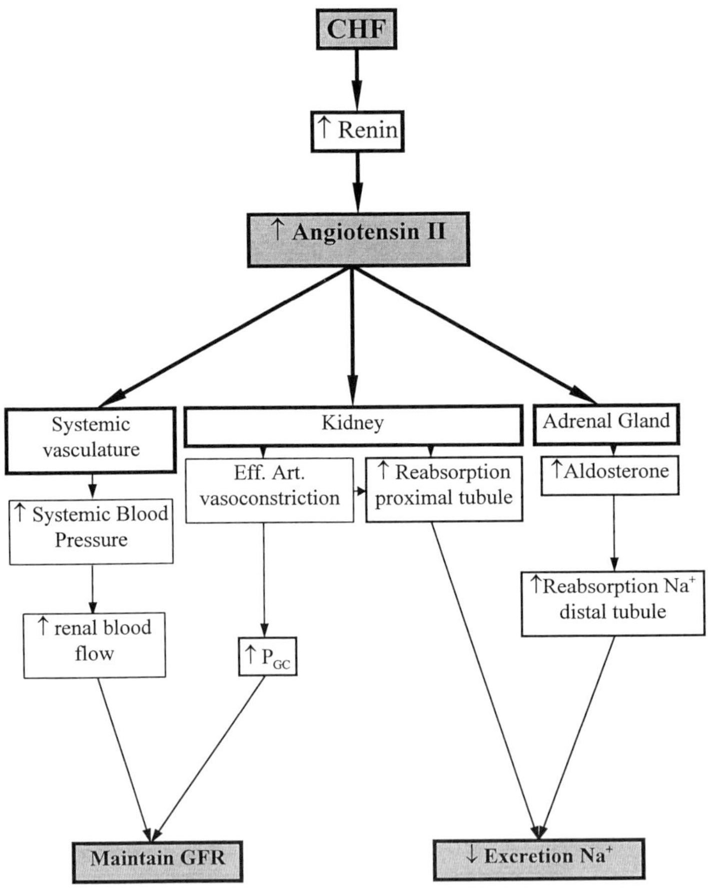

Figure 3 Effects of angiotensin II activation in CHF.

systemic blood pressure and effective arterial volume, over the long term RAA activation may have potentially deleterious effects. Several recent studies have pointed to the positive impact of the ACE inhibitor on systemic hemodynamics, renal function, and the long-term prognosis of CHF patients (44–47).

C. Atrial Natriuretic Peptide (ANP)

This octapeptide was first discovered in 1981 by De Bold (48) and belongs to a family of related peptides which include brain natriuretic peptide (BNP), urodilatin, and others (49,50). These peptides share the same receptors and have similar biological actions (51) but may have some specific functions, as their regulation differs in many pathophysiological conditions (52). In the heart, ANP is mainly produced and stored in granules localized in the atria (53), and BNP is produced by the ventricles. The most important stimulus for ANP release is atrial wall stretch and not atrial pressure (54,55). Other stimuli include the baroreceptor system (56) and intravascular sodium concentration and volume (57). There are two types of ANP receptors: a biologically active receptor coupled by guanylate cyclase the binding of which leads to ANP's various biologic actions, and a second receptor, the so-called clearance receptor, that is not coupled with guanylate cyclase and serves to internalize ANP for lysosomal degradation. ANP's principal effect on the kidney is natriuresis (58–60), which is mediated via the following actions (Fig. 4):

1. ANP constricts the efferent arteriole and dilates the afferent arteriole, thereby increasing GFR by increasing P_{GC}. It has no effect on renal glomerular blood flow (Q_A), however. Interestingly, ANP is the only known endogenous substance that may increase GFR in face of a decrease in blood pressure.
2. ANP inhibits renin secretion by increasing the sodium load to the macula densa. ANP also inhibits the secretion of aldosterone directly (61–63) as well many of the effects of AII, including sodium reabsorption (64–66).
3. ANP shifts fluid from the intravascular to the interstitial compartment by increasing capillary hydraulic permeability (67,68).

The role of ANP in normal physiology is unclear. Acute infusion of ANP in physiologic ranges has no effects on blood pressure, yet high doses induce a fall in systemic blood pressure. Chronic low-dose administration may induce reduction in systemic blood pressure by a sustained natriuretic effect. In CHF, ANP mostly acts as a counterregulatory hormone, effecting natriuresis and counteracting the efects of sympathetic and RAA stimulation. Normal plasma levels of ANP in humans range between 10 and 50 pmol/L. In CHF patients these levels may be elevated up to fivefold of normal with wide interpatient variability (69,70). ANP levels have been shown to correlate directly with right atrial pressure, and in-

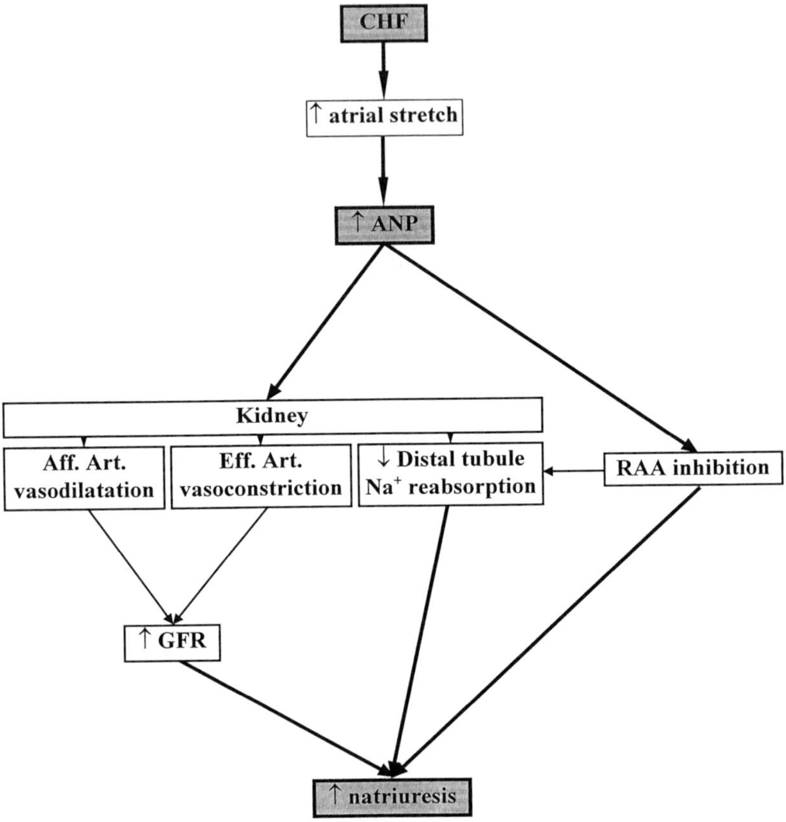

Figure 4 Glomerular hemodynamics.

versely with cardiac index and the NYHA (New York Heart Association) class (71–74). Despite elevated plasma levels, chronic CHF patients exhibit a blunted response to ANP (73,74). Nevertheless, administration of exogenous ANP was shown to have a beneficial effect in some of these patients (71,73). Anti-ANP antibodies, administered in a rat model of CHF induced by myocardial infarction, further suppressed salt and water excretion, suggesting that ANP plays a role in natriuresis and diuresis in this model of CHF (75). High ANP levels may also have a protective effect on renal function in CHF. ANP has been shown to reduce the severity of renal ischemic injury and hasten recovery from postischemic ATN in experimental models. Exogenous ANP administered to patients with established ARF increased creatinine clearance and decreased the need for dialysis as compared to controls who did not receive ANP (76).

Urodilatin is a related peptide produced by the kidneys (77,78). It is believed to have a more potent natriuretic effect than ANP. Although exogenously administered urodilatin increases GFR, endogenously it is produced by the tubules and probably exerts a paracrine effect, inhibiting tubular reabsorption of sodium (79). As in the case of ANP, urodilatin may also have a renal protective effect. Animal studies have shown that urodilatin when combined with dopamine affords protection against ischemic renal damage (80).

D. Endothelin (ET)

ET is one of the most powerful vasoconstrictors known. Three different isoforms, all 21 amino acids in length, are produced mainly by the endothelial cells. Infusion of ET into the main renal artery causes a fall in GFR and an increase in afferent and efferent arteriolar resistance (81). ET is produced in response to various stimuli including hypoxia, epinephrine, AII and endothelial damage, and vascular wall shear stress (82,83). Stimulation of ET production in turn causes the endothelial release of prostaglandins, nitric oxide, and other vasodilatory substances (84). ET levels are elevated in CHF in experimental animals (85) and in humans (86), suggesting that ET participates in the adaptive response to a fall in cardiac output. Treatment with antiendothelin antibodies infused directly into the renal artery improved the single-nephron glomerular ultrafiltration rate (SNGFR) in a rat model of postischemic ATN (81).

E. Prostaglandins

Products of cycloxygenase, lipoxygenase, and epoxygenase pathways are produced in various parts of the kidney (87). Although the precise role of all these products is not well appreciated, in balance, prostaglandins mediate cytoprotective effects in the kidney. They participate in the regulation of renal blood flow and influence tubular reabsorption of sodium and water (88). Like ANP, they behave as counterregulatory hormones to the vasoconstrictive effects of endothelin, AII, and NE. They also inhibit ADH effect on the tubules (89). The importance of prostaglandins as counterregulatory factors to the adaptive response in CHF is highlighted by the susceptibility of renal function in CHF patients to the effects of NSAIDs (90,91).

IV. MEDICAL MANAGEMENT OF RENAL FAILURE IN CCU PATIENTS

In this section we will initially highlight the implications to renal function and fluid and electrolyte balance of diuretic, dopamine, and ACE-inhibitor (ACEI) therapy in CHF, then review the use of renal replacement modalities in this patient population.

A. Drug Therapy

1. ACE Inhibitors

ACEI have been shown to improve the functional class of CHF and prolong survival of patients in several studies. As discussed previously, stimulation of RAA decreases renal blood flow, although GFR is preserved. In fact, GFR becomes dependent to some extent on AII in CHF patients. Marked stimulation of RAA, however, renders the afferent arteriole sensitive to AII, causing a drop in GFR. Therefore in many of the studies utilizing ACEI therapy (SOLVD, CONSENSUS) plasma creatinine and GFR improved after ACEI therapy (46,47,92). Furthermore, studies have shown that resistance to diuretics in CHF is diminished when ACEI are used concomitantly (93,94). AII leads to increased proximal tubular sodium re-absorption and decreased delivery of the filtrate to the distal tubule which is the main site of action of many diuretics; ACEI decrease the proximal tubular sodium reabsorption. Hyponatremia was also shown to be improved in these studies (95). ACEI could improve hyponatremia by suppression of ADH release through improved hemodynamics, as well as by the increased delivery of fluid to the distal tubule by inhibiting AII. Although hyperkalemia is a well-known side effect of ACEI therapy, patients with CHF do not usually develop dangerous levels of hyperkalemia with this therapy. CHF patients who have bilateral renal artery stenosis or are volume-depleted as a result of aggressive diuresis are at risk for developing acute renal failure due to ACEI therapy, since the maintenance of GFR in these patients is highly dependent on AII (96–98). Hypotension should be avoided when using ACEI since renal autoregulation fails when the systolic BP falls below 80 mm Hg, leading to a precipitous decline in renal blood flow and GFR.

2. Diuretics

Diuretics are an integral part of the medical regimen of CHF patients. The commonly used diuretics based on their site of action are acetazolamide and metolazone (proximal tubule), lasix, bumetamide, torsemide and ethacrynic acid (loop of Henle), thiazides and metolazone (distal tubule), amiloride, spironolactone, and triamterene (the collecting duct). A detailed discussion of diuretics is beyond the scope of this chapter; the reader is referred to reviews on this subject (99,100). The loop diuretics, particularly furosemide and bumetamide, are most commonly employed in CHF. They cause natriuresis by inhibiting the Na-K-2Cl pump in the thick ascending limb of Henle. Sodium reabsorption in this segment of the nephron contributes to the medullary concentration gradient. Because loop diuretics reduce the medullary concentration gradient, they also impair the absorption of water, so hyponatremia is unusual or less severe with these agents. Some studies have shown that continuous infusion of furosemide may be more effective than intermittent infusions (101,102). Torsemide is a newer loop diuretic with a relatively longer half-life and duration of action. It has been found to be beneficial in CHF patients in several studies, although it is unclear whether it offers any benefit over furosemide (103). Diuretic resistance is not uncommon in severe CHF (99,104). Stimulation of the RAA and sympathetic systems leads to increased proximal tubular sodium reabsorption and reduced delivery to the distal tubule, which is the main site of action of loop diuretics, thiazides, K-sparing diuretics, and endogenous natriuretic peptides such as ANP and urodilatin (105), thus rendering them less effective. Prolonged loop diuretic use can cause hypertrophy of the distal tubule with the resulting increase in sodium absorption in this segment of the tubule, another cause of diuretic resistance.

Other reasons for diuretic resistance in CHF include impaired gastrointestinal absorption of drugs in CHF (106) and decreased delivery of the active drug to the luminal site of tubular in renal failure. Diuretic resistance may be overcome by prescribing a combination of diuretics which act at different sites along the tubule, such as metolazone or thiazides in combination with loop diuretics (105). Judicious use of ACE inhibitors in combination with loop diuretics has also been shown to potentiate both diuresis and natriuresis. Hyponatremia, however, is much more likely to occur or be exacerbated with combination diuretic therapy. Hypokalemia and hypomagnesemia (except with K-sparing diuretics), elevation of BUN and uric acid, severe volume depletion, and exacerbation of prerenal azotemia are possible side effects of diuretic therapy. Concomitant use of NSAIDs with diuretics should be avoided when possible. Prostaglandins play an important role in preserving renal blood flow in volume depletion, and acute renal failure may result in NSAID-mediated inhibition prostaglandin synthesis. Finally, progressive azotemia and lack of response to diuretics necessitate ultrafiltration and dialytic therapies in some patients. These therapies are discussed in the following section.

3. *Dopamine*

The use of intravenous dopamine in the setting of CHF and renal failure continues to be a source of controversy despite its many years of clinical use. A recent randomized trial of patients with acute renal failure failed to show improvement in patient survival or in renal function after low-dose dopamine infusion (107). Nevertheless, dopaminergic agents may increase natriuresis, diuresis, and response to diuretics in some patients with CHF although it may not improve renal function or prevent the development or progression of acute renal failure (108–112).

B. Renal Replacement Therapies

As discussed above, ARF is not an uncommon complication in critically ill patients in the CCU (113). These patients often require dialytic support to maintain volume, acid/base, and electrolyte homeostasis and to decrease uremic symptoms (114). At present, three types of dialytic support are available for the patient with ARF: intermittent hemodialysis; peritoneal dialysis; and the various methods of continuous renal replacement therapies (CRRT). The advantages and disadvantages of these renal replacement therapies in the treatment of patients with ARF in the CCU will be discussed in detail in this chapter.

1. Indications for Renal Replacement Therapies

Dialysis is generally initiated in ARF for control of severe fluid or electrolyte abnormalities and for uremic symptoms. The common indications for dialysis are:

1. Volume overload refractory to medical therapy
2. Severe or refractory hyperkalemia
3. Severe metabolic acidosis
4. Uremic pericarditis
5. Symptomatic azotemia such as uremic encephalopathy
6. Uremic coagulopathy secondary to platelet dysfunction

In the absence of these definitive indications, there is much controversy as to when dialysis should be instituted. It has been suggested that a BUN of 100 mg/dl and a serum creatinine of 9 to 10 mg/dl are levels at which dialytic therapy should be initiated. In 1986, a clinical, controlled, randomized trial was undertaken in 34 patients to determine whether early and intensive dialysis might be beneficial in ARF (115). This study found no difference in morbidity or mortality between patients dialyzed daily to maintain BUN levels at less than 60 mg/dl and those dialyzed to BUN levels of 100 mg/dl. This study suggests that there is no significant benefit from early and intensive dialysis in patients with ARF. In addition, recent studies have shown that dialysis may actually exacerbate the renal injury and delay the recovery of renal function in some patients (116–118). Indeed, hemodialysis may exacerbate renal hypoperfusion as transient hypotension is a common complication of this treatment modality. Due to the lack of autoregulation of renal blood flow in ATN, repeated episodes of hypotension may result in recurrent ischemic renal tubular injury, thereby delaying the recovery of renal function. In addition, recent evidence suggests that complement activation during the blood-dialyzer interaction with bioincompatible membranes can lead to neutrophilic infiltration into the kidney and prolong the course of acute renal failure (119,120).

In a randomized, prospective study, 72 patients with ARF who required hemodialysis were assigned to therapy with either a biocompatible dialyzer membrane (synthetic polymethyl methacrylate membrane) or a bioincompatible membrane (cuprophane membrane). The patients who were treated with biocompatible membranes were found to have a higher rate of recovery of renal function, more rapid recovery as evidenced by fewer dialysis treatments, and an improvement in patient survival. These benefits were limited to patients who were nonoliguric prior to the onset of hemodialysis. It is thought that renal blood flow is generally higher in these patients (121), and their kidneys are perfused with higher concentrations of complement and neutrophil activation products. There are several mechanisms by which the activation of complement and neutrophils may lead to the delay in the recovery of renal function (122). Complement activation products have direct and indirect vasoconstrictive properties (123). Similarly, activated neutrophils secrete several vasoconstrictive compounds that can exacerbate ischemic renal tubular injury (124). The products of activated complement and activated neutrophils may also interact with glomerular endothelial cells, resulting in diminished secretion of the endothelium-derived relaxing factor nitric oxide (125). For these reasons, it has been suggested that dialysis be reserved for the management of volume overload, hyperkalemia, refractory acidosis, and treatment of symptoms or signs of uremia.

In contrast, a recent study from the Cleveland Clinic Foundation revealed that the intensity of dialysis may have an important influence on the outcome of ARF patients (126). In this study, the outcome of 58 consecutive ICU patients with ARF was analyzed. There were 34 survivors and 24 nonsurvivors, all of whom were similar with regard to age, APACHE II score, number of failed systems, and hemodynamic profile. Compared with nonsurvivors, the survivors received significantly higher dialysis dose, as assessed by Kt/V and urea reduction ratio (URR). KT/V and URR were 1.09 and 58%, respectively, in the survivor group, compared with 0.89 and 46%, respectively, in the nonsurvivor group.

At the present time, the standards for dialysis adequacy in ARF are not well-defined. Further studies evaluating the significance of dialysis dose in ARF need to be performed to resolve this issue.

2. *Hemodialysis*

Hemodialysis is the dialytic modality of choice in stable patients with acute renal failure. Solute removal during hemodialysis occurs via passive diffusion down a concentration gradient from the plasma into the dialysate fluid, and the ultrafiltration of plasma water across the dialyzer membrane. The frictional forces between water and solutes (called solvent drag) results in the convective transport of low- and middle-molecular-weight solutes. In addition to solutes, plasma water is also removed during hemodialysis by the process of ultrafiltration. Ultrafiltration is driven primarily by the hydrostatic pressure gradient across the dialyzer membrane. Vascular access for acute hemodialysis is usually achieved using a double-lumen catheter inserted into the internal jugular, subclavian, or femoral veins.

The clearance rates of urea and creatinine per unit time achieved with hemodialysis are substantially higher than those obtained with peritoneal dialysis. Hence, hemodialysis is the preferred dialytic modality in stable, hypercatabolic patients with acute renal failure. However, hemodialysis is frequently associated with episodes of hypotension, making it less useful in hemodynamically unstable patients in the CCU.

Hemodialysis-induced hypotension occurs by several mechanisms (127,128). During conventional hemodialysis, the rapid diffusive removal of urea results in an osmotic gradient favoring water movement into the cells. This osmotic shift of water along with water loss by ultrafiltration results in intravascular volume depletion and hypotension. Hypotension also occurs when the rate of intravascular volume depletion exceeds the rate of refilling of this space. Since the refilling of intravascular space is time-dependent, high ultrafiltration rates during a typical short dialytic session frequently results in hypotension, even in the setting of volume overload (129). The extracorporeal blood volume and the compliance of the dialyzer may also contribute to hemodialysis-induced hypotension. The blood volume of coil dialyzers and parallel plate dialyzers increases as transmembrane pressure increases, resulting in a larger extracorporeal blood volume (129,130). The volume of blood required to prime the extracorporeal circuit may be as high as 200 ml. The use of acetate as a buffer may also predispose to hypotension, because acetate accumulation in the blood results in both a reduction in systemic vascular resistance and a decline in myocardial contractility.

Furthermore, the frequency of dialysis-associated hemodynamic instability is greatly increased in patients with poor cardiac function and autonomic dysfunction. Patients with a prior history of congestive heart failure, cardiomyopathy, or ischemic heart disease often have poor left ventricular contractility and a diminished cardiac reserve, predisposing them to hypotension. Many dialysis patients have autonomic dysfunction which impairs their ability to maintain the systemic blood pressure following large fluid removal (131). The afferent arm of the baroreceptor reflex is believed to be blunted in these patients such that they do not mount reflex vasoconstriction during hypotensive episodes (132–135). In addition, many hemodialysis patients are taking antihypertensive medications that may interfere with the normal hemodynamic response to ultrafiltration. For example, β blockers decrease cardiac contractility and exert a negative chronotropic effect, thereby preventing a compensatory increase in cardiac output in response to hypotension. Vasodilators, on the other hand, can prevent vasoconstriction in response to ultrafiltration. And finally, the hypoxemia induced during hemodialysis results in decreased oxygen delivery to the tissues and contributes to hypotension in patients with cardiac diseases (129,130).

The time of onset of hypotension during dialysis may provide a clue to the likely cause. Pericarditis with tamponade is usually associated with early hypotension during dialysis. On the other hand, hypotension occurring late in the treatment usually results from excessive or to too rapid ultrafiltration. Therefore, prevention of hypotension during hemodialysis requires accurate assessment of the patient's dry weight to avoid excessive ultrafiltration (136). Another approach of prevention is the use of bicarbonate-based dialysate and high dialysate sodium concentration. Bicarbonate-based dialysate is associated with greater hemodynamic stability than acetate-based dialysate. The use of high dialysate sodium concentration also reduces the risk of hypotension during dialysis by mitigating the intradialytic fall in serum osmolality that occurs with rapid diffusive urea loss. The use of high dialysate calcium concentration and cool temperature dialysis is also helpful. High dialysate calcium concentration has been shown to improve myocardial contractility, whereas cooling of the dialysate to 35°C improves vascular stability by increasing systemic vascular resistance (137–140). The increasing use of biocompatible dialyzer membranes and the less compliant hollow-fiber dialyzers have also reduced the potential for hypotension. In addition, supplemental oxygen may help prevent hypotensive episodes in patients with severe cardiac diseases by improving hypoxemia and cardiac contractility. Lastly, antihypertensive medications should preferably be held for 6 to 8 h before each hemodialysis session (129,130).

Sequential ultrafiltration and dialysis has been shown to be very helpful in patients with hemodynamic instability (141,142). This sequential procedure involves isolated ultrafiltration followed by diffusive dialysis. During isolated ultrafiltration, systemic vascular resistance increases as fluid is removed, thereby maintaining the blood pressure. In addition, the plasma oncotic pressure rises during isolated ultrafiltration since proteins are not removed, resulting in continuous refilling of the intravascular space. In contrast, during conventional hemodialysis (when diffusion is added to ultrafiltration), there is either a decline or no change in systemic vascular resistance during fluid removal, resulting in a fall in blood pressure. During combined ultrafiltration and diffusion dialysis, there is osmotic shift of fluid from the plasma into the intracellular compartment as the plasma osmolality declines with rapid diffusive urea removal. Thus, the intravascular compartment loses fluid to both intracellular space and dialysate, thereby predisposing the patient to development of hypotension. For these reasons, sequential ultrafiltration and diffusion dialysis may allow large volumes of fluid removal without inducing hemodynamic instability. However, when sequential therapy is used, the total treatment time must be increased accordingly so as not to curtail the duration of diffusive dialysis to ensure adequate solute removal. Two potential complications of isolated ultrafiltration are the development of metabolic acidosis and hyperkalemia. The cause of the mild metabolic acidosis is thought to be related to the loss of bicarbonate in the ultrafiltrate resulting from the Gibbs-Donnan equilibrium. Hyperkalemia is caused by the solvent drag effect induced by the movement of intracellular fluid into the extracellular space (130,143).

As transient hypotension is a frequent complication of hemodialysis, this treatment modality may exacerbate ischemic renal tubular injury and delay the recovery of ARF. In addition, complement activation during the blood-dialyzer interaction with bioincompatible membranes may further aggravate ischemic renal injury. Biocompatible membranes should therefore be used in patients with ARF. However, caution should be exercised when using the biocompatible AN69 dialyzer in patients who are taking ACE inhibitors. There is a high incidence of anaphylactoid reactions when polyacrylonitrite (PAN) dialyzers are used in patients taking ACEI. The negatively charged surfaces of PAN membranes are able to activate Hageman factor and convert prekallikrein to kallikrein. The active kallikrein in turn is able to cleave bradykinin from its endogenous substrate, high-molecular-weight kininogen. The ensuing increase in bradykinin production is generally well tolerated unless the patient is taking an ACE inhibitor. Since ACE is a kininase, the inhibition of this converting enzyme prevents inactivation of bradykinin. The resultant increase in bradykinin levels leads to the increased likelihood of an anaphylactoid reaction (144–146). Therefore, other biocompatible dialyzers (e.g., polysulfone) should be selected in patients taking an ACE inhibitor. Alternatively, the ACE inhibitor should be discontinued if dialysis with PAN dialyzers is being contemplated. With the availability of the angiotensin II-receptor antagonist losartan, this problem may also be averted. However, there are no available data on the use of losartan in this setting.

Other complications associated with hemodialysis are hypoxemia, aggravation of coronary ischemia, precipitation of arrhythmias, and dialysis disequilibrium syndrome. Hypoxemia frequently occurs during hemodialysis and is dependent on the dialyzer membrane and the nature of the buffer used in the dialysate. Complement activation as a result of blood-membrane interactions leads to neutrophil sequestration in the pulmonary vascular bed, causing intrapulmonary diffusion abnormalities and resultant hypoxemia. A fall in arterial PO_2 also occurs when acetate-buffered dialysate is used. Since acetate has a respiratory quotient of only 0.5, its metabolism will result in less carbon dioxide production. In the setting of this decreased CO_2 production, hypoventilation occurs to prevent hypocapnia, resulting in hypoxemia. Hypoventilation is also induced by the significant loss of CO_2 by diffusion into the dialysate bath. Hypoxemia has also been associated with bicarbonate-buffered dialysate. When the dialysate bicarbonate concentration is greater than approximately 37 mEq/L, the resultant blood alkalinization frequently causes hypoventilation. However, the degree of respiratory depression is significantly less than that seen with acetate baths. In summary, the typical fall in arterial PO_2 during hemodialysis may be clinically significant in patients with underlying compromised cardiopulmonary status. Prevention of dialysis hypoxemia includes the use of supplemental oxygen, avoidance of bioincompatible membranes, and the use of bicarbonate dialysate rather than acetate bath. When bicarbonate bath is used, the bicarbonate concentration should be no more than 37 mEq/L. Correction of significant anemia with epogen also minimizes the impact of arterial hypoxemia by maximizing the blood's oxygen carrying capacity (129,130,147–150).

Hemodialysis often precipitates anginal symptoms in patients with underlying ischemic heart disease. Hemodialysis is associated with factors that either increase myocardial oxygen consumption or limit myocardial oxygen delivery. Dialysis-induced tachyarrhythmias and the reflex tachycardia that frequently accompanies ultrafiltration may precipitate angina. Coronary ischemia may also be caused by the interplay of dialysis-associated hypoxemia, hemodynamic effects of hypotension, and the increased affinity of hemoglobin for oxygen with correction of metabolic acidosis. In addition, the withholding of antihypertensive medications such as β blockers and calcium channel blockers before the dialytic session is another contributing factor. As a result, alterations in the dialysis prescription may benefit patients with ischemic heart disease. The use of biocompatible membranes and bicarbonate instead of acetate dialysate baths may reduce the frequency of angina caused by dialysis-associated hypoxemia and hypotension. Similarly, the use of sequential ultrafiltration and dialysis for fluid removal may minimize hypotensive episodes and attendant angina (129,151,152).

Hemodialysis is often associated with an increased risk of arrhythmias in patients either receiving digitalis preparations or with underlying ischemic heart disease. Factors that may precipitate arrhythmias during hemodialysis include hypoxemia, hypotension, removal of antiarrhythmic agents, and rapid changes in serum bicarbonate, magnesium, and potassium. For instance, digitalis-related arrhythmias often occur in association with hypokalemia. During hemodialysis, hypokalemia may result from either a low dialysate potassium concentration or intracellular shift of potassium induced by the administered dialysate glucose and correction of the metabolic acidosis. This risk may be minimized by increasing the dialysate potassium concentration to 3.0 to 3.5 mEq/L. Antiarrhythmic agents that are sufficiently removed by hemodialysis require supplemental dosing after dialysis. Patients with ischemic heart disease are also at high risk of arrhythmias since myocardial ischemia may be aggravated by hemodialysis by the various mechanisms previously described (129,153).

A complication unique to hemodialysis is the dialysis disequilibrium syndrome. This syndrome refers to acute symptoms that vary from nausea and vomiting, restlessness, headaches, and fatigue to seizures, coma, and even death. These symptoms usually develop during or immediately after hemodialysis and are thought to arise from rapid changes in plasma osmolality and cerebrospinal fluid (CSF) pH. The rapid lowering of plasma osmolality by urea removal during dialysis causes an osmotic shift of extracellular fluid into the intracellular compartment, resulting in cerebral edema. Moreover, the correction of the systemic metabolic acidosis during dialysis results in an associated paradoxical acidosis in the CSF due to more rapid diffusion of CO_2 than bicarbonate across the blood-brain barrier. The resultant CSF acidosis can increase the brain cell osmolality by altering osmotic activity of intracellular cations, thereby promoting water movement into the brain. Prevention of dialysis disequilibrium is the mainstay of therapy and is accomplished by slowing the rate of osmolality changes by shorter and more frequent dialyses. Low blood flow rates and small surface area dialyzers should be used initially to ensure slow urea removal. The administration of hypertonic mannitol during dialysis can be given in high-risk patients with marked azotemia to counteract the rapid changes in serum osmolality (129,130,154–156).

3. *Peritoneal Dialysis*

Peritoneal dialysis is an alternative modality to hemodialysis in patients with acute renal failure. In peritoneal dialysis, solute and water movement occur across the peritoneal membrane rather than an external dialyzer. With this modality, solute removal occurs by diffusion while water moves down an osmotic gradient created by the hyperosmotic dialysate fluid. Although the peritoneal clearance rates of urea and creatinine per unit time are substantially lower than those achieved with hemodialysis, this decreased efficiency is largely overcome by the longer time of dialysis. In addition, the clearances of middle-molecular-weight solutes are significantly higher in peritoneal dialysis.

There are several advantages to peritoneal dialysis. Peritoneal dialysis is very useful in patients with hemodynamic instability. Because of the slower rate of urea removal, hypotension is less likely to occur. Similarly, osmotic disequilibrium does not occur with this modality. Peritoneal dialysis may also facilitate recovery of residual renal function because of its associated hemodynamic stability and the lack of complement activation due to blood-membrane interaction (157–159). In addition, a major advantage to this modality is that no anticoagulation is required, making it most desirable in treating patients with active bleeding or at high risk of bleeding (160,161). However, shortcomings of this therapy are its low urea and solute clearance rates. As a result, peritoneal dialysis may not be able to control the uremic state in hypercatabolic patients and does not allow for rapid correction of significant electrolyte abnormalities (e.g., hyperkalemia).

Acute peritoneal dialysis is performed through an intraperitoneal catheter. The stiff Teflon catheter can be placed percutaneously for acute peritoneal dialysis; however, this procedure carries a high risk of infectious complications and bowel perforation. Therefore, it is preferable to place the soft Silastic catheter under direct visualization through a small minilaparotomy (161).

The major disadvantage of peritoneal dialysis is the increased risk of peritonitis. Peritoneal dialysis has also been associated with compromised pulmonary function due to elevated diaphragms and hydrothorax. The presence of dialysate in the abdomen may reduce the functional residual capacity and causes atelectasis with resultant fall in the arterial PO_2. Excessive glucose absorption may also occur, resulting in increased CO_2 production and worsening respiratory failure. On the other hand, peritoneal dialysis may have a potentially positive effect on respiratory function by increasing diaphragmatic contractility. The increased diaphragmatic contractility is thought to be related to the increased curvature of the diaphragm caused by the intraperitoneal fluid (157,162).

Hydrothorax is another potential pulmonary complication. It results from the passage of peritoneal fluid through either diaphragmatic lymphatics or diaphragmatic defects into the pleural space. This transdiaphragmatic pleural-peritoneal leak may be diagnosed by the presence of a high glucose concentration in the pleural fluid or by radionuclide scanning using technetium-labeled macroaggregated albumin. If a direct pleuro-peritoneal communication is found, peritoneal dialysis should be temporarily discontinued to allow spontaneous closure of the defect and resolution of the effusion (157,162–165). Other complications associated with peritoneal dialysis include significant protein losses and excessive glucose absorption. These problems may be circumvented by curtailing the dietary intake of carbohydrates and calories while maintaining that of protein.

4. Continuous Renal Replacement Therapies

Continuous renal replacement therapy is becoming increasingly popular in the treatment of critically ill patients with ARF. There are many variations of CRRT: CAVH, CVVH, CAVHD, and CVVHD. In CAVH, an arteriovenous access is used and solute removal is exclusively convective. With this modality, blood is driven by the patient's blood pressure through a hemofilter containing a highly permeable membrane across which fluid is ultrafiltered. Although ultrafiltration occurs isosmotically, the plasma concentrations of small solutes are lowered by dilution by the administration of replacement fluid to prevent extracellular volume depletion. The total clearance of a solute during hemofiltration is equal to the product of the ultrafiltration rate, and the ratio of the solute concentration in the filtrate is equal to that in the arterial plasma. Since the concentration of the solute in the ultrafiltrate is roughly the same as that in the plasma, the solute clearance rate is equal to the rate of ultrafiltration (166). CVVH is similar to CAVH except that the venovenous access necessitates the use of a mechanical blood pump. In hypercatabolic patients, the solute clearance may be enhanced by diffusive solute loss via the addition of countercurrent dialysate flow into the ultrafiltrate-dialysate compartment of the hemofilter (CAVHD, CVVHD). Therefore, solute removal in CRRT may occur by either passive diffusion or convective transport.

CRRT is the dialytic modality of choice in patients with hemodynamic instability. In CAVH and CVVH, the plasma oncotic pressure rises during ultrafiltration, resulting in continuous refilling of the intravascular space. In CAVH, ultrafiltration will spontaneously cease if the patient becomes hypotensive because the driving force is the mean arterial pressure. Even when there is diffusive solute loss, hypotension is less likely to occur during CRRT because of the slower rate of urea removal per unit time. The slower rate of solute and fluid removal associated with CRRT results in more gradual changes in serum osmolality and fluid volume, conferring on it greater hemodynamic stability (167). The hemodynamic advantages of CRRT may also be related to the removal of middle-molecular-weight substances with cardiodepressant or vasodilatory properties. The removal of inflammatory mediators such as tumor necrosis factor (TNF), interleukin-1 (IL-1), and interleukin-6 (IL-6) may be beneficial in the patient with sepsis since these cytokines are thought to mediate some of the detrimental hemodynamic consequences (116,168–173). In addition to the hemodynamic stability of CRRT, the lack of complement activation with the use of porous biocompatible membrane may facilitate the rate of recovery of renal function in ARF.

CRRT also offers better control of uremia and electrolyte and acid-base disturbances since these abnormalities are corrected as they are evolving (174). Urea removal during conventional hemodialysis is hindered by the multicompartment volume of urea distribution and its slow equilibration between these compartments. This resistance to urea diffusion between body compartments allows the urea concentration in the blood to fall more rapidly than urea concentrations elsewhere in the body. In contrast, the amount of urea removal in CRRT is enhanced by the continuous plasma refilling of urea from the intracellular and interstitial compartments and the constant plasma concentration profile (166). The continuous removal of fluid with CRRT also facilitates administration of parenteral nutrition and obligatory intravenous medications in oliguric patients with ARF (174,175). Lastly, CRRT is highly effective in removing fluid in patients with myocardial dysfunction and congestive heart failure (176). Fluid removal by CAVH and CVVH has been shown to result in an increase in cardiac index and a reduction of peripheral vascular resistance (166,168,177).

A major disadvantage of CRRT is the need for continuous anticoagulation and its associated risk of significant bleeding (178). Another drawback is the requirement for an arterial angioaccess in the case of CAVH and CAVHD. Arterial cannulation has been associated with significant bleeding, vessel perforation, and local thrombosis. Meticulous monitoring of fluid intake and output is mandatory and may be time-consuming when large amounts of ultrafiltrate are exchanged. Finally, the patient must be bedridden to receive this therapy. Other complications associated with CRRT include infection and sepsis due to the extracorporeal circuit, bleeding, air embolism, accidental disconnection of the extracorporeal circuit, accidental fluid overload, hypothermia, and hypophosphatemia (165).

In summary, CRRT has many advantages in the treatment of critically ill patients with ARF. Specifically, the hemodynamic stability and lack of complement activation of this modality may facilitate the rate of recovery of renal function in ARF. In addition, retrospective studies suggest that patients with ARF and multiple-organ failure may have a higher survival rate when treated with CRRT as compared to patients treated by intermittent hemodialysis. However, prospective randomized studies are clearly necessary to demonstrate these potential benefits of continuous renal replacement therapy. Pending these studies, the choice of dialytic modality will depend on a variety of factors including availability, the expertise of the clinician and ancillary personnel, hemodynamic stability and catabolic state of the patient, need for mobility, vascular access, urgency of treatment, and whether the primary need is for fluid and/or solute removal.

REFERENCES

1. D'Elia JA, Gleason RE. Am J Med 1982; 72:719.
2. Kumar S, Hull JD, Lathi S, Cohen AJ, and Pletka PG. Low incidence of renal failure after angiography. Arch Intern Med 1981; 141:1268.
3. Mangos GJ, Brown MA, Chan WY, Horton D, Trew P, Whitworth JA. Acute renal failure following cardiac surgery: incidence, outcomes and risk factors [see comments]. Aust N Z J Med 1995; 25:284.
4. Andersson LG, Ekroth R, Bratteby LE, Hallhagen S, Wesslen O. Acute renal failure after coronary surgery—a study of incidence and risk factors in 2009 consecutive patients. Thorac Cardiovasc Surg 1993; 41:237.
5. Bonventre, JV, Mechanisms of ischemic acute renal failure [clinical conference]. Kidney Int 1993; 43:1160.
6. Molitoris BA. New insights into the cell biology of ischemic acute renal failure. J Am Soc Nephrol 1991; 1:1263.
7. Burnett JC Jr, Knox FG. Renal interstitial pressure and sodium excretion during renal vein constriction. Am J Physiol 1980; 238:F279.
8. Khraibi AA. Direct renal interstitial volume expansion causes exaggerated natriuresis in SHR. Am J Physiol 1991; 261:F567.
9. Kostreva DR, Castaner A, Kampine JP. Reflex effects of hepatic baroreceptors on renal and cardiac sympathetic nerve activity. Am J Physiol 1980; 238:R390.
10. Gauer OH, Henry JP, Behn C. The regulation of extracellular fluid volume. Annu Rev Physiol 1970; 32:547.
11. Goetz KL, Hermreck AS, Slick GL, Starke HS. Atrial receptors and renal function in conscious dogs. Am J Physiol 1970; 219:1417.
12. Epstein M, Duncan DC, Fishman LM. Characterization of the natriuresis caused in normal man by immersion in water. Clin Sci 1972; 43:275.
13. Peter J. The role of sodium in the production of edema. NEJM 1948; 239:353.
14. Anderson RJ, Pluss RG, Berns AS, et al. Mechanism of effect of hypoxia on renal water excretion. J Clin Invest 1978; 62:769.
15. Zucker IH, Earle AM, Gilmore JP. The mechanism of adaptation of left atrial stretch receptors in dogs with chronic congestive heart failure. J Clin Invest 1977; 60:323.
16. Epstein F, Post R, McDowell M. Effects of an arteriovenous fistula on renal hemodynamics and electrolyte excretion. JCI 1953; 32:233.
17. Gilmore JP, Daggett WM. Response of the chronic cardiac denervated dog to acute volume expansion. Am J Physiol 1966; 210:509.
18. Knox FG, Davis BB, Berliner RW. Effect of chronic cardiac denervation on renal response to saline infusion. Am J Physiol 1967; 213:174.
19. Brenner BM, Humes HD. Mechanics of glomerular ultrafiltration. N Engl J Med 1977; 297:148.
20. Fried TA, Stein JH. Glomerular dynamics. Arch Intern Med 1983; 143:787.
21. Skorecki KL, Brenner BM. Body fluid homeostasis in man. A contemporary overview. Am J Med 1981; 70:77.
22. Ichikawa I, Brenner BM. Importance of efferent arteriolar vascular tone in regulation of proximal tubule fluid reabsorption and glomerulotubular balance in the rat. J Clin Invest 1980; 65:1192.

23. Cannon PJ. The kidney in heart failure. N Engl J Med 1977; 296:26.
24. Watkins L Jr, Burton JA, Haber E, Cant JR, Smith FW, Barger AC. The renin-angiotensin-aldosterone system in congestive failure in conscious dogs. J Clin Invest 1976; 57:1606.
25. Grassi G, Seravalle G, Cattaneo BM, et al. Sympathetic activation and loss of reflex sympathetic control in mild congestive heart failure. Circulation 1995; 92:3206.
26. DiBona GF, Herman PJ, Sawin LL. Neural control of renal function in edema-forming states. Am J Physiol 1988; 254:R1017.
27. Lilly LS, Dzau VJ, Williams GH, Rydstedt L, Hollenberg NK. Hyponatremia in congestive heart failure: implications for neurohumoral activation and responses to orthostatis. J Clin Endocrinol Metab 1984; 59:924.
28. Zucker IH, Wang W, Brandle M, Schultz HD, Patel KP. Neural regulation of sympathetic nerve activity in heart failure. Prog Cardiovasc Dis 1995; 37:397.
29. Feng QP, Carlsson S, Thoren P, Hedner T. Characteristics of renal sympathetic nerve activity in experimental congestive heart failure in the rat. Acta Physiol Scand 1994; 150:259.
30. Bell-Reuss E, Trevino DL, Gottschalk CW. Effect of renal sympathetic nerve stimulation on proximal water and sodium reabsorption. J Clin Invest 1976; 57:1104.
31. DiBona GF. Neurogenic regulation of renal tubular sodium reabsorption. Am J Physiol 1977; 233:F73.
32. Cohn JN, Levine TB, Olivari MT, et al. Plasma norepinephrine as a guide to prognosis in patients with chronic congestive heart failure. N Engl J Med 1984; 311:819.
33. Levine TB, Francis GS, Goldsmith SR, Simon AB, Cohn JN. Activity of the sympathetic nervous system and renin-angiotensin system assessed by plasma hormone levels and their relation to hemodynamic abnormalities in congestive heart failure. Am J Cardiol 1982; 49:1659.
34. Thomas JA, Marks BH. Plasma norepinephrine in congestive heart failure. Am J Cardiol 1978; 41:233.
35. Opie LH. Fundamental role of angiotensin-converting enzyme inhibitors in the management of congestive heart failure. Am J Cardiol 1995; 75:3F.
36. Kaye DM, Lefkovits J, Jennings GL, Bergin P, Broughton A, Esler MD. Adverse consequences of high sympathetic nervous activity in the failing human heart. J Am Coll Cardiol 1995; 26:1257.
37. Kastner PR, Hall JE, Guyton AC. Control of glomerular filtration rate: role of intrarenally formed angiotensin II. Am J Physiol 1984; 246:F897.
38. Schor N, Ichikawa I, Brenner BM. Glomerular adaptations to chronic dietary salt restriction or excess. Am J Physiol 1980; 238:F428.
39. Liu FY, Cogan MG. Angiotensin II stimulation of hydrogen ion secretion in the rat early proximal tubule. Modes of action, mechanism, and kinetics. J Clin Invest 1988; 82:601.
40. Schuster VL, Kokko JP, Jacobson HR. Angiotensin II directly stimulates sodium transport in rabbit proximal convoluted tubules. J Clin Invest 1984; 73:507.
41. Kon V, Hughes ML, Ichikawa I. Blood flow dependence of postglomerular fluid transfer and glomerulotubular balance. J Clin Invest 1983; 72:1716.
42. Kon V, Yared A, Ichikawa I. Role of renal sympathetic nerves in mediating hypoper-

fusion of renal cortical microcirculation in experimental congestive heart failure and acute extracellular fluid volume depletion. J Clin Invest 1985; 76:1913.

43. Ploth DW, Roy RN. Renin-angiotensin influences on tubuloglomerular feedback activity in the rat. Kidney Int Suppl 1982; 12:S114.
44. CONSENSUS Trial Study Group. Effects of enalapril on mortality in severe congestive heart failure. Results of the Cooperative North Scandinavian Enalapril Survival Study (CONSENSUS). N Engl J Med 1987; 316:1429.
45. Captopril-Digoxin Multicenter Research Group. Comparative effects of therapy with captopril and digoxin in patients with mild to moderate heart failure. JAMA 1988; 259:539.
46. SOLVD Investigators. Effect of enalapril on survival in patients with reduced left ventricular ejection fractions and congestive heart failure [see comments]. N Engl J Med 1991; 325:293.
47. SOLVD Investigators. Effect of enalapril on mortality and the development of heart failure in asymptomatic patients with reduced left ventricular ejection fractions. [published erratum appears in N Engl J Med 1992; 327(24):1768][see comments]. N Engl J Med 1992; 327:685.
48. de Zeeuw D, Janssen WM, de Jong, PE. Atrial natriuretic factor: its (patho)physiological significance in humans. Kidney Int 1992; 41:1115. Editorial.
49. Brenner BM, Ballermann BJ, Gunning ME, Zeidel ML. Diverse biological actions of atrial natriuretic peptide. Physiol Rev 1990; 70:665.
50. de Bold AJ, Borenstein HB, Veress AT, Sonnenberg H. A rapid and potent natriuretic response to intravenous injection of atrial myocardial extract in rats. Lif Sci 1981; 28:89.
51. Yoshimura M, Yasue H, Morita E, et al. Hemodynamic, renal, and hormonal responses to brain natriuretic peptide infusion in patients with congestive heart failure. Circulation 1991; 84:1581.
52. Naruse M, Takeyama Y, Tanabe A, et al. Atrial and brain natriuretic peptides in cardiovascular diseases. Hypertension 1994; 23:I231.
53. Lindop GB, Mallon EA, Hair J, Downie TT, MacIntyre G. ANF (99–126) and its propeptide, ANF (1–16), are secreted simultaneously from the human atrial myocyte. J Hypertens 1987; 5:533.
54. Ruskoaho H, Tholken H, Lang RE. Increase in atrial pressure releases atrial natriuretic peptide from isolated perfused rat hearts. Pflugers Arch 1986; 407:170.
55. Edwards BS, Zimmerman RS, Schwab TR, Heublein DM, Burnett JC Jr. Atrial stretch, not pressure, is the principal determinant controlling the acute release of atrial natriuretic factor. Circ Res 1988; 62:191.
56. Kohara K, Otsuka A, Mikami H, Katahira K, Tsunetoshi T, Ogihara T. Effects of the baroreceptor reflex system on atrial natriuretic factor secretion during volume expansion in dogs. Clin Sci 1989; 77:29.
57. Salazar FJ, Romero JC, Burnett JC Jr, Schryver S, Granger JP. Atrial natriuretic peptide levels during acute and chronic saline loading in conscious dogs. Am J Physiol 1986; 251:R499.
58. Cogan MG. Atrial natriuretic factor can increase renal solute excretion primarily by raising glomerular filtration. Am J Physiol 1986; 250:F710.

59. Burnett JC Jr, Granger JP, Opgenorth TJ. Effects of synthetic atrial natriuretic factor on renal function and renin release. Am J Physiol 1984; 247:F863.
60. Mendez RE, Dunn BR, Troy JL, Brenner BM. Modulation of the natriuretic response to atrial natriuretic peptide by alterations in peritubular Starling forces in the rat. Circ Res 1986; 59:605.
61. Metzler CH, Ramsay DJ. Physiological doses of atrial peptide inhibit angiotensin II-stimulated aldosterone secretion. Am J Physiol 1989; 256:R1155.
62. Shenker Y. Atrial natriuretic hormone effect on renal function and aldosterone secretion in sodium depletion. Am J Physiol 1988; 255:R867.
63. Richards M, Espiner E, Frampton C, et al. Inhibition of endopeptidase EC 24.11 in humans. Renal and endocrine effects. Hypertension 1990; 16:269.
64. Gomes GN, Aires MM. Interaction of atrial natriuretic factor and angiotensin II in proximal HCO_3^- reabsorption. Am J Physiol 1992; 262:F303.
65. Harris PJ, Skinner SL. Intra-renal interactions between angiotensin II and atrial natriuretic factor. Kidney Int Suppl 1990; 30:S87.
66. Harris PJ, Thomas D, Morgan TO. Atrial natriuretic peptide inhibits angiotensin-stimulated proximal tubular sodium and water reabsorption. Nature 1987; 326:697.
67. Almeida FA, Suzuki M, Maack T. Atrial natriuretic factor increases hematocrit and decreases plasma volume in nephrectomized rats. Life Sci 1986; 39:1193.
68. Huxley VH, Tucker VL, Verburg KM, Freeman RH. Increased capillary hydraulic conductivity induced by atrial natriuretic peptide. Circ Res 1987; 60:304.
69. Shenker Y, Sider RS, Ostafin EA, Grekin RJ. Plasma levels of immunoreactive atrial natriuretic factor in healthy subjects and in patients with edema. J Clin Invest 1985; 76:1684.
70. Ding J, Thibault G, Gutkowska J, et al. Cardiac and plasma atrial natriuretic factor in experimental congestive heart failure. Endocrinology 1987; 121:248.
71. Cody RJ, Atlas SA, Laragh JH, et al. Atrial natriuretic factor in normal subjects and heart failure patients. Plasma levels and renal, hormonal, and hemodynamic responses to peptide infusion. J Clin Invest 1986; 78:1362.
72. Raine AE, Erne P, Burgisser E, et al. Atrial natriuretic peptide and atrial pressure in patients with congestive heart failure. N Engl J Med 1986; 315:533.
73. Saito Y, Nakao K, Nishimura K, et al. Clinical application of atrial natriuretic polypeptide in patients with congestive heart failure: beneficial effects on left ventricular function. Circulation 1987; 76:115.
74. Burnett JC Jr, Kao PC, Hu DC, et al. Atrial natriuretic peptide elevation in congestive heart failure in the human. Science 1986; 231:1145.
75. Awazu M, Imada T, Kon V, Inagami T, Ichikawa I. Role of endogenous atrial natriuretic peptide in congestive heart failure. Am J Physiol 1989; 257:R641.
76. Rahman SN, Kim GE, Mathew AS, et al. Effects of atrial natriuretic peptide in clinical acute renal failure. Kidney Int 1994; 45:1731.
77. Drummer C, Fiedler F, Konig A, Gerzer R. Urodilatin, a kidney-derived natriuretic factor, is excreted with a circadian rhythm and is stimulated by saline infusion in man. J Am Soc Nephrol 1991; 1:1109.
78. Goetz KL. Renal natriuretic peptide (urodilatin?) and atriopeptin: evolving concepts. Am J Physiol 1991; 261:F921.
79. Goetz K, Drummer C, Zhu JL, Leadley R, Fiedler F, Gerzer R. Evidence that

urodilatin, rather than ANP, regulates renal sodium excretion. J Am Soc Nephrol 1990; 1:867.

80. Shaw S, Weidmann P, Zimmermann A. Urodilatin, not nitroprusside, combined with dopamine reverses ischemic acute renal failure. Kidney Int 1992; 42:1153.
81. Kon V, Yoshioka T, Fogo A, Ichikawa I. Glomerular actions of endothelin in vivo. J Clin Invest 1989; 83:1762.
82. Kourembanas S, Marsden PA, McQuillan LP, Faller DV. Hypoxia induces endothelin gene expression and secretion in cultured human endothelium. J Clin Invest 1991; 88:1054.
83. Luscher TF, Boulanger CM, Dohi Y, Yang ZH. Endothelium-derived contracting factors. Hypertension 1992; 19:117.
84. Chou SY, Dahhan A, Porush JG. Renal actions of endothelin: interaction with prostacyclin. Am J Physiol 1990; 259:F645.
85. Margulies KB, Hildebrand FL Jr, Lerman A, Perrella MA, Burnett JC Jr. Increased endothelin in experimental heart failure. Circulation 1990; 82:2226.
86. Cavero PG, Miller WL, Heublein DM, Margulies KB, Burnett JC Jr. Endothelin in experimental congestive heart failure in the anesthetized dog. Am J Physiol 1990; 259:F312.
87. Schlondorff D, Ardaillou R. Prostaglandins and other arachidonic acid metabolites in the kidney. Kidney Int 1986; 29:108.
88. Dworkin LD, Ichikawa I, Brenner BM. Hormonal modulation of glomerular function. Am J Physiol 1983; 244:F95.
89. Grantham JJ, Orloff J. Effect of prostaglandin E1 on the permeability response of the isolated collecting tubule to vasopressin, adenosine 3′,5′-monophosphate, and theophylline. J Clin Invest 1968; 47:1154.
90. Clive DM, Stoff JS. Renal syndromes associated with nonsteroidal antiinflammatory drugs. N Engl J Med 1984; 310:563.
91. Dunn MJ, Zambraski EJ. Renal effects of drugs that inhibit prostaglandin synthesis. Kidney Int 1980; 18:609.
92. Dzau VJ, Colucci WS, Williams GH, Curfman G, Meggs L, Hollenberg NK. Sustained effectiveness of converting-enzyme inhibition in patients with severe congestive heart failure. N Engl J Med 1980; 302:1373.
93. Dzau VJ, Hollenberg NK. Renal response to captopril in severe heart failure: role of furosemide in natriuresis and reversal of hyponatremia. Ann Intern Med 1984; 100:777.
94. Motwani JG, Fenwick MK, Morton JJ, Struthers AD. Furosemide-induced natriuresis is augmented by ultra-low-dose captopril but not by standard doses of captopril in chronic heart failure. Circulation 1992; 86:439.
95. Riegger AJ. ACE inhibitors in congestive heart failure. Cardiology 1989; 76(suppl 2):42.
96. Oster JR, Materson BJ. Renal and electrolyte complications of congestive heart failure and effects of therapy with angiotensin-converting enzyme inhibitors. Arch Intern Med 1992; 152:704.
97. Mandal AK, Markert RJ, Saklayen MG, Mankus RA, Yokokawa K. Diuretics potentiate angiotensin converting enzyme inhibitor-induced acute renal failure. Clin Nephrol 1994; 42:170.

98. Dzau VJ. Renal effects of angiotensin-converting enzyme inhibition in cardiac failure. Am J Kidney Dis 1987; 10:74.
99. Brater DC. The use of diuretics in congestive heart failure. Semin Nephrol 1994; 14:479.
100. Cody RJ, Kubo SH, Pickworth KK. Diuretic treatment for the sodium retention of congestive heart failure. Arch Intern Med 1994; 154:1905.
101. Martin SJ, Danziger LH. Continuous infusion of loop diuretics in the critically ill: a review of the literature. Crit Care Med 1994; 22:1323.
102. Singh NC, Kissoon N, al Mofada S, Bennett M, Bohn DJ. Comparison of continuous versus intermittent furosemide administration in postoperative pediatric cardiac patients. Crit Care Med 1992; 20:17.
103. Fowler SF, Murray KM. Torsemide: a new loop diuretic. Am J Health Syst Pharm 1995; 52:1771.
104. Abraham WT, Schrier RW. Body fluid volume regulation in health and disease. Adv Intern Med 1994; 39:23.
105. Ellison DH. The physiologic basis of diuretic synergism: its role in treating diuretic resistance [see comments]. Ann Intern Med 1991; 114:886.
106. Beermann B, Groschinsky-Grind M. Pharmacokinetics of hydrochlorothiazide in patients with congestive heart failure. Br J Clin Pharmocol 1979; 7:579.
107. Chertow GM, Sayegh H, Allgren RL, Lazarus JM. Is the administration of dopamine associated with adverse or favorable outcomes in acute renal failure? Auriculin Anaritide Acute Renal Failure Study Group. Am J Med 1996; 101(1):49–53.
108. Cosentino F. Drugs for the prevention and treatment of acute renal failure. Cleve Clin J Med 1995; 62(4):248–253.
109. Duke GJ, Briedis JH, Weaver RA. Renal support in critically ill patients: low-dose dopamine or low-dose dobutamine? Crit Care Med 1994; 22(12):1919–1925.
110. Vendegna TR, Anderson RJ. Are dopamine and/or dobutamine renoprotective in intensive care unit patients? Crit Care Med 1994; 22(12):1893–1894.
111. Parks RW, Diamond T, McCrory DC, Johnston GW, Rowlands BJ. Prospective study of postoperative renal function in obstructive jaundice and the effect of preoperative dopamine. Br J Surg 1994; 81(3):437–439.
112. Baldwin L, Henderson A, Hickman P. Effect of postoperative low-dose dopamine on renal function after elective major vascular surgery. Ann Intern Med 1994; 120(9): 744–747.
113. Kikeri D, Mitch WE. The heart and kidney disease. In: Schlant RC, Alexander RW, eds. The Heart, Companion Handbook. New York: McGraw-Hill 1995:317–328.
114. Kellerman PS. Perioperative care of the renal patient. Arch Intern Med 1994; 154: 1674–1688.
115. Gillum DM, Dixon BS, Yanover MJ. The role of intensive dialysis in acute renal failure. Clin Nephrol 1986; 25:249–255.
116. Mehta RL. Therapeutic alternatives to renal replacement for critically ill patients in acute renal failure. Semin Nephrol 1994; 14(1):64–82.
117. Conger JD. Does hemodialysis delay recovery from acute renal failure? Semin Dial 1990; 3:146–148.
118. Conger JD, Robinette JB, Hammond WS. Differences in vascular reactivity in models of ischemic acute renal failure. Kidney Int 1991; 39:1087–1097.

119. Hakim RM, Wingard RL, Parker RA. Effect of the dialysis membrane in the treatment of patients with acute renal failure. N Engl J Med 1994; 331(20):1338–1342.
120. Schulman G, Fogo A, Gung A, Badr K, Hakim RM. Complement activation retards resolution of acute ischemic renal failure in the rat. Kidney Int 1991; 40:1069–1074.
121. Myers BD, Moran SM. Hemodynamically-mediated acute renal failure. N Engl J Med 1986; 314:97–105.
122. Hakim RM. Clinical implications of hemodialysis membrane biocompatibility. Kidney Int 1993; 44:484–494.
123. Cheung AK, LeWinter M, Chenoweth DE, Lew WY, Henderson LW. Cardiopulmonary effects of cuprophane-activated plasma in the swine. Kidney Int 1986; 29:799–806.
124. Strasser T, Schiffl H. Generation of leukotriene B4 by hemodialyzer membranes: a novel index of biocompatibility. Klin Wochenschr 1991: 69:808–812.
125. Brezis M, Heyman SN, Dinour D, Epstein FH, Rosen S. Role of nitric oxide in renal medullary oxygenation: studies in isolated and intact kidneys. J Clin Invest 1991; 88:390–395.
126. Leblanc M, Tapolyai M, Paganini EP. What dialysis dose should be provided in acute renal failure? A review. Adv Renal Replace Ther 1995; 2(3):255–264.
127. Henrich WL. Hemodynamic instability during hemodialysis. Kidney Int 1986; 30: 605–612.
128. Daugirdas JT. Dialysis hypotension: a hemodynamic analysis. Kidney Int 1991; 39: 233–246.
129. Schulman G, Hakim RM. Complications of hemodialysis. In: Jacobson HR, Striker GE, Klahr S, eds. The Principles and Practice of Nephrology. St. Louis: Mosby–Year Book, 1995:673–683.
130. Ahmad S, Blagg CR, Scribner BH. Center and home chronic hemodialysis. In: Schrier RW, Gottschalk CW, eds. Diseases of the Kidney. Boston: Little, Brown, 1993:3031–3068.
131. Ewing DJ, Winney R. Autonomic function in patients with chronic renal failure on intermittent hemodialysis. Nephron 1975; 15:424–429.
132. Lilley JJ, Golden J, Stone RA. Adrenergic regulation of blood pressure in chronic renal failure. J Clin Invest 1976; 57:1190–1200.
133. Nies AS, Robertson D, Stone WJ. Hemodialysis hypotension is not the result of uremic peripheral neuropathy. J Lab Clin Med 1979; 94:395–402.
134. Friess U, Rascher W, Ritz E, Gross P. Failure of arginine-vasopressin and other pressor hormones to increase in severe recurrent dialysis hypotension. Nephrol Dial Transplant 1995; 10:1421–1427.
135. Daul AE, Wang XL, Michel MC, Brodde OE. Arterial hypotension in chronic hemodialyzed patients. Kidney Int 1987; 32:728–735.
136. Kouw PM, Kooman JP, Cheriex EC. Assessment of postdialysis dry weight: a comparison of techniques. J Am Soc Nephrol 1993; 4:98–104.
137. Maggiore Q, Pizzarelli F, Zocalli C. Effect of extracorporeal cooling on dialytic arterial hypotension. Proc Eur Dial Transplant Assoc 1981; 18:597–602.
138. Sherman RA, Rubin MP, Cody RP, Eisinger RP. Amelioration of hemodialysis-associated hypotension by the use of cool dialysate. Am J Kidney Dis 1985; 5: 124–127.

139. Jost CM, Agarwal R, Khair-el-din T. Effects of cooler temperature dialysate on hemodynamic stability in "problem" dialysis patients. Kidney Int 1993; 44: 606–612.
140. Mahida BH, Dumler F, Zasuwa G. Effect of cooling dialysate on serum catecholamines and blood pressure stability. Trans Am Soc Artif Intern Organs 1983; 29: 384–389.
141. Hampl H, Paeprer H, Unger V. Hemodynamic changes during hemodialysis, sequential ultrafiltration and hemofiltration. Kidney Int 1980; 18:S83–S88.
142. Wehle B, Asaba H, Castenfors J. Hemodynamic changes during sequential ultrafiltration and dialysis. Kidney Int 1979; 15:411–418.
143. Caruana RJ, Keep D, Kozeny GA, Ing TS. Isolated ultrafiltration. In: Nissenson AR, Fine RN, eds. Dialysis Therapy. Philadelphia: Hanley and Belfus, 1993: 104–107.
144. Parnes EL, Shapiro WB. Anaphylactoid reactions in hemodialysis patients treated with the AN69 dialyzer. Kidney Int 1991; 40:1148–1152.
145. Schulman G, Hakim R, Arias R, Silverberg M, Kaplan AP, Arbeit L. Bradykinin generation by dialysis membranes: possible role in anaphylactic reaction. J Am Soc Nephrol 1993; 3:1563–1569.
146. Verresen L, Fink E, Lemke HD. Bradykinin is a mediator of anaphylactoid reactions during hemodialysis with AN69 membranes. Kidney Int 1994; 45:1497–1503.
147. Ross EA, Nissenson AR. Dialysis hypoxemia. In: Nissenson AR, Fine RN, eds. Dialysis Therapy. Philadelphia: Hanley and Belfus, 1993:130–132.
148. Cardoso M, Vinay P, Vinet B. Hypoxemia during hemodialysis: a critical review of the facts. Am J Kidney Dis 1988; 11:281–297.
149. Hunt JM, Chappell TR, Henrich WL, Rubin LJ. Gas exchange during dialysis: contrasting mechanisms contributing to comparable alterations with acetate and bicarbonate buffers. Am J Med 1984; 77:255–260.
150. Patterson RW, Nissenson AR, Miller J. Hypoxemia and pulmonary gas exchange during hemodialysis. J Appl Physiol 1981; 50:259–264.
151. Rostand SG. Management of ischemic heart disease, heart failure and pericarditis in hemodialysis patients. In: Nissenson AR, Fine RN, eds. Dialysis Therapy. Philadelphia: Hanley and Belfus, 1993:252–259.
152. Rostand SG, Rutsky EA. Cardia diseases in dialysis patients. In: Nissenson AR, Fine RN, Gentile DE, eds. Clinical Dialysis. South Norwalk, CT: Appleton and Lange, 1990:409–446.
153. Rutsky EA. Arrhythmias in hemodialysis patients. In: Nissenson AR, Fine RN, eds. Dialysis Therapy. Philadelphia: Hanley and Belfus, 1993:116–123.
154. Arieff AI. Dialysis disequilibrium syndrome: current concepts on pathogenesis and prevention. Kidney Int 1994; 45:629–635.
155. Rodrigo F, Shideman J, McHugh R. Osmolality changes during dialysis. Ann Intern Med 1977; 86:554–561.
156. Silver SM, DeSimone JA, Smith DA, Stern RH. Dialysis disequilibrium syndrome in the rat: role of the "reverse urea effect." Kidney Int 1992; 42:161–166.
157. Burkart JM, Nolph KD. Peritoneal dialysis. In: Brenner BM, ed. The Kidney. Philadelphia: W.B. Saunders, 1996:1507–2575.

158. Rottembourg J. Residual renal function and recovery of renal function in patients treated by CAPD. Kidney Int 1993; 43:S106–S110.
159. Lysaght MJ, Vones EF, Gotch F. The influence of dialysis treatment modality on the decline of remaining renal function. Trans ASAIO 1991: 37:598–604.
160. Diaz-Buxo JA. Clinical use of peritoneal dialysis. In: Nissenson AR, Fine RN, Gentile DE, eds. Clinical Dialysis. Connecticut: Appleton and Lange, 1990: 256–300.
161. Ash SR, Bever SL. Peritoneal dialysis for acute renal failure: the safe, effective and low-cost modality. Adv Renal Replace Ther 1995; 2(2):160–163.
162. Breyer JA. Complications of peritoneal dialysis. In: Jacobson HR, Striker GE, Klahr S, eds. The Principles and Practice of Nephrology. St. Louis: Mosby–Year Book, 1995:700–712.
163. Spinowitz BS, Charytan C, Gupta B. Hydrothorax and peritoneal dialysis. In: Nissenson AR, Fine RN, eds. Dialysis Therapy. Philadelphia: Hanley and Belfus, 1993:189–191.
164. Mestas D, Wauquier JP, Escande G. Diagnosis of hydrothorax complicating CAPD and demonstration of successful therapy by scintigraphy. Perit Dial Int 1991; 11: 283–285.
165. Saillen P, Mosimann F, Wauters JP. Hydrothorax and end-stage chronic renal failure. Chest 1991; 99:1010–1011.
166. Ronco C. Continuous renal replacement therapies for the treatment of acute renal failure in intensive care patients. Clin Nephrol 1993; 40(4):187–198.
167. Sigler MH, Teehan BP. Continuous arteriovenous hemodialysis in acute renal failure. In: Glassock RJ, ed. Current Therapy in Nephrology and Hypertension. St. Louis: Mosby–Year Book, 1992:281–285.
168. Kaplan AA. Continuous renal replacement therapies—whom, how and why. ASAIO J 1994; 40:940–942.
169. Goldfarb S, Golper TA. Tumor necrosis factor-alpha and interleukin-1 selectively sieve through and bind to hemofilter membranes. J Am Soc Nephrol 1993; 4:316.
170. Stein B, Pfenninger E, Grunert A. Influence of continuous hemofiltration on hemodynamics and central blood volume in experimental endotoxic shock. Intens Care Med 1990; 16:494–499.
171. Gomez A, Wang R, Unruh H. Hemofiltration reverses left ventricular dysfunction during sepsis in dogs. Anesthesiology 1990; 73:671–685.
172. Barzilay E, Kessler D, Berlot G. Use of extracorporeal supportive techniques as additional treatment for septic-induced multiple organ failure patients. Crit Care Med 1989; 17:634–637.
173. Bellomo R, Tipping P, Boyce N. Tumor necrosis factor clearances during venovenous hemodiafiltration in the critically ill. ASAIO Trans 1991; 37:M322–M323.
174. Sigler MH, Teehan BP, Daugirdas JT, Ing TS. Slow continuous therapies. In: Daugirdas JT, Ing TS, eds. Handbook of Dialysis. Boston: Little, Brown, 1994: 169–197.
175. Sigler MH, Manns M. Continuous renal replacement therapy in the critically ill patient with acute renal failure—pros and cons. ASAIO J 1994; 40(4):928–930.
176. Biasioli S, Barbaresi F, Barberio M. Intermittent venovenous hemofiltration as a

chronic treatment for refractory and intractable heart failure. ASAIO J 1992; 38: M658–M663.

177. Lauer A, Alvis R, Avram M. Hemodynamic consequences of continuous arterio-venous hemofiltration. Am J Kidney Dis 1988; 12:110–115.
178. Kaplan AA. Renal replacement therapy for acute renal failure. In: Glassock RJ, ed. Current Therapy in Nephrology and Hypertension. St. Louis: Mosby–Year Book, 1992:264–274.

15

Diabetic Ketoacidosis

PHILIP BARNETT

Cedars-Sinai Medical Center and University of California, Los Angeles, School of Medicine, Los Angeles, California

The major acute metabolic complications occurring in patients with diabetes mellitus include diabetic ketoacidosis (DKA), hyperglycemic hyperosmolar nonketotic syndrome (HHNK), lactic acidosis, and hypoglycemia. This chapter will deal predominantly with the management of DKA, the commonest of these complications, although diabetic patients within the cardiac care unit (CCU) may present with or develop any of these. They may also present with one of a number of other acute metabolic complications or they may have one or more of the many chronic complications of diabetes. The chronic complications of diabetes may require monitoring and management because of progressive deterioration, or as a result of an acute on chronic problem that develops within the CCU. In general, patients within the CCU are older and probably already have some of the chronic complications of diabetes: namely, macrovascular diseases such as ischemic heart disease, cerebrovascular and peripheral vascular disease, and microvascular diseases represented by nephropathy, neuropathy, or retinopathy.

Of the numerous types of diabetes, the main ones are type 1 (pancreatic islet β-cell destruction, usually leading to absolute insulin deficiency, and prone to ketoacidosis. In most cases the process is immune mediated; in some it remains idiopathic), and type 2 (most prevalent form of diabetes, resulting from variable insulin resistance and insulin secretory defect). Although DKA develops more commonly in type 1 patients, it does also present in those with type 2, especially during acute illness, when it may portend the onset of insulin deficiency.

A host of other medical conditions may coexist in patients with diabetes, but it is important to remember the endocrine associations (both autoimmune and non-autoimmune) such as acromegaly, Cushing's syndrome, Addison's disease, and thyroid dysfunction. These will also require recognition and treatment, either as ongoing chronic diseases or due to acute crises that may complicate a patient's CCU admission.

Diabetic patients, especially those with poorly controlled blood glucose levels, often have associated hyperlipidemia, which may be a contributing risk factor for the underlying cause of their current reason for admission to the CCU, e.g., myocardial infarction. This may require separate attention and therapy in addition to the acute management of blood glucose levels.

Various aspects of the definition, pathogenesis, and management of DKA remain controversial and will be discussed briefly where appropriate. I have adopted practical definitions and principles of management for the purpose of this discussion.

I. DIAGNOSIS OF DKA

There is as yet no consensus on the exact definition of DKA, of which there are mild to severe forms (1). DKA resides at one end of the spectrum of diabetic metabolic decompensation with HHNK at the other end.

Diabetic ketoacidosis may be generally defined as being present in patients with relative or absolute insulin deficiency when the following criteria are met:

1. *Hyperglycemia*: blood glucose > 250 mg/dl. For population-based studies, hyperglycemia is defined as > 200 mg/dl (2). Other authors use a value of $\geqslant 300$ mg/dl, stating that patients with glucose values $\leqslant 350$ mg/dl (15% of DKA patients) have "euglycemic DKA" (3,4).
2. *Ketosis*: moderate to severe ketonemia (ketone levels positive at a serum dilution of $\geqslant 1{:}2$, or serum β-hydroxybutyrate concentration > 0.5 mmol/L [5] and moderate ketonuria (2–3+ by the nitroprusside method).
3. *Acidosis*: pH $\leqslant 7.3$ and/or bicarbonate $\leqslant 15$ mEq/L (6–8).

Associated metabolic and plasma abnormalities include: dehydration requiring intravenous fluid replacement; increased osmolality, usually less than 320 mOsm/kg; elevated anion gap > 12 mEq/L (5–7); increased serum amylase; increased white blood cell count, not $> 25{,}000/mm^3$; and hypertriglyceridemia.

The diagnosis of DKA is made when the three conditions of hyperglycemia, ketosis, and acidosis coexist (9). Each of the above three components may, however, be separately associated with other conditions.

Hyperglycemic states include diabetes mellitus, HHNK, impaired glucose tolerance, and stress hyperglycemia. Metabolic acidosis, with increased anion gap, may be due to lactic acidosis, salicylate overdose, methanol ingestion, or other drugs; and with normal anion gap, may be due to hyperchloremic acidosis, uremia, or gastrointestinal disease. Ketosis may exist during hypoglycemia, acute alcoholism (10), and starvation (1).

DKA is an extremely serious acute metabolic condition, which, despite advances in our understanding of the pathophysiology and improvements in management, is still associated with considerable morbidity and mortality.

The incidence of DKA, derived from population-based studies, is approximately 5–8/1000 diabetic persons/year. DKA is more common in young diabetic persons, 13–54/1000 persons aged < 15 years/year. DKA occurs in approximately 2–3/1000 persons/year in people > 30 years of age (2). Although approaching neutrality, DKA is still more prevalent in females, 1.5–1.8:1 (11). Figures for CCU admissions are not available.

Between 1989 and 1991, 100,000 hospital discharges were coded to DKA annually. The most recent mortality rates for DKA in the United States have been approximately 9–14% (11,12) with rates exceeding 20% for people > 65 years (2,13). Death often results not from the ketoacidosis itself, but from one of the comorbid conditions such as myocardial infarction or other cardiovascular pathology, pulmonary complications such as pneumonia or other infections, or from complications induced by the treatment regimen per se (6,7,8). For patients in the CCU, the coexistence of DKA and cardiac disease often complicated by sepsis or pulmonary pathology increases the risk of death.

II. PRECIPITATING FACTORS

In the general population, the most common precipitating factor in the development of DKA is infection (30%), which is often minor, with origin usually in the respiratory or urinary tracts. This is followed in decreasing order of frequency by cases of new-onset diabetes (25%) (14), problems with insulin administration (20%), and then a collection of miscellaneous causes (15). In as many as 25% of cases a precipitating cause may not be identified (16).

Patients with DKA may be in the CCU for one of several reasons:

1. A diabetic patient presenting with DKA may be found to have myocardial ischemia, infarction, or other cardiac event as the precipitating cause. Myocardial ischemia may be painful but frequently is silent and only diagnosed by electrocardiogram and cardiac enzyme criteria.
2. A patient with a myocardial infarction or other cardiac event already in the CCU may develop DKA. These patients may have previously diagnosed diabetes or this acute event may be the first manifestation of diabetes. This latter possibility serves to emphasize the importance of obtaining a de-

tailed history from both the patient and family or chaperone, including a history of previous DKA (22% of patients have had more than one DKA [17]). A full physical examination may also alert the physician to the possibility of diabetes in a previously undiagnosed individual and raise awareness of the risk of development of DKA and other metabolic complications.

All patients with type 2 diabetes admitted to the CCU, if not already taking insulin, should be converted to insulin therapy, at least for the duration of their stay in the CCU, irrespective of their metabolic and diabetic status.

In almost one-quarter of patients with newly diagnosed type 1 diabetes, DKA may be the presenting illness (18). Thirty percent of patients older than 65 years may have no previous history of diabetes (13). Patients on continuous subcutaneous insulin infusion (CSII) via an insulin pump are more vulnerable to DKA. This may develop within hours following unrecognized pump failure or other reason for interrupted insulin delivery. Only regular, short-acting, insulin is used in the pump and there is thus no safety cushion of a depot of intermediate- or long-acting insulin.

The importance of education and patient empowerment to assume responsibility for their own disease management cannot be overemphasized. Trials such as the DCCT (19) have demonstrated a lower incidence of DKA in patients receiving intensive diabetes education. Lack of, or inadequate, health insurance and limited access to reasonable health care are important factors in the development of DKA (20).

III. PATHOPHYSIOLOGY

Absolute or relative insulin deficiency is central to the development of DKA. The concurrent increase in the insulin counterregulatory hormones (ICRH) glucagon, growth hormone, cortisol, and catecholamines together interact to produce the metabolic decompensation of DKA. The net effects are as follows:

1. Hyperglycemia is the end result of several simultaneous processes;
   a. Increased rate of hepatic glucose production by gluconeogenesis, driven by increased circulating concentrations of both amino acids and free fatty acids, which result from increased skeletal muscle proteolysis and adipose tissue lipolysis, respectively, in the insulin-deficient state.
   b. Increased hepatic glycogenolysis stimulated by glucagon.
   c. Decreased peripheral glucose uptake predominantly by skeletal muscle and adipose tissue.
   d. Diminished glomerular filtration rate due to progressive dehydration (see below).

2. Ketosis results from:
   a. Increased hepatic production of ketone bodies (ketogenesis) by the β-oxidation of excess free fatty acids. Loss of inhibition of insulin-sensitive lipase results in increased lipolysis and triglyceride breakdown releasing free fatty acids, a process enhanced by glucagon (21).
   b. Diminished peripheral utilization of ketones during insulin deficiency.
3. Metabolic acidosis arises from a failure to adequately buffer the excess ketoacids with a resultant increase in the plasma anion gap and an equivalent decrease in plasma bicarbonate concentration (1). The acidosis and elevated prostaglandins found in this state (22) result in loss of vascular tone, which together with the marked fluid loss (osmotic diuresis; see below) may lead to vascular collapse and shock.
4. Dehydration is the result of the osmotic diuresis produced when the proximal renal tubule glucose threshold of 180 mg/dl is exceeded during hyperglycemia, leading to glycosuria and polyuria. This results in urinary loss also of electrolytes and ketone bodies (which exacerbates the osmotic diuresis) with subsequent volume depletion (intravascular, intracellular, and extracellular) and hyperosmolarity of the extracellular fluid. This may lead to impairment of renal function and exacerbate the hyperglycemia (above). The actual fluid loss incurred may be as great as 10% of the body weight (23).
5. Electrolyte abnormalities resulting from the osmotic diuresis are:
   a. Hyponatremia: This may reflect a total-body Na deficit of 7–10 mEq/kg body weight. Water loss usually exceeds NaCl loss (24,25), and together with osmotic shifts, plasma Na concentrations may initially be normal or low.
   b. Hypokalemia: This may be profound with a total-body deficit usually of about 3–5 mEq/kg body weight, but which may be as high as 10 mEq/kg (1,6,23). Plasma concentrations of potassium, which reflect only 2% of body potassium stores, although occasionally low, are usually normal or elevated at the time of presentation, owing to a combination of acidosis, increased osmolality in the extracellular fluid, and increased intracellular proteolysis. Insulin deficiency retards the intracellular movement of potassium.
   c. Hypophosphatemia: Total-body deficit ranges from 0.15 to 1.5 mmol/kg body weight (23). At presentation, serum concentrations may be high, normal, or low and will fall with treatment following cellular uptake of phosphate. Respiratory failure, rhabdomyolysis, hemolytic anemia, decreased red cell 2,3-diphosphoglycerate levels, and impaired cardiac and skeletal muscle function have all been associated with hypophosphatemia. Numerous authors have failed to demonstrate any positive effect of phosphate supplementation during the

treatment of DKA (26–29) but no studies have addressed this issue in patients specifically with cardiopulmonary disease, especially those within the CCU, in whom replacement may prove beneficial or in fact be essential.

d. Hypomagnesemia: Total-body deficit ranges from 1 to 2 mEq/kg body weight. There are no data to support routine replacement of this electrolyte but it may be necessary following phosphate therapy.
e. Hypocalcemia: Total-body deficit ranges from 1 to 2 mEq/kg body weight. This electrolyte is not routinely replaced but it may become necessary if clinical signs and symptoms dictate, or following phosphate therapy.
f. Hypochloremia: Total-body deficit ranges from 3 to 5 mEq/kg body weight (1).

Patients presenting early in the course of development of DKA or who have managed to maintain adequate NaCl and fluid intake and have good renal function usually have increased urinary ketone loss and a relatively smaller anion gap and may present with hyperchloremic acidosis (1).

In summary, insulin deficiency and raised ICRH result in increased hepatic glucose production and decreased peripheral glucose utilization leading to hyperglycemia and hyperosmolarity with consequent osmotic diuresis with electrolyte loss and dehydration. Activation of lipase stimulates free fatty acid release from adipose tissues, which are oxidized in the liver to produce ketone bodies. These spill over into the circulation resulting in ketosis and metabolic acidosis.

IV. PRESENTATION

DKA may not be obvious at presentation because signs and symptoms are subtle and may be overshadowed by those of acute macrovascular disease or infection or because they may not be recognized in patients presenting for the first time with DKA. Patients may also be admitted with a primary diagnosis other than diabetes mellitus. DKA usually develops within hours to days, and in contrast to patients presenting with HHNK, the hyperglycemia and hyperosmolality are usually not as severe because the metabolic acidosis makes these patients feel ill and leads them to seek early medical attention. Prevention of DKA is the best policy, and within the CCU heightened awareness and regular patient monitoring with appropriate fluid and insulin therapy will hopefully result in early detection of metabolic decompensation, possibly even before the patient starts exhibiting classical symptoms and signs. Although usually obvious within the CCU setting, a search for the precipitating cause(s) (see above) must be initiated at the time of diagnosis, as early treatment will obviously facilitate the rapid resolution of DKA.

The following are the most commonly experienced symptoms of DKA, listed in decreasing order of frequency. Not all of these will be evident in patients within the CCU.

Nausea/vomiting
Thirst/polydipsia
Polyuria
Weight loss
Abdominal pain
Weakness
Fatigue
Anorexia

The following are the commonly observed signs of DKA. Diagnosis in patients within the CCU may be made well before many of these manifest themselves.

Tachycardia
Orthostatic hypotension
Dehydration
Warm, dry skin and mucous membranes
Flushed appearance
Hyperventilation → Kussmaul's respiration
Hypothermia/normothermia
Ketones on the breath
Altered mental status → coma

V. SIGNS AND SYMPTOMS

The signs and symptoms (listed above) reflect the presence of dehydration, hyperglycemia, and metabolic acidosis.

Dehydration, if severe enough, may result in thrombosis and thromboembolism. Although more common in patients with HHNK, this complication may be relevant in patients immobilized in the CCU.

Abdominal pain, often mimicking an acute abdomen, occurs in 25–30% of cases of DKA and may be due to mesenteric thrombosis, pancreatitis in patients with severe hypertriglyceridemia, or some other underlying abdominal disease, especially in the population of patients found in the CCU. Elevated serum amylase, which is found in as many as 80% of patients with DKA (30), originates from both salivary (parotid) glands and pancreas. Isoenzymes will help differentiate the source and exclude pancreatitis. If this is not available, a normal serum lipase level will usually rule out pancreatitis. More commonly, the abdominal pain is related to the DKA per se and remains unexplained in two-thirds of episodes (21,31). The abdominal pain of DKA resolves rapidly with treatment of the underlying metabolic abnormalities.

As many as 80% of patients at some time during the episode of DKA have a degree of mental obtundation, which is proportional to the increase in serum osmolality (29). Ten percent may, in fact, proceed to coma.

Hypothermia or normal body temperature may be present in the face of infection (32,33) and reflect the degree of dehydration and intravascular volume depletion with hypotension and peripheral vascular shutdown. True temperature values will be seen following fluid replacement.

VI. LABORATORY INVESTIGATIONS

Diabetic ketoacidosis is a life-threatening condition and it is important not to take any shortcuts in the diagnosis and monitoring of patients with this condition. Patients within the CCU are probably more vulnerable than those managed in other settings because of their comorbid conditions, and extra vigilance is needed to ensure that all abnormalities are detected and treated appropriately.

Patient history and physical examination will determine the range of initial investigations (Table 1), and response to therapy will dictate the appropriateness of further tests. Patients in the CCU will require a complete baseline metabolic/biochemical profile, and lack of an obvious precipitating cause may require an early comprehensive workup including the spectrum of tests listed.

Hyperglycemia in DKA, on average, is approximately 500 mg/dl (34) compared to the average of > 1000 mg/dl in patients with HHNK. Early detection of DKA may yield blood glucose values between 200 and 300 mg/dl, so-called "euglycemic" ketoacidosis. Prior ineffective use of insulin in an attempt to prevent DKA may result in partial lowering of elevated blood glucose levels. Raised serum lipids may result in falsely low blood glucose values, within the euglycemic range.

Serum Na concentrations are usualy low or normal (approximately 130–140 mEq/L) and serum K values normal or elevated (approximately 5–6 mEq/L). Hyperglycemia itself may result in a spuriously low plasma Na concentration. The actual sodium concentration can be calculated by adding 1.6 mEq to the reported Na value for every 100 mg/dl of glucose above 100 mg/dl (35). Hypertriglyceridemia, through a dilutional effect (displacement of plasma water by elevated lipids) is also responsible for falsely low serum Na values. This may be suspected by the lipemic appearance of the serum sample, which should be appropriately processed to avoid delay in diagnosis and treatment.

Serum osmolality rarely exceeds 320 mOsm/kg in patients with DKA although it is usual to record values greater than this in HHNK. The anion gap is increased on average by 17–29 mEq/L (36), because of unmeasured anions, which in DKA are due to the ketone bodies β-hydroxybutyrate, acetoacetate, and acetone. The nitroprusside test, commonly used to detect ketones, only measures acetoacetate and acetone but not β-hydroxybutyrate. In all patients, but particularly older ones with comorbid conditions in the CCU, certain drugs may influence laboratory values; e.g., urine ketones may be falsely elevated in patients taking captopril (6).

Elevated serum ketones are responsible for factitiously elevated serum creatinine values. This results in a reversal of the expected ratio in which BUN is elevated out of proportion to creatinine in dehydration. Creatinine values will return to their true concentrations following rehydration and a decrease in ketones. Urea concentrations, therefore, should be used as a guide to the severity of renal dysfunction. They will, however, also be influenced by the degree of dehydration.

It is important to be aware that numerous other acid-base abnormalities, in addition to ketoacidosis, may be present in patients with DKA, especially in patients in the CCU. Limitation of space prevents any discussion of these besides listing just a few:

- Mixed metabolic acidosis, which is influenced by volume status, e.g., ketoacidosis and hyperchloremic acidosis in patients with mild dehydration. Hypotension or shock will result in increased lactate production during anaerobic metabolism and accentuate any acidosis already present.
- Respiratory alkalosis in a patient with pneumonia.
- Metabolic alkalosis resulting from vomiting or prior use of diuretics, associated with hypokalemia and hypochloremia.
- Primary respiratory acidosis, which may be acute, as in cardiopulmonary arrest, neuromuscular diseases, or drug-induced or cerebral disorders that depress the respiratory center. It may be chronic, as in chronic emphysema or bronchitis or due to extreme obesity (Pickwickian syndrome).

The white blood cell count is commonly nonspecifically elevated but not more than 20–25,000 mm^3 unless an infection is present, when left shift or toxic granulation may also be apparent.

The importance of a thorough physical examination cannot be overemphasized especially in the CCU where changes in cardiovascular, respiratory, and other systems need to be detected early and treated. Failure to improve clinically and metabolically following initiation of therapy indicates the need for repeat physical examination and review of the history. The presence and status of comorbid conditions and complications in patients with diabetes require regular reappraisal.

VII. TREATMENT

DKA is characterized by ICRH-stimulated hepatic glucose production combined with severe resistance to the action of insulin in both liver and peripheral tissues (primarily muscle) (37). The presence in the plasma of acidosis, hypertonicity, increased levels of ketones, free fatty acids, amino acids, and lactate and decreased total-body phosphate together with the elevated ICRHs all exacerbate the inhibition of insulin-mediated glucose disposal in peripheral tissues.

Table 1 Recommended Baseline Investigations for the Diagnosis of DKA and Establishment of a Precipitating Cause

- Blood glucose
- Plasma urea, creatinine, and electrolytes
- Plasma bicarbonate
- Liver function
- Lipid profile
- Plasma ketones
- Serum amylase/lipase
- Full blood count with differential
- Arterial blood gas[a]
- Blood cultures
- Culture of abscess or infected site
- Urine glucose and ketones
- Urine microscopy and culture
- Chest x-ray
- Abdominal x-ray (in presence of abdominal pain)
- Electrocardiogram
- Cardiac enzymes (if appropriate)
- Lumbar puncture (if appropriate)
- Acute illness/stress
  - Infection (30–40%)
    - Respiratory
    - Urinary tract
    - Sepsis
    - Other (otitis media, vaginitis)
  - Myocardial infarction
  - Cerebrovascular accident
  - Acute pancreatitis
  - Trauma
  - Surgery
  - Gastrointestinal disease
    - Gastroenteritis
    - Nausea/vomiting
- Pregnancy
- Hypokalemia
  - Diuretics
  - Nasogastric suction
  - Vomiting
- Alcohol abuse
- Renal failure
- Endocrine
  - Acromegaly
  - Thyrotoxicosis
  - Cushing's syndrome

Table 1 Continued

New-onset diabetes (25% of patients with type 1 diabetes)
Insufficient Insulin
Failure to meet increasing insulin requirements (15–20%)
Missed injection/cessation of insulin therapy
Mechanical failure (pen/pump/syringe)/poor technique
Inadequate glucose monitoring
Lack of diabetes education and training
Poor communication
Psychological
Noncompliance
Poor self-care
Insulin antibodies with resistance to insulin
Use of continuous subcutaneous insulin infusion (CSII) by insulin pump
Medication
Thiazide diuretics
Beta blockers
Calcium channel blockers
Steroids
Pentamidine
Precipitating factors for DKA in patients with established diabetes mellitus (11,18,20,21, 45,94–96)
Indeterminate cause
Mismanagement of diabetes including poor compliance and poor self-care
Unrecognized subclinical illness
Lack of health insurance
Lack of access to appropriate health care
Serum osmolality[b]
Anion gap[c]

[a]If venous blood is used, a factor of 0.03 should be added to the pH value. Venous blood should not be used for blood gas evaluation.

[b]Calculation of osmolality:

$$2[\mathrm{Na}^{2+}\ (\mathrm{mEq/L})] + 2\ [\mathrm{K}^{+}\ (\mathrm{mEq/L})] + \frac{\text{glucose (mg/dl)}}{18} + \frac{\text{BUN (mg/dl)}}{2.8}$$

[c]Calculation of anion gap:

$$\mathrm{Na}^{2+} - (\mathrm{Cl}^{-} + \mathrm{HCO}_3^{-})$$

Most important in the therapy of DKA is the restoration of circulating volume, maintenance of cardiac output and renal function, and improvement of tissue perfusion. This will automatically result in lowering of blood glucose, lipids, osmolality, ketones, and ICRHs (38,39), as well as improvement in the peripheral utilization of ketones and glucose. Insulin administration will facilitate the peripheral uptake of ketones and glucose, stop the urinary glucose loss, and most important, inhibit hepatic glucose production (40). Initial fluid therapy also lowers blood glucose levels by enhancing glucose loss in the urine and diluting it in the serum. Correction of electrolyte imbalances is the third component in the therapeutic triad, which includes fluid and insulin replacement. Identification of a precipitating cause will dictate specific treatment that should complement that of the DKA.

General therapeutic principles will be discussed below and specific elements will be expanded in a set of guidelines. Therapy may be divided into four phases, which tend to blend into one another. The first usually consists of making the diagnosis and initiating treatment commonly in the emergency department. For the purpose of this discussion it will be presumed that the patient is already in the CCU where the diagnosis is suspected and confirmed by examination and appropriate laboratory investigations. At this stage a precipitating cause should be sought. Other causes of acidosis should be explored if serum acetone and acetoacetic acid levels are normal. Intravenous fluids, insulin, and potassium replacement should be commenced immediately. The urgency to initiate treatment following the diagnosis is supported by data that reflect an increased risk of morbidity and mortality in these patients based on the length of time from diagnosis to commencement of therapy (7,8,13). Knowledge of fluid status is crucial when rehydrating patients, especially those with cardiac pathology, in whom overvigorous replacement can be catastrophic. Ideally, all patients in the CCU should have a central venous line or Swan-Ganz catheter for assessment of fluid status and central pressures in addition to adquate venous access for fluid replacement. In severely ill and acidotic patients, consider a peripheral arterial catheter for frequent arterial blood gas (ABG) and other laboratory measurements. All fluid intake and output should be charted, preferably on a flow chart together with all other therapies, laboratory values, and vital signs. It may be necessary to insert a Foley catheter into the bladder to monitor urinary output if there has been none 2 hr after initiation of therapy. At this time, a urine sample should be sent for culture. Comatose patients, those with absent or diminished gag and/or cough reflexes, vomiting, and the presence of a succussion splash or dilated stomach should be nil per mouth and have nasogastric suction. Oxygen therapy should be considerd for hypoxic ($po_2 < 80$ mmHg) and comatose patients and all those with cardiopulmonary diseases. In patients without cardiopulmonary disease, the po_2 at the time of presentation is usually normal but may decline with therapy due to progressive pulmonary edema (41). It may be prudent to deliver supplemental oxygen to all patients with DKA in the CCU at a rate of 4–6 L/min by face mask or 2 L/min by nasal prongs. The oxygen saturation should be maintained above 90% and can be monitored by a peripheral pulse oximeter.

Following these initial steps, the treatment regimen moves into the acute phase. The therapy already initiated continues together with frequent monitoring of laboratory values (Table 2) and continued reevaluation of the patient response.

Table 2 Monitoring Frequency Guidelines to Track Treatment Sequelae of DKA in CCU Patients Following Initial Baseline Assessments

Hourly
Vital signs (until stable; then 2–4 hourly)
Fluid intake/output (until eating/drinking; then 4–6 hourly)
Blood glucose (for first 4–6 hr or until stable; then 2–4 hourly until conversion to subcutaneous insulin)
Arterial blood gas (until stable or improving; then as indicated)
ECG (preferably continuous monitoring)
Temperature (until stable; then 4 hourly)
1–2 hourly
Serum potassium (for approximately first 8 hr; then 2–4 hourly)
Serum electrolytes (Na, Cl, HCO_3) (until K and HCO_3 normal; then 4–6 hourly)
4 hourly
Serum electrolytes (PO_4, Mg, Ca)
BUN/creatinine
6 hourly
Mental status (until stable; then 12 hourly)

The frequency of some of these investigations may be questioned on the basis of cost benefit (97–99), but in medically unstable patients within the CCU, extra vigilance requires that these parameters be constantly reevaluated. These estimations may not need to be as frequent outside the CCU setting.

Potassium and phosphate values tend to reach a nadir at approximately 4–6 hours after initiation of treatment.

Serum and urine ketones are not used as indices of improvement of DKA, following initiation of therapy, but may be measured before therapy to help confirm the diagnosis and, at the end, to establish resolution of DKA.

Changes in electrolyte and fluid levels are most marked within the first 4 hr of therapy. Vital signs (pulse, blood pressure, respiration, temperature) and mental status should be monitored frequently. Capillary blood glucose monitoring is performed hourly and serum electrolytes measured every 2 hr. Phosphate levels should be assessed every 4 hr. Within the CCU it is advisable to measure ABG hourly until the acidosis shows signs of continued resolution (pH > 7.35). In this regard, it is important to note that the peripheral utilization of ketones occurs through acetoacetic acid. The usual ratio of β-hydroxybutyrate to acetoacetate is about 3:1, but may increase in DKA to 7–8:1 (1). Following insulin and fluid therapy, the concentrations of both of these ketones decrease in the plasma due to decreased hepatic production, increased peripheral utilization, and increased urinary losses. However, the ratio of these two ketone bodies changes as β-hydroxybutyrate is converted to acetoacetate. Measurement of ketones by the nitroprusside method, which detects only acetoacetate, will reflect a factitious and misleading transient elevation in ketones (29). A more accurate assessment of resolution of DKA after initiation of therapy is to follow the decrease in the anion gap. Ketones should not be used to monitor therapy; they should be used only for diagnosis and to verify final control of DKA.

If the patient is able to eat, he/she should be prescribed an individualized diabetic diet with appropriate calories taking into consideration the precipitating illness, activity level, and probable catabolic state. If appropriate, diabetes education may also be started.

Transition to the stable phase occurs as soon as the primary metabolic acidosis has resolved, gag and cough reflexes have returned, orthostatic vital signs are within normal limits, the systolic blood pressure differential is < 10 mmHg, blood glucose is < 200 mg/dl, and mental status has returned to the premorbid level. Serum biochemical parameters should then be measured every 4 hr. Conversion from intravenous to subcutaneous insulin should be considered. At this stage, capillary blood glucose monitoring should be performed before meals and before bedtime. Fluid intake and output should still be monitored.

Continued diabetes education should consist of dietary advice, discussion of medication regimen and self-care skills, including insulin dosing, preparation and administration, self-monitoring of blood glucose, exercise routine, and demonstration of glucagon injection technique. The important central role that education plays in patient management cannot be stressed often enough. Through education patients should be able to reduce complications by earlier detection or prevention of DKA. Hospital admission provides an ideal setting in which to review patient knowledge and skills. Analysis of the cause of the current admission may help focus this education. It is also an opportune time to review the therapeutic regimen and make the necessary changes to achieve good blood glucose control with a view to improving long-term prospects by preventing the onset of complications and retarding the progression of those already present.

At all times the comorbid conditions may determine the rate at which therapeutic changes are made and the DKA resolves. The patient may be transferred to a general medical ward during the stable phase of DKA therapy, provided the cardiopulmonary status is sufficiently stable to allow this.

At the end of this phase and in preparation for discharge from the hospital, patients should have had a home health consultation and have an outpatient follow-up appointment. Ensure that they have the following: insulin, syringes, alcohol swabs, oral medication if appropriate, urine Ketodiastix, Glucotabs, a glucose meter with test strips, and glucagon for intramuscular injection. They should also be advised to wear a Medic-Alert bracelet.

Patients should be drinking adquate amounts of fluid without vomiting, have normal arterial or venous pH with a serum bicarbonate concentration > 15 mEq/L, serum sodium between 135 and 145 mEq/L (or attainment of the stable prehospitalization level), and potassium concentration between 3.5 and 5.0 mEq/L. By this stage the urinary Foley catheter should have been removed. The discharge phase occurs when the above criteria are met, the patient has resumed subcutaneous insulin therapy, and the patient or caregiver is able to demonstrate the self-care skills of medication administration, self-monitoring of blood glucose, dietary knowledge, and prevention of DKA.

Guidelines for the three main therapeutic components, fluid, insulin, and electrolyte replacement, will now be separately discussed although ideally in practice they should all be occurring concurrently. The search for and management of the precipitating cause forms the fourth component but will not be discussed further besides noting that some physicians prescribe broad-spectrum antibiotics if infection is suspected, before results of cultures are reported.

A. Fluid Therapy

The importance of rehydration has already been stressed. This is the first step in the initiation of DKA therapy. Hydration alone replaces fluid and electrolytes, restores intravascular volume, reduces the levels of insulin counterregulatory hormones, and lowers blood glucose concentrations (1). The issues concerning type of fluid replacement (colloid versus crystalloid), concentration or osmolality, rate of infusion, and total volume (34,41–43) remain controversial and will not be discussed further. Fluid therapy in DKA can theoretically be divided into three phases, which in practice blend into one another. Initially, there is a short period of rapid normal saline infusion. This is followed by a slower infusion of normal saline with additional electrolytes, mainly potassium. The third phase occurs when glucose levels have stabilized and before patients can eat and drink normally. This consists of a dextrose infusion usually with added electrolytes, again mainly potassium (7). For practical purposes the following schedule is recommended:

1. Type of fluid
   a. If serum sodium is 135–145 mEq/L and the patient has orthostatic hypotension, administer NS.
   b. If serum sodium is 135–145 mEq/L and the patint has no orthostatic hypotension, administer 1/2 NS.
   c. If serum sodium is $<$ 135 mEq/L, administer NS (irrespective of orthostasis).
   d. If serum sodium is $>$ 145 mEq/L, administer 1/2 NS (irrespective of orthostasis).
2. Rate of administration
   a. Initial rate = "wide open." Use NS unless serum Na concentration is $>$ 150 mEq/L. Give 1 L/hr for the first 1–2 hr. Decrease to 250–500 cc/hr as orthostatic changes disappear. Very rapid rehydration of patients within the CCU may not be appropriate and needs to be closely monitored. Concerns regarding cerebral and pulmonary edema are

discussed below. In general, very rapid rehydration may be associated with complications and slower resolution of biochemical and clinical abnormalities (6,44). The rate of initial replacement is based on calculated fluid deficit [body weight on admission subtracted from last known stable weight (assume 10% weight loss if these figures are not available)], corrected serum Na concentration and calculated serum, osmolality, assessment of circulatory sufficiency (requiring CVP in the CCU setting), and renal function. Aim to replace approximately 50% of the estimated fluid deficit by 8 hr. Replacement of the total deficit should proceed over 12–24 hr unless otherwise indicated.

b. If the patient is in shock, use a plasma expander (albumin) and consider dopamine. Rule out myocardial infarction and sepsis.
c. If after 2–4 hr volume status has improved, consider changing from NS to 1/2 NS to prevent hypernatremia. Monitor sodium closely.
d. Switch to 5% dextrose containing solution when plasma glucose is < 250 mg/dl. Continue intravenous insulin infusion (below).
e. Continue intravenous fluid therapy until vital signs are normal, acidosis has resolved, and the patient is able to eat and drink freely.

Fluid therapy in patients in the CCU needs to be tempered by their comorbid conditions, e.g., renal insufficiency or impaired left ventricular function, and requires individual prescriptions guided by vital signs, physical examination, invasive (e.g., CVP, arterial line, Swan-Ganz catheter) and noninvasive (ECHO, ECG, CXR, urine output) monitoring. Although careful intravenous therapy in CCU patients is recommended by most practicing physicians, there are some who argue that for those patients in cardiac failure and/or who have sustained a myocardial infarction, low-dose intravenous insulin infusion is sufficient as the sole therapeutic regimen without the use of intravenous hydration and potassium supplementation as these patients may already have normal or excessive hydration (62).

Patients developing DKA are generally not as dehydrated as those developing HHNK. However, within the CCU these patints may be at increased risk of thrombosis, and heparin prophylaxis (8000 U heparin subcutaneously every 8 hr) should be considered (45).

B. Insulin Therapy

It is now well established that low-dose (5–10 U/hr or 1.2–2.4 U/kg/min) continuous intravenous insulin therapy effectively lowers blood glucose levels in a smooth and timely fashion, thus minimizing rapid fluctuations in plasma osmolality (46–48). The infusion rates used result in relatively high but physiological plasma insulin levels (100–200 μU/ml), which represent maximal or near-maximal levels (49–51) for the suppression of hepatic glucose production and glycogenolysis, stimulation of peripheral glucose uptake, and inhibition of lipolysis and ketogenesis (18,52). Plasma insulin concentration increases by 20 μU/ml for every unit of regular insulin given hourly. In addition to treating the hyperglycemia, insulin also importantly reduces the ketoacidosis with regeneration of bicarbonate. Maximal cellular uptake of glucose and potassium occurs at insulin levels much greater than these, thus accounting for the increased incidence of hypoglycemia and hypokalemia that complicates high-dose insulin therapy. Blood glucose levels usually respond rapidly to intravenous insulin, decreasing optimally at a rate no faster than 60–120 mg/dl/hr (15,46). More rapid resolution of hyperglycemia may be dangerous. The improvement of ketoacidosis takes longer, usually in the order of 12–24 hr, and it is because of this that the intravenous infusion of insulin is prolonged. Blood glucose should not be allowed to fall much below 250 mg/dl within the first 24 hr or until the ketoacidosis has cleared and may be maintained by a 5% dextrose infusion together with the insulin infusion. The development of hypoglycemia during treatment, which has been a concern in the past with high-dose regimens, is uncommon in patients treated with low-dose insulin infusions, provided close monitoring detects the need to maintian glucose levels with a dextrose infusion.

In the CCU, subcutaneous or intramuscular insulin should not be used in the initial management of these patients as peripheral circulation may be compromised (vasoconstriction/hypotension) thus limiting insulin absorption and the effectiveness of this therapy. The recommended practice is:

1. Loading dose of insulin: 10 U regular insulin bolus IV or calculated at 0.1 U/kg body weight. This loading dose may hasten the resolution of ketosis (53). Although used by this author and others (4,34,54,55), and even larger loading doses of up to 20 U, or 0.4 U/kg regular insulin by yet others (56), its importance remains in dispute (1,57).
2. Follow this immediately with a continuous IV insulin infusion (1 U insulin/5 ml normal saline) at 0.1 U/kg/hr if weight is known, otherwise at an initial rate of 6 U/hr (58). Insulin has a very short intravenous half-life of 5–7 min and biological half-life of $<$ 20 min (59). This makes it necessary to start the continuous IV insulin infusion immediately following the IV bolus. It is also the reasoning behind the absolute necessity of maintaining a constant IV insulin infusion and not discontinuing it when sugar levels drop, as there will be a very rapid rebound in the hyperglycemia. Instead, the rate of the insulin infusion can be slowed to 0.5 U/kg/hr and a glucose infusion started to maintain adequate glucose levels.
3. If the glucose concentration has not decreased by $\geqslant$ 10% in 2 hr, provided hydration is appropriate, double the insulin infusion rate (60). The infusion rate may be doubled every 1–2 hr thereafter if the blood glucose concentration fails to fall by 10% of the initial level (4). Ensure that there are no technical reasons for lack of insulin effect, e.g., failure to flush the IV line

with insulin/saline mixture prior to starting the infusion, inadquate mixing of insulin in NS, leaking or blocked tubing or venipuncture site, etc.. Beware of possible increased occurrence of hypoglycemia and/or hypokalemia at these higher insulin infusion rates.

4. During the stable phase, with continued improvement in the serum glucose levels it will be necessary to change from the initial fixed intravenous insulin infusion to a variable one to maintain the blood glucose at approximately 250 mg/dl as long as the acidosis is present. A sliding scale for this purpose is shown below. This is only a guide and must be reviewed regularly (hourly) and the rate of infusion changed as insulin requirements vary. The blood glucose bracketing may also require revision.

Blood glucose (mg/dL)	Human regular insulin intravenous infusion rate (U/hr)
0–70	0.5
71–140	1.0
141–200	2.0
201–270	4.0
271–350	6.0
> 351	8.0

An alternative and possibly simpler scheme is as follows:

Blood glucose (mg/dL)	Human regular insulin intravenous infusion rate (U/hr)
<120	Decrease by 2 U every hour
121–180	Maintain same IV rate
>181	Increase by 1 U every hour

Both of these regimens require hourly blood glucose monitoring with hourly correction of the insulin infusion rate.

When the blood glucose concentration reaches 250 mg/dl, the rehydration fluid should be changed to 5% dextrose (occasionally 10% is needed) as a separate infusion or combined with saline (isotonic or hypotonic depending on serum Na concentration) to support the glucose level. At this time it may be advisable to slow the glucose infusion rate to 150 ml/hr.

As the glucose concentration improves long before the acidosis clears, on average 4–6 hr (46), it is important to maintain the insulin infusion to correct the acidosis, which may take up to 12–24 hr. As the acidosis resolves, the insulin infusion rate should be gradually reduced together with the glucose infusion and may be safely maintained at 1–2 U/hr.

Prior to converting to subcutaneous insulin, the blood glucose levels should ideally be 150–200 mg/dl. Tight glucose control in hospital is not recommended as patients may develop hypoglycemia following discharge when their activity levels increase and dietary habits change. However, if patients are to remain in the hosptial for any length of time, tight control may be improtant to promote healing or recovery from infection and the stringency can be relaxed prior to discharge.

If the patient cannot eat or drink because of an ongoing medical reason, despite resolution of the acidosis, dehydration, and hyperglycemia, some authors advocate 4–6-hourly subcutaneous regular insulin cover while maintaining 5% dextrose infusion (5,55). For this purpose, a sliding scale for 4-hrly subcutaneous regular insulin is required. When the patient starts eating, this sliding scale can then be used premeals and at bedtime, in addition to NPH insulin BID or ultralente insulin once daily (see below). However, these patients may not yet be stable, and particularly for those in the CCU, it is prudent to continue both the insulin and dextrose intravenous infusions. Important points to note are:

1. The new rapid-acting insulin Lispro has exactly the same intravenous pharmacokinetic profile as regular insulin. The two differ only when injected subcutaneously.
2. Insulin resistance may reflect inadequate hydration. However, if hydration is adequate, failure of blood glucose levels to fall following initiation of insulin therapy will require increased concentrations of insulin to overcome it.
3. Infection may increase resistance to insulin and slow the rate of fall of blood glucose by up to 50%.

C. Potassium and Phosphate Replacement

The main electrolyte requiring urgent attention is potassium. Both hypo- and hyperkalemia have deleterious cardiac effects including arrhythmias, cardiac arrest, and paralysis. Close monitoring to prevent either of these extremes is essential. Initial plasma concentrations of potassium may be normal (74%), increased (22%), or decreased (4%), despite a total-body deficit (61). Replacement of potassium, which is required in all patients, should begin as soon as the recorded value falls below 5 mEq/L or is in the normal range, as the subsequent rate of fall may be quite rapid provided renal function and urine output are normal. If not, then the replacement scheme below needs to be adjusted to avoid hyperkalemia. In this setting hyperkalemia may be treated with insulin and bicarbonate very judiciously. These patients will subsequently still require K supplementation although substantially less than those with normal renal function (62). Ideally, potassium replacement to maintain levels between 4.0 and 5.0 mEq/L should be based on 2-hourly serum measurements, with dosing as follows:

	KCl replacement	
Serum K level (mEq/L)	mEq/hour	mEq/L replacement fluid
< 3.5	10	40–60
3.6–4.0	7.5	30–40
4.1–5.0	5.0	20
>5.1	0	0

This schema may need to be revised if serum potassium values fall faster than replacement infusion is able to match. The guidelines for potassium replacement are given as both mEq/hr and mEq/L of infusate. When the patient is ready to eat, K replacement can be continued orally depending on the serum concentration.

Some authors advocate serial ECG recordings to monitor potassium levels and its replacement. This is, however, a very crude method, as ECG changes may lag behind the more rapid plasma fluctuations in potassium, and not all patients demonstrate the classical ECG changes of hypo- or hyperkalemia. Furthermore, in the CCU setting, acute or chronic cardiac pathology may result in ECG changes that mask the classic ECG criteria for the diagnosis of potassium abnormalities. However, if laboratory results are not available and there is no current or prior reason for ECG abnormalities, potassium replacement therapy may be guided by the following ECG criteria:

1. With reference to the initial rhythm strip (lead II, V1, or V2) use the T wave as baseline.
2. Follow T waves on the ECG hourly.
3. If the T wave is peaked or if the patient is not passing urine, do not add K to the IV.
4. If the T wave is normal and the patient is passing urine, add 5 mEq KCl/hr.
5. If the T wave is low and/or U waves are present, add 10 mEq KCl/hr.

In any event, ECG monitoring should be performed hourly, if not monitored continuously, in every patient in the CCU.

If serum PO_4 falls below 1.5 mg/dl with treatment, consider changing K replacement to 2/3 KCl and 1/3 K_2HPO_4. Supplementation should be at the rate of 10–20 mEq/hr (27,28). K_2HPO_4 in an IV precludes use of other medications through the same line as it precipitates many other substances. During phosphate supplementation be alert to the possibility of hypocalcemia (28), which may present as circumoral and finger paraesthesiae, muscle cramps, facial grimacing, tetany, and in severe cases with laryngeal spasm and seizures. Chvostek's and Trousseau's signs are used clinically to predict incipient tetany. Hypomagnesemia may also be unmasked.

Despite the failure to demonstrate improved outcome in controlled studies of phosphate replacement during DKA therapy (28,63,64), which included only patients without "severe medical problems," the known actions and importance of this electrolyte still argue in favor of cautious replacement when serum concentrations fall with therapy due to intracellular shifts, especially in patients compromised by cardiopulmonary complications, anemia, or other causes of hypoxia.

D. Bicarbonate Therapy

Metabolic acidosis in patients in the CCU is a very real hazard as it decreases the threshold of cardiac irritability, exerts a negative inotropic effect on the heart, and depresses the respiratory drive in patients who are already compromised by comorbid illness. However, many authors flatly condemn the use of bicarbonate therapy because of its toxic potential (65) and most studies fail to show a definite benefit in the therapy of patients with DKA (66–69). The resolution of ketosis results in the regeneration of bicarbonate and normalization of the pH. Sodium bicarbonate should only be used in extreme circumstances and may be considered if:

1. pH is 6.9–7.0 and the patient is in impending cardiovascular collapse or intractable shock, after adequate fluid replacement.
2. Significant cardiac dysrhythmias are present (67).
3. pH < 6.9 in most patients.

The following recommendations concerning bicarbonate therapy should be followed:

1. NEVER give an IV bolus. Patient death secondary to hypokalemia has been reported even in the presence of an elevated initial K level.
2. For pH 6.9–7.0: Infuse 44 mEq $NaHCO_3$ in 1 L of 0.45% saline (or 5% dextrose) at 1 L/hr.
3. For pH < 6.9: Infuse 88 mEq $NaHCO_3$ in 1 L of 0.45% saline (or 5% dextrose) at 1 L/hr.

If bicarbonate is used, the fall in K will be enhanced and additional potassium replacement will be required; 15 mEq KCl may be added to each liter of the infusions above, depending on serum K levels and other K-containing infusions currently running. Close monitoring for potential metabolic alkalosis and hypoxia is also advocated. Bicarbonate infusion should be stopped when the pH is > 7.0 and improving.

E. Resumption of Subcutaneous Insulin Therapy

When glucose levels are below 250 mg/dl and preferably between 150 and 200 mg/dl, acidosis has resolved and patients can drink and eat light foods without difficulty, they may be converted from continuous insulin infusion to a subcutaneous regimen, provided all other medical conditions are stable. This usually occurs after 24–36 hr.

This change should be made before breakfast, at the latest before lunch, but never any later.

1. Insulin dose: Restart subcutaneous insulin at one-half to two-thirds of prior maintenance dose. However, patients who are still ill at the time of conversion often require 10–20% more insulin than usual. This is an opportune time, in conjunction with patient education, to improve and intensify insulin therapy. Ideally, patients should inject insulin four times daily (short-acting TID with meals and intermediate-acting at bedtime). There are many variations on this theme and different physicians have their preferences. If the patient was not previously on insulin, calculate the approximate dose based on the preceeding 24-hr requirements, and administer four times daily, equally divided. Alternatively, some physicians use the latest hourly insulin infusion rate multiplied by 24 to calculate daily requirements. If subcutaneous insulin is only going to be given twice daily, the calculated 24-hr requirements can be divided into thirds with two-thirds administered before breakfast and one-third before supper. The morning insulin should consist of two-thirds NPH and one-third regular, while the evening dose should be one-half to two-thirds NPH and one-third to one-half regular. Whichever regimen is used, the insulin requirements can then be fine-tuned based on regular capillary blood glucose monitoring, the optimal dose being realized only after the patient is active and back at home.
2. Administration time of subcutaneous insulin: 30 min prior to the meal.
3. Feed the patient.
4. Discontinue insulin infusion 30–60 min after the meal. If NPH or lente insulin is used without regular, then the insulin infusion should be continued for 4 hr after the subcutaneous injection.

VIII. COMPLICATIONS OF THERAPY OF DKA

Potential complications during and after treatment of DKA, although relatively infrequent, are numerous and varied ranging from hypoglycemia, hypernatremia, and fluid overload, to death from hypokalemia, aspiration, thromboembolism, disseminated intravascular coagulation, and cerebral edema. Problems with comorbid conditions and precipitating factors such as myocardial infarction and untreated infection may also be encountered.

Patients with DKA require expert and personalized care with attention to detail and strict monitoring to predict, recognize, and treat some of these common complications.

The complications of cerebral edema, adult respiratory distress syndrome, and hyperchloremic metabolic acidosis are described in more detail below.

A. Cerebral Edema

This rare complication has a high mortality rate (approximately 90%) and occurs predominantly in young patients, < 20 years (22,70,71). Subclinical asymptomatic cerebral edema, demonstrated by CT scans, echoencephalograms, and direct pressure measurements, has been documented within the first 24 hr of treatment of DKA in both adults and children (4,72,73). It has also been demonstrated to occur prior to initiation of therapy for DKA (74).

During the development of DKA, the intracellular tonicity of brain cells is maintained by the production of idiogenic osmoles including sorbitol (75,76). Some of the factors implicated in the development of cerebral edema by promoting an intracellular fluid shift in brain cells include:

1. Reduced plasma osmolality following resolution of hyperglycemia.
2. Movement of osmotically active particles into the intracellular space, promoted by insulin.
3. Further lowering of plasma osmolality by water replacement.
4. Activation of the Na/H plasma membrane transporter.
5. A defect in the blood-brain barrier.

Rapid sodium replacement may contribute to the increase in interstitial fluid volume in the brain independent of changes in plasma osmolality. Other theories suggest that the responsible mechanism may be a paradoxical CNS acidosis with altered tissue oxygenation resulting from a change in the extracellular pH and a shift of the oxygen-hemoglobin dissociation curve. New-onset diabetes and prolonged duration of ketoacidosis are also possible risk factors. Although all of these mechanisms may be influential in the development of cerebral edema, none have been definitely proven. They may not be mutually exclusive and, in fact, support a multifactorial etiology (34).

Symptoms present suddenly with progressive deterioration in mental status (77). It is not possible at present to predict who will develop this complication (71, 76, 78) and therapy that consists of dexamethasone and mannitol (77,79) is usually ineffective. Care should, however, be exercised in the rate of water and sodium replacement and blood glucose normalization in patients with DKA (15,78).

B. Adult Respiratory Distress Syndrome (ARDS)

Another rare complication, ARDS consists of diffuse noncardiogenic pulmonary edema and reduced lung compliance resulting from an alveocapillary leak in patients with severe acidosis (15,78,80). Patients present with progressive dyspnea, hypoxemia, a classic chest x-ray, and are usually less than 50 years old. ARDS is an extreme manifestation of pulmonary edema and may be predicted to occur in patients with widened alveolar to arterial O_2 gradients and who have crepitations on chest examination at the time of presentation. Increased cardiac filling pressures, particularly left atrial, and decreased colloid osmotic pressure with normal cardiac output, occurring during therapy of DKA, are possible factors in the development of ARDS. This suggests that attention to the nature (crystalloid versus colloid) and rate of fluid replacement may reduce the risk of the development of this complication (15,78). Treatment is via mechanically assisted ventilation.

Cerebral edema and ARDS probably represent the extreme end of a spectrum of tissue changes occurring throughout the body that develop with treatment of DKA. These tissue responses are related to rapid changes in osmotic pressures in different fluid compartments with varied abilities of different tissues to respond quickly and appropriately (41). These different reaction times will dictate the clinical and biochemical manifestations of response to therapy.

C. Hyperchloremic Metabolic Acidosis

This transient, clinically relatively insignificant, state occurs commonly in the course of the resolution of DKA (24). It may be present at the time of presentation in well-hydrated patients. Although acidosis tends to resolve initially with therapy of DKA, the HCO_3 may remain at approximately 18 mEq/L and pH at approximately 7.3 for up to 48 hr.

The indicators of DKA, decreased HCO_3 and increased anion gap, may mask the increased urinary loss of the important buffers of bicarbonate, namely the ketone bodies. Treatment of DKA may initially promote further loss of ketone bodies thus further reducing the necessary substrate for regeneration of HCO_3 and resulting in a hyperchloremic state that resolves within a few days in patients with normal renal function, through enhanced renal acid excretion (25).

Mechanisms other than relative ketone body deficits that may contribute to the hyperchloremic acidosis following initiation of therapy include:

1. Infusion of high concentration chloride fluids
2. Infusion of bicarbonate-free fluids
3. Intracellular shifts of $NaHCO_3$

In DKA, Na loss exceeds that of Cl, and with ketonuria, there is Cl retention. Thus NaCl infusion results in relative hyperchloremia, which is noted within the first 2–4 hr of therapy (1) and is evident in most patients within 8 hr (24).

D. Other Diabetic Emergencies

This section provides a brief description of the other severe acute complications of diabetes mellitus, viz., hyperglycemic hyperosmolar nonketotic syndrome (HHNK), hypoglycemia, and lactic acidosis.

1. Hyperglycemic Hyperosmolar Nonketotic Syndrome (HHNK)

This acute life-threatening complication of diabetes represents one end of the spectrum of diabetic decompensation with DKA at the other (36). It occurs almost exclusively in patients with type 2 diabetes, who are usually elderly and dependent and may be distinguished from DKA by the marked hyperglycemia (> 600 mg/dl), the relative absence of acidosis (pH > 7.3; HCO_3 > 15 mEq/L) and ketonemia (negative at 1:2 dilution), and the excessive dehydration (serum osmolality > 320 mOsm/kg; Na 145–155 mEq/L; blood urea nitrogen 20–40 mg/dl; K 4–5 mEq/L). Insulin resistance is usually present with normal or elevated levels of serum insulin.

Occasional patients with DKA may present with features of HHNK and there are records of HHNK and DKA occurring on different occasions in the same patient. Many patients have features of both conditions (33%) while DKA occurs in 22% and HHNK in 45% of patients presenting with decompensated diabetes (8).

There are no good figures on the incidence and prevalence of this condition but many patients developing HHNK may have previously undiagnosed diabetes (30–40% of patients >65 years) (13,81,82). Mortality still remains high in patients with HHNK, approximately 15% (81–83).

The pathogenesis of HHNK is probably similar to that of DKA but these patients develop more severe hyperglycemia and hyperosmolality with definite but mild ketoacidosis (84). Increased serum lactic acid levels result from poor tissue perfusion and oxygen delivery and are more marked than in DKA.

HHNK usually develops insidiously (days to weeks) and may only present some time after admission to the CCU for a comorbid illness. Precipitating factors include those listed for DKA as well as pulmonary embolus, intestinal obstruction, peritoneal dialysis, mesenteric thrombosis, heat stroke, hypothermia, subdural hematoma, severe burns, and an extensive list of drugs (36,85–87). Some of these factors, however, may themselves also result from the severe dehydration, hemoconcentration, and poor tissue perfusion in HHNK.

Patients within the CCU are particularly at risk for the development of HHNK (elderly, obese, limited access to fluid, diminished thirst) and the complications of dehydration (thrombosis, thromboembolism, hypotension, poor tissue perfusion). As HHNK occurs in a large percentage of patients with no prior history of diabetes, it is important to have a high index of suspicion. A search for precipitating factors must be instigated as soon as the diagnosis is suspected. Physical examination is crucial and assessment of abdominal pain, as in DKA, is complicated. Mesenteric thrombosis may be the cause of abdominal pain, as a presenting feature.

The laboratory investigations in HHNK reveal a marked hyperglycemia and hyperosmolality with mild acidosis. Acid-base disturbances may be present especially in this older patient population with comorbid vomiting or thiazide diuretic use (metabolic alkalosis), for example. Fluid deficits in HHNK may be as great as 15% of body weight in patients with a long prodrome who present with hypernatremia. Electrolyte deficits are similar to those in DKA and hypertriglyceridemia is also present.

Therapy of HHNK follows the same general principles as that of DKA with particular emphasis on hydration and potassium replacement. Insulin therapy is the same as in DKA and should be started only after rehydration is in progress. Blood glucose levels fall rapidly and 75% of this fall reflects the dilution of glucose and the urinary loss (glycosuria) that occurs with rehydration (88). Fluid replacement should follow the same pattern as in patients with DKA but a larger total volume of fluid may need to be replaced.

The elderly and those with cardiac pathology and other comorbid conditions require careful monitoring of the rate and volume of fluid replacement. The restoration of the entire fluid deficit should proceed more slowly than in DKA, ideally over 36–72 hr, bearing in mind that this condition has developed over a relatively protracted time interval.

Vascular thrombosis is a serious complication in patients with both DKA and HHNK. A common site appears to be the cerebral vessels (89). Predisposing factors include dehydration, with contracted intravascular volume, decreased cardiac output and presence of atherosclerosis (both likely in patients within the CCU), increased blood viscosity, and increased procoagulant clotting factors (90). These patients should receive heparin prophylaxis of intravascular thrombosis (8000 U heparin subcutaneously every 8 hr).

Complications of therapy of HHNK are also similar to those for DKA. Mortality rates for HHNK have not fallen as low as those for DKA over the years and may be related to the increased incidence of associated medical conditions in this older population. Again, there is an absolute need to exercise great care, attention to detail, and regular monitoring of the clinical and laboratory parameters in each patient.

2. *Hypoglycemia*

This potentially serious acute complication of diabetes occurs in patients with both type 1 and type 2 diabetes for different reasons. The potential for its development in the CCU must be constantly borne in mind. Discussion of the various types of hypoglycemia and their causes and management is beyond the scope of this chapter.

Precipitating factors common to all patients with diabetes include missed meals, alcohol consumption, nonselective β-blocking drugs, increased physical activity, renal failure, hypothyroidism, hypoadrenalism, hypopituitarism, autonomic neuropathy, impaired gastric emptying, insulin antibodies, insulin overdosage, and intensity of glycemic control. More than 30% of episodes remain unexplained. With the relatively recent increased emphasis on intensified treatment regimes to achieve "tight control" in patients with diabetes, there has been a marked increase (at least threefold) in the incidence of hypoglycemic events (19). The severity of these will depend on the rate at which they develop, the presence of warning signs and symptoms (25% of patients with longstanding disease have lost warning symptoms), and the precipitating event. Patients within the CCU who experience hypoglycemia are more susceptible to myocardial ischemia and infarction as well as cerebrovascular accidents during hypoglycemia. Most hospital-reported hypoglycemic episodes occur in diabetic patients >65 years of age (91).

In patients with NIDDM, long-acting sulfonylurea agents are a common cause of hypoglycemia especially in the elderly. The other oral agents used in the management of diabetes, viz., biguanides, α-glucosidase inhibitors, and thiazolidinediones, by themselves do not generally precipitate hypoglycemia. However, if any are taken together with a sulfonylurea or insulin, the risk of hypoglycemia from these combinations may be enhanced.

Symptoms of hypoglycemia include tremor, sweating, anxiety, nausea, dizziness, confusion, tiredness, difficulty with speech and concentration, headache, hunger, thirst, and blurred vision. Signs are manifest by tachycardia, diplopia, pallor, tremor, motor disturbances, and altered mental status through to convulsions and coma.

The diagnosis is readily confirmed by blood glucose testing; a figure below 70 mg/dl being generally accepted as significant of hypoglycemia. Patients with mild hypoglycemia (60–70 mg/dl) may have very few symptoms, whereas those with severe hypoglycemia (<40 mg/dl) will probably have neurological impairment. Patients' subjective assessment of hypoglycemia is often inaccurate and those patients with poorly controlled diabetes may experience hypoglycemic symptoms when their blood glucose levels approach the normal range.

Treatment will depend on the level of consciousness of the patient and his or her ability to swallow. Generally, patients with blood glucose values of 40–70 mg/dl are treated with oral carbohydrates. Although severe hypoglycemia (<40 mg/dl) usually requires intravenous glucose or glucagon (intravenous or intramuscular) , patients may still be sufficiently alert to take oral carbohydrates. If they are able to swallow, carbohydrates (15 g) should be given by mouth [4 oz (½ glass) unsweetened fruit juice, ½ regular soda, 2–3 glucose tablets (4 g glucose/tab), 10 Lifesavers, or 4 oz nonfat milk.] A snack in the form of milk and crackers or half a sandwich provides carbohydrate for quick relief of symptoms and elevation of blood glucose, as well as protein and fat, which delay gastric emptying, producing a less prompt but more sustained glucose response. Blood glucose should be checked again within 10–15 min. A follow-up snack should be taken within 30 min of the initial treatment, unless it is time for the next meal. Be wary of giving too much carbohydrate and causing rebound hyperglycemia. In patients unable to swallow, it may be necessary to infuse glucose. Start with 50 ml 50% dextrose IV. For patients not in the CCU, 1 mg glucagon may be given SC or IM.

In patients in whom the hypoglycemia is due to relative or absolute insulin overdose, the duration of the hypoglycemia may be predicted from the type of insulin administered and the site of injection. Overdose of sulfonylureas is usually inadvertent due to use of first-generation long-acting agents such as chlorpropamide. This occurs most commonly in patients >60 years who may have mild renal insufficiency. Therapy may include a constant dextrose infusion, which in some patients may need to be maintained for up to 7–10 days especially if there is any degree of renal failure because of delayed renal excretion of the sulfonylurea.

For all patients with type 2 diabetes admitted to the CCU, it is advisable to maintain them on insulin (SC, IM, or IV depending on their illness) at least for the duration of their stay irrespective of their previous therapeutic regimen.

Identifying the cause and offering appropriate education (discussed above) are important aspects in the management of these patients to prevent future episodes.

3. *Lactic Acidosis*

Lactic acidosis is the most common type of metabolic acidosis. The production (by erythrocytes, skin, intestines, and muscle) and utilization (by liver and kidney) of lactate are normally in balance. Development of hypoxia will result in lactate generation by any tissue.

Lactic acidosis should be suspected in any patient with circulatory insufficiency. The diagnosis is made by demonstrating a serum lactic acid level $\geqslant$ 2.0 mmol/L, with an acidosis, pH $\leqslant$ 7.3, without significant ketoacidosis. Low ketone levels ($\leqslant$ 1:4 on serum dilution, or β-hydroxybutyrate 0.4–0.6 mmol/L) may be detected.

In patients with diabetes, there is often increased lactate production by skeletal muscle and utilization for gluconeogenesis by the liver. Fifty percent of cases of lactic acidosis occur in patients with diabetes mellitus and it may coexist with DKA, where it may be the result of hemodynamic rather than metabolic factors. Lactic acidosis may mask an associated or underlying DKA because excess lactate results in a decreased production of acetoacetate without effecting the elevated β-hydroxybutyrate. Thus the ratio of β-hydroxybutyrate to acetoacetate is increased and the routinely used method for detecting ketone bodies (above) will not record the ketoacidosis.

Most patients developing lactic acidosis are >45 years and female. Precipitating factors, many of which are pertinent to patients being admitted to or already in the CCU, include acute myocardial infarction with hypoxia, septic shock, massive hemorrhage, respiratory arrest, severe hepatic failure, and drugs such as sodium nitroprusside, epinephrine, and norepinephrine. The oral antihyperglycemic agent phenformin is no longer approved by the Food and Drug Administration for use in patients with diabetes because of the unacceptably high incidence of lactic acidosis associated with it. Metformin, the only other approved biguanide, is an effective oral agent in type 2 diabetes patients. Lactic acidosis occurs rarely in patients taking it (0.03 cases/1000 patient-years) (2) and almost always when prescribed inappropriately such as in patients with renal or hepatic disease, a history of alcohol abuse, or other acute or chronic metabolic acidoses. Poorly controlled diabetes is not usually associated with lactic acidosis unless there is an associated condition responsible for hypoxia.

Treatment of the underlying cause, which is usually associated with circulatory collapse or respiratory failure, generally results in correction of the acidosis by improving hydration and tissue perfusion. Restoration of electrolytes and treatment of the hyperglycemia are also important (see above). Rapid correction of these abnormalities has been associated with cerebral edema.

The use of bicarbonate in the therapy of this condition is controversial. The generation of lactate and H^+ is very rapid, resulting in a relative resistance to alkali therapy and necessitating very large amounts of bicarbonate to correct the acidosis. This may paradoxically increase lactate production. However, as severe acidosis may perpetuate the underlying cause of the lactic acidosis by exacerbating the circulatory collapse, it may be necessary to use bicarbonate. Intravenous bicarbonate should be infused at a rate sufficient to maintain the bicarbonate level between 8 and 10 mmol/L and $pH > 7.10$.

Recognition of lactic acidosis, often in conjunction with DKA, and appropriate management are challenges for the CCU physician. Mortality rates in lactic acidosis are proportional to the level of lactic acid. Lactic acidosis is responsible for only a small percentage of the total mortality in diabetic patients.

IX. OTHER ENDOCRINOLOGY IN CCU PATIENTS

It has already been mentioned that other endocrine disorders may coexist in patients with diabetes. Awareness of these possibilities and elicitation of their existence during history taking cannot be stressed highly enough.

Thyroid dysfunction may be misdiagnosed during acute illness, in both myocardial infarction and DKA, and is termed the sick-euthyroid syndrome. Generally, thyroid function tests in these patients show a low FT_3 and variable FT_4 (low in severe illness) with a normal TSH. Reverse T_3, if measured, will be elevated in contrast to patients with genuine thyroid dysfunction. Unless specifically indicated, the evaluation of thyroid function in acute illness is not recommended. Acute illness may, however, precipitate thyroid storm in poorly controlled patients with hyperthyroidism (previously undiagnosed). Excess amounts of iodine in radiographic contrast medium used during angiography or in the antiarrhythmic drug amiodarone may also induce hyperthyroidism (Jod Basedow phenomenon) in susceptible individuals. In addition, uncontrolled hyperthyroidism in patients with diabetes may lead to DKA.

X. CONCLUSION

DKA is a serious, acute state of metabolic decompensation that is still associated with considerable morbidity and mortality. Precipitating causes are numerous, but infection, incorrect insulin therapy, and new-onset diabetes account for over 50% of presentations. Therapy, although now fairly standard in format and content in most centers, consisting of fluid, insulin, and electrolyte replacement in addition to treatment of the precipitating cause, remains controversial with respect to the finer points of each of these components.

Of patients developing DKA, those within the CCU are at greatest risk of mortality. These patients are vulnerable because of their age, cardiac pathology, and susceptibility to infection, the three leading causes of death in DKA (61,92–94).

Patients in the CCU may exhibit acute or chronic complications of diabetes or other illnesses and require expert and individual full-time monitoring to anticipate, prevent, and treat the rapid fluctuations in metabolic and clinical parameters that are recognized accompaniments of their unstable condition. Continued vigilance in this patient population will hopefully help reduce morbidity and mortality.

Finally, comprehensive diabetes education should continue to form the central focus of patient care both within and outside the hospital setting. The fine tuning of medical therapeutics will continue but it will only be through increased patient awareness and empowerment to take control of their own disease that we can hope to improve the poor health statistics of patients with diabetes mellitus.

ACKNOWLEDGMENTS

Special thanks to Brenda Gilmore for her expert assistance in the preparation of this manuscript.

REFERENCES

1. Kitabchi AE, Wall BM. Diabetic ketoacidosis. Med Clin North Am 1995; 79(1):9–37.
2. Fishbein H, Palumbo PJ. Acute metabolic complications in diabetes. In: Harris MI, Cowie CC, Stern MP, Boyko EJ, Reiber GE, Bennett PH, eds. Diabetes in America, 2nd ed. National Diabetes Data Group, Bethesda: NIH/NIDDK, 1995:293–291.

3. Munro JF, Campbell IW, McCuish AC, Duncan LJF. Euglycaemic diabetic ketoacidosis. Br Med J 1973; 2:578–580.
4. Jenkins D, Close CF, Krentz AJ, Nattras M, Wright AD. Euglycemic diabetic ketoacidosis: does it exist? Acta Diabetol 1993; 30:251–253.
5. Rumbak MJ, Kitabchi AE. Diabetic acidosis: Etiology, pathophysiology and treatment. Compr Ther 1991; 17:46–49.
6. Keller U. Diabetic ketoacidosis: current views on pathogenesis and treatment. Diabetologia 1986; 29:71–77.
7. Hamblin PS, Topliss DJ, Stockigt JR. Practical management of diabetic ketoacidosis and hyperosmolar coma. Aust NZ J Med 1990; 20(6):836–841.
8. Wachtel TJ, Tetu-Mouradjian LM, Goldman DL, Ellis SE. Hyperosmolarity and acidosis in diabetes mellitus: a three-year experience in Rhode Island. J Gen Intern Med 1991; 6(6):495–502.
9. Kitabchi AE, Fisher JN. Diabetes Mellitus. In: Glow RH, Peters SP, eds. Clinical Studies in Medical Biochemistry. New York: Oxford University Press, 1987:95–149.
10. Fulop M, Hoberman HD. Alcoholic ketosis. Diabetes 1975; 24(9):785–790.
11. Faich GA, Fishbein HA, Ellis SE. Epidemiology of diabetic acidosis: a population-based study. Am J Epidemiol 1983; 117:551–558.
12. Johnson PD, Palumbo PH, Chu CP. Diabetic ketoacidosis in a community based population. Mayo Clin Proc 1980; 55:83–88.
13. Malone ML, Ennis V, Goodwin JS. Characteristics of diabetic ketoacidosis in older versus younger adults. J Am Geriatr Soc. 1992; 40:1100–1104.
14. Lebovitz ME. Diabetic ketoacidosis. Lancet 1995; 345:767–772.
15. Kitabchi AE, Fisher JN, Murphy MB, Rumbak MJ. Diabetic ketoacidosis and hyperglycemic hyperosmolar nonketotic state. In: Kahn CR, Weir G, eds. Joslin's Diabetes Mellitus Textbook, 13th ed. Philadelphia: Lea & Febiger, 1994:753–760.
16. Schade DS, Eaton RP. Diabetic ketoacidosis-pathogenesis, prevention and therapy. Clin Endocrinol Metab 1983; 12(2):321–338.
17. Chapman J, Wright AD, Nattrass M, Fitzgerald MG. Recurrent diabetic ketoacidosis. Diabetic Med 1988; 5:659–661.
18. DeFronzo RA, Matsuda M, Barrett EJ. Diabetic ketoacidosis: a combined metabolic-nephrologic approach to therapy. Diabetes Rev 1994; 2:209.
19. DCCT Research Group: The diabetes control and complications trial research group. The effect of intensive treatment of diabetes on the development and progression of long-term complications in insulin-dependent diabetes mellitus. N Engl J Med 1993; 329:977–986.
20. Weissman JS, Gatsonis C, Epstein AM. Rates of avoidable hospitalization by insurance status in Massachusetts and Maryland. JAMA 1993; 2388–2394.
21. Siperstein MD. Diabetic ketoacidosis and hyperosmolar coma. Endocrinol Metab Clin North Am 1992; 21:415–432.
22. Walker M, Marshall SM, Albertick GM. Clinical aspects of diabetic ketoacidosis. Diabetes Metab Rev 1989; 5(8):651–663.
23. Foster DW, McGarry JD. The metabolic derangements and treatment of diabetic ketoacidosis. N Engl J Med 1983; 309:159–169.
24. Androgue H, Wilson H, Boyd AE III, Suki WN, Eknoyan G. Plasma acid-base patterns in diabetic ketoacidosis. N Engl J Med 1982; 26:1603–1610.

25. Oh MS, Carroll MJ, Uribarri J. Mechanism of normochloremic and hyperchloremic acidosis in diabetic ketoacidosis. Nephron 1990; 54:1–6.
26. Keller U, Berger W. Prevention of hypophosphatemia by phosphate infusion during treatment of diabetic ketoacidosis and hyperosmolar coma. Diabetes 1980; 29:87–95.
27. Wilson HK, Keuer SP, Lea AS, Boyd AE, Eknoyan G. Phosphate therapy in diabetic ketoacidosis. Arch Intern Med 1982; 142(3):517–520.
28. Fisher JN, Kitabchi AE. A randomized study of phosphate therapy in the treatment of diabetic ketoacidosis. J Clin Endocrinol Metab 1983; 57(1):117–180.
29. Israel RS. Diabetic ketoacidosis. Emerg Med Clin North Am 1989; 7(4):859–871.
30. Vinicor F, Lehrner LM, Karn RC, Merritt AD. Hyperamylasemia in diabetic ketoacidosis: sources and significance. Ann Intern Med 1979; 91(2):200–204.
31. Campbell IW, Duncan LJ, Innes JA, MacCuish AC, Munro JR. Abdominal pain in diabetic metabolic decompensation, clinical significance. JAMA 1975; 233(2): 166–168.
32. Gale AE, Tattersall RB. Hypothermia: a complication of diabetic ketoacidosis. Br Med J 1978; 2:1387–1389.
33. Johnson DG, Alberti KG. Diabetic emergencies: practical aspects of the management of diabetic ketoacidosis and diabetes during surgery. Clin Endocrinol Metab 1980; 9:437(3):437–460.
34. Ennis ED, Kreisberg RA. Diabetic ketoacidosis and the hyperglycemic hyperosmolar syndrome. In: LeRoith D, Taylor SI, Olefsky JM, eds. Diabetes Mellitus. Philadelphia: Lippincott-Raven, 1996:276–286.
35. Katz MA. Hyperglycemia-induced hyponatremia: calculation of expected serum sodium depression. N Engl J Med 1973; 289:843–844.
36. Ennis ED, Stahl EJvB, Kreisberg RA. The hyperosmolar hyperglycaemic syndrome. Diabctcs Rev 1994; 2:115.
37. Barrett EJ, DeFronzo RA, Bevilacqua S, Ferrannini E. Insulin resistance in diabetic ketoacidosis. Diabetes 1982; 31:923–928.
38. Waldhausl W, Kleingerger G, Korn A, Dudczak R, Bratusch-Marrain P, Nowotny P. Severe hyperglycaemia: effects of rehydration on endocrine derangements and blood glucose concentration. Diabetes 1979; 28:577–584.
39. Owen OE, Licht JH, Sapir DG. Renal function and effects of partial rehydration during diabetic ketoacidosis. Diabetes 1981; 80:510–518.
40. Luzi L, Barrett EJ, Groop LC, Ferrannini E, DeFronzo R. Metabolic effect of "low dose" insulin therapy on glucose metabolism in diabetic ketoacidosis. Diabetes 1988; 37:1470–1477.
41. Fein IA, Rackow EC, Sprung CL, Grodman R. Relation of colloid osmotic pressure to arterial hypoxemia and cerebral edema during crystalloid volume loading of patients with diabetic ketoacidosis. Ann Intern Med 1982; 96:570–575.
42. Hillman K. Fluid resuscitation in diabetic emergencies—a reappraisal. Intensive Care Med 1987; 13:4–8.
43. Rotter KI, Schwank WF. Effect of rehydration fluid with 75 mmol/L of sodium on serum sodium concentration and serum osmolality in young patients with diabetic ketoacidosis. Mayo Clin Proc 1994; 69:1149–1153.
44. Androgue HJ, Barrero J, Eknoyan G. Salutary effects of modest fluid replacement in the treatment of adults with diabetic ketoacidosis. JAMA 1989; 262:2108–2113.

45. Clements RS, Jr., Vourganti B. Fatal diabetic ketoacidosis: major causes and approaches to their prevention. Diabetes Care 1978; 1:314–425.
46. Kitabchi A, Ayyagari V, Guerra S. The efficacy of low dose versus conventional therapy of insulin for treatment of diabetic ketoacidosis. Ann Intern Med 1976; 84:633–638.
47. Alberti KGMM. Low-dose insulin in the treatment of diabetic ketoacidosis. Arch Intern Med 1977; 137:1367–1276.
48. Gwilt DJ, Nattrass M, Pentecost BL. Use of low-dose insulin infusions in diabetes after myocardial infarction. Br Med J 1982; 285:1402–1404.
49. Guerra SMO, Kitabchi AE. Comparison of the effectiveness of various routes of insulin injection: insulin levels and glucose response in normal subjects. J Clin Endocrinol Metab 1976; 42(5):869–874.
50. Schade DS, Eaton RP. Dose response to insulin in man: differential effects on glucose and ketone body regulation. J Clin Endocrinol Metab 1977; 44(6):1038–1053.
51. Kitabchi AE, Sacks HS, Young RT, Morris LR. Diabetic ketoacidosis: reappraisal of therapeutic approach. Annu Rev Med 1979; 30:339–357.
52. Kitabchi AE. Low dose insulin in the treatment of diabetic ketoacidosis. In: Stollerman GH, ed. Advances in Internal Medicine. Chicago: Year Book Medical Publishers, 1978:115–135.
53. Kitabchi AE. Low dose insulin therapy in diabetic ketoacidosis: fact or fiction? Diabetes Metab Rev 1989; 5(4):337–363.
54. Fish LH. Diabetic ketoacidosis: insulin treatment strategies to avoid complications. Postgrad Med 1994; 96(3):75–96.
55. Lipsky MS. Management of diabetic ketoacidosis. Am Fam Phys 1994; 49(7):1607–1612.
56. Chouhan SP, Perry KG. Management of diabetic ketoacidosis in the obstetric patient. Obstet Gynecol Clin North Am 1995; 22(1):143–155.
57. Burghen GA, Etteldorf JN, Fisher JN. Comparison of high dose and low dose insulin by continuous intravenous infusion in the treatment of diabetic ketoacidosis in children. Diabetes Care 1980; 3:15–20.
58. Rayfield EJ, Giegerich EW. Diabetic ketoacidosis. In: Krieger, Bardin, eds. Current Endocrinologic Therapy. St. Louis: CV Mosby, 1983:175–180.
59. Hersch IB, McGill JB. Role of insulin in management of surgical patients with diabetes mellitus. Diabetes Care 1990; 13(9):980–991.
60. Berger W, Keller U. Treatment of diabetic ketoacidosis and nonketotic hyperosmolar diabetic coma. Baillieres Clin Endocrinol Metab 1992; 6:1–22.
61. Beigelman PM. Severe diabetic ketoacidosis (diabetic coma): 482 episodes 257 patients; experience of three years. Diabetes 1971; 20(7):490–500.
62. Jolobe OMP. Characteristics of diabetic ketoacidosis in older patients. J Am Geriatr Soc 1993; 41(8):888.
63. Becker DJ, Brown DR, Steranka BH, Drash AL. Phosphate replacement during treatment of diabetic ketosis: effects on calcium and phosphorus homeostasis. Am J Dis Chil 1983; 137(3):241–246.
64. Kebler R, McDonald FD, Cadnapaphoruchai P. Dynamic changes in serum phosphorus levels in diabetic ketoacidosis. Am J Med 1985; 79(5):571–576.
65. Lever E, Jaspan JB. Sodium bicarbonate therapy in severe diabetic ketoacidosis. Am J Med 1983; 75(2):263–268.

66. Hale PJ, Crase J, Nattrass M. Metabolic effects of bicarbonate in the treatment of diabetic ketoacidosis. Br Med J 1984; 289:1035–1038.
67. Morris LR, Murphy MB, Kitabchi AE. Bicarbonate therapy in severe diabetic ketoacidosis. Ann Intern Med 1986; 836–840.
68. Riley LR Jr, Cooper M, Narims RG. Alkali therapy of diabetic ketoacidosis: biochemical, physiological and clinical perspectives. Diabetes Metab Rev 1989; 5: 627–636.
69. Gamba G, Oseguera J, Castrejon M, Gomez-Perez FJ. Bicarbonate therapy in severe diabetic ketoacidosis: a double blind, randomized, placebo controlled trial. Rev Invest Clin 1991; 43:234–248.
70. Duck SC, Weldon VV, Pagliara AS, Haymond MW. Cerebral edema complicating therapy for diabetic ketoacidosis. Diabetes 1976; 25(2):111–115.
71. Rosenbloom AL. Intracerebral crises during treatment of diabetic ketoacidosis. Diabetes Care 1990; 13(1):22–33.
72. Clements RS, Blumenthal SA, Morrison AD, Winegrad AI. Increased cerebrospinal-fluid pressure during treatment of diabetic ketosis. Lancet 1971; 2:671–675.
73. Krane EJ, Bockoff MA, Wallman JK, Wolfsdorf JI. Subclinical brain swelling in children during treatment of ketoacidosis. N Engl J Med 1985; 312(18):1147–1151.
74. Hoffman WH, Steinhart CM, Gammal TE, Steele S, Cuadrado AR, Morse PK. Cranial CT in children and adolescents with diabetic ketoacidosis. AJNR 1988; 9: 733–739.
75. Arieff AI, Kleeman CR. Studies on mechanisms of cerebral edema in diabetic comas: effects of hyperglycemia and rapid lowering of plasma glucose in normal rabbits. J Clin Invest 1973; 52:571–583.
76. Harris GD, Fiordahsi I, Harris WL. Minimizing the risk of brain herniation during treatment of diabetic ketoacidemia: a retrospective and prospective study. J Pediatr 1991; 118(1):22–166–167.
77. Hammond P, Wallis S. Cerebral edema in diabetic ketoacidosis. Br Med J 1992; 305: 203–204.
78. Kreisberg RA. Diabetic Ketoacidosis. In: Rifkin M, Porte D, eds. Diabetes Mellitus: Theory and Practice, 4th ed. New York: Elsevier Science, 1990:591–603.
79. Bello FA, Sotos JF. Cerebral edema in diabetic ketoacidosis in children. Lancet 1990; 336:64.
80. Carroll P, Matz R. Adult respiratory distress syndrome complicating severe uncontrolled diabetes mellitus: report of nine cases and a review of the literature. Diabetes Care 1982; 5(6):574–580.
81. Arieff AI, Carroll HJ. Nonketotic hyperosmolar coma with hyperglycaemia. Clinical features, pathophysiology, renal function, acid-base balance, plasma-cerebrospinal fluid equilibria and the effects of therapy in 37 cases. Medicine 1972; 51(2):73–94.
82. Wachtel TJ, Silliman RA, Lamberton P. Predisposing factors for the diabetic hyperosmolar state. Arch Intern Med 1988; 148(3):747 (letter).
83. Khardori R, Soler NG. Hyperosmolar hyperglycemic non-ketotic syndrome. Am J Med 1984; 77(55):899–904.
84. Halperin ML, Marsden PA, Sniger GG, West ML. Can marked hyperglycaemia occur without ketosis? Clin Invest Med 1986; 8:253–256.
85. Lorber D. Non-ketotic hypertonicity in diabetes. Endocrinologist 1995; 79(1):39–52.

86. Levin SN, Sanson TH. Treatment of hyperglycemic hyperosmolar nonketotic syndrome. Drugs 1989; 38(3):462–472.
87. Matz R. Hyperosmolar nonacidotic diabetes (HNAD). In: Rifkin H, Porte D, eds. Ellenberg and Rifkin's Diabetes Mellitus, Theory and Practice, 4th ed. New York: Elsevier, 1990:604–616.
88. Halperin M, Goldstein M, Richardson R, Robeson L. Quantitative aspects of hyperglycemia in the diabetic. A theoretical approach. Clin Invest Med 1980; 2:127.
89. Timperly WR, Preston FE, Ward JD. Cerebral intravascular coagulation in diabetic ketoacidosis. Lancet 1974; 1:952–956.
90. Paton RC. Haemostatic changes in diabetic coma. Diabetologia 1981; 21:172–177.
91. Centers for Disease Control and Prevention: Diabetes Surveillance 1993. Atlanta, GA: CDC, Division of Diabetes Translation, 1994.
92. Beardwood JT, Rouse GP. Diabetic acidosis: a study of two hundred and twenty consecutive cases. JAMA 1941; 117:1701–1704.
93. Cohen AS, Vance VK, Runyan JW, Hurwitz D. Diabetic acidosis: an evaluation of the cause, course and therapy of 73 cases. Ann Intern Med 1960; 52:55–86.
94. Johnson D, Palumbo P, Chu C. Diabetic ketoacidosis in a community-based population. Mayo Clin Proc 1980; 55:85–88.
95. White K, Kolman ML, Wexler P, Polin G, Winter RJ. Unstable diabetes and unstable families: a psychosocial evaluation of diabetic children with recurrent ketoacidosis. Pediatrics 1984; 73:749–755.
96. Keller AS, Link RN, Bickell NA, Charap MH, Kalet AL, Schwartz MD. Diabetic ketoacidosis in prisoners without access to insulin. JAMA 1993; 269(5):633–634.
97. Eisenberg JM. An educational program to modify laboratory use by housestaff. J Med Educ 1977; 52:578–584.
98. Griner PL, Liptzin B. Use of laboratory tests in a teaching hospital. Long term trends: reduction in use and relative costs. Ann Intern Med 1979; 90:243–248.
99. Moss JM. Diabetic ketoacidosis: effective low-cost treatment in community hospital. South Med J 1987; 80(7):875–881.

16

Imaging Issues in the Cardiac Care Unit

CAROLINE CHIA-LIN CHOW and CHARLES S. WHITE

University of Maryland Medical Center, Baltimore, Maryland

I. INTRODUCTION

A majority of imaging studies performed in the critical care patient are portable chest radiographs. Several studies have shown that new or unsuspected findings that affect patient management are found in 37% to 65% of portable chest radiographs (1–3). Of unexpected findings, 30% are potentially life-threatening (4). The abnormalities are evenly divided between cardiopulmonary disease and malposition of monitoring devices. Bekemeyer et al. (5) found that 27% of catheters and support devices were improperly positioned and that 6% of patients demonstrated other complications such as pneumothorax or pleural effusion (5). Therefore, use of daily radiographs to monitor these critically ill patients is imperative.

The quality of portable radiographs contributes substantially to proper interpretation of these studies. Patients should be centered in relation to the radiographic plate and not rotated. The film should be appropriately labeled with the name of the patient, hospital number, date, time, patient position, tube-film distance, and exposure technique. Since comparison of the films from day to day is of primary importance, radiographic consistency must be assured with regard to both film quality and patient position. The radiographic exposure should be adequate to provide faint visualization of the vertebral bodies (6). Optimally, the patient should be in an upright position and in inspiration to avoid an erroneous impression of pulmonary hypertension from prominent pulmonary vessels (7), atelectasis or lower lobe pneumonia secondary to low lung volumes, or mediastinal pathology from a widened mediastinum (6).

Portable chest radiographs are often compromised by technical factors. In such cases, computerized tomography (CT) can contribute significantly to patient management. Mirvis et al. (8) found that 70% to 75% of CT scans in critically ill patients showed findings that affected diagnosis, assessment of disease extent, or patient management. Roddy et al. (9) reported that information on CT altered management in 26% of patients. CT may be useful if portable chest radiographs fail to reveal the cause of unexplained fevers, clinical deterioration, or lack of response to treatment. Other indications for CT include detection of subtle pneumothoraces, differentiation of pleural fluid from parenchymal processes, evaluation of mediastinal and chest wall pathology, and guidance of therapeutic procedures (8). With the recent development of spiral CT, images can be attained more quickly, decreasing scanning time and limiting motion artifact.

Magnetic resonance imaging (MRI) is useful to evaluate cardiovascular diseases of the thoracic aorta, para- or intracardiac masses, congenital heart disease (CHD), and pericardial disease (10). However, MRI of the chest in the critically ill patient can present a challenge because of incompatibility of supportive devices and the magnetic field and difficulty in monitoring the patient. Development of MRI-compatible devices and faster imaging sequences are strategies that may extend applications of MRI.

II. MONITORING LINES AND TUBES

Evaluation of placements of catheters, tubes, and support equipment and complications caused during their placement are an essential part of the assessment of the ICU radiograph.

A. Endotracheal Tubes

The endotracheal tube (ET) should be positioned with its tip 5 to 7 cm above the carina (11,12). The carina is located between the T5 and T7 vertebrae in 95% of patients on portable chest radiographs, and the tip of the ET should be positioned at the level of T4 if the carina is difficult to visualize (12). This permits movement of 4 cm due to neck flexion or extension without bronchial intubation or inadvertent extubation (11). Malposition of the endotracheal tube occurs in 12% of intubated patients (2). Placement into the right main bronchus is most common (9% of intubated patients) (13), and can result in obstruction of the left main bronchus and left lung atelectasis, hyperinflation of the right lung, and leftward shift of the mediastinum (14).

Placement of the ET into the esophagus is a serious complication that can be difficult to detect on a frontal radiograph. Indirect findings include a distended stomach, positioning of the ET lateral to the tracheal air column, or location of the distal tip of the ET below the carina. Placement that is too proximal in the trachea can lead to extubation or injury of the vocal cords (14). Other complications from ET placement include aspiration pneumonia, tracheal or laryngeal injury, pneumothorax or mediastinal hemorrhage. After weaning a patient from ventilatory support, the chest radiograph may initially appear worse than on previous radiographs because of decreased positive end-expiratory pressure (PEEP) (15).

B. Thoracostomy Tubes, Thoravents, Pigtail Catheters

Thoracostomy tubes, thoravents, or pigtail catheters are tubes placed into the pleural space to evacuate either air or fluid. Removal of air or fluid is accomplished by anterosuperior or posteroinferior positioning, respectively. Malposition of these tubes can result in placement in the extrapleural soft tissue, in the lung parenchyma causing lung laceration or bronchopleural fistula, or in the pleural fissures (6). If suspicion arises that the tube is malpositioned or malfunctioning, a lateral radiograph or CT of the thorax may be helpful in demonstrating the relationship of the air or fluid collection and the chest tube (15). Other complications include kinking of the tube, loculated air or fluid collections that do not communicate with the tube, formation of a subcutaneous air or fluid collection due to a superficial location of the side port of the tube, infection secondary to incomplete drainage, and development of tube tracks with resultant atelectasis and focal inflammation (6).

C. Nasogastric Tubes and Feeding Tubes

The tip of a nasogastric (NG) tube should terminate in the stomach beyond the cardia, and its side hole should also be in the stomach. A feeding tube should terminate in the second portion of the duodenum (16). The former has a radiopaque stripe, and the latter a radiopaque tip. Malposition can occur due to coiling of the tube in the esophagus or pharynx, or placement into the trachea or bronchus (Fig. 1) (6). Initiation of feeding through a tube placed into the airways can lead to severe pneumonitis, emphysema, pneumothorax, hydrothorax, or hemothorax (6). A feeding tube or NG tube whose tip is in the hypopharynx can predispose to aspiration (15). Traumatic insertion can lead to perforation or laceration of the GI tract (15).

D. Central Venous Catheter

A central venous catheter (CVC) should be placed with its tip in the superior vena cava and oriented parallel to the lumen (6). The tip should be 2 to 3 cm above the right atrium at the level of the first anterior intercostal rib on the chest radiograph. Malposition of CVCs occurs in 23% to 38% of cases (17–19). Abnormal locations

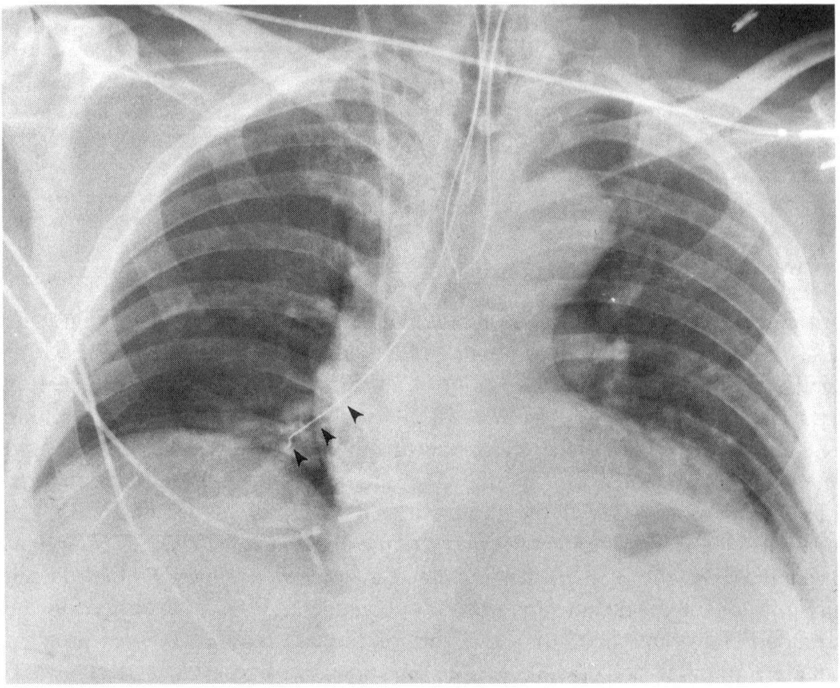

Figure 1 Supine AP view of an intensive care unit patient demonstrates the NG tube to be coiled in the trachea with the tip terminating distally in the right mainstem bronchus (arrowheads).

include the right ventricle, inferior vena cava, internal mammary veins, left pericardiophrenic vein, left superior intercostal vein, aorta, great vessels, azygous vein, contralateral innominate and subclavian vein, right atrium, and retrograde in the internal jugular vein from a subclavian approach. Malposition can increase the risk of arrhythmias (20) and perforation (21). Infusion of fluid into extravascular spaces of the mediastinum or pleura occurs most often from a subclavian approach (15). If radiographs suggest a malpositioned line, fluoroscopy following injection of water-soluble contrast into the catheter or CT can localize the position. The most common complication of CVC insertion is pneumothorax (1% to 12%) (16), which can occur immediately or several days after line placement (22). Vascular injury is suggested by the development of an apical pleural cap, pleural effusion (hemothorax), or mediastinal widening (hemomediastinum). An angled catheter whose tip is embedded in the wall of the vessel increases the risk for perforation (15). Other complications include thrombus formation, infection, kinking of the catheter, shearing off of wire fragments that embolize to the pulmonary arteries (Fig. 2), arrhythmias, or perforation (6). Fragments can be retrieved using percutaneous techniques (23).

E. Pulmonary Artery Catheter

A pulmonary artery (Swan-Ganz) catheter is inserted through a barely opaque, short, wide-bore sheath (cordis). The tip of the Swan-Ganz catheter should be in the proximal right or left pulmonary artery with the balloon deflated as visualized on the radiograph (24). Catheters placed too distally in the pulmonary circulation can result in infarction (25) or pneumothorax. Redundant coiling within the heart can lead to a variety of arrhythmias and even complete heart block (15). Other complications include thrombosis of the catheter, pulmonary artery rupture, pseudoaneurysm formation (26), and intracardiac catheter knotting (27).

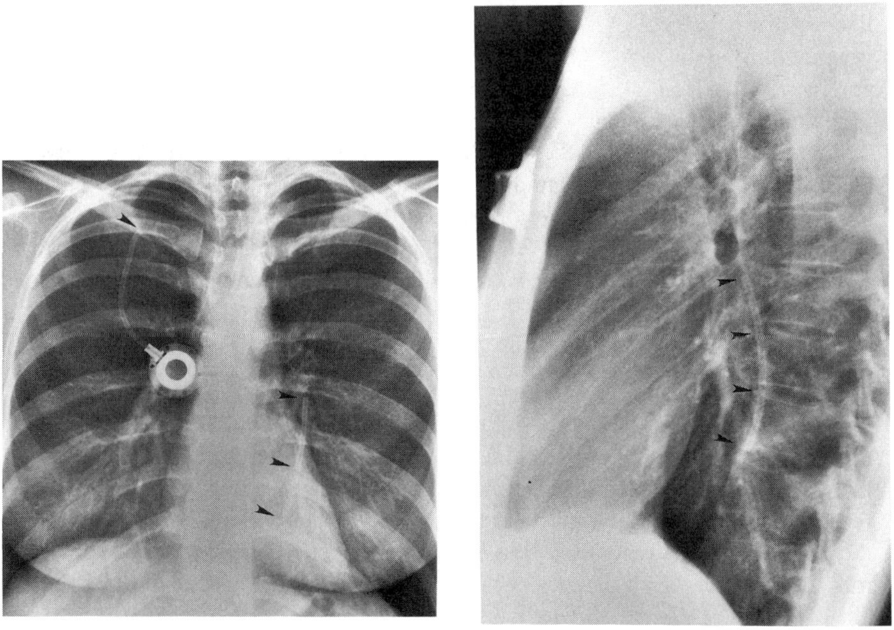

A B

Figure 2 PA and lateral views of the chest demonstrate embolized tip of the central line into the lung after being sheared off (arrowheads).

F. Intra-Aortic Counterpulsation Balloon Pump

The tip of an intra-aortic counterpulsation balloon pump (IABP) should be positioned immediately distal to the origin of the left subclavian artery in the aorta. The balloon inflates during diastole to increase the coronary perfusion, and deflates during systole. If the radiograph is obtained during diastole, air within the balloon can be seen as a long tubular structure within the descending aorta. An IABP that is positioned too proximally in the aorta can occlude the left subclavian artery or cause emboli to the cerebral circulation (15). An IABP that is too distal loses efficacy. Complications of IABP placement include aortic injury, red blood cell fragmentation, and balloon rupture causing gas emboli (15).

G. Transvenous Cardiac Pacemakers

Transvenous cardiac pacemakers should be located with the pacer tip in the right ventricle for ventricular pacemakers or the right atrium and right ventricle for atrioventricular sequential pacemakers (6). On the frontal view, the tip should extend to the apex of the right ventricle. On the lateral view it should lie 3 to 4 mm behind the epicardial fat stripe (28). If the tip is more anteriorly located on the lateral view or projects outside the cardiac silhouette on the frontal view, perforation should be suspected (16). Malposition of the pacemaker can occur in the coronary sinus, right atrium, pulmonary artery, or pulmonary outflow tract (15). Malposition in the coronary sinus is the most difficult to diagnose on a frontal radiograph. When placed in the coronary sinus, the pacemaker wire shows upward deflection of the tip (15). This finding can be confirmed on the lateral view because the tip is located along the posterior heart border, rather than anteriorly. In addition to risks of pneumothorax and vascular injury, pacemaker leads may fracture. Fracture typically occurs near the pacemaker box, at the venous insertion site, and at sharp angulations of the wire (6).

H. Patch Defibrillators

Other cardiac devices include automatic implantable cardioverter defibrillator ("patch" defibrillator) (AICD) which is used to treat life-threatening ventricular tachyarrythmias (29). An AICD patch can be recognized radiographically by its rectangular wires (peripheral marking wires of the defibrillator) on the surface of the heart (15). More recently, a transvenous approach has been used for defibrillators that obviates such patches.

III. ASSESSMENT OF ACUTE MYOCARDIAL INFARCTION

A. Acute Myocardial Infarction

In assessing a patient with suspected acute myocardial infarction (MI), the chest radiograph is a vital component and should be used in conjunction with clinical history, physical exam, ECG, and CPK-MB measurements. Chest radiography allows for assessment of cardiac size, individual chamber enlargement, interstitial or alveolar edema, pulmonary vascular redistribution, and exclusion of other diagnostic possibilities (15). It is essential as a tool for follow-up assessment and for evaluating complications of acute myocardial infarction (AMI). Such complications include left ventricular aneurysm, papillary muscle rupture, perforated ventricular septum, postinfarction pericardial inflammation (Dressler syndrome), or myocardial rupture (30,31).

B. Cardiac Enlargement

Evaluation of cardiac size is usually limited on a portable AP film due to magnification; however, comparison of sequential daily radiographs can be helpful to determine changes in cardiac size. On an upright PA chest radiograph, the largest transverse diameter of the normal-size heart should be less than half the width of the chest. In clinical practice, however, the size of the heart is usually estimated (32).

C. Cardiac Calcifications

Cardiac calcifications occur in the coronary arteries, cardiac valves, ventricular aneurysms, and pericardium. Coronary artery calcification has a tubular tram track appearance on chest radiography and is associated with significant coronary artery disease (33). Valvular calcification is usually aortic (indicating aortic stenosis) and infrequently mitral (indicating rheumatic mitral valve disease with stenosis or prolapse). Calcification of the mitral annulus exhibits a "C" or "J" configuration and usually has no physiological significance. To localize specific valvular calcifications, a line is drawn on the lateral radiograph from the left main bronchus to the anterior costophrenic angle. The mitral valve is below and posterior to the line, and the aorta is above and anterior to the line.

D. Pulmonary Edema

The chest radiograph is often used to assess the severity of an AMI (15). Many of the chest radiographic findings in a patient with an AMI are nonspecific, and often no abnormality is found. The most common abnormality is pulmonary edema due to left ventricular failure. The heart size may be normal because of the acute nature of AMI (15). When present, cardiac enlargement and pleural effusions are useful to distinguish cardiogenic from noncardiogenic edema. Several studies have shown a correlation between pulmonary capillary wedge pressures (PCWP) and radiographic findings of pulmonary venous hypertension and edema (34–36).

Cardiogenic edema is classified into four radiographic categories. Stage I refers to pulmonary venous hypertension that is radiographically demonstrated as engorgement of upper lobe vessels (cephalization). This stage corresponds to PCWP measurements of approximately 12 to 18 mm Hg. Stage II occurs at higher PCWP and is characterized radiographically by indistinctness of pulmonary vessels and development of Kerley B lines (Fig. 3). Kerley B lines are thickened interlobular septae that are due to fluid. They are typically 1 mm thick, 1 cm long, and manifest as horizontal peripheral lower lobe densities (37). Stage III denotes greater pulmonary venous hypertension in which patchy perihilar alveolar edema develops. Dense diffuse bilateral alveolar edema is classified as stage IV (Fig. 4) (38).

Resolution of the radiographic findings of pulmonary edema usually lags behind that of clinical improvement by 24 to 48 h due to delay required for the lymphatics to resorb large amounts of extravascular fluid (39). In patients who have underlying chronic left-sided heart failure, radiographic findings include cephalization of pulmonary vessels, interstitial edema, septal lines, and cardiomegaly (40). Atypical patterns of pulmonary edema can be seen in patients with underlying pulmonary parenchymal disease such as COPD, fibrosis, postsurgical changes, atelectasis, or pneumonia. Gravity (dependent positioning) is the major cause of unilateral pulmonary edema (41,42).

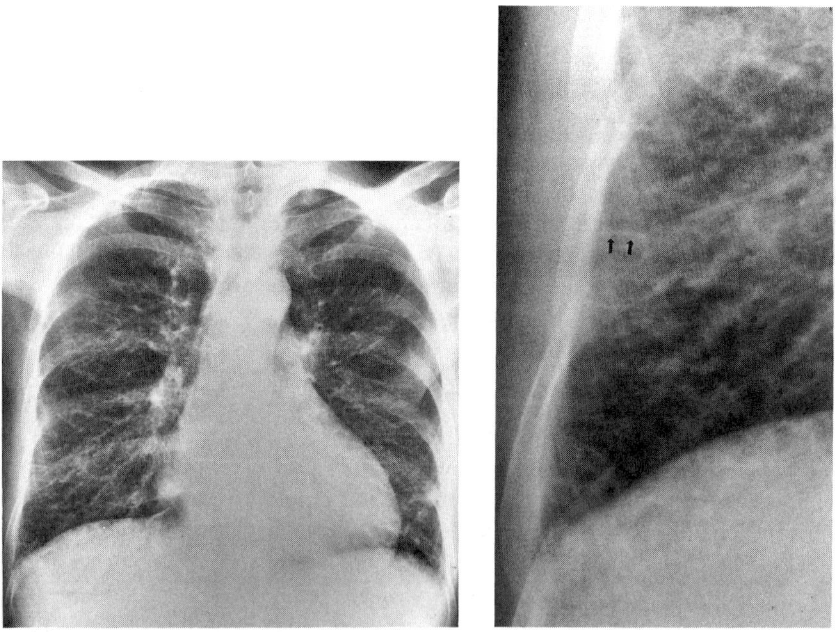

A B

Figure 3 PA view of the chest demonstrates increased interstitial markings with presence of Kerley B lines (arrows) in a patient with interstitial edema.

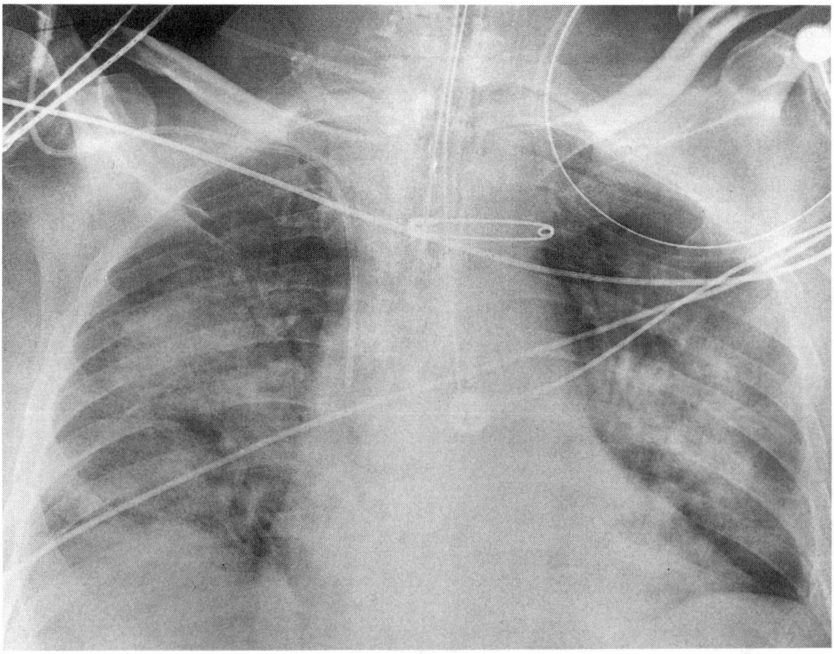

Figure 4 Upright AP view of the chest demonstrates diffuse air space disease which is consistent with alveolar pulmonary edema. This radiographic appearance is not specific and can also be seen with pneumonia as well as ARDS.

E. Complications

In uncomplicated AMI, serial chest radiographs show rapid resolution of the pulmonary edema with treatment. If edema persists, post-MI complications should be suspected (15). Mitral valve insufficiency, perforated ventricular septum, and myocardial rupture can result in cardiac failure that is manifested radiographically as persistent pulmonary edema. If chest radiographs demonstrate a developing focal bulge near the cardiac apex, further workup with echocardiography, CT, or MRI should be performed to evaluate for a left ventricle aneurysm. Calcification in the wall of the left ventricle indicates a healed infarction or an aneurysm that often contains organized thrombus (Fig. 5) (47). An enlarging globular cardiac silhouette should prompt evaluation for pericardial fluid.

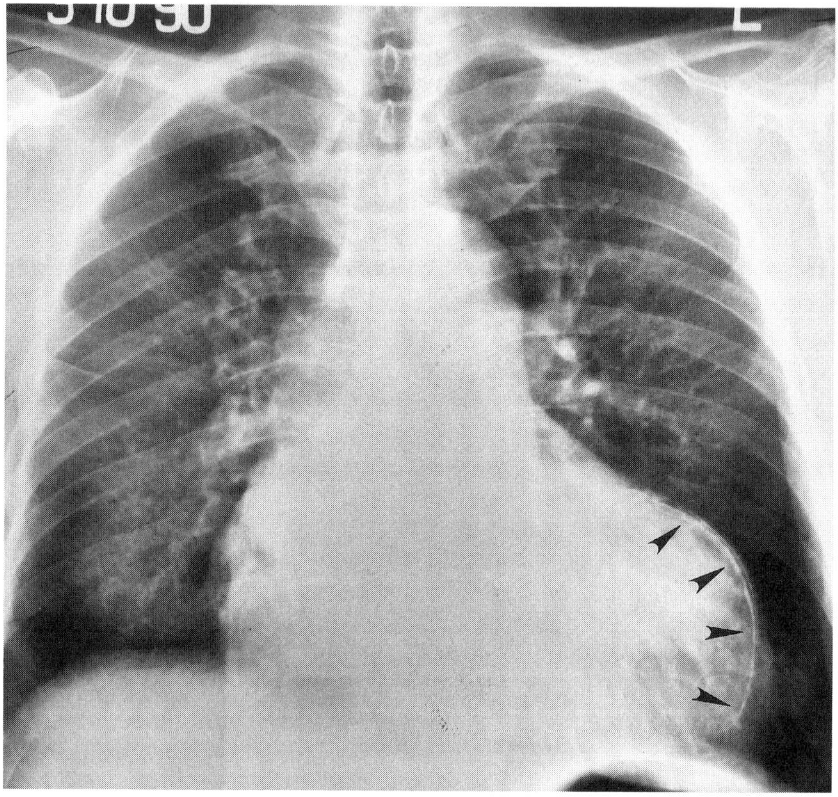

Figure 5 Calcification is seen along the wall of the left ventricle (arrowheads) in a patient with an aneurysm.

IV. IMAGING OF MEDIASTINAL PATHOLOGY IN THE CCU

A. Pericardial Effusion

The normal pericardium is usually not visualized on the frontal view because of its thinness and its close proximity and similar density to the heart (15). The most common pericardial abnormality is pericardial effusion. Causes of pericardial effusions are usually infectious (viral, TB); however, other considerations include renal failure, systemic lupus erythematosus, cardiogenic pulmonary edema, and postmyocardial infarction syndrome (Dressler's syndrome). Findings on chest radiographs that may indicate pericardial effusion include: globular or flask-shaped configuration of the cardiac silhouette (48); an epicardial fat pad sign (visible in 52% of pericardial effusions) which is a separation of > 2 mm of the epicardial and anterior mediastinal fat planes on the lateral view (49); and an increase in lucency of the margin of the cardiac shadow due to differences in tissue attenuation of the heart and the pericardial fluid (50). However, chest radiographs are not reliable for detecting pericardial effusions, and cross-sectional imaging is required for confirmation.

B. Pneumomediastinum and Pneumopericardium

Pneumopericardium can be difficult to differentiate from pneumomediastinum and medial pneumothorax. Pneumomediastinum can be detected radiographically as air outlining mediastinal structures. It is distinguished from pneumopericardium because air extends above the azygous arch whereas air in pneumopericardium is limited at the root of the great vessels by the pericardial reflection. To distinguish a medial pneumothorax from a pneumomediastinum, the patient can be placed in a lateral decubitus position with the side of the suspected pneumothorax in the nondependent position. The distribution of air does not change with pneumomediastinum whereas in a pneumothorax, the air shifts to the lateral aspect of the pleural space.

C. Aortic Dissection

Aortic disease is a common occurrence in the ICU. Aortic dissection and aneurysms are most common. Chest radiographs are occasionally useful. In patients with dissection, mediastinal widening, displacement of intimal calcifications of more than 6 mm (43), indistinct aortic contour, and disparity in size of the ascending and descending aorta may be found but are not specific (15). A normal chest radiograph does not exclude aortic dissection. The diagnosis relies on cross-sectional techniques. MRI can be valuable in detecting the intimal flap and evaluating flow in the true and false lumen and has an accuracy of nearly 100% (Fig. 6) (44). However, in the unstable patient, MRI may not be feasible, and CT of the thorax or transesophageal echocardiography (TEE) can be used. CT has an accuracy rate of 95% (45) and is as accurate as angiography in detecting and classifying aortic dissections (46). If CT is used for diagnosis of dissection, administration of intravenous contrast with dynamic scanning is mandatory to identify the intimal flap. Spiral CT, a newer CT technology, is likely to provide improved capabilities. TEE is also a valuable technique and has the advantage of portability. Optimal use of TEE depends on the skill of the operator.

D. Thoracic Aortic Aneurysm

Thoracic aortic aneurysms are usually atherosclerotic in etiology. A thoracic aortic aneurysm is diagnosed if the AP diameter of the thoracic aorta is > 4.5 cm. The aneurysm may contain intraluminal thrombus. Radiographically, there is

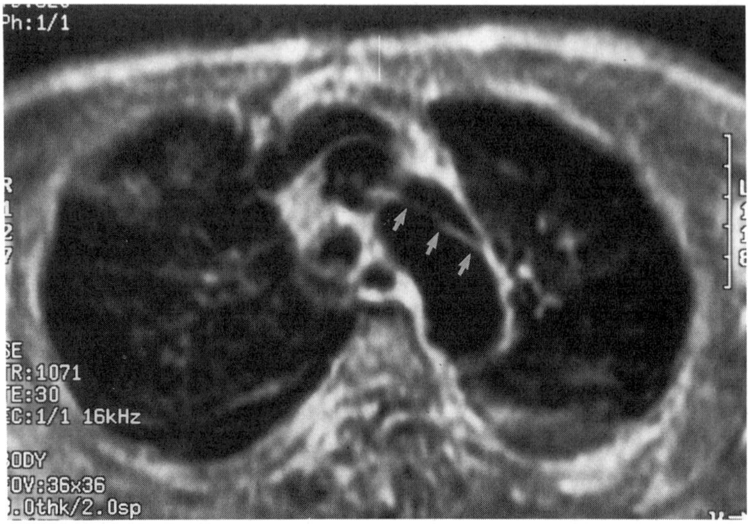

Figure 6 Axial T1-weighted MR image of the aorta demonstrates the intimal flap (arrow) in a patient with aortic dissection.

dilatation of the aorta. If progressive enlargement of the aorta, widening of the mediastinum, pleural or pericardial effusions occur, rupture of the aneurysm should be suspected (15).

V. IMAGING OF PULMONARY PATHOLOGY IN THE CCU

A. Atelectasis

Atelectasis is the most frequent chest radiographic abnormality in the critical care setting (15). Factors that contribute to the development of atelectasis include hypoventilation due to CNS depression, pain causing shallow respiratory excursions, endobronchial intubation, and decreased ability to cough and clear secretions (6). Lobar or segmental atelectasis can result from either extrinsic bronchial compression by adenopathy, a mass lesion or the heart, or from endobronchial occlusion by mucous, an endobronchial lesion or foreign body.

Radiographically, atelectasis can have a variety of appearances. Chest radiographs can be normal or can show mild linear basilar shadowing or broad bands of segmental or lobar consolidation with volume loss (6). Secondary signs of volume loss include ipsilateral shift of adjacent structures such as fissures, the mediastinum, trachea, or diaphragm. Atelectasis can sometimes mimic pneumonia and the distinction may rest on clinical grounds. Serial radiographs may reveal rapid change if consolidation is caused by atelectasis.

The most common location of atelectasis is the left lower lobe (Fig. 7). This predilection is presumably due to compression of the left lower lobe bronchus by the heart in supine bedridden patients (51). Radiographically, there is opacification of the retrocardiac area, loss of definition of the left hemidiaphragm and descending aorta, elevation of the left hemidiaphragm, depression of the left hilum, mediastinal shift, and hyperlucency of the left upper lobe (6).

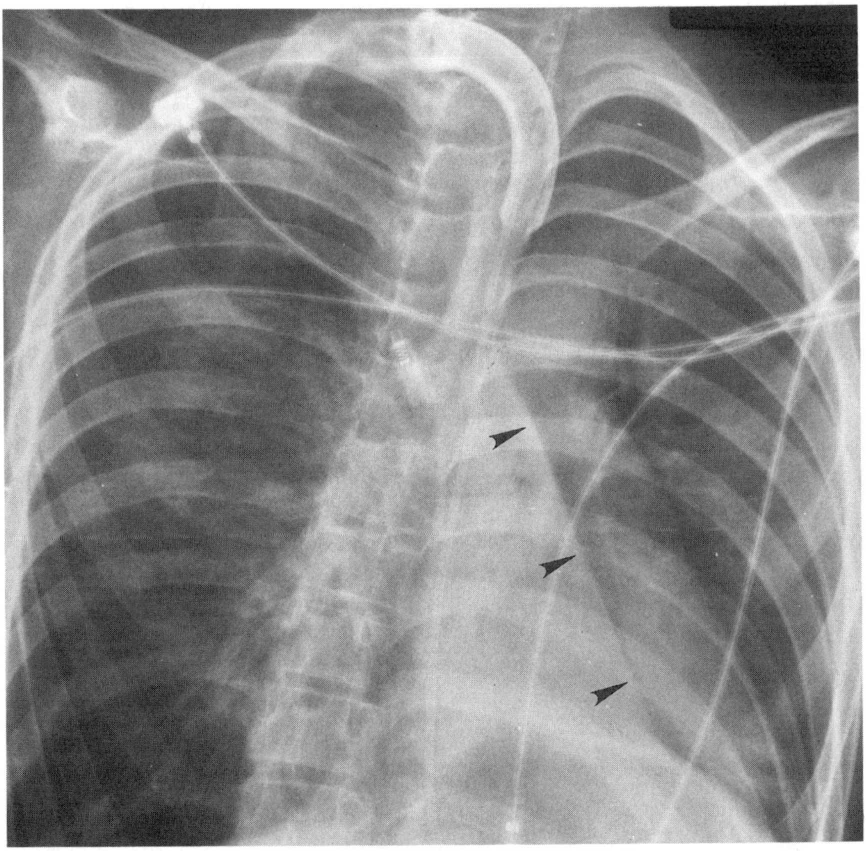

Figure 7 Increased density of the left lower lobe (arrowheads) on the PA chest radiograph is consistent with left lower lobe collapse (atelectasis).

B. Pneumonia

Prolonged hospitalization increases the risk for nosocomial infection. Nosocomial pneumonias occur in 1% of patients in the general hospital population and 12% in the intensive care unit and are the leading infectious cause of death in hospitals (15). In the critical care setting, mortality from nosocomial pneumonia is 20% to 35% (15). Chest radiographs usually show consolidation or patchy air space changes that are nonspecific. Atelectasis, edema, aspiration, ARDS, or pulmonary embolism can cause a similar appearance. A normal radiograph does not completely exclude infection. When clinical suspicion remains, CT, either using standard or high-resolution technique, or gallium scan may be contributory. Serial radiographs in patients with pneumonia may detect complications including pulmonary abscess, pleural effusions, empyema, or bronchopleural fistula. In such cases, chest CT is often useful.

C. Aspiration Pneumonia

Aspiration pneumonia is another common inflammatory condition in the critically ill patient. Predisposing factors include mechanical devices and conditions that reduce consciousness or cause dysphagia (NG and ET tubes) (6). The type of aspirate also plays a role. Aspiration of nasal, oral, or tracheal secretions usually clears in several days with appropriate antibiotic treatment (52). Aspiration of gastric contents (Mendelson's syndrome) can lead to severe hypoxia, fever, rales, and homogeneous or patchy and nodular areas of consolidation on radiographs (6). The most common sites of aspiration pneumonia are the posterior segments of upper lobes and superior and basal segments of lower lobes because these locations are gravity-dependent. The right side is affected more than the left. Usually there is clearing clinically after 1 to 2 days and radiographic clearing after 3 days with complete resolution after 1 to 2 weeks (15). In patients who show deterioration or lack of improvement, superimposed infection, abscess formation, or empyema should be suspected. Aspiration of bland fluids or solids such as blood, barium, or water is less serious because of the lack of chemical pneumonitis. Radiographs in such patients are either normal or show atelectasis or focal hyperinflation that clears rapidly with coughing or suction.

D. Adult Respiratory Syndrome

The adult respiratory distress syndrome (ARDS) is due to a variety of pulmonary and nonpulmonary insults. ARDS is characterized by acute severe and progressive respiratory distress, hypoxemia unresponsive to oxygen treatment, increase stiffness of lungs leading to acute respiratory failure, and diffuse radiographic opacifications (53). Predisposing factors include sepsis (38% developed ARDS), aspiration of gastric contents (30%), multiple emergency transfusions (24%), and pulmonary contusions (17%) (54). Most patients with ARDS require endotracheal intubation (55). Four stages of ARDS are described: initial injury, apparent stability, respiratory insufficiency, and terminal stage. The injury phase occurs up to 6 h after the inciting event and usually demonstrates no clinical or radiographic findings. Major radiographic abnormalities usually do not occur until respiratory insufficiency is evident. These findings often persist during the terminal phase (15). Radiographs are nonspecific and should be evaluated in serial fashion. Usually the chest radiograph is normal in the first 12 to 24 h. After 24 h development of bilateral perihilar haze occurs with ill-defined linear opacifications extending from the hilum due to interstitial edema. If there is abnormal opacification within the first 8 to 12 h, aspiration pneumonia, congestive heart failure, or fluid overload should be suspected. Between 24 and 48 h, the linear opacifications coalesce to form focal areas of alveolar edema. There is absence of cardiomegaly, pleural effusions, Kerley B lines, and pulmonary vascular redistribution—findings that help to differentiate ARDS from cardiac failure. The radiographic appearance of alveolar edema remains unchanged for several days to weeks and then may either clear slowly or show focal areas of scarring due to fibrosis (15). Sudden apparent improvement may be produced with use of PEEP because of increase in lung volumes (52).

E. Pulmonary Embolism

The chest radiograph in a patient with pulmonary embolism is usually normal. The most important role of the chest radiograph is to exclude other diseases that mimic pulmonary embolism. In patients with abnormal chest radiographs, the findings are often nonspecific. Nonspecific findings include atelectasis, pleural effusions, and an elevated hemidiaphragm. More suggestive abnormalities are peripheral patchy, wedge-shaped density, indicating either pulmonary hemorrhage or infarct, and paucity of lung markings (Westermark sign). The initial study of choice is a ventilation-perfusion (VQ) lung scan. A diagnostic (high-probability) perfusion study in a patient with pulmonary embolism demonstrates multiple wedge-shaped peripheral photopenic areas that correspond to areas of normal ventilation. If diagnosis is equivocal, pulmonary angiography is the standard reference technique. Abnormal areas of perfusion on the VQ scan can be used to guide angiography. Venous stasis in the deep veins of legs can result in thrombus formation that predisposes to pulmonary embolism. Vascular ultrasound is valuable to evaluate for lower-extremity thrombus. Sensitivity of this study is 90% to 95%; specificity is 85% to 95% (56). If the study is equivocal or if calf thrombosis is suspected, venography can be performed. If anticoagulation therapy is contraindicated, an inferior vena cava filter can be inserted percutaneously.

F. Pleural Effusion

Disease of the pleural space is initially evaluated on chest radiographs. Pleural effusion is the most common abnormality; however, detection on portable supine radiographs is difficult because of posterior layering of fluid (57). Useful radiographic findings to detect effusions are homogeneous opacification at the bases with preservation of pulmonary vessel shadows, loss of normal hemidiaphragm silhouette, meniscoid appearance of opacification at the lateral costophrenic sulcus, apical capping, apparent elevation of the hemidiaphragm, and thickening of the fissure with fluid (38,52). Atelectasis, aspiration pneumonitis, pneumonia, overlying soft tissue, and abdominal pathology can mimic pleural effusions. Lateral decubitus views, CT, or ultrasound can be helpful to diagnose pleural effusions. CT or ultrasound can also provide guidance for obtaining fluid for diagnostic or therapeutic purposes. In the patient with clinically suspected infected pleural fluid, chest CT with intravenous contrast media is recommended to evaluate for an empyema. The “split pleura” sign is a characteristic finding of empyema and appears as an enhancing pleural rim that corresponds to thickened parietal and visceral pleura (58).

G. Pneumothorax

Pneumothorax is often the result of line or tube placement or barotrauma. Typically a thin white visceral pleural line is seen without peripheral lung markings in an apicolateral location on erect radiographs. The majority of pneumothoraces in supine patients are anteromedial and subpulmonic, in the least dependent pleural recesses. Subpulmonic pneumothoraces manifest as hyperlucency over the upper abdomen and deep costophrenic sulcus (59). Occasionally, a medial pneumothorax can be difficult to differentiate from pneumomediastinum. Skin folds can mimic pneumothoraces; however, parenchymal vascular markings are usually seen lateral to the fold. In cases of uncertainty, CT may be helpful for further evaluation. If an air-fluid level is present, hydropneumothorax should be suspected (60). Tension pneumothorax occurs when intrapleural pressure equals atmospheric pressure, resulting in decreased venous return to the right heart (6). Radiographically, there are contralateral mediastinal shift, flattening of the cardiomediastinal contour, inversion of hemidiaphragm, and ipsilateral lung compression (6). Patients with ARDS on PEEP who have noncompliant lungs may not demonstrate contralateral mediastinal shift. In patients whose pneumothorax does not respond to chest tube placement, a bronchopleural fistula should be suspected.

VI. IMAGING THE ABDOMEN IN THE CCU PATIENT

A. Bowel Obstruction

A common clinical situation found in the critical care patient is abdominal distension and pain. Supine and upright abdominal films are necessary to evaluate for free intraperitoneal air, obstruction, or adynamic ileus. On abdominal radiographs, complete small-bowel obstruction is characterized by lack of colonic air after 24 to 28 h, disproportionate distension of small-bowel loops, and air-fluid levels on the upright film (15). Partial small-bowel obstruction can be difficult to distinguish from adynamic ileus (absent peristalsis without mechanical obstruction). The radiographs in adynamic ileus demonstrate uniform diffuse dilatation of the small bowel and air within the colon. A localized area of dilatation and air-fluid levels are more typical of partial small-bowel obstruction. A small-bowel barium study can be helpful to find a "transition zone" between normal and abnormal bowel in partial small-bowel obstruction. Similarly, a barium enema can be performed to exclude a colonic obstruction.

B. Pneumoperitoneum

Pneumoperitoneum is caused by rupture of an abdominal viscus or by dissection of air from the thorax. The upright abdominal film should be evaluated for lucency beneath the hemidiaphragms. Other indirect findings of pneumoperitoneum include prominent outline of the bowel wall due to air on both sides (Rigler's sign), delineation of the falciform ligament, lucency anterior to the liver, or a triangular gas collection under the liver margin (61). If the patient is unable to maintain an upright position, a left lateral decubitus view of the abdomen may demonstrate air along the lateral liver margin.

C. Hemorrhage

If patients are receiving anticoagulants or urokinase for AMI and there is clinical suspicion for peritoneal or retroperitoneal hemorrhage, an abdominal CT is the study of choice.

D. Acalculous Cholecystitis

During prolonged hospitalization, patients can develop acalculous cholecystitis. The cystic duct is obstructed by inflammation and edema. Ultrasound and CT may be normal or may demonstrate wall thickening, a dilated gallbladder, dilated ducts, or pericholecystic fluid. Hepatobiliary scintigraphy scan is probably the most useful study. In acalculous cholecystitis, nonfilling of the gallbladder occurs in association with normal uptake by the liver and normal excretion through the common bile duct.

E. Conclusion

Radiographic imaging of intensive care patients is often challenging because of the unstable condition of many of these patients. Evaluation of monitoring and supportive devices is essential. The chest radiograph is typically the first study used to evaluate cardiac, pulmonary, or pleural pathology. Other modalities such as echocardiography, nuclear medicine, CT, and MRI play important supplemental roles in evaluation of critically ill patients.

REFERENCES

1. Greenbaum DM, Marschall KE. The value of routine daily chest x-rays in intubated patients in the medical intensive care unit. Crit Care Med 1982; 10:29–30.
2. Henschke CI, Pasternack GS, Schroeder S, Hart KK, Herman PG. Bedside chest radiography: diagnostic efficacy. Radiology 1983; 149:23–26.
3. Janower ML, Jennas-Nocera Z, Mukai J. Utility and efficacy of portable chest radiographs. AJR 1984; 142:265–267.
4. Horst HM, Fagan B, Beute GH. Chest radiographs in surgical intensive care patients: a valuable "routine." Henry Ford Med 1986; 34:84–86.
5. Bekemeyer WB, Crapo RO, Calhoon S, Cannon CY, Clayton PD. Efficacy of chest radiography in a respiratory intensive care unit; a prospective study. Chest 1985; 88(5):691–696.
6. Templeton PA, Diaconis JN. Critical care chest imaging. In: Mirvis SE, Young JW, eds. Imaging in Trauma and Critical Care. Baltimore: Williams & Wilkins, 1992: 516–567.
7. Minagi H, Jeffrey RB Jr. Radiologic techniques in the treatment of the critically ill trauma patient. Crit Care Clin 1986; 2(4):821–838.
8. Mirvis SE, Tobin KD, Kostrubiak I, Belzberg H. Thoracic CT in detecting occult disease in critically ill patients. AJR 1987; 148:685–689.
9. Roddy LH, Unger KM, Miller WC. Thoracic computed tomography in the critically ill patient. Crit Care Med 1981; 9(7):515–518.
10. Higgins CB, Caputo GR. Role of MR imaging in acquired and congenital cardiovascular disease. AJR 1993; 161:13–22.
11. Goodman RL, Putnam CE. The SICU chest radiograph after massive blunt trauma. Radiol Clin North Am 1981; 19(1):111–123.
12. Goodman LR, Conrardy PA, Laing F, Singer MM. Radiographic evaluation of endotracheal tube position. AJR 1976; 127:433–434.
13. Stauffer JL, Olson DE, Petty TL. Complications and consequences of endotracheal intubation and tracheotomy. Am J Med 1981; 70:65–76.
14. Zwillich CW, Pierson DJ, Creagh CE, Sutton FD, Schatz E, Petty TL. Complications of assisted ventilation; a prospective study of 354 consecutive episodes. Am J Med 1974; 57:161–170.
15. Goodman LR, Putman CE. Critical Care Imaging, 3rd ed. Philadelphia: W. B. Saunders, 1983.
16. Wechsler RJ, Steiner RM, Kinori I. Monitoring the monitors; the radiology of thoracic catheters, wires and tubes. Semin Roentgenol 1988; 23(1):61–84.
17. Langston C. The aberrant central venous catheter and its complications. Radiology 1971; 100:55–59.
18. Deitel M, McIntyre JA. Radiographic confirmation of site of central venous pressure catheters. Can J Surg 1971; 14:42–52.

19. Gilday DL. The value of chest radiography in the localization of central venous pressure catheters. Can Med Assoc J 1969; 101:363–364.
20. Dunbar RD, Mitchell R, Lavine M. Aberrant locations of central venous catheters. Lancet 1981; 1:711–714.
21. Huyghens L, Sennesael J, Verbeelan D, Deraemaecker R, Corne L. Cardiothoracic complications of centrally inserted catheters. Acute Care 1985; 11:53–56.
22. Sivak SL. Late appearance of pneumothorax after subclavian venipuncture. Am J Med 1986; 80:323–324.
23. Mirvis SE. Imaging of thoracic trauma. In: Turney S, Rodriquez A, Cowley RA, eds. Management of Cardiothoracic Trauma. Baltimore: Williams and Wilkins, 1990.
24. Swan HJC, Ganz W. Use of a balloon flotation catheter in critically ill patients. Surg Clin North Am 1975; 55:501–509.
25. Sise MJ, Hollingsworth P, Brimm JE, Peters RM, Virgilio RW, Shackford SR. Complications of the flow-directed pulmonary-artery catheter: a prospective analysis in 219 patients. Crit Care Med 1981; 9(4):315–318.
26. Dieden JD, Friloux LA III, Renner JW. Pulmonary artery false aneurysms secondary to Swan-Ganz pulmonary artery catheters. AJR 1987; 149:901–906.
27. Lipp H, O'Donoghue K, Resnekov L. Intracardiac knotting of a flow-directed balloon-tipped catheter. N Engl J Med 1971; 284:220.
28. Ormond RS, Rubenfine M, Anbe DT, Drake EH. Radiographic demonstrations of myocardial penetration by permanent endocardial pacemakers. Radiology 1971; 98: 35–37.
29. Lehmann MH, Steinman RT, Schuger CD, Jacson K. The automatic implantable cardioverter defibrillator as antiarrhythmic treatment, modality of choice for survivors of cardiac arrest unrelated to acute myocardial infarction. Am J Cardiol 1988; 62:803–805.
30. Feigenbaum H. Echocardiography. 4th ed. Philadelphia: Lea & Febiger, 1986.
31. Kisslo JA, Abrams DB, Leech GJ. Essentials of Echocardiography: Heart Muscle Disease. New York: Medi Cine Prod, 1988.
32. Walker JM, Margouleff D. A Clinical Manual of Nuclear Medicine. South Norwalk, CT: Appleton-Century-Crofts, 1984.
33. Thompson PL, Fletch EE, Katavatis V. Enzymatic indices of myocardial necrosis: influence on short and long-term prognosis after myocardial infarction. Circulation 1979; 59:113–119.
34. Hamosh P, Cohen JN. Left ventricular function in acute myocardial infarction. J Clin Invest 1971; 50:523–533.
35. McHugh TJ, Forrester JL, Adler L, Zion D, Swan HJC. Pulmonary vascular congestion in acute myocardial infarction; hemodynamic and radiologic correlations. Ann Intern Med 1972; 76:29–33.
36. Sjoigren A. Left heart failure in acute myocardial infarction: a clinical hemodynamic and therapeutic study. Acta Med Scand 1970; 188:(suppl 510)1–87.
37. Kerly P. Radiology in heart disease. Br Med J 1933; 2:594–597.
38. Underwood GH Jr, Newell JD. Pulmonary radiology in the intensive care unit. Med Clin North Am 1983; 67(6):1305–1324.
39. Nakahara K, Nanjo S, Maeda M, Kawashima Y. Dynamic insufficiency of lung lymph

from the right lymph duct with acute infiltration edema. Am Rev Respir Dis 1983; 127:67–71.
40. Chen JTT. Essentials of Cardiac Roentgenology. Boston: Little, Brown, 1987.
41. Leeming BWA. Gravitational edema of the lungs observed during assisted respiration. Chest 1973; 64:719–722.
42. Zimmerman JE, Goodman LR, Andre AC, Wyman AC. Radiographic detection of mobilizable lung water: the gravitational shift test. AJR 1982; 138:59–64.
43. Eyler WR, Clark MD. Dissecting aneurysms of the aorta; roentgen manifestations including a comparison with other types of aneurysms. Radiology 1965; 85:1047–1057.
44. Nienaber CA, Spielman RP, von Kodolitsch Y, et al. Diagnosis of thoracic aortic dissection: magnetic resonance imaging versus transesophageal echocardiography. Circulation 1992; 85:434–447.
45. Thorsen MK, Lawson TL, Foley WD. CT of aortic dissections. CRC Crit Rev Diagn Imaging 1986; 26:291–324.
46. Moncada R, Salinas M, Churchill R, et al. Diagnosis of dissection aortic aneurysm by computed tomography. Lancet 1981; 1:238–241.
47. Elliott LP. Introduction to disease showing normal vascularity and normal size heart. In: Taveras JM, Ferrucci JT, eds. Radiology, Diagnosis-Imaging-Intervention. Philadelphia: Lippincott, 1991:1–4.
48. Ellis K, King DL. The pericardium. In: Haskin M, Teplick G, eds. Surgical Radiology. Philadelphia: W.B. Saunders, 1981.
49. Carsky EW, Mauceri RA, Azimi F. The epicardial fat pad sign: analysis of frontal and lateral chest radiographs in patients with pericardial effusions. Radiology 1980; 137(2):303–308.
50. Tehranzadeh J, Kelley MJ. Differential density sign of pericardial effusion. Radiology 1979; 133:23–30.
51. Shevland J, Hirkman MT, Huang KA, Kealey GP. Lobar collapse in the surgical intensive care unit. Br J Radiol 1983; 56:531–534.
52. Good LR, Putnam CF. Intensive Care Radiology: Imaging of the Critically Ill. 2nd ed. Philadelphia: W.B. Saunders, 1983.
53. Greene R. Adult respiratory distress syndrome: acute alveolar damage. Radiology 1987; 163:57–66.
54. Pepe PE, Potkin PT, Reus DH, Hudson LD, Carrico CJ. Clinical predictors of the adult respiratory distress syndrome. Am J Surg 1982; 144:124–130.
55. Ashbaugh DG, Bigelow DB, Petty TL, Levine BE. Acute respiratory distress in adults. Lancet 1967; 2:319–323.
56. Cronan JJ, Dofman GS, Scola FH, Schappo B, Alexander J. Deep venous thrombosis: US assessment using vein compression. Radiology 1987; 162:191–194.
57. Ruskin JA, Gwiney JW, Thorsen MK, Goodman LR. Detection of pleural effusions on supine chest radiographs. AJR 1987; 148:681–684.
58. Stark DD, Federle MP, Goodman PC. CT and radiographic assessment of tube thoracostomy. AJR 1983; 141:253–258.
59. Gordan R. The deep sulcus sign. Radiology 1980; 136:25–27.
60. Chiles C, Raven CE. Radiographic recognition of pneumothorax in the intensive care unit. Crit Care Med 1986; 14(8):677–680.
61. Ravin CE, Cooper C. Review of Radiology. Philadelphia: WB Saunders, 1990.

Index

About the Editors

ZAB MOHSENIFAR is Director of the Division of Pulmonary and Critical Care at Cedars-Sinai Medical Center, Los Angeles, California, as well as Professor of Medicine at the University of California, Los Angeles, School of Medicine. The author or coauthor of over 100 journal publications, he is a Fellow of the American College of Chest Physicians and the American College of Physicians, among others. Dr. Mohsenifar received the M.D. degree (1974) from the University of Tehran, Iran, and the New Jersey College of Medicine Hospitals.

P. K. SHAH is Director of the Division of Cardiology and of the Atherosclerosis Research Center at Cedars-Sinai Medical Center, Los Angeles, California, where he holds the Shapell and Webb Chair in Cardiology. Dr. Shah is also a Professor of Medicine at the University of California Los Angeles (UCLA) School of Medicine. The editor of one book and the author or coauthor of over 130 journal publications and book chapters, he is a Fellow of the American College of Cardiology, the American College of Chest Physicians, and the American College of Physicians, among others. Dr. Shah received the M.D. degree from the Medical School, Medical College, Srinagar, Kashmir, India, and his cardiology training from the Montefiore Hospital of Albert Einstein College of Medicine, Bronx, New York.